Diagnostic and Therapeutic Cardiac Catheterization

Edited by

Carl J. Pepine, M.D.

Professor of Medicine
Department of Medicine
University of Florida
Gainesville, Florida

and Associates

James A. Hill, M.D.

Associate Professor of Medicine
Department of Medicine
University of Florida
Gainesville, Florida

Charles R. Lambert, M.D., Ph.D.

Assistant Professor of Medicine
Department of Medicine
University of Florida
Gainesville, Florida

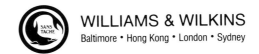

WILLIAMS & WILKINS
Baltimore • Hong Kong • London • Sydney

Editor: Jonathan W. Pine
Associate Editor: Carol Eckhart
Copy Editors: Klemie Bryte, Stephen Siegforth
Design: Dan Pfisterer
Illustration Planning: Ray Lowman
Production: Barbara Felton

Library of Congress Cataloging-in-Publication Data

Diagnostic and therapeutic cardiac catheterization / edited by Carl J. Pepine, James A. Hill,
Charles R. Lambert
    p.   cm.
  Includes index.
  ISBN 0-683-06851-2
  1. Cardiac catheterization. I. Pepine, Carl J. II. Hill, James A., 1950– . III. Lambert,
Charles R., 1951–
  [DNLM: 1. Heart Catheterization—methods. 2. Heart Diseases—diagnosis 3. Heart
Diseases—therapy. WG 141.5.C2 D536]
RC683.5.C25D53 1989
616.1'20754—dc19

                    88–20852
                      CIP

            89 90 91 92 93
            1 2 3 4 5 6 7 8 9 10

To our wives and families
The time that was taken from them
enabled us to develop this book.
In this way, they are
very special contributors to this work.

Preface

INTRODUCTION

Cardiac catheterization comprises a number of specific procedures that require introduction of special catheters into the central arterial and/or venous circulation in order to obtain information or apply treatment related to the heart and vascular system. Very few procedures in medicine have provided more excitement and contributions to research, diagnosis, and treatment of disease than those encompassed by cardiac catheterization. This benchmark has brought about substantial change in the approach to patients with either known or suspect cardiovascular disease of all types.

Specifically, cardiac catheterization procedures, such as coronary angiography, left ventriculography, pressure and flow recordings, and oximetry, give graphic descriptions of the anatomy and physiology of the heart and great vessels and of circulatory function. Catheter-obtained endomyocardial biopsy provides tissue for histologic diagnosis of a variety of disease states and is an objective method to document responses to specific treatment. More recently, the rapid growth of a number of therapeutic procedures has given the cardiovascular catheterization specialist a direct method of intervention in the treatment of many patients with a variety of cardiac disorders. These interventions range from creation of atrial septal defects to dilation of vascular obstructions and from induction of arrhythmias to introduction of prosthetic devices. These cardiac catheterization-based procedures, their theory, and clinical application are the subject of this text.

PURPOSE

The general aims of this book are as follows: to provide the reader with background material needed to make appropriate decisions concerning the role, value, and application of diagnostic cardiac catheterization (e.g., right and left heart catheterization, coronary angiography) and related therapeutic interventions (e.g., percutaneous transluminal coronary angioplasty, intracoronary thrombolytic agents, valvuloplasty).

The first chapter reviews the historical background of diagnostic and therapeutic cardiac catheterization. The chapters in Section 2 introduce and describe specific indications and contraindications for the procedures used in cardiac catheterization. The chapters in Section 3 provide background and technical information for catheterization, radiological techniques, and procedures used in the catheterization laboratory. Those in Section 4 describe the theoretical and practical aspects of the various physiological measurements made in the catheterization laboratory. The chapters in Section 5 represent a unique feature of this text. These chapters are designed to guide the reader in selecting the approach to specific clinical states through integration of cardiac catheterization data. Each clinical state is reviewed in terms of natural history and clinical presentation in view of the cardiac catheterization data, stressing correlation or lack of correlation. Noninvasive laboratory data, obtained to supplement cardiac catheterization data, obviate the need for cardiac catheterization, or aid in selection of patients for catheterization, is reviewed. Catheterization data critical to providing optimal management are discussed in detail. Finally, the use of specific cardiac catheterization data in determining medical, surgical, or catheter-directed interventional therapy is evaluated. From this information dealing with specific patients, the reader will learn what to expect from diagnostic and therapeutic catheterization procedures when applied to patients with suspect or known disease states and how to use this information in the optimal management of these patients.

This book is intended for physicians at all levels of training who care for patients with cardiovascular disease, refer patients for cardiac catheterization, and/or perform catheterization. Nonphysicians (e.g., nurses, physician assistants, technicians, students) working in cardiovascular care areas (catheterization laboratories, coronary care units, critical care units, etc.) will also find this text very useful.

With an understanding of this information, the reader should be able to make appropriate decisions concerning the precise role, value, and application of the diagnostic and therapeutic techniques that comprise the field of cardiac catheterization.

Acknowledgments

We are indebted to our collaborators for their invaluable contributions to this book. Special thanks are directed to those individuals who have helped to provide the opportunity for each of us to develop a career in the catheterization laboratory and the environment that enabled us to write about it. We are deeply obliged to Ava DeLorenzo for expert editorial assistance, helpful suggestions and untiring effort. We have made unreasonable demands upon the time and temperament of these individuals in order that this book might reflect what we feel represents the current state of cardiac catheterization.

Contributors

George S. Abela, M.D.
Assistant Professor of Medicine
Division of Cardiology
Director, Cardiovascular Laser Laboratory
Department of Medicine
University of Florida
Gainesville, Florida

Michael E. Assey, M.D.
Assistant Professor of Medicine
Director, Adult Cardiac Catheterization
    Laboratory
Division of Cardiology
Department of Medicine
Medical University of South Carolina
Charleston, South Carolina

Arnold Auger, M.D.
Administrator
Department of Diagnostic Radiology
Hahnemann University College of Medicine
Philadelphia, Pennsylvania

Jeffrey A. Brinker, M.D.
Associate Professor of Medicine
Director, Cardiac Catheterization and
    Pacemaker Laboratory
Department of Medicine
The Johns Hopkins Hospital
Baltimore, Maryland

Blase A. Carabello, M.D.
Professor of Medicine
Division of Cardiology
Department of Medicine
Medical University of South Carolina
Charleston, South Carolina

C. Richard Conti, M.D.
Professor of Medicine
Chief, Division of Cardiology
Department of Medicine
University of Florida
Gainesville, Florida

J. Michael Criley, M.D.
Professor of Medicine and Radiological
    Science
Chief, Division of Cardiology
Harbor-UCLA Medical Center
Torrance, California

Ira H. Gessner, M.D.
Professor of Medicine
Chief, Pediatric Cardiology
Department of Pediatrics
University of Florida
Gainesville, Florida

Leonard S. Gettes, M.D.
Professor of Medicine
Chief, Division of Cardiology
Department of Medicine
University of North Carolina
Chapel Hill, North Carolina

Sheldon Goldberg, M.D.
Professor of Medicine
Division of Cardiology
Department of Medicine
Director, Cardiac Catheterization Laboratory
Thomas Jefferson University Hospital
Philadelphia, Pennsylvania

Frank J. Hildner, M.D.
Professor of Medicine
University of Miami School of Medicine
Director, Cardiac Catheterization Laboratory
Mt. Sinai Medical Center
Miami Beach, Florida

James A. Hill, M.D.
Associate Professor of Medicine
Director, Adult Cardiac Catheterization
  Laboratory
Shands Hospital
Department of Medicine
University of Florida
Gainesville, Florida

L. David Hillis, M.D.
Professor of Internal Medicine
Medical Director, Cardiac Catheterization
  Laboratory
Parkland Memorial Hospital
Department of Cardiology
University of Texas Southwestern Medical
  School
Dallas, Texas

John W. Hirshfeld, M.D.
Associate Professor of Medicine
Director, Cardiac Catheterization Laboratory
Hospital of the University of Pennsylvania
Philadelphia, Pennsylvania

David R. Holmes, Jr., M.D.
Professor of Medicine
Mayo Medical School
Mayo Clinic
Rochester, Minnesota

Paul R. Julsrud, M.D.
Assistant Professor of Radiology
Consultant
Department of Diagnostic Radiology
Mayo Medical School
Rochester, Minnesota

Stephen L. Kaufman
Professor of Radiology
Director, Division of Vascular and
  Interventional Radiology
Emory University School of Medicine
Atlanta, Georgia

Stephen Keim, M.D.
Division of Cardiology
Department of Medicine
University of Florida
Gainesville, Florida

J. Ward Kennedy, M.D.
Professor of Medicine
Chief of Cardiology
Division of Cardiology
University of Washington School of Medicine
Seattle, Washington

J. Patrick Kleaveland, M.D.
Assistant Professor of Medicine
Director, Cardiac Catheterization
  Laboratory
Temple University Hospital
Philadelphia, Pennsylvania

W. Peter Klinke, M.D.
Associate Professor of Medicine
Chief of Cardiology
Royal Alexandra General Hospital
Edmonton, Alberta, Canada

Charles R. Lambert, M.D., Ph.D.
Assistant Professor of Medicine
Director, Cardiac Catheterization
  Laboratory
VA Regional Medical Center
Department of Medicine
University of Florida
Gainesville, Florida

Richard A. Lange, M.D.
Assistant Professor of Internal Medicine
University of Texas Southwestern Medical
  School
Dallas, Texas

Robert G. Macdonald, M.D.
Assistant Professor of Medicine
Maritime Heart Center
Victoria General Hospital
Dalhousie University
Halifax, Nova Scotia, Canada

Tomas D. Martin, M.D.
Division of Cardiothoracic Surgery
Department of Surgery
University of Florida
Gainesville, Florida

Wilmer W. Nichols, Ph.D.
Associate Professor of Medicine
Division of Cardiology
Department of Medicine
University of Florida
Gainesville, Florida

Carl J. Pepine, M.D.
Professor of Medicine
Chief of Cardiology
VA Regional Medical Center
Department of Medicine
University of Florida
Gainesville, Florida

Barry Rose, M.D.
Clinical Associate
Memorial University of Newfoundland
    Medical School
Cardiology Division
General Hospital
Health Science Center
St. John's, Newfoundland, Canada

Allan M. Ross, M.D.
Professor of Medicine
Director, Division of Cardiology
George Washington University Medical
    Center
Washington, D.C.

Michael Savage, M.D.
Assistant Professor of Medicine
Thomas Jefferson University
Philadelphia, Pennsylvania

Florence H. Sheehan, M.D.
Research Associate Professor of Medicine
Director, Quantitative Angiocardiographic
    Laboratory
University of Washington
Seattle, Washington

Robert J. Siegel, M.D.
Associate Professor of Medicine
UCLA School of Medicine
Cardiology Division
Cedars Sinai Medical Center
Los Angeles, California

James F. Spann, Jr., M.D.
Professor of Medicine
Director, Division of Cardiology
Department of Medicine
Medical University of South Carolina
Charleston, South Carolina

Richard S. Stack, M.D.
Assistant Professor of Medicine
Department of Medicine
Director, Interventional Cardiac
    Catheterization Program
Duke Medical Center
Durham, North Carolina

Bruce W. Usher, M.D.
Associate Professor of Medicine
Division of Cardiology
Department of Medicine
Medical University of South Carolina
Charleston, South Carolina

George N. Vetrovec, M.D.
Professor of Medicine
Director, Cardiac Catheterization Laboratory
Medical College of Virginia
Richmond, Virginia

Benjamin E. Victorica, M.D.
Professor of Medicine
Director, Pediatric Cardiac Catheterization
    Laboratory
Department of Pediatrics
University of Florida
Gainesville, Florida

Alan G. Wasserman, M.D.
Assistant Professor of Medicine
Department of Medicine
George Washington University Medical
    Center
Washington, D.C.

Michael D. Winniford, M.D.
Assistant Professor of Medicine
Department of Internal Medicine
Director, Cardiac Catheterization Laboratory
University of Iowa Hospital
Iowa City, Iowa

Alan Woelfel, M.D.
Assistant Professor of Medicine
Division of Cardiology
Department of Medicine
The University of North Carolina
Chapel Hill, North Carolina

Merrill A. Wondrow
Associate, Division of Cardiovascular
    Disease and Internal Medicine
Mayo Clinic and Mayo Foundation
Rochester, Minnesota

Contents

Section *4*
PHYSIOLOGICAL MEASUREMENT 281

Section **5**

SPECIFIC CLINICAL STATES: THEIR ASSESSMENT AND INTERVENTION BY CATHETER TECHNIQUES

Section

1

INTRODUCTION

1

History of the Development and Application of Cardiac Catheterization

Carl J. Pepine, M.D.
James A. Hill, M.D.
Charles R. Lambert, M.D., Ph.D.

HISTORICAL BACKGROUND

In order to practice cardiac catheterization and make use of the results of the procedure to its full extent in the management of patients, some knowledge of its development is useful. Like many diagnostic and therapeutic techniques catheterization evolved through several phases before it reached the position that it now occupies in the practice of medicine. The development and application of cardiac catheterization can be traced through four distinct phases. These are (*a*) development of a technique for measuring intracardiac physiologic events in animals, (*b*) application of these techniques for catheterization of humans, (*c*) development of techniques for selective coronary angiography, and (*d*) development of catheter-based therapeutic procedures.

Development of a Technique for Measuring Intracardiac Physiologic Events in Animals

Claude Bernard is given credit for developing a technique for catheterization of the heart of living animals from the peripheral vessels (1). His initial work in this area began in 1844 when he inserted a mercury thermometer into the carotid artery of a horse and advanced it through the aortic valve into the left ventricle. He also advanced a thermome-

ter from the jugular vein to the right ventricle. The purpose of these experiments was to determine the temperature difference between blood returning from the lungs and that returning from the remainder of the body. His work continued for almost 40 years. During this period, he described in great detail the procedures for venous and arterial catheterization of many animals, crossing the aortic valve and measuring intracardiac pressures. He refined these techniques and then used them as tools to gather data and to solve many scientific problems. From his work the catheter became the accepted reference standard of physiologists for cardiovascular hemodynamic study. The next important milestone came with Adolph Fick's brief but famous single-page note on calculation of blood flow in 1870 (2). Thus, with the measurement of intracardiac pressures and blood flow by cardiac catheterization, detailed studies of the heart and circulation of animals followed.

Development of Techniques for Catheterization of Humans

Credit for human cardiac catheterization is not as easy to assign. Several years before Claude Bernard, J.F. Dieffenbach published his experience with an elastic catheter used to remove extra blood from the central circulation of a dying patient with cholera (3). He described

3

introduction of the catheter into the brachial artery approximately as far as the heart, but we do not know if the heart chambers were actually entered. Frizt Bleichroeder, E. Unger, and W. Loeb published descriptions of human catheterization as early as 1912 and were among the first workers to insert catheters into the blood vessels without x-ray visualization (4). They assigned no specific purpose to these experiments other than to document that catheters could be passed through human veins from the forearm to axilla and from the thigh to the vena cava without problems. During one attempt, Unger and Loeb catheterized Bleichroeder, who reported a stabbing pain in his chest, suggesting that they may have reached his heart.

The advent of chemotherapy apparently stimulated interest in catheterization for the purpose of injecting drugs directly into the central circulation. Bleichroeder and colleagues examined the effects of inserting catheters into dog arteries and leaving the catheters in place for several hours (4). They reported no clot formation or other complications. A clinical trial was done in four patients with puerperal sepsis. They were injected with Collargol through a catheter inserted into the femoral artery and advanced to the bifurcation of the aorta.

In 1929, Werner Forssmann, a 25-year-old surgical trainee in Eberswalde, Germany, apparently unaware of Bleichroeder's work, became interested in catheterization of the heart (5). After an experiment on a human cadaver Forssmann realized how easy it was to guide a urological catheter from an arm vein into the right atrium (6). Apparently, he had the same objective as Bleichroeder et al. of intracardiac injection of drugs, but recognized the potential for diagnosis. Against the advice of his colleagues he dissected the veins of his own forearm and guided a urological catheter to his right atrium using fluoroscopic control and a mirror. He then walked to the x-ray department with the catheter in place, without discomfort or other ill effects to have chest x-rays filmed. Thus, Forssmann was the first to document right heart catheterization using radiographic techniques in humans. Over the next 2 years Forssmann studied a technique in which radiographic contrast material was injected directly into the right atrium through a catheter for radiologic examination of the

right heart (7, 8). He also injected 40% Uroselectan through a catheter that he had positioned in his own right heart (8, 9).

In 1929 dos Santos and colleagues performed abdominal aortography (10). In 1930 Jimenez Diaz and Sanchez-Cuenca advanced a urethral catheter through a cannula into an arm vein of a moribund patient and provided x-ray confirmation of its location in the right atrium. They also suggested its many diagnostic and therapeutic possibilities (11). In the same year they measured the oxygen content in peripheral veins and the right atrium and also the arteriovenous difference (12). At about the same time O. Klein, in Prague, sampled venous blood from the right ventricle and applied the Fick principle to determine cardiac output in several patients with chronic disease (13). Similar studies were done in 1932 by Padilla and associates in Buenos Aires (14). Except for the development of pulmonary angiography, these cardiac catheterization procedures were performed sporadically over the next decade. This "limbo" status was possibly due to severe criticism because of lack of understanding of the full clinical and research applications of the information that could be obtained from cardiac catheterization.

Finally, in the early 1940s Andre Cournand and Hilmert Ranges (15), working in New York with Dickinson Richards, began a systematic and comprehensive investigation of cardiac function in normal and disease patients using **right heart catheterization.** They made many technical advances which included design and construction of catheters with features resembling those used today. These features included balance between flexibility and rigidity to enhance maneuverability, coating with a nonwettable radiopaque material, and a preformed tip. They also designed a special needle cannula with the assistance of Richard Riley. This needle could be inserted percutaneously into either the brachial or femoral artery and left in place for long periods of time. They even developed a mobile recording system capable of recording multiple pressures from fluid-filled manometers along with the electrocardiogram (ECG). They clearly popularized the procedure of right heart catheterization by demonstrating that it was safe and useful, and it subsequently won widespread application. Cournand and his collaborators and trainees moved cardiac catheterization to a level where it became a reference standard for precise anatomical and physiological studies for the evaluation of heart disease in patients. Later, Andre Cournand, Dickinson Richards, and Werner Forssmann shared a Nobel Prize (1956) in physiology and medicine in recognition of their contributions to cardiac catheterization.

By 1947 Zimmerman, working in Cleveland, developed a completely intravascular technique for human **left heart catheterization** (16). This procedure, which was carefully planned, involved retrograde catheterization of the left ventricle from the ulnar artery in a patient with severe aortic insufficiency. This condition was chosen to allow rather easy retrograde passage of the catheter across the incompetent aortic valve. Soon Zimmerman and his colleagues performed simultaneous catheterization of both the right and left heart. Thus, they are credited with the development of **combined heart catheterization** (17).

In 1953 Seldinger described a percutaneous approach to introduce catheters for either right or left heart catheterization (18). An extension of this approach led to the **transseptal approach** to the left heart that was developed independently in 1959 by John Ross (19) and Constantin Cope (20). Later Brockenbrough and Braunwald (21) modified the apparatus so that the last centimeter of the transseptal needle was narrower (21-gauge instead of 18-gauge). Thus, if the needle puncture was done in the wrong place, the resulting hole was not as large. By 1960 Charles Dotter and Goffredo Gensini had adapted the Seldinger technique to special catheters which were more practical for left heart catheterization (22). In the 1950s with the introduction of cardiopulmonary bypass, which made open heart surgery possible, diagnostic catheterization became established for confirmation of clinical findings prior to cardiac surgery for valvular or congenital heart disease.

Development of a Technique for Coronary Angiography in Humans

During the late 1940s and early 1950s, many investigators were working to develop nonselective techniques to visualize the coronary arteries (23). These indirect methods included simply flooding the aortic root with a large quantity of contrast material that flowed into the coronary arteries in diastole. In most instances, only the proximal portions of the left and right coronary arteries were adequately visualized using conventional cineradiographic techniques. Opacification of distal vessels and collaterals was poor, and assessments of coronary obstruction, based upon this method of visualization, were limited. Because most coronary blood flow occurs in diastole, attempts to develop a method of injecting contrast material during diastole were made using electronic devices to activate pressure injectors at selected phases of the cardiac cycle (24, 25). These methods improved opacification, but there were still limitations in visualizing the mid and distal portions of major coronary vessels. While the nonselective methods have been obsolete for more than 20 years, they are presently being revived for use with digital subtraction coronary angiography, cine-computed tomography, three-dimensional computed tomography, and magnetic resonance imaging.

Another example of the indirect method was advanced by Arnulf and Chacornac (26). They observed excellent opacification of coronary arteries in dogs with contrast material injected during cardiac arrest, which was produced accidentally as a complication of anesthesia. This prompted them to arrest an animal's heart deliberately using acetylcholine. Resumption of the heartbeat was usually spontaneous but could always be induced, if necessary, by atropine. In animal experiments in this country, Lehman and colleagues, using this technique, were able to visualize most of the left coronary system (27). It is interesting to note that intracoronary acetylcholine injection has recently been used in humans during coronary angiography to evaluate endothelial function and to provoke coronary artery constriction in patients with variant angina and other conditions (28) (see Chapter 13). Another novel indirect method was advanced by Boerema and Bickman (29). They caused tamponade of the superior vena cava to limit right heart filling by intrabronchial pressure elevation to levels above venous pressure. This maneuver reduced both cardiac output and coronary flow and improved opacification of coronary vessels with nonselective injections. The technique was standardized by Nordenstrom et al. and applied clinically in the early 1960s (30).

In further attempts to improve opacification of coronary arteries, Dotter and Frische utilized a double-lumen, balloon occlusion catheter (31). The soft balloon on this catheter occluded the ascending aorta above the coronary ostia, and a port was provided for contrast material injection below the balloon and just above the aortic valve. General anesthesia was used, and the catheter was introduced through the surgically exposed right brachial artery. Gensini and associates combined this method with either acetylcholine arrest or intrabronchial pressure elevation to improve coronary artery visualization (24).

Bellman and colleagues introduced a specially designed catheter to direct the stream of injected contrast material laterally toward the walls of the aorta to improve opacification of coronary arteries (32). The catheter was preformed into a loop configuration slightly smaller in diameter than the aortic root diameter which was judged by chest x-ray. Side holes along the outer periphery of the loop were oriented to point toward the coronary ostia. Success in dogs prompted Williams and co-workers to apply this technique to human coronary angiographic studies (33).

In 1958 Mason Sones, working in Cleveland, began to develop a **selective coronary angiography** procedure that used appropriate image amplification and optical amplification with high speed cinetechnique. In 1959, while Sones was developing these methods for use in animals, he and his colleagues accidentally injected approximately 40 cc of 90% Hypaque into the right coronary artery of a patient with aortic valve disease during a planned aortogram (34). Although asystole occurred, the patient was resuscitated using coughs and had an uneventful recovery. Sones and Shirey then developed a catheter to selectively enter the coronary arteries. The catheter body was relatively rigid for good torque control but tapered at the tip to facilitate formation of a curve as the tip was advanced against the left aortic valve leaflet (35). They also demonstrated that the selective procedure using this type of catheter was very safe. Thus, selective coronary angiography became the reference standard to assess the coronary arteries for both diagnostic and research purposes (see Chapter 13).

Ricketts and Abrams introduced a **percutaneous technique for selective coronary angiography** in 1962 (36). By 1967 Melvin Judkins (37) and Kurt Amplatz et al. (38) had applied preformed catheters that actually "sought" each coronary ostium from the percutaneous femoral artery approach. A single catheter technique, using a modified Sones-type catheter for use from the percutaneous femoral approach, was introduced in 1966 by Schoonmaker and King (39). Again, with introduction of a safe and effective surgical procedure for coronary artery bypass by Favalaro (40) in 1968, selective coronary angiography grew to become the most frequently performed cardiac catheterization procedure.

Development of Therapeutic Catheterization

Use of catheterization for therapeutic purposes, although clearly in the mind of early workers for the purpose of delivering drugs and withdrawing blood, was delayed until 1950 when Rubeo-Alvarez and Limon-Lason suggested that a catheter method might be used to treat pulmonic stenosis (41). Practical therapeutic catheterization was then realized with the work of William Raskind, working in Philadelphia, who developed a successful procedure to enhance pulmonary blood flow by creation of or enlargement of an atrial septal defect using a balloon (42). Since then, **balloon atrioseptostomy** has continued to have widespread acceptance. **Catheter embolectomy technique** was developed using a small balloon catheter which is now very popular for routine clinical use. Catheter-mounted balloons were also used to test occlude the pulmonary artery for preoperative evaluation of separate lung function (43, 44). Pressure recordings distal to the pulmonary artery balloon occlusion suggested the potential for obtaining pulmonary-capillary pressure from the balloon occlusion pressure. This is the technology which Lategola and Rahn used to develop a **"self-guiding" catheter** for cardiac and pulmonary artery catheterization and occlusion in dogs (45). Swan and Ganz then adapted the concept into a fast, safe, and reliable technique to monitor left ventricle filling pressure and cardiac output in the critical care setting using a **balloon flotation catheter** (46) (see Chapter 6). Moulopoulos et al. introduced (47) adapted catheter-mounted balloon technology in the form of an **intraaortic balloon pump** (IABP) for use as a circulatory assist device.

Independently, several groups developed methods to close congenital cardiac defects with devices delivered by catheters. With further advances in technique, some of the devices are now in use (see Chapter 28). Likewise, techniques to partially interrupt the inferior vena cava with catheter delivered devices (umbrellas, caval filters, etc.) to prevent recurrent pulmonary embolization evolved.

Dotter and Judkins in 1964 were the first to extend interventional catheter techniques to the area of atherosclerosis (48). Intraluminal catheter angioplasty was first performed using serial coaxial catheters to puncture soft thromboatheroma and stretch the lumen of peripheral arteries. Balloons were later applied to the peripheral angioplasty technique by Portsmann (49) and Zeitler et al. (50) in the early 1970s. The balloon technique was further modified and subsequently popularized by Andreas Gruentzig (51). He developed cylindrical, thin-walled, relatively nondistensible balloons for peripheral angioplasty. The balloon was mounted on a double-lumen catheter with equipment for high pressure inflation of the balloon with fluid. Several years later he constructed miniaturized balloons on very small double-lumen catheters for application in the proximal coronary arteries. This technique was applied to the first patient by Gruentzig in Zurich in 1977 (52, 53). His concept of protecting the artery by flexible, small guidewires and using balloons that maintained a relatively uniform preselected size and shape resulted in high success rates and very low occlusion rates. Over the course of several years Gruentzig and others refined the balloon catheter approach to coronary arteries that is now firmly established as **percutaneous transluminal coronary angioplasty (PTCA).** Its success has stimulated the development of a host of other catheter-based interventional vascular procedures which include atherectomy devices, lasers, sparks, and rotary drills. Further evolution of the interventional coronary artery techniques referred to above is discussed in detail in Chapters 15 and 16.

The balloon catheters used for peripheral angioplasty were then enlarged and modified for dilation of stenotic pulmonary valves of children and adults in 1982 (54, 55) (see Chapter 17). Later these balloons were applied to stenotic mitral and aortic valves (56, 57). These **balloon valvuloplasty** techniques continue to evolve (see Chapter 17).

A large number of implantable devices for **cardiac pacing** and **control of arrhythmias** have also been developed which depend upon insertion of catheter-mounted electrodes. Since 1969, when a technique for His' bundle recording was introduced (58), the diagnostic application of catheter techniques to sense intracardiac electrical activity and induce arrhythmias has advanced rapidly. This has developed into a catheter laboratory-based field of clinical electrophysiology (see Chapter 29). This field also now includes catheter directed His' bundle and arrhythmia foci ablation procedures.

SUMMARY

Cardiac catheterization was developed and applied to humans over 5 decades ago. Over these years it has evolved through four major phases. Each phase has led to far-reaching advances in our knowledge and practice of medicine. In its current phase catheterization is a highly specialized discipline encompassing more and more therapeutic procedures that promise to further expand our abilities to manage many problems. Continued advances in the fields of material science and miniaturization are only likely to yield new applications.

References

1. Buzzi A. Claude Bernard on cardiac catheterization. Am J Cardiol 1959;4:405–409.
2. Fick A. Uber die Messung des Blutquantums in den Herzventrikeln'. Phys-med Ges. Wurzburg, July 9, 1870.
3. Dieffenbach JF. Physiologish-chirurgish beobachtigen bie cholera-kranken. Cholera Arch 1832;1: 86–105.
4. Bleichroeder F, Unger E, Loeb W. Intraterielle therapy. Klin Wochenschr 1912;49:1503.
5. Forssmann W. Die sondierung des rechten Herzens. Klin Wochenschr 1929;8:2085–2087.
6. Benatt AJ. Cardiac catheterization: a historical note. Lancet 1949;746–747.
7. Forssmann W. Uber Kontrastdarstellung der Hohlen des lebenrden rechten Herzens und der Lungenschlagader. Munchen Med Wochenschr 1931;78:489–492.

8. Forssmann W. Experiments on myself. Memoirs of a surgeon in Germany. New York: Saint Martin's Press, 1974:84–85.

9. Cournand A. Cardiac catheterization: development of the technique, its contributions to experimental medicine and its initial applications in man. Acta Med Scand 1975;579:7–32.

10. dos Santos R, Lamas AC, Pereira-Caldas J. Arteriografia da aorta e dos vasos abdnominais. Med Contemp 1929;47:93–96.

11. Jimenez-Diaz C, Sanchez-Cuenca B. El sondage del corazon derecho. Arch Cardioly Hemat 1930; 11:105–108.

12. Jimenez-Diaz C, Sanchez-Cuenca B. Estudios de insuficiencia circulatoria: investigaciones sobre los gases en la sangra arterial y venosa en reposo y en el esfuerzo. Arch Cardioly Hemat 1930;11:531–550.

13. Klein O. Determining human cardiac output (minute volume) using Fick's principle (extraction of mixed venous blood by cardiac catheterization). Med Wochenschr 1930;77:1311–1312.

14. Padilla T, Cossio P, Berconsky I. Sondeo del Corazon: determinacion del volumen minuto circulatorio. Semana Medica 1932;2:445–448.

15. Cournand A, Ranges HA. Catheterization of the right auricle in man. Proc Soc Exp Biol Med 1941;46:462–466.

16. Zimmerman HA, Scott RW, Becker NO. Catheterization of the left side of the heart in man. Circulation 1950;1:357–359.

17. Zimmerman HA, ed. Intra vascular catheterization. Springfield, IL: Charles C Thomas, 1959.

18. Seldinger SI. Catheter replacement of the needle in percutaneous arteriography. Acta Radiol 1953;39:368–376.

19. Ross J. Transseptal left heart catheterization: a new method of left atrial puncture. Ann Surg 1959; 149:395–401.

20. Cope C. Technique for transseptal catheterization of the left atrium: preliminary report. J Thorac Surg 1959;37:482–486.

21. Brockenbrough EC, Braunwald E. A new technic for left ventricular angiocardiography and transseptal left heart catheterization. Am J Cardiol 1960;6:1062–1064.

22. Dotter CT, Gensini GG. Percutaneous retrograde catheterization of left ventricle and systemic arteries of man. Radiology 1960;75:171–184.

23. Radner S. An attempt at the roentgenologic visualization of coronary blood vessels in man. Acta Radiol 1945;26:497–502.

24. Gensini GG, Di Giorgi S, Black A. New approaches to coronary arteriography. Angiology 1961;12:223–238.

25. Richards LS, Thal, AP. Phasic dye injection control system for coronary arteriography in the human. Surg Gynecol Obstet 1958;107:739–743.

26. Arnulf G, Chacornac R. L'arteriographie methodique des arteres coronaires grâce a l'utilisation de l'acetylcholine. Donnees experimentales et cliniques. Bull Acad Natl Med (Paris) 1958;25, 26:661–673.

27. Lehman JS, Boyer RA, Winter FS. Coronary arteriography. Am J Roentgenol 1959;81:749–763.

28. Yasue H, Horio Y, Nakamura N, et al. Induction of coronary artery spasm by acetylcholine in patients with variant angina: possible role of the parasympathetic nervous system in the pathogenesis of coronary artery spasm. Circulation 1987;74:955–963.

29. Boerema I, Blickman JR. Reduced intrathoracic circulation as an aid in angiocardiography: an experimental study. J Thorac Surg 1955;30:129–142.

30. Nordenstrom B, Ovenfors C, Tornell G. Coronary angiography in 100 cases of ischemic heart disease. Radiology 1962;78:714–724.

31. Dotter CT, Frische LH. Visualization of the coronary circulation by occlusion aortography: a practical method. Radiology 1958;71:502–523.

32. Bellman S, Frank HA, Lambert PB, Littmann D, Williams JA. Coronary arteriography. I. Differential opacification of the aortic stream by catheters of special design—experimental development. N Engl J Med 1960;262:325–328.

33. Williams JA, Littmann D, Hall JH, Bellman S, Lambert PB, Frank HA. Coronary arteriography. II. Clinical experiences with the loop-end catheter. N Engl J Med 1960;262:328–332.

34. Sones MF, Shirey EK, Proudfit WL, Westcott RN. Cine coronary arteriography (abstr). Circulation 1959;20:773.

35. Sones FM, Shirey EK. Cine coronary arteriography. Mod Concepts Cardiovasc Dis 1962;31:735–738.

36. Ricketts HJ, Abrams HL. Percutaneous selective coronary cine arteriography. JAMA 1962;181:620–624.

37. Judkins MP. Selective coronary arteriography. Part I. A percutaneous transfemoral technic. Radiology 1967;89:815–824.

38. Amplatz K, Formanek G, Stanger P, Wilson W. Mechanics of selective coronary artery catheterization via femoral approach. Radiology 1967:89:1040–1047.

39. Schoonmaker FW, King SB. Coronary arteriography by the single catheter percutaneous femoral technique. Experience in 6800 cases. Circulation 1974;50:735–740.

40. Favaloro RG. Saphenous vein autograft replacement of severe segmental coronary artery occlusion: operative technique. Ann Thorac Surg 1968;5:334–339.

41. Rubeo-Alvarez V, Limon-Lason J. Treatment of pulmonary valvular stenosis and tricuspid stenosis with a modified cardiac catheter. Washington, DC, Proceedings of the First National Conference on Cardiovascular Diseases, 1950.

42. Rashkind WJ, Wagner HR, Tait MA. Historical aspects of interventional cardiology: past, present and future. Texas Heart Inst J 1986;13:363–367.

43. Carlens E, Hanson HE, Nordenstrom B. Temporary unilateral occlusion of the pulmonary artery. J Thorac Surg 1951;22:527–536.

44. Dotter CT, Lukas DS. Acute cor pulmonale. An experimental study utilizing a special cardiac catheter. Am J Physiol 1951;164:254–262.

45. Lategola M, Rahn H. A self-guiding catheter for cardiac and pulmonary arterial catheterization

and occlusion. Proc Soc Exp Biol Med 1953;84: 667–668.

46. Swan HJC, Ganz W, Forrester JS, Marcus H, Diamond G, Chonette D. Catheterization of the heart in man with use of a flow-directed balloon-tipped catheter. N Engl J Med 1970; 283:447–451.

47. Moulopoulos SD, Topaz S, Kolff WJ. Diastolic balloon pumping (with carbon dioxide) in the aorta: mechanical assistance to the failing circulation. Am Heart J 1962;63:669–675.

48. Dotter CT, Judkins MP. Transluminal treatment of arteriosclerotic obstruction: description of a new technique and a preliminary report of its application. Circulation 1964;30:654–670.

49. Porstmann W. Ein neuer korsett-ballonkatheter fur transluminalen rekanalisation nach dotter unter besonderer berucksichtigung von obliterationen an den beckenarterien. Radiol Diagn (Berl) 1973;14:239–244.

50. Zeitler E, Schmidtke J, Schoop W. Die perkutane Behandlung von arteriellen Durchblutungsstorungen der extremitaten mit katheter. Vasa 1973;2:401–408.

51. Gruentzig A. Die perkutane Rekanalisation chronischer arterieller Verschlusse (Dotter-Prinzip) mit einem doppellumigen Dilatationskatheter. Fortschr Roentgenstr 1976;124:80–86.

52. Gruentzig A, Senning A, Siegenthaler WE. Nonoperative dilatation of coronary-artery stenosis: percutaneous transluminal coronary angioplasty. N Engl J Med 1979;301:61–68.

53. Gruentzig A. Transluminal dilatation of coronary-artery stenosis (letter to editor). Lancet 1978; I:263.

54. Kan JS, White RI, Mitchell SE, Gardner TJ. Percutaneous balloon valvuloplasty: a new method for treating congenital pulmonary valve stenosis. N Engl J Med 1982;307:540–542.

55. Pepine CJ, Gessner IH, Feldman RL. Percutaneous balloon valvuloplasty for pulmonic valve stenosis in the adult. Am J Cardiol 1982;50:1442–1445.

56. Cribier A, Saoudi N, Berland J, Savin T, Rocha P, Letac B. Percutaneous transluminal valvuloplasty of acquired aortic stenosis in elderly patients: an alternative to valve replacement? Lancet 1986; 1:178–179.

57. Inoue K, Owaki T, Nakamura T, Kitamura F, Miyamoto N. Clinical application of transvenous mitral commissurotomy by a new balloon catheter. J Thorac Cardiovasc Surg 1984;87:394–402.

58. Damato AN, Lau SH, Berkowitz WD, Rosen KM, Lisi KR. Recording of specialized conducting fibers (A-V nodal, His bundle, and right bundle branch) in man using an electrode catheter technique. Circulation 1969;39:435–447.

Section

2

INDICATIONS/ CONTRAINDICATIONS/ RISKS/BENEFITS

2

Indications and Contraindications

Carl J. Pepine, M.D.
James A. Hill, M.D.
Charles R. Lambert, M.D., Ph.D.

GENERAL GOALS

The general goal of a cardiac catheterization procedure is **to precisely define patho-anatomic and pathophysiologic alterations caused by various disease or treatment processes.** These data provide information to aid in subsequent management of patients with cardiovascular disorders.

Subjective data (patient symptoms) should be correlated with objective anatomical and physiological data obtained during catheterization. This information is then used to answer a number of clinically important questions. Who is normal? Who is abnormal? If abnormal, how severe is the abnormality? It must be determined whether or not the clinical findings are due to a specific etiologic form of heart disease. This information is then used in the management of the patient regarding prognosis determination and selection of the type of treatment, whether it be drugs alone, catheterization intervention, or surgical. Cardiac catheterization aids in the determination of candidates for application of specific therapeutic interventions such as percutaneous transluminal coronary angioplasty (PTCA), intracoronary thrombolysis, and valvuloplasty. The results of treatment may also be evaluated at cardiac catheterization. This includes atherosclerosis regression or progression, deterioration or improvement in left ventricular function, and restenosis following PTCA or graft occlusion following surgery.

Decisions relative to precise diagnosis, formulation of prognosis, and specific therapeutic interventions can be applied based upon objective data. Since the introduction of cardiac catheterization, science and technology in this area have rapidly developed. Some catheterization procedures are unique. For example, coronary angiography is the only means by which one can adequately visualize the coronary arteries in a living patient. There is no other technique short of pathologic dissection to precisely identify and assess the extent and degree of coronary obstruction. In addition, other obstructive lesions (e.g., coronary spasm and thrombus) and congenital variations within arteries supplying the heart may be documented. Cardiac catheterization can be performed very safely; therefore, if patients are carefully selected, the benefit obtained from the information gathered far outweighs the relatively low risk and cost.

INDICATIONS
General Considerations

Specific situations where cardiac catheterization is indicated will vary depending upon the specific catheterization procedure under consideration. One should also appreciate that the need for a specific cardiac catheterization procedure appears to be variable within different practice settings, even when similar patients are evaluated. For example, the need for coronary angiography was examined by physicians from University, Community, and Health Maintenance Organization practices (1). These physicians all reviewed the same case histories and then recorded their opinions relative to a perceived need for coronary angiography using a semiquantitative scale ranging from definitely not indicated to definitely indicated. Results of their assessments are shown in Figure 2.1. Although the median values agree closely, there is a wide range of opinion among the different settings on the need for this catheterization procedure. The important point is that any list of indications for cardiac catheterization is not absolute. One should not expect to refer every patient seen with a specific condition or situation that might be listed in a table of indications for catheterization. There are special aspects related to every case that demand clinical judgment.

Specific Considerations

There are situations within the various forms of heart disease where there is sufficient general agreement to provide some guidelines to help make decisions about the need for catheterization (2, 3). Specific situations where there is agreement on the application of coronary angiography have been summarized by the ACC/AHA Task Force (2). We are in agreement with these guidelines and use them in our laboratory. Since coronary angiography is by far the most frequently performed catheterization procedure, we have summarized these guidelines below in slightly modified form.

Classification of Applications of Coronary Angiography

In considering the use of coronary angiography in specific disease states, the Task Force Committee used the following classification.

Class I: Conditions for which there is **general agreement that coronary angiography is justified**. A Class I indication should not be taken to mean that coronary angiography is the only acceptable diagnostic procedure.

Class II: Conditions for which coronary angiography is **frequently performed, but**

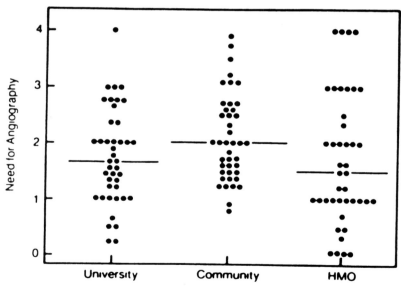

Figure 2.1 Variability of the need for cardiac catheterization procedures. Given the same case histories, the need for coronary angiography was rated by physicians in three practice settings (university, community, and health maintenance organization) on a scale from 0 (definitely not indicated) to 4 (definitely indicated). Each *black circle* relates to a single case, and the *horizontal lines* indicate median ratings. The data suggest that patients with medical problems are evaluated differently in different settings relative to the need for catheterization. Thus, the indications for catheterization are not to be taken as absolute. (From Hlatky MA, Lee KL, Botvinick EH, Brundage BH. Diagnostic test use in different practice settings. A controlled comparison. Arch Intern Med 1983;143:1886-1889.

there is a divergence of opinion with respect to its justification in terms of value and appropriateness.

Class III: Conditions for which there is general agreement that coronary angiography is not ordinarily justified.

Known or Suspect Coronary Heart Disease

Asymptomatic Patients

Asymptomatic patients with **known** coronary artery disease (CAD) generally are those who have had previous myocardial infarction, coronary bypass surgery, or angioplasty (asymptomatic patients within 8 weeks of an acute myocardial infarction are considered under convalescent myocardial infarction listed later). Asymptomatic patients with **suspected** CAD generally are those who have rest or exercise-induced ECG abnormalities suggesting "silent myocardial ischemia," often in association with other risk factors.

Class I includes those with:

1. Evidence of "high risk" (see Table 2.1) on noninvasive testing (4, 5).
2. An occupation that involves safety of others, for example, airline pilots, bus drivers, truck drivers, air traffic controllers. Also certain occupations that frequently require sudden vigorous activity, for example, firefighters, police officers, athletes.
3. Successful resuscitation from cardiac arrest that occurred without obvious precipitating cause when a reasonable suspicion of CAD exists.

Class II includes those with:

1. The presence of ≥ 1 but <2 mm of ischemic ST depression during exercise, confirmed as ischemia by an independent noninvasive stress test (thallium or ventriculographic study by radionuclide, contrast, or two-dimensional echocardiography), but without criteria for high risk as listed in classes I.1, I.2, and I.3).
2. Two or more major risk factors and evidence for ischemia by noninvasive testing in a man without known coronary heart disease.
3. Prior myocardial infarction with normal left ventricular function at rest and evidence for ischemia by noninvasive testing, but without high risk criteria (class I.1).
4. Coronary bypass surgery or PTCA, after which there is evidence for ischemia by noninvasive testing.
5. Evidence for ischemia by noninvasive testing in patients who need to undergo high-risk noncardiac surgery.
6. Cardiac transplantation undergoing yearly evaluation.

Table 2.1
High-Risk Indicators by Noninvasive Testing for Patients with Known or Suspect Coronary Artery Disease

A. Exercise ECG Testing
  Abnormal horizontal or downsloping ST segment depression:
    Onset at HR <120 min or ≤ 6.5 METS
    Magnitude ≥ 2.0 mm of depression
    Postexercise duration ≥ 6 min
    Depression in multiple leads
  Abnormal systolic blood pressure response during progressive exercise:
    With sustained decrease of >10 mm Hg *or*
    Flat response (≤ 130 mm Hg), associated ECG evidence of ischemia
  Other potentially important determinants:
    Exercise-induced ST segment elevation in leads other than aVR
    Exercise-induced ventricular tachycardia
B. Thallium Scintigraphy
  Abnormal thallium uptake in more than one vascular region either at rest or with exercise that shows redistribution.
  Increased lung uptake of thallium produced by exercise.
C. Radionuclide Ventriculography or Quantitative Two-Dimensional Echocardiography
  A fall in left ventricular ejection fraction of 0.10 or more during exercise, or a resting or exercising left ventricular ejection fraction of less than 0.50 when suspected to be due to coronary artery disease (CAD).

Class III includes those with:

1. Need for a screening test for coronary artery disease without appropriate noninvasive testing.
2. Coronary bypass surgery or PTCA after which there is no evidence of ischemia, unless with informed consent for institutionally approved research purposes.
3. An abnormal ECG exercise test alone, excluding the categories listed in classes I and II.

Symptomatic Patients

Symptomatic patients are those with symptoms thought to be due to CAD. Symptoms are defined in accordance with the Canadian Cardiovascular Society classification (6) (Table 2.2).

Class I includes those with:

1. Angina pectoris that is inadequately responsive to medical treatment, PTCA, thrombolytic therapy, or coronary bypass surgery. "Inadequately responsive" is taken to mean that both patient and physician feel that angina significantly interferes with a patient's occupation or ability to perform his or her usual activities and therefore results in an unacceptable life-style.

Table 2.2
Grading of Effort Angina by the Canadian Cardiovascular Society[a]

I. **Ordinary physical activity, such as walking and climbing stairs, does not cause angina.** Angina occurs with strenuous or prolonged exertion at work or recreation.

II. **Slight limitation of ordinary activity.** Angina occurs with walking or climbing stairs rapidly, walking uphill, walking or stair climbing after meals, or in cold, or in wind, or under emotional stress, or only during the few hours after awakening. Walking more than two blocks on the level and climbing more than one flight of ordinary stairs at a normal pace and in normal conditions.

III. **Marked limitation of ordinary physical activity.** Angina occurs with walking one to two blocks on the level and climbing one flight of stairs in normal conditions and at normal pace.

IV. **Inability to carry on any physical activity without discomfort.** Angina may be present at rest.

[a] Campeau L. Grading of angina pectoris (letter to editor). Circulation 1976;54:522-523.

2. Unstable angina pectoris
   a. Acceleration with increased severity and frequency of chronic angina pectoris within the past 2 months, despite medical management, including onset of angina at rest (Canadian Cardiovascular Society class IV, Table 2.2).
   b. New onset (within 2 months) of angina pectoris that is either severe or increases despite medical treatment.
   c. Acute coronary insufficiency, with pain at rest (Canadian Cardiovascular Society class IV), that is usually 15 min or longer in duration, associated with ST-T wave changes, within the preceding 2 weeks.
3. Prinzmetal's or variant angina pectoris
4. Angina pectoris (even of Canadian Cardiovascular Society class I or II severity) in association with any of the following:
   a. Evidence of "high risk" as outlined in Table 2.1.
   b. Coexistence of a history of either myocardial infarction or hypertension with ST segment depression.
   c. Intolerance to medical therapy because of uncontrollable side effects.
   d. An occupation or life-style that involves either unusual risk, or "need to know" for insurance or job-related purposes.
   e. Episodic pulmonary edema or symptoms of left ventricular failure without obvious cause.
5. Before major vascular surgery, such as repair of an aortic aneurysm, iliofemoral bypass, or carotid artery surgery, if angina pectoris is present or there is objective evidence of myocardial ischemia.
6. After resuscitation from cardiac arrest (ventricular fibrillation or standstill) or from sustained ventricular tachycardia in the absence of acute myocardial infarction.

Class II includes those with:

1. Angina pectoris in the following groups:
   a. Female patients <40 years of age with objective evidence of myocardial ischemia by noninvasive testing.
   b. Male patients <40 years of age.
   c. Patients <40 years of age with previous myocardial infarction.
   d. Patients requiring major nonvascular surgery (intraabdominal, intrathoracic, and so on) if there is objective evidence of myocardial ischemia.
   e. Patients who show a progressively more abnormal exercise ECG or other noninvasive stress test on serial testing.
2. The presence of Canadian Cardiovascular Society class III or IV angina which, with

medical management, changes to class I or II when other studies suggest absence of high risk (see above).

3. Patients who cannot be risk-stratified by other means; for example, those unable to exercise because of amputation, arthritis, limb deformity, or peripheral vascular disease.

Class III includes those with:

1. Mild, clinically stable angina pectoris who do not have impaired ventricular function or exercise studies suggesting high risk.
2. Well-controlled angina pectoris who are clearly not candidates for either coronary artery bypass surgery or angioplasty because of age or a life expectancy limited by other illnesses.

Atypical Chest Pain of Uncertain Origin

Atypical chest pain is defined as single or recurrent episodes of chest pain suggestive but not typical of the discomfort usually associated with transient myocardial ischemia. The discomfort may have some features of ischemic pain together with features of noncardiac pain. Chest pain that has no features of cardiac pain, as well as typical angina as determined by a careful history, is excluded from this definition.

Class I includes those with:

1. Atypical chest pain when stress tests indicate that high-risk CAD may be present (see Table 2.1).
2. Atypical chest pain thought to be due to coronary artery spasm.
3. Associated symptoms or signs of abnormal left ventricular function or heart failure.

Class II includes those with:

1. Atypical chest pain when noninvasive studies are either equivocal or cannot be adequately performed.
2. Noninvasive tests that are negative but whose symptoms are severe and management requires that significant CAD be excluded.

Acute Myocardial Infarction

The management of acute myocardial infarction is rapidly changing. Therefore, indications for coronary angiography and its timing after acute myocardial infarction are topics of controversy and continue to change as

experience evolves. Acute infarction will be considered in three phases. The phase of **evolving myocardial infarction** encompasses the initial hours after the onset of chest pain and is the period when intravenous or intracoronary fibrinolytic agent use has been shown to reduce mortality and the amount of tissue necrosis. The phase of **completed infarction** begins after the initial hours lasting up to, but not including, predischarge evaluation; during this period a relatively small percentage of patients suffer additional complications. The phase of **convalescent infarction** is the ensuing period of up to 8 weeks, when predischarge and postdischarge assessment, progressive ambulation, and rehabilitation take place.

Evolving Myocardial Infarction

The evolving myocardial infarction phase is limited to the initial hours of myocardial infarction.

Class I includes when coronary angiography, and possible PTCA can be performed within the first 6 hr after onset of chest pain in patients who are not candidates for intravenous thrombolytic therapy due to contraindication related to possible bleeding (recent stroke, coagulation disorder, gastrointestinal bleeding, recent surgery, etc.)

Class II includes:

1. When coronary angiography can be performed within the first 6 hours after the onset of chest pain in patients who are candidates for revascularization therapy (PTCA, coronary bypass surgery, and intracoronary thrombolysis).
2. After early intravenous thrombolytic therapy when immediate PTCA or coronary artery bypass grafting is being contemplated.

Completed Myocardial Infarction

The completed myocardial infarction phase begins after the initial 6 hr and continues up to but not including predischarge evaluation.

Class I includes those with:

1. Recurrent episodes of ischemic chest pain, particularly if accompanied by ECG changes.
2. Suspected mitral regurgitation or ruptured interventricular septum causing heart failure or shock.
3. Suspected subacute cardiac rupture (pseudoaneurysm).

Class II includes those with:

1. Thrombolytic therapy during the evolving phase, particularly with evidence of reperfusion.
2. Congestive heart failure and/or hypotension while receiving intensive medical therapy.
3. Recurrent ventricular tachycardia and/or ventricular fibrillation while receiving intensive antiarrhythmic therapy.
4. Cardiogenic shock.
5. Infarction suspected to be a consequence of coronary embolization.

Class III includes those with uncomplicated infarction without prior thrombolytic therapy.

Convalescent Myocardial Infarction

The convalescent myocardial infarction phase includes the immediate predischarge evaluation up to approximately 8 weeks after discharge.

Class I includes those with:

1. Angina pectoris occurring either at rest or with minimal activity.
2. Either heart failure during the evolving phase or left ventricular ejection fraction <45%, primarily when associated with some manifestation of recurrent myocardial ischemia or with significant ventricular arrhythmias.
3. Evidence of myocardial ischemia on laboratory testing: exercise-induced ischemia (with or without exercise-induced angina pectoris), manifested by ≥1 mm of ischemic ST segment depression or exercise-induced reversible thallium-201 perfusion defect or defects, or exercise-induced reduction in the ejection fraction or new wall motion abnormalities on radionuclide ventriculographic studies.
4. Non-Q wave myocardial infarction.

Class II includes those with:

1. Mild angina pectoris.
2. Asymptomatic status at <50 years of age.
3. The need to return to unusually active and vigorous physical employment.
4. A past history of documented myocardial infarction or stable angina pectoris, or both, present for >6 months before the current infarction.
5. Thrombolytic therapy during the evolving phase, particularly with evidence of reperfusion.

Class III includes those with:

1. Presence of advanced physiologic age.
2. Coexisting disease, judged to be primarily responsible for prognosis, with a greatly shortened life expectancy.
3. Presence of very advanced left ventricular dysfunction in the absence of angina pectoris or evidence of ischemia.
4. Ventricular arrhythmias but no evidence of ischemia (symptomatically or on exercise testing), well-preserved exercise tolerance and no suggestion of aneurysm formation

Valvular Heart Disease

Class I is indicated:

1. When valve surgery is being considered in the adult patient with chest discomfort or ECG changes, or both, suggesting CAD.
2. When valve surgery is being considered in male patients ≥35 years of age.
3. When valve surgery is being considered in female patients who are postmenopausal.

Class II is indicated:

1. During left heart catheterization when aortic or mitral valve surgery is being considered in male patients <35 years of age.
2. During left heart catheterization when aortic or mitral valve surgery is being considered in female patients ≥40 years of age.
3. When one or more major risk factors for CAD are present (heavy smoking history, diabetes mellitus, hypertension, hyperlipidemia, strong family history of premature CAD) in adult patients of any age being considered for valve surgery.
4. During left heart catheterization when reoperation for aortic or mitral valve disease is being considered in patients who have not had coronary angiography for ≥1 year.
5. In the presence of infective endocarditis when there is evidence of coronary embolization.

Class III is indicated:

1. When cardiac surgical treatment is planned for infective endocarditis in patients who are <35 years of age and have no evidence of coronary embolization.
2. When aortic or mitral valve surgery is being considered in female patients <40 years of age who have no evidence suggesting ischemic heart disease.

Known or Suspected Congenital Heart Disease

Class I is indicated in:

1. Evaluation of patients with congenital heart disease who have signs or symptoms suggesting associated atherosclerotic CAD.
2. Suspected congenital coronary anomalies such as congenital coronary artery stenosis, coronary arteriovenous fistula, supravalvular aortic stenosis, and anomalous origin of the left coronary artery, provided that aortography is not diagnostic.
3. When corrective open heart surgery for congenital heart disease is being planned in male patients >35 years or in postmenopausal female patients.

Class II is indicated by the presence of forms of congenital heart disease frequently associated with coronary artery anomalies that may complicate surgical management (including tetralogy of Fallot, truncus arteriosus, transposition complexes, corrected (levo) transposition), provided that aortography is not diagnostic.

Class III is appropriate in the routine evaluation of congenital heart disease.

Other Conditions

Class I is indicated:

1. In diseases affecting the aorta when knowledge of the presence or extent of coronary artery involvement is necessary for management (for example, the presence of aortic aneurysm or ascending aortic dissection), arteritis or homozygous type II hypercholesteremia in which coronary artery involvement is suspected. The latter includes the presence of Kawasaki's disease in patients who have angina and other evidence of myocardial ischemia or infarction.
2. When there is left ventricular failure without obvious cause and adequate left ventricular systolic function (see section on high risk above).
3. When male patients who are ≥35 years of age or female patients who are postmenopausal with hypertrophic cardiomyopathy have angina pectoris uncontrolled by medical therapy or are to undergo surgery for outflow tract obstruction.

Class II is indicated in:

1. The presence of dilated cardiomyopathy.
2. Recent blunt trauma to the chest and evidence of acute myocardial infarction or ischemia in patients who have no evidence of preexisting CAD.
3. Male patients >35 years or postmenopausal female patients who are to undergo other cardiac surgical procedures, such as pericardiectomy or removal of chronic pulmonary emboli.
4. Prospective immediate cardiac transplant male donors >35 or females >40 years of age.
5. Evaluation of asymptomatic patients with Kawasaki's disease who have coronary artery aneurysm or echocardiography.

Application of Other Catheterization Procedures

The indications for other cardiac catheterization procedures are not as easily summarized as those for coronary angiography. Those used in our laboratory are outlined below. In our opinion these all would be class I. As the indications for coronary angiography are detailed above, these indications are in most cases for **right and left heart catheterization** unless otherwise noted.

Patients with Known or Suspected Valvular Heart Disease

1. Preoperative evaluation of all patients with signs and symptoms suggesting moderately severe or severe valvular stenosis or incompetence.
2. Evaluation of certain patients with mitral or aortic valve disease when symptoms are severe and out of proportion to noninvasive laboratory findings.

Patients with Known or Suspected Congenital Heart Disease

1. Preoperative evaluation of all patients with signs or symptoms suggesting moderately severe disease.
2. All cyanotic patients.

Patients with Known or Suspected Miscellaneous Cardiovascular Disorder

1. Aortic root dissection.
2. Hypertrophic cardiomyopathy prior to surgical correction.
3. Constrictive pericarditis.

4. Cardiac or pericardial tumors.
5. Heart failure of undetermined origin.
6. Pulmonary hypertension.
7. Transluminal retrieval of intravascular foreign bodies.
8. As an investigative tool for Institutional Review Board-approved research projects.

CONTRAINDICATIONS

All contraindications to cardiac catheterization are relative except, perhaps, for those of the rare patient with lack of vascular access to the heart (Table 2.3). However, a number of patients may have an increased risk and/or debilitation at some point in time from other diseases. Some could benefit from correction of the other illness prior to cardiac catheterization. In this sense, catheterization may be relatively contraindicated at a certain point in time. These patients include: those with recent stroke (within 1 month); progressive renal insufficiency; active gastrointestinal bleeding; fever which may be due to infection; known active infection; severe electrolyte imbalance; severe anemia (e.g., hematocrit <30%); severe uncontrolled hypertension (e.g., BP 180/100); and lack of available emergency cardiac surgical backup for patients who are particularly unstable. For example, a patient in cardiogenic shock in the course of an acute myocardial infarction with suspected mitral insufficiency due to papillary muscle rupture would best be stabilized with an intraaortic balloon pump and nitroprusside infusion. The patient could then be transferred to a center where emergency cardiac surgery is available both during and immediately after cardiac catheterization. Also included are patients with conditions which limit the patient's life span to a greater degree than the suspected cardiac illness, such as cancer, advanced physiologic age (perhaps greater than 80 years) but not chronologic age, end-stage pulmonary, or liver disease. Finally, we include patients who refuse intended therapeutic procedures for which the catheterization is being performed, for example, those refusing coronary bypass surgery, PTCA, or other potential forms of treatment. Also included are patients with general systemic or psychologic illnesses for which the outcome is so unpredictable that catheterization would be associated with an undue risk.

Table 2.3
Relative Contraindications to Cardiac Catheterization

Conditions which may temporarily increase risks so that when possible they should be corrected before cardiac catheterization.

    Recent cerebral vascular accidents (within 1 month)

    Progressive renal insufficiency

    Active gastrointestinal bleeding

    Fever which may be due to infection

    Known active infection

    Severe anemia

    Severe uncontrolled hypertension

    Lack of available emergency cardiac surgical backup

Conditions which may limit patients' survival or function

    Cancer and/or other disease that limits the patient's life to a greater degree than the suspected cardiac illness

    End-stage pulmonary or liver disease

    Advanced physiologic age >80 years

    General systemic or severe psychiatric illness

Patients who refuse therapeutic procedures to be directed by catheterization results

    Those refusing cardiac surgery

    Those who either can not or will not undergo cardiac surgery and who also refuse other potential forms of treatment (e.g., PTCA, valvoplasty)

All of the above problems, however, are only **relative contraindications** because they may be reversible or temporary in certain patients. Hence, a relatively safe or safer catheterization could be performed when or if the condition is corrected. However, in the event of a life-threatening cardiac emergency, which could be corrected by information obtained by catheterization, the high-risk procedure may be justified.

In summary, from a practical standpoint the patient's physician must make the best estimate possible of the potential risks and benefits in either recommending or not recommending a specific cardiac catheterization procedure to any given patient. In many patients this decision is relatively straightforward, but in some others it may be very difficult. The guidelines presented in this chapter are intended to assist in this important task.

References

1. Hlatky MA, Lee KL, Botvinick EH, Brundage BH. Diagnostic test use in different practice settings. A controlled comparison. Arch Intern Med 1983;143:1886–1889.
2. ACC/AHA Task Force on Assessment of Diagnostic and Therapeutic Cardiovascular Procedures (Subcommittee on Coronary Angiography). Guidelines for coronary angiography. J Am Coll Cardiol 1987;10:935–950.
3. Willerson JT. Selection of patients for coronary angiography. Circulation 1985;72:V3–V8.
4. ACC/AHA Task Force on Assessment of Cardiovascular Procedures. Guidelines for exercise testing. J Am Coll Cardiol 1986;8:725–738.
5. ACC/AHA Task Force on Assessment of Cardiovascular Procedures. Guidelines for clinical use of cardiac radionuclide imaging. J Am Coll Cardiol 1986;8:1471–1483.
6. Campeau L. Grading of angina pectoris (letter to editor). Circulation 1976;54:522–523.

3

Risks of Cardiac Catheterization

Frank J. Hildner, M.D.

COMPLICATIONS, RISKS, AND PREVENTION

The practice of cardiac catheterization and angiography has continued to evolve throughout its 60 years of existence. Current practices are substantially different from those of the 1950s and early 1960s when congenital and valve diseases were primarily studied, and technical advances such as direct current (DC) defibrillation, closed chest cardiac massage, and temporary pacemakers were being introduced. The late 1960s and 1970s saw monumental changes in catheter design; electronic, hemodynamic and angiocardiographic recording devices; and knowledge of cardiovascular physiology. These, in turn, permitted invasive procedures to focus on coronary artery disease (CAD) and catheter-delivered therapeutic interventions. Initially, sick or unstable patients were not studied. Now, because of the advances noted above, neither acute myocardial infarction (AMI) nor unstable angina are contraindications for study. The possibility of salvaging ischemic myocardium has revolutionized indications and the practice of invasive cardiology. As a result of this evolution, the complications associated with cardiac catheterization and angiography have changed. They reflect the skills and technologic advances achieved through the years, as well as challenges of treating patients who have more complex problems and are at higher risk. The purpose of this chapter is to review these complications and specifically focus on factors that relate to risk of complication and prevention.

MAJOR STUDIES OF CATHETERIZATION-RELATED COMPLICATIONS

General Catheterization Procedures

Many reports chronicle complications which have occurred over the years during general cardiac catheterization procedures that usually include left heart catheterization and left ventriculography (1-4). Experience has shown, however, that proper perspective and precise knowledge are best derived from prospective studies, encompassing a wide variety of pathologic conditions in very large groups and subsets of patients. Four studies (Table 3.1) that meet these criteria and present a clear picture of contemporary catheterization practice are the: (*a*) Coronary Artery Surgery Study (CASS) report of complications of coronary arteriography in 1979 (5); (*b*) CASS report of coronary arteriography and bypass surgery of 1983 (6); (*c*) Society for Cardiac Angiography (SFCA) Registry report of 1982 (7); and (*d*) SFCA registry data accumulated from July 1984 through June 1987 that have not been previously reported (8).

The CASS study enrolled approximately 25,000 patients beginning in 1974 and continuing through 1979. The report included 7553 consecutive patients undergoing coronary arteriography at 15 institutions (5). The report of 1983 included data on 19,309 patients undergoing coronary angiography (6). The 1982 report of the Registry Committee of the SFCA was based on 53,581 studies performed by 66 laboratories over a 14-month period

Table 3.1
Comparison of Demographic Data from Major Studies of Catheterization Related Complications (%)

(*n*) a	CASS 1979 (7553)	CASS 1983 (19,309)	SFCA 1982 (53,581)	SFCA 1987 (156,853)
Patient description				
Age (yr)				
<1	- b	0.0	0.9	0.2
1-29	-	0.9	3.0	0.9
30-45	-	17.5	15.0	11.2
46-60	-	57.3	49.0	39.2
60 +	-	24.3	33.0	48.5
Sex				
Male	-	75	56	66
Female	-	25	44	34
Functional class				
I	-	6	16	14
II	-	29	36	29
III	-	36	32	34
IV	-	18	16	23
Ejection fraction				
<30%	-	-	6	4
30–49%	-	27	21	20
50 + %	-	73	73	76
Coronary anatomy				
No stenosis	27	21	28	28
1 Vessel	20	21	16	-
2 Vessel	22	25	19	-
3 Vessel	31	33	30	-
Left main	9	9	9	6

[a] *n*, number of patients.
[b] -, not available.

ending in 1981 that reported their experience after entering the registry at various times. The 1987 report from the SFCA includes data from 199,176 patients, of whom 156,853 had coronary angiographic procedures reported by 70 laboratories according to a protocol established by the Registry Committee of the SFCA. These prospective studies represent the largest numbers of patients reported thus far. They are identical neither in design nor composition, but the subgroups created are so large that valid comparisons may be made.

Analysis of Complications

In the CASS patients, who had only CAD, the total complication rate was 1.76 in the 1979 report and 1.67% in the 1983 report (Table 3.2). The SFCA studies included all diagnoses and indications for catheterization and considered all possible complications. Nevertheless, the rate of complications was a little higher at 1.82 in the 1982 report and 1.70% in the 1987 report. These total complication rates are remarkably similar and are low in comparison with previously published reports. They do, nevertheless, accurately indicate the incidence of complications in a very large series and probably represent **acceptable reference standards.**

Mortality

Previous studies ranging in size from under 50 to over 46,000 patients have reported mortality rates ranging from 0.03 to 2.6% (9). The CASS and SFCA mortality rates range from 0.07 to 0.14% and reflect a large patient sample and a very large variety of laboratory conditions. Risk factors associated with death include left main and multivessel CAD, recent unstable angina, a high New York Heart

Table 3.2
Complications of Cardiac Catheterization (%)

Complication $(n)^a$	CASS 1979 (7553)	CASS 1983 (19,309)	SFCA 1982 (53,581)	SFCA 1987 (156,853)
Death	0.11	0.07	0.14	0.10
MI	0.25	0.34	0.07	0.07
CVA	0.03	0.13	0.07	0.06
Arrhythmia	0.63	0.38	0.56	0.44
Vascular	0.74	0.83	0.57	0.44
Other	$-^b$	-	0.41	0.26
Total	1.76	1.67	1.82	1.70

^{a} CVA, cerebrovascular accident; MI, myocardial infarction; n, number of patients.
^{b} -, not available.

Association (NYHA) or Canadian Heart Association class, low ejection fraction, recent myocardial infarction, complex congenital anomalies, cardiogenic shock, critical aortic stenosis, severe mitral valve disease, severe ventricular arrhythmias, hypertension, and age over 65 years. Previously, brachial artery catheterization was thought to have a higher mortality than femoral artery catheterization. However, more experience and a larger survey indicate that, overall, no significant difference exists. More specifically, there is no difference in mortality rates between these approaches when the laboratory utilizing the brachial method performs more than 80% of its procedures by this method. Death from technical errors and misadventures from inexperience have become very infrequent. Mortality related to cardiac catheterization occurs most often in patients with severe cardiovascular disease, usually of an advanced degree.

Myocardial Infarction

The rate of myocardial infarction ranges from 0.07 to 0.34% (Table 3.2). Higher rates would be expected to occur in patients with severe CAD, acute ischemic syndromes, angina, or prior infarction, and this may account for the difference between CASS and SFCA reports. Also, diligence in detecting acute myocardial injury will affect the **documented** rate of occurrence. Frequently, isoenzyme evaluations are omitted either before or after procedures. Acute myocardial ischemia secondary to mishandling of catheters appears to be infrequent as skills and equipment have improved, although particle or air embolism,

coronary dissections, and sudden occlusions are still reported. When detected, severe myocardial ischemic injury, occurring during catheterization, is now usually treated very aggressively with an attempt to identify the artery and process involved and by proceeding with acute revascularization.

Cerebrovascular Accidents

Cerebrovascular accidents vary widely in presentation, etiology, and duration, depending on location and size of the affected brain area. Their rate of occurrence ranges from 0.03 to 0.13% related to cardiac catheterization. While most emboli are probably atheromatous or thrombotic particles, air and foreign bodies from catheters and wires have also been implicated during catheterization. Contrast agent administration alone may result in seizures, neurologic deficits, or transient blindness, even without excessive dosage. Fortunately, most studies report that the incidence of cerebrovascular accidents is lower than most other complications (Table 3.2). Patients with signs and symptoms of cerebrovascular disease and those with hypertension are at greatest risk. Treatment for embolic stroke usually includes systemic heparinization. When air embolus occurs, hyperbaric oxygenation has been used with success. Control of hypertension is also important.

Arrhythmias

Arrhythmias occur in 0.38 to 0.63% of catheterization procedures. Prior to availability of DC defibrillation and newer antiarrhythmic drugs, ventricular tachycardia and fibrillation were usually fatal. Contemporary drug therapy and DC electronic conversion units now make these arrhythmias little more than potentially serious inconveniences. If they occur in association with severe disease, such as critical aortic stenosis, left main or triple-vessel CAD, low ejection fraction or heart failure, resuscitative efforts may be unsuccessful. Rapid supraventricular arrhythmias are usually treated successfully with electrical conversion and/or drugs. By themselves they seldom result in severe consequences. However, when rapid supraventricular tachycardia occurs in combination with severe CAD or valvular abnormalities like aortic stenosis or mitral stenosis, myocardial infarction, pulmonary edema, and death may result. Bradycardia, atrioventricular (AV) block, and asystole are usually treated with inhaled ammonia, intravenous atropine, or temporary pacing. The newer transcutaneous pacers offer very rapid control, and some laboratories apply these electrodes to the skin routinely in high-risk cases. The speed with which treatment is instituted frequently determines outcome.

Vascular Incidents

Most vascular incidents result from and near the sites of catheter insertions, but these complications may also result from embolic debris generated by catheter or wire manipulation. These complications result in 0.44 to 0.83% of cases. Vascular occlusions away from the site of entry are infrequent compared with those which result from brachial or femoral entry (Table 3.3). Major incidents after brachial artery entry are thrombosis or local vascular obstruction from flaps, dissections, subintimal hemorrhage, or clotting at traumatized areas (10-14). These brachial artery complications can usually be treated with local revision in the laboratory, often by the catheterizing physician. Percutaneous femoral artery puncture is more likely to result in hemorrhage or hematoma requiring open surgical correction in the operating room with general anesthesia. AV fistulae, pseudoaneurysms, local nerve damage, infection, and persistent pain may occur with either technique. The incidence of local vascular complications in most studies appears to be somewhat higher for procedures done from brachial entry, as compared with those done from the femoral artery. Use of less familiar techniques results in increased mortality and morbidity rates.

Other Complications

The variety of other possible complications related to cardiac catheterization is enormous. Among these are acute pulmonary edema, hypotension, shock, vascular or cardiac perforation, cardiac tamponade, endocarditis, internal hemorrhage, allergic and anaphylactic reactions, pyrogenic reactions, error in drug dosage, loss of limb, coronary spasm, aortic dissecting aneurysm, renal failure, and pulmonary infarction. Taken as a group, these occurrences are infrequent and individually are seldom tabulated. However, their occurrence must be considered part of any report regarding catheterization complications. The

Table 3.3
Complications According to Arterial Entry Site (%)

Complication (n)[a]	CASS 1979 Brachial (1187)	Femoral (6328)	SFCA 1982 Brachial (18,123)	Femoral (23,075)	SFCA 1987 Brachial (49,720)	Femoral (99,440)
None	_[b]	–	–	–	98.00	98.40
Death	0.51	0.14	0.10	0.12	0.09	0.11
Infarction	0.42	0.22	–	–	0.06	0.07
CVA	–	–	–	–	0.06	0.06
Arrhythmia	–	–	–	–	0.45	0.45
Vascular	2.78	0.36	–	–	0.91	0.22
Contrast	–	–	–	–	0.20	0.29
Hemorrhage	–	–	–	–	0.01	0.12
Other	–	–	–	–	0.22	0.28

[a] CVA, cerebrovascular accident; *n*, number of patients.
[b] -, not available.

analysis performed by CASS specifically excluded these complications from consideration, whereas the SFCA registry specifically provided for their inclusion. Thus, the overall rate of complications as noted in both SFCA reports is somewhat higher and probably more accurate than those reported in CASS (Table 3.2).

Electrophysiologic Procedures

Complications related to electrophysiologic studies seldom receive individualized attention, probably because these procedures are limited, for the most part, to only the venous system. The underlying disease processes in patients requiring these studies include severe CAD, dilated and hypertrophic cardiomyopathies, and valvular and congenital heart diseases, as well as patients with no obvious cardiac structural abnormalities (see Chapter 29).

The incidence of complications associated with electrophysiologic studies in a report of 1000 patients appears in Table 3.4 (15). The frequency of complications in 2210 electrophysiologic procedures was 1.8%. Hypotension from vasovagal reaction or administration of antiarrhythmic drugs was the most frequent complication. But these complications were easily treated in most cases without sequelae. Venous injury resulting in pulmonary embolism or phlebitis represents the cause of significant clinical disability. Pericardial tamponade, necessitating pericardiocentesis, occasionally resulted from perforation by venous catheters

despite their small size. In this report, there was one death of a patient with recent myocardial infarction, heart failure, pericarditis, sepsis, and recurrent ventricular tachycardia unresponsive to initial drug therapy.

Coronary Angioplasty Procedures

Angioplasty of the coronary arteries and peripheral vessels has revolutionized catheterization. The value of these procedures is now commonly derived from an analysis of their potential risks and benefits when compared with risks associated with coronary or peripheral artery bypass surgery. The National Heart Lung and Blood Institute's (NHLBI) Coronary Angioplasty Registry, begun in 1979 (16, 17), documented a relatively high incidence of complications (Table 3.5). The NHLBI PTCA registry was comprised mostly of patients with single-vessel CAD (Table 3.6), and PTCA was performed with equipment of limited capabilities. The SFCA Coronary Angioplasty registry, begun in 1984 and completed in 1988 (18), chronicled results of a larger number of patients, many of whom were subjected to multivessel angioplasty performed with more varied and newer techniques. As a result of these technical advances and operator experience, fewer complications were noted. A comparison of the two reports (Tables 3.5 and 3.6) reveals what progress has been made.

Despite numerous publications regarding complications and untoward events related to PTCA, standard definitions of all individual occurrences are not available. Also, less

Table 3.4
Complications of Electrophysiologic Catheterization Studies [a]

Complication	Incidence/1,000 Patients Exposed	Incidence/Procedure
Death	1 (0.1%)	1/2210 (0.05%)
Vascular	12 (1.2%)	12/1782[b] (0.7%)
Arterial injury	4 (0.4%)	4/1782 (0.2%)
Thrombophlebitis	6 (0.6%)	6/1782 (0.3%)
Severe hematoma	2 (0.2%)	2/1782 (0.1%)
Embolism	4 (0.4%)	4/2210 (0.2%)
Systemic arterial	1 (0.1%)	1/2210 (0.05%)
Pulmonary	3 (0.3%)	3/2210 (0.15%)
Cardiac perforation	2 (0.2%)	2/1782 (0.1%)
Hypotension	20 (2.0%)	20/2210 (1%)
Total		39/2210 (1.76%)

[a] From Horowitz LN, Kay HR, Kutalek SP, et al. J Am Coll Cardiol 1987;1261-1268. Reprinted with permission from the American College of Cardiology.
[b] The number of studies in which catheter insertion occurred.

Table 3.5
Complications of Coronary Angioplasty

(n)	PTCA [a] Registry			
	NHLBI (1,500)		SFCA (20,417)	
	n	%	n	%
Patients with complications	314	21.0	3112	15.2
Prolonged angina	121	8.0	684	3.4
Myocardial infarction	72	4.8	369	1.8
Coronary occlusion	70	4.7	534	2.6
Coronary spasm	63	4.2	- [b]	-
Dissection/tear	43	2.9	677	3.3
Hypotension/bradycardia	56	3.7	452	2.2
VF/VT	32	2.1	941	4.6
Local vascular injury	22	1.5	583	2.9
Hospital death	16	1.1	212	1.0
Excessive blood loss	11	0.7	291	1.4
Coronary embolism	2	0.1	176	0.9
Neurologic events	5	0.3	200	1.0
Other	24	1.6	154	0.8
Emergency surgery	102	6.8	980	4.8
Elective surgery	293	19.5	715	3.5

[a] n, number of patients; PTCA, percutaneous transluminal coronary angioplasty; VF, ventricular fibrillation; VT, ventricular tachycardia.
[b] -, not available.

Table 3.6
Coronary Angioplasty Complications—Patient Description

	PTCA Registry	
	NHLBI [a]	SFCA
No. of patients	1500	20417
Male/female (%)	78/22	73/27
Age (mean yr)	52.5	- [b]
Coronary disease		
1 Vessel	79%	68%
Multivessel	19%	32%
Left main	2	1.5%
Angina classes III and IV	62% [c]	78% [d]
Ejection fraction		
<30%	-	2.5%
30-49%	-	17.7%
50%	93%	79.8%
Vessels attempted		
Left anterior descending	64%	44.6%
Right coronary artery	26%	28.8%
Left circumflex	6%	18.4%
Left main	2%	0.7%
Bypass grafts	2%	7.5%

[a] From 1979-1981 study.
[b] - , not available.
[c] Canadian Cardiovascular Society classification.
[d] American Heart Association classification.

serious events are frequently equated with life-threatening events. For example, easily corrected ventricular fibrillation is listed with paralytic stroke or acute myocardial infarction requiring surgery. Also, there is a vast difference between emergency bypass surgery for sudden vessel reclosure and elective coronary bypass graft surgery performed several days later because a lesion could not be crossed or dilated. Clear distinction between minor and major events has not yet been made. Ultimately, the value of individual techniques may be determined by just such an analysis.

Both NHLBI and SFCA PTCA registries list a wide variety of untoward events that are not mutually exclusive. It is therefore not possible to determine the true incidence of complications of these procedures. Nevertheless, important conclusions may be made. Patients included in the NHLBI report had less multivessel disease, higher left ventricular ejection fractions, and less severe angina (Table 3.6). Despite an increased severity of underlying disease and higher percentages of multivessel procedures, the SFCA registry reveals lower rate of death, subsequent bypass surgery, myocardial infarction, hypotension/bradycardia, and coronary occlusions. Other important complications occurred with somewhat higher frequencies, including vessel dissection/tear, blood loss, and neurologic events. It is likely that the differences between these reports resulted, during recent years, from attempts to achieve more complete revascularization with the use of newer equipment and better selection of procedures for specific lesions and patients, which is part of the "learning curve."

PSEUDOCOMPLICATIONS

Because of concern for patient welfare, all laboratories performing cardiac catheterization must investigate the underlying causes of untoward events. While investigation is frequently rewarding, some complications remain unexplained. All so-called complications are not necessarily complications of the catheterization procedure. For example, it is not unusual for heart disease patients to die at home awaiting hospitalization for cardiac catheterization. The frequency of these "preadmission" events is not known and cannot be established confidently. However, once a

patient is scheduled for catheterization, accurate records may be kept of the eventual disposition of the case.

Accordingly, we undertook two studies of complications occurring in patients scheduled for catheterization. These studies were performed 10 years apart, and similar conclusions were obtained on each occasion (18, 19). Patients entered included all those who were officially scheduled to have cardiac catheterization procedures having been given a specific date and time. All untoward events occurring in these individuals from 24 hr before the time the procedure was scheduled to 72 hr thereafter were recorded. Three classes of events were recorded. **Pseudocomplications** were defined as either spontaneous medical or surgical events that occurred in hospitalized patients during the 24-hr period before the time catheterization was scheduled, or actually were performed if a delay had occurred. These complications were of such a type that they would have been attributed to the procedure had it been performed during this 24-hr period or on schedule if the procedure had been delayed. **Time-related complications** were defined as those occurring in patients who were seriously ill before and after catheterization. Despite intensive medical treatment, these complications occurred and were related to the procedure in time but probably not in cause. By definition, however, these were considered to have been caused by the procedure and were so recorded. **Procedure-related complications** were defined as those occurring during or after catheterization and were probably associated causally. The definition of complications was identical to that subsequently adopted by the SFCA.

During a 24-month period, 1606 cardiac catheterizations were performed (Table 3.7). There were 13 (0.81%) procedure-related complications with no deaths. There were 17 (1.06%) pseudocomplications, including 4 deaths (0.24%). In this latter group, 7 events occurred within 2 hr prior to the time the procedure was done. One patient whose procedure was delayed 3 hr experienced severe chest pain and died 2 hr before the rescheduled time. Another patient developed right bundle branch block associated with an acute myocardial infarction while in his room before the scheduled time of the procedure. Four patients developed major complications in the waiting area within 30 min of entering the laboratory. These events included one patient with slurred speech; one with diplopia, slurred speech, and paresthesias; another with ventricular tachycardia; and a fourth with an acute myocardial infarction related to symptom-free massive gastrointestinal bleeding. The other pseudocomplication occurred suddenly and without warning while the patient was awaiting catheterization in his room.

Attention should be focused on the types of occurrences included in the list of pseudocomplications. Usually, a thrombus or vascular occlusion occurring in the arm after brachial cutdown is assumed to be procedure-related. In at least two instances, sudden brachial occlusions occurred before the procedures were performed. One similar episode occurred in a femoral artery. Ordinarily, cardiac tamponade is considered procedure-related when found after catheterization. Tamponade was also found before a procedure was begun.

Time-related complications, as noted above, also are not necessarily caused by catheter procedures or manipulations. For example, in one instance, a large apical left ventricular thrombus was found incidentally during filming after a pulmonary angiogram. Within 48 hr a femoral artery embolus occurred that required surgical removal. Subsequent left heart study confirmed the absence of the previously seen ventricular mass.

In the study described above, the incidence of complications would have doubled if these catheterizations had been performed on time or 24 hr earlier. The four deaths are evidence that pseudocomplications may be more severe than those which are procedure-related. Pseudocomplications are frequently indistinguishable from those occurring either during or after a procedure. But for the patient, injury has occurred, and assignment of blame and a causal relationship are frequently demanded by our litigious social structure. Nevertheless, there can be no doubt that events occurring before catheterization are related to the underlying disease process. It is reasonable to assume that such events may also occur after a cardiac procedure has begun and are not necessarily always caused by it.

IDENTIFICATION OF PATIENTS AT HIGH RISK FOR COMPLICATIONS

Numerous reports have identified risk factors for catheterization. Conflicting opinions have been expressed concerning the importance of many variables. Conflict occurs because reports of this information (*a*) varied widely in size from less than 100 patients to over 100,000, (*b*) focused on a limited patient population, (*c*) selected a certain subset of patients, (*d*) failed to survey a wide spectrum of laboratories, or (*e*) were unable to accumulate sufficient numbers of certain occurrences to achieve significance. Nevertheless, certain clinical features are unequivocally recognized as being associated with higher patient risk. Strategies to improve catheterization safety

Table 3.7
Comparison of Procedure-Related and Pseudocomplications in 1606 Patients

	Procedure-Related Complications	Pseudocomplications
Acute myocardial infarction	4	6
Ventricular arrhythmia	1	1
Hypotension/shock	1	2
Hemorrhage	2	1
Septicemia	0	1
Cerebrovascular accident	2	2
Local vascular injury	3	0
Death	0	4 (0.24%)
Total	13 (0.81%)	17 (1.06%)

must include identification of these conditions before the study is attempted so that by modification of the procedure, complications may be avoided or their severity reduced. The newer nonionic and/or low osmolality contrast agents may help reduce risks in some of these patient subsets (see Chapter 10). Situations in which use of nonionic low osmolality agents may reduce the risk of complications include:

1. Acute myocardial infarction.
2. Acute or chronic renal disease.
3. Congestive heart failure.
4. Ejection fraction of 30% or less.
5. Previous coronary bypass surgery.
6. Coronary angioplasty procedures.
7. Anticipated use of large volumes of contrast agent.
8. Complex or multiple ventricular arrhythmias.
9. Anticipated left main or multivessel disease

Left Main and Triple-Vessel Disease

Catheterization study of patients with unrecognized left main CAD has resulted in mortality rates ranging from 1 to 16% and equally high morbidity rates. Catheter placement within 6 mm of a lesion or catheterization study of left main CAD in a patient having experienced angina within the previous 24 hr appears to have an unusually high incidence of lethal consequences (20). Noninvasive identification of patients highly suspect for either left main or triple-vessel disease can be accomplished with high rates of sensitivity and specificity during stress testing (21, 22). Addition of stress thallium-201 scintigraphy to exercise ECG testing improves identification of patients with coronary disease in general, although identification of subsets is less specific. However, markedly positive scintigraphic results (e.g., new defects at low workload, multiple defects with redistribution, and increased lung uptake) correlate closely with the presence of severe ischemia due to either left main or multivessel disease (23).

Unstable Angina and High New York or Canadian Heart Association Classification

Although only a symptom of coronary artery disease, unstable angina or a high NYHA or Canadian Heart Association classification for angina usually indicates patients with severe CAD. In this group the frequency of left main CAD may be as high as 13% and multivessel disease as high as 80%, while the frequency of normal coronary arteries may be as high as 10%. Retrospective analyses of procedure-related deaths in patients with left main, triple-vessel, or combined high left anterior descending and high circumflex lesions (left main equivalent) reveal a very high incidence of unstable angina frequently reaching 85% (9, 24, 25). Deaths in class IV (rest angina) patients may approach the high procedure-related death rates (<1 to 10%) seen in patients with left main disease. Even when the mortality rates reported in class IV patients are low, these mortality rates are four times higher than in class III and 13 times higher than in class II patients.

Reduced Ejection Fraction and Congestive Heart Failure

It is difficult to prove that poor left ventricular function is an independent risk factor during catheterization since it cannot be separated from its etiology. Nevertheless, an ejection fraction of <30% is associated with a mortality rate approximately 15 times that associated with an ejection fraction of ≥50%. When echocardiographic or other noninvasive studies demonstrate a low ejection fraction and catheterization is required, an appropriately modified study should be used.

Mitral and Aortic Valve Disease

Statistically, mortality as a result of cardiac catheterization in the presence of mitral valve disease, either stenosis or insufficiency, is almost double that associated with aortic valve disease. The presence of either, however, is associated with a mortality substantially higher than for patients with no valve disease (9). In recent studies, many mitral valve abnormalities have been associated with CAD and papillary muscle dysfunction. Thus, the contribution of myocardial ischemia cannot be ignored. Earlier studies dealing primarily with rheumatic or nonischemic mitral and aortic diseases ascribed similar or worse implications to the presence of either condition. Inadvertent overhydration or underhydration, catheter valve obstruction, major arrhythmia, or even vasovagal episodes leading to hypotension and ischemia would frequently result in pulmonary edema, shock, or even death. In many instances, the presence of a valve abnormality indicates the need for more extensive investigation at catheterization, thereby compounding the risk. A large volume contrast load may depress myocardial function, temporarily increase circulating volume, and begin the cascade of events noted above.

Female Sex

By itself, female sex does not appear to represent an independent risk factor. However, when combined with certain other elements of invasive procedures, subsets are created that apparently represent markedly increased risk. Even in a laboratory which performs catheterization predominately by the brachial approach, a complication rate of over 16% is found in women but only 3.8% in men (13). Use of anticoagulants or the presence of aortic regurgitation in elderly women results in an unusual incidence of false aneurysms when procedures are performed by the percutaneous femoral approach. Similarly, although infrequent, femoral artery occlusion is thought to occur almost exclusively in women who presumably have small vessels that are totally occluded by the catheter.

Renal Insufficiency

Renal insufficiency, advanced age, dehydration, recent use of contrast material, myeloma, decreased renal arterial perfusion, and hypertension increase the risk of significant renal damage.

NONDIAGNOSTIC STUDIES

When a patient is subjected to the risk and expense of a diagnostic or therapeutic cardiac catheterization procedure, satisfactory completion of the procedure should be achieved in >99% of patients. Restudy must be considered unacceptable unless originally planned as part of a "staged" procedure for patient safety, a change in patient condition prompted premature termination of the original attempt, or a new event required reassessment. It is incumbent upon the physician to continuously monitor results of the catheterization study as it progresses, assuring that results will yield conclusive information during final reporting.

The complexity of contemporary equipment is such that even with proper preventive maintenance and operation, component failure may occur. At these times a well-run laboratory should be able to call upon its resources to achieve a complete study. Sudden failure of radiographic equipment can frequently be corrected by local personnel, resulting only in temporary delay. More commonly, one encounters failure of the hemodynamic recording system. This situation is less apt to result in complete loss of data because spare transducers should be readily available. A computer is not essential for measurement of either pressure or cardiac output. Malfunction of a physiologic recorder may not be serious if only a single channel or bank are involved (see Chapter 21). Total power supply failure may necessitate recruitment of a backup system, usually an obsolete machine that is still functional and is retained for such emergencies. Videotape backup is mandatory in studies performed primarily for anatomic evaluation, such as in congenital anomalies or CAD. Lack of required diagnostic catheters, guidewires, or other equipment because of stock depletion should be discovered and corrected before the patient is initially anesthetized or instrumented. Proper maintenance, calibration, periodic inspection, and replacement of all devices utilized during catheterization must be an ongoing, routine function with responsibility shared by the chief technologist and medical director.

Nondiagnostic studies may also be the result of physician errors of omission or commission. Once credentialed for independent practice in the laboratory, the catheterization physician accepts the responsibility of completing a procedure successfully. A physician not trained in all major methods of catheterization will not be able to care for those few patients requiring a special approach. For example, if femoral pulses are absent and brachial cutdown is required, that procedure should be referred to another physician who does brachial procedures regularly. It is not unreasonable to expect that someone experienced in invasive techniques, such as brachial artery cutdown, femoral artery puncture, transseptal puncture, left ventricular puncture, and all methods of coronary angioplasty should be available among the laboratory's physician staff or from within the surrounding community.

"Routine" Right Heart Catheterization

Controversy still exists concerning the necessity and propriety of right heart catheterization in a patient being studied because of suspected CAD. There is agreement that every study should be individualized and based on needs and circumstances of the patient. Furthermore, right heart catheterization is considered acceptable when indications or circumstances exist that make it potentially useful in evaluation of preexisting congenital heart disease, valvular heart disease, myocardial infarction, cardiomyopathy, heart failure, pulmonary hypertension, or other suspected problems. However, Greene et al., representing the SFCA, stated that routine performance of right heart catheterization is unwarranted and use without a specific indication is potentially abusive because of the risk and additional cost involved (26). A contrary opinion is held by Samet, who claims that risks of right heart catheterization are minimal, and coronary arteriography without right and left cardiac study may miss unsuspected, albeit very infrequent, problems such as pulmonary hypertension (27). He emphasizes that omission of right heart catheterization because of busy laboratory schedules or lack of attention to hemodynamics or physiologic parameters in favor of angiography may interfere with consistently complete patient evaluations. In a report of this subject by Shanes et al., 585 patients who underwent right and left cardiac catheterization were analyzed (28). A total of 63% had indications sufficient to warrant right heart catheterization. But the remaining 37% did not and thereby became the subject of subgroup analysis. In this subgroup, 3 to 11% of hemodynamic variables detected by right heart catheterization were found to be moderately-to-severely abnormal. Four patients had a patent foramen ovale, and at least one had a hydrogen curve positive for left to right shunt. They concluded that the results obtained did not justify routine performance of right heart catheterization procedures. While controversy regarding right heart catheterization remains

unsettled, the principle of providing complete data, while avoiding unnecessary cost and risk, remains unchanged.

MEASURES TO MINIMIZE RISKS

General Considerations

In laboratory practice, experience and discipline have no substitute. So it is easier for active laboratories to maintain high-quality studies and low complication rates than for those with small caseloads. Time has shown that the recommendation of a minimum of 300 cases per year for a single laboratory is an acceptable standard. Because pediatric laboratories operate with other constraints, such as somewhat longer procedures, a smaller number of cases, and specialized equipment, an annual caseload of at least 150 is recommended. Any physician who does not perform 50 cases per year should strive to increase the number of cases that he is involved with, or consider withdrawing from laboratory practice. On the other hand, more than 500 to 600 cases per year per physician may represent a maximum level of practice which saturates an individual's ability to render personalized care and meticulous attention to detail required for high-quality study results.

Supportive Services

Close cooperation with ancillary services within the institution occupied by the catheterization laboratory must be maintained. Prior commitment to assist in emergency conditions must be obtained from vascular surgery, cardiothoracic surgery, anesthesia, operating room, respiratory therapy, and other specialized areas. The ability to secure immediate assistance is crucial to the management of any untoward event. This consideration alone militates against performance of catheterization in freestanding facilities or at least suggests that the margin of safety is less. Similarly, higher risk procedures such as transseptal catheterization, left ventricular puncture, or coronary angioplasty must not be performed under less than optimal conditions. Outpatient catheterization has been shown to be acceptable if complete emergency assistance is available and if the patient can be admitted for satisfactory follow-up care (see Chapter 4). Adherence to established local rules, based upon experience, must be enforced by the laboratory medical director. In turn, an active peer review system must regularly examine all mortality and morbidity statistics, the number of incomplete cases, and excessive use of catheters, wires, and other equipment and ultimately decide whether acceptable standards are being maintained. Removal of physicians' privileges or dismissal of technical staff may prove necessary when complication rates exceed established norms. Perhaps, it would be advantageous to require yearly renewal of all catheterization privileges rather than granting them on an indefinite basis.

Patient Condition

Cardiac catheterization, which was once primarily diagnostic, has now also become therapeutic. Patients who previously would not have entered the laboratory with conditions such as acute myocardial infarction, cardiogenic shock, or chronic renal failure are now considered suitable candidates for invasive procedures. These expanded indications should neither obscure nor circumvent the principle that every patient should be in optimal condition prior to any procedure. Thus, workup for all patients, and particularly for those undergoing purely diagnostic procedures, must include a complete evaluation of hematologic and biochemical parameters, as well as coagulation parameters, when necessary. Abnormalities detected should be corrected whenever possible. For example, recognition of early renal compromise permits appropriate consultation and pretreatment which may prevent further deterioration as a result of contrast or fluid loads. Cardiac surgical standby may be necessary during catheterization of certain patients if their condition is poor or deteriorating.

Conduct of the Procedure

Procedure and Arterial Time

Of itself, speed has no value. However, a procedure that is conducted expertly with each element successfully completed on the first try will be swift and expeditious. Procedures with arterial time exceeding 60 min have been incriminated as potentially more hazardous than those which are shorter. Once this time

has been reached, the physician should deliberately decide whether or not to continue a procedure that is going well or terminate one that is going poorly.

Catheters

Selection of catheters is a highly subjective issue and depends on an individual physician's training, experience, and preference. Which catheter a physician chooses is less important than whether it will be used safely and successfully. It is more important to refrain from use of a catheter in a situation for which it was not intended and in which there is a low or unknown probability for success. Of equal importance is the proper use of the catheter. Without attention to initial back-bleeding, flushing, and constant pressure-assisted drip, any catheter may become a source of thrombus and embolism (29). Catheters with both end and side holes (e.g., particularly pigtail) permit dissipation of fluid through their side holes, often leaving the distal tip stagnant unless forcefully flushed frequently (e.g., every 2 min). Clot formation in these areas is common, particularly if the catheters are constructed of polyurethane, even in heparinized patients (30). Although single end-hole catheters should not clot as easily, they may be the cause of endothelial trauma resulting from a relatively sharp edge at the tip. The incidence of vessel dissection, subintimal burrowing, and contrast injection around coronary orifices and in larger vessels is quite small. Although new catheters with malleable tips are available, careful and meticulous handling of all catheters is essential.

Heparin

The use of intraarterial heparin during brachial cutdown procedures is mandatory to avoid clot formation in a vessel with limited flow. Full systemic heparinization is required in addition to installation into the distal vessel. Use of systemic heparin for percutaneous femoral puncture is widely practiced by more than 60% of laboratories. Since thromboembolic complications carry the potential for greater morbidity and mortality than bleeding complications, many laboratories prefer to use heparin anticoagulation, which is then reversed by protamine. However, other laboratories are more fearful of potential bleeding complications even if the heparin is eventually reversed. Analyses of complication rates fail to reveal any difference whether or not heparin is used, but large, controlled prospective studies have not been performed (31-33). Administration of heparin during angioplasty is mandatory because of the coaxial configuration of catheters resulting in stagnant flow. Whenever heparin is utilized in fixed doses, the physician must not assume its efficacy since certain patients appear to be resistant to drugs of porcine origin. When this is suspected, a bleeding time which takes only several minutes should be employed, and beef heparin substituted if necessary.

Details related to catheter entry site and contrast agents relative to prevention of complications are discussed elsewhere in this text (see Chapters 6 and 10). I want to emphasize that special efforts to limit the volume of contrast material and catheter manipulation in critically ill patients will permit biplane ventriculography with ≤25 ml of contrast material and biplane coronary angiography to yield a diagnostic study with ≤90 ml of contrast material (34).

LABORATORY STAFFING AND EQUIPMENT

Staffing

To assure excellence in invasive diagnostic and therapeutic procedures, every laboratory must employ well-trained personnel capable of performing all routine and emergency procedures. The total number of individuals needed will be determined by laboratory caseload, physical layout, and individual experience and training (35). Although no specific number has been established, it is expected that the staff size should be sufficient to perform all functions peculiar to a catheterization facility operating at its expected maximum load. While patient care is the job of all staff members, a registered nurse is invaluable when drugs are to be administered or mixed, particularly during emergencies or difficult situations. A radiologic technician brings expertise in use and maintenance of radiographic equipment as well as radiation physics and safety. Graduate cardiovascular technologists are valuable because they have acquired skills in most aspects of laboratory practice, including pressure monitoring, operation of physiologic recording equipment, cardiopulmonary resuscitation, basic ECG interpretation, blood gas analysis, and even operation of the intraaortic balloon pump (IABP) and other emergency equipment. Film processing is best handled by an individual who is capable of operating and maintaining the film processor and performing darkroom functions such as sensitometry, densitometry, and quality control. Cross-training of all staff members is mandatory for cost containment and assuring that in someone's absence, another staff member will be able to perform a vital service.

Equipment

In addition to basic radiographic, angiographic, and hemodynamic recording equipment, every laboratory should have immediately available, specialized devices for handling any emergency or complication. Oxygen and suction must be available at tableside. A "crash cart," including emergency drugs, DC defibrillator, and intubation tray with ventilation bag, must be kept in the room near the patient. A temporary pacemaker power pack, sterile pacing wires, and introducers must be prepared for use literally within seconds and must be kept in each procedure room. Automatic mechanical ventilators should be available in the hospital on request. A thoracotomy tray and pericardial aspiration equipment should always be available in the room. Many laboratories, particularly those performing angioplasty, now keep an IABP in the catheterization suite and regard it as an integral part of advanced cardiovascular life support measures. Even if it is stored in the operating or emergency room, it should be available in the hospital for immediate use.

Once an emergency arises, specialized assistance, including the operating room, anesthesiology, cardiovascular surgery, and neurology, must be available on short notice. These working arrangements must be prearranged and periodically reaffirmed. Special services such as these are as important as any piece of emergency equipment, and they must also be maintained in good working order.

QUALITY ASSURANCE AND RISK PREVENTION

High-quality performance of all laboratory functions results in successful procedures with few complications. Successful operation requires a disciplined efficient administrative structure. Organization begins with an institutional cardiac catheterization laboratory committee that is authorized by the governing board to set qualifications for credentialing physicians and to establish standards of practice and to periodically monitor the performance of all physicians, staff, and equipment (36).

Laboratory Director

The medical director should be a respected, licensed medical staff member who is Board-certified or eligible in the subspecialty of the laboratory, be it adult cardiology, pediatric cardiology, or cardiovascular radiology (37). If both pediatric and adult patients are to be studied, the medical director must be conversant with both disciplines, or two directors should be appointed. The director must have extensive experience, including at least 2 years of formal training in catheterization in addition to the usual 3 years of cardiology fellowship and 5 years of active practice during which he has spent at least 50% of his time in pursuits related to invasive cardiology. He should maintain a personal minimum of 200 cases per year with which he demonstrates proficiency and competence. He should have a wide knowledge of laboratory equipment, including cineangiographic devices, film processing, radiographic imaging, computer technology for hemodynamic recording and reporting, electronic measuring instruments, and other technologies peculiar to this type of invasive cardiology.

The director guides daily administrative functions, consulting and working with the technical staff. He oversees efficient scheduling and optimal utilization of laboratory facilities. In cooperation with the chief technologist he assures adequate staffing and reviews training and the performance of all staff. He is ultimately responsible for all operations relative to the catheterization laboratory, including maintenance of equipment, provision of supplies, preparation of an annual budget, and other financial matters to assure that professional goals are met. His responsibilities also include review of applications for laboratory privileges either as a primary reviewer or as a member consultant of institutional committees. As part of an ongoing oversight process he must review performance of all personnel, including other physicians, assuring that a daily log of procedures is kept, including morbidity, mortality, indicators of quality, and other data valuable to safe and successful ractices. He should be responsible to an oversight committee such as the cardiac catheterization laboratory committee to whom he reports current performance and to whom he recommends changes or modifications of policy.

Quality Assurance

Quality of laboratory performance is elusive and easily lost if not deliberately maintained. Constant monitoring of all laboratory activities may be performed by designated individuals, but ultimately it is the laboratory director who bears responsibility. Evaluation of physician performance must be ongoing with periodic conferences. The quality of studies, number of complications, their handling, and adherence to accepted laboratory practice standards must be monitored. A recorded daily log of procedures must be kept to assure accurate statistics. This should include patient age, sex, NYHA class, procedures performed, length of procedure, fluoroscopic and arterial times, general coronary anatomy, and special statistics such as previously operated patients or emergency situations. Regular staff conferences should be held to maintain and upgrade skills and performance. A discussion of cases encourages both medical and technical staff to analyze hemodynamic and angiographic results better and serves to upgrade their ability to recognize unusual circumstances. Conferences should be used to discuss complications and monitor performance as well as indications for procedures. Discussions should include adherence to laboratory standards, including the percent of normal studies, excessive or inappropriate use of equipment, on-time starts, scheduling, cancellations, and other administrative as well as technical details.

Oversight and Peer Review

Intradepartmental peer review is mandated by the Joint Commission on Accreditation of Healthcare Organizations and is needed if high-quality procedures with low morbidity and mortality are to be maintained. Quarterly reports with periodic close inspection are useful. This may be the function of the cardiac catheterization laboratory committee in cooperation with the director and representatives of groups working in the laboratory. The committee should include not only physicians but also other professional staff with interest in imaging technology, cost containment, personnel utilization, and care of cardiovascular patients.

Grievance Protocol

Disputes that arise from either the medical or technical staff are best handled by the director if at all possible. After suitable investigation, he should be able to resolve most difficulties if he has the respect of his associates and authority from the institution. If this cannot be achieved, the next level of appeal should be the cardiac catheterization laboratory committee or an ad hoc committee of the medical staff. If complaints concerning the director arise, these should be taken to the cardiac catheterization laboratory committee. If disputes cannot be resolved through the mechanism outlined, the protocol for due process established by institutional bylaws should be followed.

References

1. Edemas DF, Fraser DB, Abrams HL. The complications of coronary arteriography. Circulation 1973;48:609–618.
2. Bourassa MG, Noble J. Complication rate of coronary arteriography. Circulation 1976;53:106–114.
3. Takaro T, Hultgren H, Littmann D, Wright EC. An analysis of deaths occurring in association with coronary arteriography. Am Heart J 1973;86:587–597.
4. Ross RS, Gorlin R. Cooperative study on cardiac catheterization: coronary arteriography. Circulation 1968;38:III–67–73.
5. Davis K, Kennedy JW, Kemp HG, et al. Complications of coronary arteriography from the collaborative study of coronary artery surgery (CASS). Circulation 1979;59:1105–1112.
6. Gersh J, Kronmal RA, Frye RL, et al. Coronary arteriography and coronary artery bypass surgery: morbidity and mortality in patients ages 65 years or older. Circulation 1983;67:483–491.
7. Kennedy JW, Registry Committee of Society for Cardiac Angiography. Complications associated with cardiac catheterization and angiography. Cathet Cardiovasc Diagn 1982;8:5–11.
8. Registry Committee Annual Report, Society for Cardiac Angiography, December, 1987.
9. Kennedy JW, Registry Committee of Society for Cardiac Angiography. Mortality related to cardiac catheterization and angiography. Cathet Cardiovasc Diagn 1982;8:323–340.
10. Armstrong PW, Parker JO. The complications of brachial arteriotomy. Am Heart J 1971;61:424–429.
11. McMillan I, Murie JA. Vascular injury following cardiac catheterization. Br J Surg 1984;71:832–835.
12. McCollum CH, Mavor E. Brachial artery injury after cardiac catheterization. J Vasc Surg 1986;4:355–359.
13. Harris JM. Coronary angiography and its complications. Arch Intern Med 1984;144:337–341.
14. Green GS, McKinnon M, Rosch J, Judkins MP. Complications of selective percutaneous transfemoral coronary arteriography and their prevention. Circulation 1972;45:552–557.
15. Horowitz LN, Kay HR, Kutalek SP, et al. Risks and complications of clinical cardiac electrophysiologic studies: a prospective analysis of 1,000 patients. J Am Coll Cardiol 1987;9:1261–1268.
16. Dorros G, Cowley MJ, Simpson J, et al. Percutaneous transluminal coronary angioplasty: report of complications from the National Heart Lung and Blood Institute PTCA registry. Circulation 1983;76:723–730.
17. Cowley MJ, Dorros G, Kelsey SF, Van Radden M, Detre KM. Acute coronary events associated with percutaneous transluminal coronary angioplasty. Am J Cardiol 1984;53:12C–16C.
18. Hildner FJ, Javier RP, Ramaswamy K, Samet P. Pseudocomplications of cardiac catheterization. Chest 1973;63:15–17.
19. Hildner FJ, Javier RP, Tolentino A, Samet P. Pseudo complications of cardiac catheterization: update. Cathet Cardiovasc Diagn 1982;8:43–47.
20. Carabello BA, Gordon PR. Risk factors for cardiac catheterization in left main coronary artery stenosis. Cardiol Board Rev 1987;4:63–69.
21. Goldschlager N, Selzer A, Cohn K. Treadmill stress tests as indicators of presence and severity of coronary artery disease. Ann Intern Med 1976;85:277–286.
22. Cheitlin MD, Davia JE, de Castro CM, Barrow EA, Anderson WT. Correlation of "critical" left coronary artery lesions with positive submaximal exercise tests in patients with chest pain. Am Heart J 1975;89:305–310.
23. Dash H, Massie BM, Botvinick EH, Brundage BH. The noninvasive identification of left main and three-vessel coronary artery disease by myocardial stress perfusion scintigraphy and treadmill exercise electrocardiography. Circulation 1979;60:276–284.
24. Alison HW, Russell Jr RO, Mantle JA, Kouchoukos NT, Moraski RE, Rackley CE. Coronary anatomy and arteriography in patients with unstable angina pectoris. Am J Cardiol 1978;41:204–209.

25. Wolfson S, Grant D, Ross AM, Cohen LS. Risk of death related to coronary arteriography: role of left coronary arterial lesions. Am J Cardiol 1976;37: 210–216.

26. Greene DG, Society for Cardiac Angiography Officers and Trustees. Right heart catheterization and temporary pacemaker insertion during coronary arteriography for suspected coronary artery disease. Cathet Cardiovasc Diagn 1984;10:429–430.

27. Samet P. The complete cardiac catheterization. Cathet Cardiovasc Diagn 1984;10:431–432.

28. Shanes JG, Stein MA, Dierenfeldt BJ, Kondos GT. The value of routine right heart catheterization in patients undergoing coronary arteriography. Am Heart J 1987;113:1261–1263.

29. Page HL, Campbell B. Percutaneous transfemoral coronary arteriography: prevention of morbid complications. Chest 1975;76:221–225.

30. Rashid A, Hildner FJ, Fester A, Javier RP, Samet P. Thromboembolism associated with pigtail catheters. Cathet Cardiovasc Diagn 1975;1:183–194.

31. Broders AC, Wilson JW. Heparin: help or hindrance? a commentary and review. J Reprod Med 1973;10:269–271.

32. Novak E, Sekhar NC, Dunham NW, Coleman LL. A comparative study of the effect of lung and gut heparins on platelet aggregation and protamine neutralization in man. Clin Med 1972;79:22–27.

33. Dehmer GJ, Haagen D, Malloy CR, Schmitz JM. Anticoagulation with heparin during cardiac catheterization and its reversal by protamine. Cathet Cardiovasc Diagn 1987;13:16–21.

34. Hildner FJ, Furst A, Krieger R, et al. New principles for optimum left ventriculography. Cathet Cardiovasc Diagn 1986;12:266–273.

35. Friesinger GC, Adams DF, Courassa MG, et al. Optimal resources for examination of the heart and lungs: cardiac catheterization and radiographic facilities. Circulation 1983;68:893A–930A.

36. Judkins MP, LabStandards Committee, Society for Cardiac Angiography. Guidelines for organization and quality assurance in cardiovascular laboratories. Cathet Cardiovasc Diagn 1983;9:327–328.

37. Judkins MP, Lab Standards Committee, Society for Cardiac Angiography. Guidelines regarding qualifications and responsibilities of a catheterization laboratory director. Cathet Cardiovasc Diagn 1983;9:619–621.

4

Outpatient Cardiac Catheterization

W. Peter Klinke, M.D.

INTRODUCTION

Cardiac catheterization and coronary angiography have become important and integral components in the investigation of patients with known or suspected cardiovascular disease. The advent of therapeutic catheterization procedures such as angioplasty and valvuloplasty and the advances made in the surgical treatment of coronary artery disease (CAD), valvular heart disease, and arrhythmias have significantly increased the need for cardiac catheterization procedures. Many patients will now undergo more than one cardiac catheterization during the course of their illness. In a busy hospital, this increase in the frequency of cardiac catheterization can place a significant burden on bed utilization and budgets. Outpatient cardiac catheterization has evolved, in part, as a response to these concerns. Cardiac catheterization, for the purposes of this chapter, will include right and left heart catheterization and left ventricular and coronary angiography, whether or not all procedures are performed singly or in combination.

Since its inception, cardiac catheterization has been considered to be primarily an inpatient procedure. However, in an attempt to more efficiently utilize facilities and beds, outpatient cardiac catheterization has become an accepted alternative. **Outpatient** or **ambulatory cardiac catheterization** refers to performance of cardiac catheterization **without overnight hospitalization**. Outpatient cardiac catheterization may be performed in a number of settings: (*a*) the same in-hospital

cardiac catheterization laboratory which performs inpatient catheterizations; (*b*) catheterization laboratories specifically designated for outpatients but still physically within or adjacent to a hospital; or (*c*) a facility which is physically separate from the hospital (i.e., freestanding). The Health Care Financing Administration distinguishes between a hospital-affiliated ambulatory surgical center and an independent ambulatory surgical center regardless of physical location (1). Freestanding facilities lack geographic proximity to a hospital such that emergency transport of patients requires the use of an ambulance or similar vehicle. Additionally, freestanding facilities are not subject to a given hospital's credentialing or peer review procedures. These are important when considering freestanding cardiac catheterization laboratories.

When addressing the question of the optimal site for performance of cardiac catheterization, it is necessary to review both the complexity and variety of procedures performed in the catheterization laboratory, as well as the wide diversity and severity of cardiac disease.

Data from a large prospective study by the Registry Committee of the Society for Cardiac Angiography (SFCA) illustrate the wide diversity of diagnoses that can be expected in the general population of patients undergoing catheterization (2, 3). The majority (77%) of patients had coronary disease, 12% valvular heart disease, 2.8% congenital heart disease, and 1.5% myocardial disease. Considering the severity of disease present in these patients, a large proportion (48%) were found to be in New York Heart Association (NYHA) class III or IV. Of the patients reported, 28% had at least a moderate decrease in left ventricular function defined as an ejection fraction ≤49%. At the time of their report, one-third of the patients were older than 60 years of age, but with the increasing age of the general population, the percentage of elderly patients undergoing catheterization will certainly rise. In this large study, data of the procedures performed reveal that more than 75% of patients had both left heart catheterization and coronary angiography and more than 90% of patients had left ventricular angiography. Transseptal catheterization was relatively rare (0.9%). Procedure time was regularly less than 1 hour. Selective coronary angiography is the most commonly performed diagnostic cardiac angiographic procedure performed in the United States today (4). An estimated 1 million coronary angiograms are performed each year (C.J. Pepine, personal communication). Thus, based upon the above consideration there are several hundred thousand patients each year who are not class III or IV, not in heart failure, or not elderly who will have had a coronary angiographic procedure and may be candidates for outpatient catheterization.

A comparison of outpatient vs. inpatient studies will be presented in detail. The argument for outpatient cardiac catheterization can only be sustained as long as the risks of the procedure for a given patient in an ambulatory setting are not greater than those for the hospitalized setting. The efficacy and potential benefits must also be addressed. Potential cost savings and better utilization of beds are the two most apparent benefits, but better patient compliance and satisfaction can also be anticipated. Recommendations as to the type of facility (i.e., hospital-affiliated or freestanding), equipment, and personnel required and a general profile of patients most likely to benefit from outpatient catheterization will be discussed.

RESULTS OF OUTPATIENT CARDIAC CATHETERIZATION

Since 1977, 11 reports on the results of outpatient catheterization (5–15) have appeared. Two of these describe the results for freestanding laboratories (10, 11). Ideally, any valid comparison of inpatient and outpatient cardiac catheterization results must deal with patients who would be candidates for either type of catheterization. A second best estimate should at least involve patients matched for age, sex, extent of heart disease and complexity of the procedure. However, only five of the reports provide data on the extent of heart disease and the complications of outpatient catheterization in detail (5-8, 10) (Table 4.1). Normal coronary arteries were detected in 11 to 28.9% of patients (average 17.3%). This range is consistent with the 20% reported by Kennedy et al. (2) from hospitalized patients in the SFCA Registry and the 27% of normal coronary arteries reported in the Coronary Artery Surgery Study (CASS) study (16). The incidence of left main CAD of 5% in the studies by Klinke et al. (7) and Mahrer et al.(8) and of 6.3% in a study by Diethrich et al. (11) are comparable to the 9% reported in the CASS study (16) and the 6% reported by Kennedy et al. (2) for hospitalized patients. In another study by Mahrer and Eshoo (6) of 308 patients the high prevalence of left main CAD (20%)

Table 4.1
Cardiac Pathology Found in Patients Undergoing Outpatient Catheterization (%)

Author	No. of Patients	Normal	CAD Extent				CAD	CHD	VHD	CM
			3-Vessel	2-Vessel	1-Vessel	LM				
Fierens	5,107	16.5	–[b]	-	-	-	61.0	-	4.0	2.8
Baird[c]	620	28.9	-	-	-	-	59.7	0.6	9.5	1.3
Mahrer[c]	308	16.3	37	30	13	20	74.0	6.8	2.6	-
Klinke	3,071	13.6	27	32	36	5	70.4	-	12.5	3.5
Mahrer	3,537	11.0	-	-	-	5	74.0	-	15.0	-
Total	12,643	17.3					67.8		8.7	

[a]*LM*, left main coronary artery disease; *CHD*, congenital heart disease; *CM*, cardiomyopathy; *VHD*, valvular heart disease.
[b]–, not available.
[c] Includes patients with congenital heart disease.

was attributed to the rigid screening of patients prior to cardiac catheterization in their institution. Significant CAD was detected in 59.7 to 74% (average 67.8%) of patients undergoing outpatient catheterization (Table 4.1). Again, data figures are comparable to the incidence of significant CAD (77%) reported by Kennedy et al. (2) in hospitalized patients. Other cardiac diseases, including congenital heart disease, valvular heart disease, and cardiomyopathy, were seen in the remainder of the patients. It is apparent from these results that patients undergoing outpatient cardiac catheterization in the various institutions had significant heart disease, primarily consisting of CAD. However, the decision to perform outpatient catheterization was not randomized. This introduces the possibility of bias that is well known when comparing results of two different procedures. Furthermore, the lack of detailed data on baseline characteristics, noted with many of the reports, results in important limitations to the interpretations of complications that are reviewed below.

COMPLICATIONS

Major complications of cardiac catheterization are discussed in detail in Chapter 3. The incidence of complications of catheterization in an inpatient setting has been well documented in many large retrospective and prospective studies (2, 3, 16-20). Complication rates from all 11 reported studies of outpatient cardiac catheterization are shown in Table 4.2. All of the deaths reported occurred in patients with severe CAD. The causes included cerebrovascular accidents, anaphylactic shock, out-of-hospital cardiac arrest after an otherwise uncomplicated procedure, and coronary artery dissection. The overall complication rates (Table 4.2) for mortality (0.11%), nonfatal myocardial infarction (0.18%), peripheral vascular problems (1.24%), cerebral vascular events (0.09%), and significant arrhythmias (0.84%) approximate the rates reported for inpatient cardiac catheterization (1, 2, 16-19). Vascular complications were higher in those institutions using the Sones technique (5, 9, 10, 11, 15). Other than this, there does not appear to be a major difference in complication rates between the Judkins and Sones techniques in patients undergoing outpatient catheterization.

Only one report has been published comparing inpatients and outpatients done in the same institution. Fighali et al. reported in 1985 on a consecutive series of patients in their institution over a 2-year period. There were 676 outpatients and 1106 inpatients (9). The Sones approach was used in the majority of cases.

Table 4.2
Summary of Complications Reported During Outpatient Catheterization (%)

Author	No. of Patients	Death	MI[a]	Vasc	CNS	Arrhythmias	Total Complications
Fierens[b]	5107	0	0	2.04	0.02	0.14	2.20
Mahrer	308	0.30	0.97	0.65	0.32	-[c]	2.24
Klinke	3071	0.13	0.07	0.35	0.14	0.42	1.11
Mahrer[d]	3537	0.32	0.05	0.30	0.05	1.10	1.82
Fighali[b,e]	676	0	-	0.44	-	-	1.5[e]
Baird[b]	620	0.16	0.16	2.00	-	0.16	2.48
Diethrich[b]	254	0	0	3.10	0	0.80	3.90
Oehlert	100	0	0	0	0	1.00	1.00
Gavin	>100	-	-	-	-	-	4-8[f]
Beauchamp	596	-	-	-	-	-	1.1[g]
Rogers[b]	89	-	-	2.25	-	2.25	4.50
Total	14,458	0.11	0.18	1.24	0.09	0.84	2.67

[a] MI, myocardial infarction; CNS, central nervous system; Vasc, vascular.
[b] Primarily Sones technique.
[c] -, not available.
[d] 2,011 elective outpatients and 1330 transfer patients.
[e] Total complications include three patients admitted for angina and one patient for anaphylactic reaction.
[f] Hypotension, nausea, and vomiting.
[g] Data incomplete—1.1% admitted.

Results of this nonrandomized study suggested that the patients were comparable in terms of severity and extent of CAD. An important difference was that inpatients were more likely to be functional class IV. There were no major complications, including deaths, in the outpatient group. One death and three other major complications occurred in the inpatient group for an incidence of 0.4%. Minor complications occurred infrequently and were similar in both groups (approximately 1.5%). Although a relatively small number of patients were reported, these results suggest that major complications arising from the performance of cardiac catheterization are not related to whether or not overnight hospitalization is involved.

The outpatient catheterization reports listed in Table 4.2 describe complication rates primarily for middle-aged adult patients. The results of elderly patients, children, and adolescents undergoing outpatient catheterization are less well documented. Cumming reported on his experience with 2113 children studied over a 12-year period (21). Of these, 1358 catheterizations were performed as an outpatient procedure (64%). Over 45% of newborns and 80% of patients older than one year underwent outpatient catheterization. All patients required catheterization for diagnosis of cyanotic or acyanotic congenital heart disease. No specific exclusions were used. Some patients with severe pulmonary hypertension and severe cyanotic heart disease were included in the outpatient group. No deaths occurred, and only 1% suffered a major complication. The majority of these complications were vascular problems, such as thrombophlebitis, hematomas, and arterial thrombosis. One patient had transient aphasia 24 hr following catheterization, and two patients with tetralogy of Fallot were admitted following a severe cyanotic spell. Further evaluation of outpatient catheterization in children and adolescents is necessary to confirm its safety and effectiveness. Data for elderly patients are also needed.

By analyzing the data from just those studies which provide the most complete information on patient characteristics and complication rates (5-10), certain conclusions concerning the risk of outpatient cardiac catheterization can be made. Overall, the complication rate in a large number of patients having outpatient cardiac catheterization does not seem to vary significantly from that reported for inpatient cardiac catheterization.

Patients undergoing outpatient catheterization appear to have the same extent of heart disease as seen in previously reported inpatient series. However, as more patients undergo cardiac catheterization and more aggressive use of these procedures occurs in unstable patients, the inpatient population consisting of patients with unstable angina, acute myocardial infarction (AMI), and NYHA class III and IV may well have a slightly higher complication rate.

Given the variability and extremely low mortality rates, a significant difference in complication rates between inpatient and outpatient catheterization will be detectable only if there is a large difference in mortality rates, or if very large comparable sample sizes are studied. Ideally, a prospective randomized study comparing the results of patients suitable for outpatient catheterization but randomized to either outpatient catheterization or inpatient catheterization should be conducted. Because of the very low overall mortality rate, it is estimated that a sample size of 362,835 outpatients would be necessary to demonstrate a 50% difference in mortality rate (20). It is highly unlikely that a study this large can be undertaken.

EFFICACY

The major advances in cardiology in the last century were dependent upon the concurrent development of cardiac catheterization techniques, coronary angiography, and open-heart surgery. Recent advances such as percutaneous transluminal coronary angioplasty (PTCA), percutaneous balloon valvoplasty, electrophysiological surgery, and thrombolysis in the treatment of AMI have depended on the safe performance of and access to high-quality cardiac catheterization. The question remaining is not whether cardiac catheterization has a major role in diagnosis and management of cardiac diseases, but rather if any of the benefits are lost or risks increased by moving the procedure into an ambulatory setting. No randomized control trial of patients having clearly defined, specific cardiac diseases has evaluated the efficacy of cardiac catheterization either as an inpatient or outpatient procedure. The efficacy of outpatient cardiac catheterization depends on determining the potential patient and institutional benefits, as well as the best and most cost-effective manner for detecting and defining heart disease in order to aid in clinical decision-making.

There is no reason to believe that efficacy for certain hospital-based outpatient catheterization would not be equivalent to that of inpatient catheterization, especially if laboratories maintain recommended utilization rates. Approximately 80% of all patients undergoing cardiac catheterization were eligible for an outpatient procedure in both the reports by Klinke et al. (7) and Mahrer et al. (8). Over 96% of patients were discharged following an uncomplicated cardiac catheterization while 2.3% were admitted for prolonged observation for a variety of reasons, including severity of disease, hypotension, hemorrhage, vasovagal reactions, allergic reactions, and social reasons (7).

COST

The fixed cost for cardiac catheterization includes general and cardiac catheterization laboratory fees, hospitalization room-and-board charges, and professional fees. Less obvious costs incurred by the patients include loss of income while away from work, loss of productivity, transportation costs, and room and board if not hospitalized.

Hansing reported on the cost of inpatient cardiac catheterization in 15 hospitals surveyed in the state of Washington in 1977 (22, 23). The costs ranged between $774 and $1988. The average charge for the cardiac catheterization laboratory was $623 and an additional $481 for professional fees. Two-thirds of the total cost of cardiac catheterization was attributable to catheterization laboratory charges.

Levin, in 1982, reported on the results of a questionnaire completed by 54 cardiac catheterization laboratories affiliated with the SFCA (4). The mean catheterization laboratory charge was reported as $760, with a mean professional fee of $640, for a total procedural cost of $1400. This is comparable to that reported by Hansing (22, 23) in 1979, after adjusting for inflation. Levin felt that hospital-related costs reported both by Hansing and

the SFCA were inappropriately low and calculated a total hospital-related cost in his own institution of $1200. This would yield a total procedural cost in his institution of between $1800 and $2000. Additionally, he estimated the average charge for a hospital bed in his own institution to be only $130 per day. Even using this low figure and making adjustments to account for intervening inflation, one can calculate a potential cost savings of $300 million a year based on 75% of all patients undergoing cardiac catheterization having the procedure performed on an outpatient basis (75% × 1,000,000 catheterizations per year x $400 savings in hospital charge).

In theory, the cost savings of outpatient cardiac catheterization should be limited to the charges for hospital room and board and pharmacy fees. However, additional savings may be realized if precatheterization data from patient records can reduce or eliminate redundant tests performed in hospitals, for example, admission blood work, chest x-ray, and ECG. The cost to the patient for transportation and room and board before an outpatient procedure must also be considered.

Cost savings for outpatient cardiac catheterization were reported in seven studies (5, 6, 9, 10, 11, 13, 14). Savings range from a low of $276 to a high of $1000 per patient. Mahrer et al., in 1987, estimated that the cost savings in their institution would amount to over $1 million (8). They speculated that a potential $200 million a year might be saved by performing outpatient catheterization. A direct comparison of inpatient catheterization vs. outpatient catheterization was made by Fighali et al. (9). Their average cost for an outpatient cardiac catheterization, including preliminary blood work, ECG, and radiological studies, was $744, whereas the average cost for inpatient catheterization based on a 2-night stay in a semiprivate room was $1050. The average savings by patients studied on an outpatient basis was $276, representing a 27% reduction in hospital-related costs for the procedure. Therefore, it seems reasonable to estimate cost savings of approximately 30% in a study performed in an outpatient facility. The Inter-Society Commission for Heart Disease also considers the procedural costs for repeated studies due to nondiagnostic or incomplete studies as hidden but important costs for any evaluation of the efficacy of cardiac catheterization (24). Unfortunately, these costs have not been described in most reports. It is imperative, therefore, that outpatient facilities maintain the same quality for angiographic and catheterization studies as inpatient facilities in order to achieve these savings.

Other benefits to patients will be in allaying anxiety associated with a procedure formerly requiring hospitalization and greater flexibility in arranging time off from work and away from family. Patients who have already undergone outpatient cardiac catheterization invariably prefer this approach to hospitalization.

CATHETERIZATION SITE

In comparing the risks and benefits of outpatient cardiac catheterization, one must also consider the access to emergency facilities in case of major complications. If facilities and personnel are equivalent, complications should depend primarily on the severity of cardiac diseases. Hospital-associated facilities are most likely to have adequate volume and the ability to handle acutely ill patients. Utilization rates and experience of personnel are also major factors in the safe performance of outpatient cardiac catheterization. A large number of cardiac catheterization laboratories at present do not meet the expected utilization rate of 300 adult cases per year. Considering these factors, with the anticipated leveling off of the number of cardiac catheterizations performed and the decrease in the mortality of heart disease, the establishment of many new and/or freestanding units does not appear justified (25).

Freestanding units have introduced at least two major problems. First, access to emergency care may be compromised if a complication occurs or if the procedure documents disease requiring emergency hospitalization. A study of catheterization-related deaths by Kennedy and co-workers showed that one-third of the patients with left main disease who died, died after an uneventful catheterization (2). This suggests that for some patients immediate access to a hospital or to a cardiovascular surgical team would be helpful. The number of patients who would benefit from such access is small (estimated at approximately 14 per 10,000 patients). It is unlikely

that in an emergency (rather than an average situation) access could be equivalent in the freestanding unit (26). Even hospitals performing cardiac catheterization without on-site surgical facilities would be better equipped for emergency cardiac care. The second important problem relating to freestanding units is quality control and peer review. Most hospital-affiliated cardiac catheterization laboratories are required to maintain accurate statistics on the numbers and types of cardiac procedures performed, diagnosis of cardiac diseases, and complications occurring during and immediately following catheterization. Hospital-based laboratories are under the same review as that seen in other areas of the hospital. Directors of cardiac catheterization laboratories have a responsibility to assure that only qualified and experienced medical personnel are permitted to perform cardiac catheterization procedures.

ESTABLISHING AN OUTPATIENT CARDIAC CATHETERIZATION FACILITY

It is strongly recommended that all ambulatory facilities for cardiac catheterization be closely affiliated with a hospital. This facility may be within or physically adjacent to the hospital. In most cases, it will likely be the facility that is also used for inpatients and more complex procedures such as valvuloplasty, coronary angioplasty, and electrophysiological studies. This will give the facility the proper case mix and utilization rates to maintain expertise. Where no on-site cardiac surgery is available, a formalized, carefully delineated relationship to a nearby cardiac surgical program is essential.

Equipment and Room

The outpatient facility must have the same quality and standard of radiographic equipment required in an inpatient facility. Space requirements and backup for radiographic and other equipment failures should be the same. The facility should be capable of providing excellent angiographic studies in all types of patients. Standard multichannel ECG and hemodynamic monitoring are mandatory. Resuscitation equipment, including defibrillator, temporary pacemakers, intubation equipment, intraaortic balloon pumps (IABP), and appropriate emergency drugs, must be readily available. The facility must be integrated with the hospital in such a manner as to provide immediate emergency access to a coronary care unit and cardiac surgery. The ability to perform emergency PTCA is desirable but may not be feasible in all laboratories.

Observation Room

Electrocardiographic monitoring is optional, but immediate access to resuscitation equipment, oxygen, and suction is mandatory. Patient beds should be comfortable enough for patients to be able to lay flat for 4 to 6 hr. All beds should be visible from a central nursing station. Facilities for precatheterization preparation may be in the observation room or, alternately, in a staging area adjacent to the cardiac catheterization laboratory. It is desirable that the observation room be adjacent to the cardiac catheterization laboratory, as this will allow for much easier transfer of patients and also more ready access to the catheterization laboratory if problems develop.

Educational and instructive materials such as heart diagrams and heart models are useful in explaining procedures and the results of the catheterization to patients and relatives. The observation room should be organized so that patients will feel comfortable and relaxed before and after their procedure. A waiting room for relatives should be provided.

Staff

The nursing staff assigned to the outpatient laboratory observation room should be fully trained in advanced cardiac life support and preferably have coronary care and cardiac catheterization experience. Nursing coverage must be continuous so that patients are never left alone in the room. In addition, these nurses will require training to evaluate puncture or incision sites; to detect early signs of bleeding, thrombosis, and vasovagal reactions; and to diagnose angina pectoris and evolving myocardial infarction. Medication should be available to treat angina pectoris, bradyarrhythmias, and tachyarrhythmias. Clear lines of communication must be established so that a physician is immediately available if problems arise.

CATHETERIZATION PROCEDURE

Our own experience at the Royal Alexandra Hospital has been previously reported (7), but now includes nearly 6000 diagnostic outpatient cardiac catheterizations on adult patients. This represents 75% of all catheterizations performed in our laboratory. The majority of patients have had CAD (70%) and less than 15% have a normal study. Essentially, all of our procedures are done using 7 or 8 French (Fr) Judkins catheters with or without sheaths. Complication rates for femoral or brachial techniques should not differ greatly, but earlier ambulation is possible for patients having a brachial procedure. However, the femoral percutaneous approach is usually quicker and easier to perform.

Right and left heart catheterization, with left ventricular and coronary angiography, are performed as required. The use of heparin is controversial. However, frequent aspiration and flushing of catheters with heparinized solution is mandatory. Standard 7 or 8 Fr catheters are usually used. Smaller 5 or 6 Fr catheters have potential advantages for outpatients in that trauma to the femoral artery may be less. But difficulty with manipulation of these catheters and poor control and stability during injection continue to be drawbacks with certain designs. At present, no controlled studies have documented an improvement in vascular complication rates using these smaller catheters in either outpatient or inpatient procedures. Our own experience has shown an increase in both procedure and fluoroscopic time when comparing 5 Fr with 7 or 8 Fr catheters. Time to obtain hemostasis was significantly reduced, but there was no difference in incidence of hematoma formation (W.P. Klinke, unpublished data). The increased procedure and fluoroscopic time required to use these catheters may outweigh the small advantage they have over larger catheters. Additionally, the quality of the angiogram and the fluoroscopic image is often suboptimal. It is anticipated that future developments in the construction of these catheters may improve their handling characteristics.

In our experience use of nonionic or low osmolality contrast agents can be expected to result in less hemodynamic response to injection of contrast and has also tended to decrease procedure duration. Nausea and vomiting are reduced with use of these agents. Important ventricular arrhythmias and bradyarrhythmias appear to occur much less frequently. Patients with severe coronary disease, moderate-to-severe left ventricular dysfunction, and aortic stenosis will benefit from use of these more expensive contrast agents. Although not mandatory, their use in outpatient cardiac catheterization will help to facilitate the procedure.

Precatheterization Preparation

The cardiologist performing the procedure must not be an itinerant angiographer technician, but must be involved in the medical care of the patient. A few days prior to catheterization, the procedure should be explained, the risks outlined, and informed consent obtained. Precatheterization data at this time would include blood work (CBC, BUN, creatinine, electrolytes, blood glucose), ECG, chest x-ray, exercise stress test, echocardiogram, and radionuclide studies when appropriate. Any special patient problems, such as insulin-dependent diabetes, anticoagulant therapy, or severe hypertension, should be evaluated and specific instructions given to the patient and nursing staff prior to the catheterization. Insulin-dependent diabetics should be scheduled as the first case of the day, following which insulin can be resumed at a reduced dose. Alternately, an intravenous drip of insulin (0.5 to 1 unit/hr in 5% Dextrose and water at 100 cc/hr) can be utilized.

Standard precatheterization orders for outpatients may include the following:

1. No food for 6 to 8 hr prior to procedure. Fluids only. NPO x 4 hr prior to procedure.
2. Consent signed for: "Cardiac Catheterization and Coronary Angiogram."
3. ECG done prior to procedure. Send ECG and chart to catheterization laboratory with patient.
4. Start IV 5% D/W, 500 ml in left arm to keep vein open.
5. Skin shave prep both groins.
6. Patient to void prior to procedure.
7. Record height and weight.
8. List medications:
9. List allergies:
10. Precatheterization sedation, typically Valium 10 mg po 1 hr before catheterization.

Educational booklets and videos on outpatient cardiac catheterization have proven useful and often help to allay anxiety. Written instructions are given to patients indicating the time they should arrive at the facility, which medications are indicated or contraindicated, and that they be accompanied by a relative or responsible person before and after the procedure (Fig. 4.1).

Day of the Catheterization

The patient usually comes to the facility 1 or 2 hr before the time of catheterization, having fasted for 6 to 8 hr. Standard orders will then be undertaken by the nursing staff. After the usual preparation and insertion of intravenous lines, the patient is then transferred to the cardiac catheterization laboratory. The proposed procedure is undertaken, and then postcatheterization hemostasis is obtained by manual or mechanical means. A sandbag is then applied to the puncture site, and peripheral pulses are checked and noted if any discrepancy is present. It is helpful to mark palpable pedal pulses with an ink marker prior to catheterization. Intravenous fluid orders and other medication orders, such as insulin requirements and prescriptions for antihypertensive or antianginal medications, should be written at this time by the cardiologist. The patient is then transferred back to the observation room. Direct communication with the nurses in the observation room by the cardiologist performing the procedure will facilitate care of the patient.

The following postcatheterization procedures should be observed:

1. Check groin for bleeding and hematoma q. 15 min x 1 hr, then q. 1/2 hr x 1 hr, then q. 1 hr x 4 hr; blood pressure, radial pulse and circulation of limb (i.e., color, warmth, and pedal pulses) q. 1/2 hr x 1 hr, then q. 1 hr x 5 hr. Temperature p.r.n.
2. Sand bag 3 hr and remove if no signs of bleeding, thrombosis, or limb ischemia occur. **Note:** If color change occurs in the leg, remove sandbag and notify physician immediately.
3. Check for orthostatic and vasovagal reactions. These usually respond to the patient resuming the supine position and to the use of intravenous fluids and atropine.
4. Complete bed rest x 4 hr then allow patient to be up for 2 hr before discharge.
5. ECG postcatheterization.
6. Warm fluids p.o. following procedure. Direct agglutination test (DAT).

7. IV to keep vein open until postambulation. If patient is nauseated or not tolerating fluids, check with physician regarding rate of IV.
8. Catheterize the bladder if patient is unable to void and is uncomfortable.
9. Remove dressing before discharge.
10. Call attending catheterization physician p.r.n.
11. Discharge after 6 hr if no bleeding. If bleeding occurs, reapply sand bag for 4 hr.

The patient is then allowed to ambulate for 2 hr, and if there are no signs of bleeding, thrombosis, or hypotension, the patient may be discharged. The cardiologist should check each patient prior to release and confirm a follow-up visit for the patient in the next few days. In most cases, a preliminary report can be given to the patient and relatives at this time. This is also an opportune time to initiate or change medical therapy. Patients requiring elective angioplasty, valvoplasty, or heart surgery are given an admission appointment. The patient is then given both verbal and written instructions to return immediately to the hospital if signs of bleeding, thrombosis, or any other serious symptoms occur. A follow-up telephone call the following day by the nurse is useful. Patients are not allowed to drive postcatheterization and undertake any heavy lifting or stair climbing for at least the first 24 hr. It is recommended that patients do only a limited amount of walking after the procedure until the next morning. The patient is told not to take a bath or shower that evening and not to wash groin area until the

---

Cardiac Catheterization And Coronary Angiogram
Outpatient Information Sheet

*Important - Bring This Sheet To The Hospital With You

1. Please arrive at the hospital "**ADMITTING DEPARTMENT**" at
   _____ AM on _____. Your Cardiac Catheterization will be done at _____ AM/PM.
2. No food or drink is to be taken after midnight on the day of the test. Do not smoke or consume alcoholic drinks of any kind on the day of your test.
3. Stop taking all **ANTICOAGULANTS** (blood thinners) 48 hours prior to your Cardiac Cath (or as directed by your physician). These Anticoagulants include: Aspirin; Entrophen; Coumadin; Asasantine and Persantine.
4. On admission please list all **DRUGS** or **MEDICINES** that you have been taking.
5. Please report any **ALLERGIES** you have and how they affect you. Please tell us if you have a tendency to **BLEED** excessively.
6. Your case may be canceled due to any acute medical condition, for example, flu, cold, infection, very sore back. If in doubt, please contact your doctor prior to the day of the test.
7. You may **NOT** drive your own vehicle or travel home by bus. You **MUST** be accompanied home by a responsible adult who can be contacted at any time after your test.
8. You will be detained at least 6 hours after completion of the test and in certain cases may be kept overnight in the hospital.
9. Consent for the test must be signed by the patient, if an adult, or by the parent or legal guardian for a patient under 18 years of age. This will be done while you are on Station 63 of the Hospital.
10. At least one parent or a responsible adult must remain at the hospital with children under 12 years of age.
11. Please do not wear makeup, nail polish, jewelry, or bring large sums of money or valuables.
12. Please bring your own slippers.

FOR NURSING UNIT ONLY
Precatheterization Sedation Order:
Valium _____ po on call from Cath Lab
Signed: _____

Figure 4.1 Form given to patients at the Royal Alexandra Hospitals, Edmonton, Alberta, Canada, to be filled out before cardiac catheterization.

next morning. He or she may resume medications, except for antiplatelet or anticoagulant drugs, which may be resumed 48 hr later. In most cases, patients will be discharged to their own home. The patient is told to apply firm and direct pressure and return to the hospital immediately by ambulance if bleeding from the puncture site occurs. Patients from out of town, if stable and accompanied by a relative, can stay overnight in a nearby hotel. If bruising to the groin site seems to increase in size or hardness, the patient is told to consult with his or her doctor. It is important to keep an accurate logbook and record any postcatheterization complications. The most common problem after discharge is related to late bleeding, resulting in hematoma formation or ecchymosis. In most cases, cold compresses with elevation of the affected leg is sufficient. No accurate data for this complication are currently available, but from our own series it is probably less than 1%. Over 90% of the patients should be eligible for release to home the same day. Depending on the case mix and referral patterns at each institution, approximately 60 to 80% of all cardiac catheterization patients can be considered for outpatient cardiac catheterization. The reasons for prolonged observation and/or admission to hospital are outlined in Table 4.3.

Table 4.3
Reasons for Prolonged (Overnight) Observation or Admission of Outpatients After Cardiac Catheterization

1. Social-patients living excessive distance from hospital; patients unable to follow instructions
2. Left main coronary artery disease
3. Severe three-vessel coronary artery disease requiring urgent surgery
4. Severe aortic stenosis
5. Other unexpected disease requiring surgery, e.g., atrial myxoma, aortic dissection
6. Prolonged angina or ST segment changes during or following procedure
7. Occurrence of potentially lethal ventricular arrhythmias.
8. Heart block requiring pacemaker insertion
9. Severe pulmonary hypertension
10. Severe vasovagal reactions or prolonged hypotension
11. Major complications due to catheterization
12. Rebleeding with large hematoma

PRESENT RECOMMENDATIONS

The Health and Public Policy Committee of the American College of Physicians, in a policy statement in 1985, recommended that outpatient cardiac catheterization be performed only in the setting of an outpatient facility affiliated with a hospital (26). Eligible patients should have a history of stable symptoms and no significant comorbid factors (bleeding, diathesis, renal insufficiency, uncontrolled diabetes, or uncontrolled systolic hypertension). All outpatient facilities must have immediate access to emergency medical and surgical care and must provide a setting wherein adequate observation for 4 to 6 hr can be provided. Patients who have complications during cardiac catheterization or who are found to have significant left main CAD or severe aortic stenosis should be immediately hospitalized following the procedure, even if no complications have occurred. Additionally, other patients with adverse psychosocial characteristics may benefit from hospitalization. The American College of Cardiology (ACC) and American Heart Association (AHA), in a policy statement in 1985 (27), concurred with the recommendations of the American College of Physicians. The American College of Cardiology and American Heart Association did not approve the use of freestanding, nonhospital-based or mobile cardiac catheterization laboratories for either ambulatory or hospitalized patients because of uncertainty regarding quality control and continuity of care. A task force of the ACC and AHA is now preparing a revised position paper on ambulatory cardiac catheterization to be published soon (28).

Criteria for outpatient catheterization are up to each cardiologist, but in most cases, the only reason for not performing an outpatient catheterization is that the patient is already in the hospital because of unstable or acute events of cardiovascular disease such as unstable angina, myocardial infarction, congestive heart failure, or lethal cardiac arrhythmias. Greater than 96% of our patients are released the same day following an uncomplicated cardiac catheterization. The total complication rate is 1.4%. Reasons for patients being admitted to the hospital for observation after catheterization (1.7%) are in Table 4.3.

SUMMARY

Adult patients of NYHA class III or less are possible candidates for outpatient catheterization, providing they do not meet certain exclusion criteria (Table 4.4). The facility performing outpatient cardiac catheterization should be hospital-affiliated, either on-site or adjacent, and have easy and ready access to emergency facilities and the ability to readily admit patients for observation. Laboratories doing less than 300 cardiac catheterizations per year probably will not have the experience or expertise to consider outpatient cardiac catheterization. The benefits of freestanding or mobile cardiac catheterization laboratories for outpatient cardiac catheterization are not proven and, therefore, cannot be recommended.

Outpatient cardiac catheterization can play a major role in the more efficient use of hospital beds and financial resources. Significant cost savings can be achieved for hospitals, third-party payers, and patients. One can expect utilization rates of 60 to 80% of all patients undergoing cardiac catheterization, depending upon the case mix and referral patterns of the institutions. Same-day discharge is possible in 95% of appropriately selected outpatients. Complication rates should be comparable to inpatient catheterization. Provided that outpatient cardiac catheterization laboratories maintain adequate workloads, quality control and peer review, and have provisions for immediate access to emergency care and prolonged observation as required, the performance of outpatient cardiac catheterization should involve no more risk than inpatient catheterization.

Table 4.4
Exclusion Criteria for Outpatient Cardiac Catheterization

A. Absolute
1. Unstable angina
2. Recent myocardial infarction (14 days)
3. Suspected left main coronary disease
4. Potentially lethal ventricular arrhythmias
5. NYHA class IV heart failure
6. Severe pulmonary hypertension
7. Severe uncontrolled hypertension
8. Severe renal disease
9. Active infective endocarditis
10. Coagulation disorder or coumadin use
11. Complex procedures (e.g., PTCA, valvuloplasty)
12. Cyanotic or complex congenital heart disease
13. Unaccompanied or elderly patients

B. Relative
1. Suspected three-vessel coronary disease with markedly positive stress test
2. Aortic stenosis
3. NYHA class III heart failure
4. Transseptal left heart catheterization needed
5. History of severe contrast reaction
6. Other significant medical disease

References

1. Proposed Rules. Federal Regulations. 1982;47:12574–12593.
2. Kennedy J, Registry Committee of the Society for Cardiac Angiography. Complications associated with cardiac catheterization and angiography. Cathet Cardiovasc Diagn 1982;8:5–11.
3. Kennedy JW, Registry Committee of the Society for Cardiac Angiography. Mortality related to cardiac catheterization and angiography. Cathet Cardiovasc Diagn 1982;8:323–339.
4. Levin DC. Invasive evaluation (coronary arteriography) of the coronary artery disease patient: clinical, economic and social issues. Circulation 1982;66:III–71–III–79.
5. Fierens E. Outpatient coronary arteriography. Cathet Cardiovasc Diagn 1984;10:27–32.
6. Mahrer PR, Eshoo N. Outpatient cardiac catheterization and coronary angiography. Cathet Cardiovasc Diagn 1981;7:355–360.
7. Klinke WP, Kubac G, Talibi T, Lee SSK. Safety of outpatient cardiac catheterizations. Am J Cardiol 1985;56:639–641.
8. Mahrer PR, Young C, Magnusson T. Efficacy and safety of outpatient cardiac catheterization. Cathet Cardiovasc Diagn 1987;13:304–308.
9. Fighali S, Krajcer Z, Gonzales-Camid F, Varda M, Edelman S, Leachman R. Safety of outpatient cardiac catheterization. Chest 1985;88:349–351.
10. Baird C. The trend to outpatient care: ambulatory cardiac catheterization. Va Med Mon 1980;107:621–622.
11. Diethrich EB, Kinard SA, Pierce SA, Koopot R. Outpatient cardiac catheterization and arteriography: twenty-month experience at the Arizona Heart Institute. Cardiovasc Dis Bull Texas Heart Inst 1981;8:195–204.
12. Oehlert WH. Outpatient coronary arteriography. Oklahoma State Med Assoc 1981;74:314–315.
13. Gavin VA, Stewart DK, Murray JA. Outpatient coronary arteriography (editorial). Cathet Cardiovasc Diagn 1981;7:347.

14. Beauchamp PK. Ambulatory cardiac catheterization cuts costs for hospital and patients. Hospitals 1981;62–63.

15. Rogers WF, Moothart RW. Outpatient arteriography and cardiac catheterization: effective alternatives to inpatient procedures. AJR 1985;144:233–234.

16. Davis K, Kennedy JW, Kemp HG Jr, Judkins MP, Gosselin AJ, Killip T. Complications of coronary arteriography from the collaborative study of coronary artery surgery (CASS). Circulation 1979;59:1105–1112.

17. Bourassa MG, Noble J. Complication rate of coronary arteriography: a review of 5250 cases studied by a percutaneous femoral technique. Circulation 1976;53:106–114.

18. Adams DF, Abrams HL. Complications of coronary arteriography: a follow-up report. Cardiovasc Radiol 1979;2:89–96.

19. Adams DF, Fraser DB, Abrams HL. The complications of coronary arteriography. Circulation 1973;48:609–618.

20. Kahn KL. The efficacy of ambulatory cardiac catheterization in the hospital and free-standing setting. Am Heart J 1986;111:152–167.

21. Cumming GR. Cardiac catheterization in infants and children can be an out-patient procedure. Am J Cardiol 1982;49:1248–1253.

22. Hansing CE. The risk and cost of coronary angiography. I. Cost of coronary angiography in Washington State. JAMA 1979;242:731–738.

23. Hansing CE. The risk and cost of coronary angiography. II. The risk of coronary angiography in Washington State. JAMA 1979;242:735–738.

24. Judkins MP, Abrams HL, Bristow JD, et al. Report of the Inter-Society Commission for Heart Disease Resources: optimal resources for examination of the chest and cardiovascular system: a hospital planning and resource guideline. Circulation 1976;53:A1–37.

25. Kennedy RH, Kennedy MA, Fige RL, et al. Cardiac catheterization and cardiac surgical facilities. N Engl J Med 1982;307:986–993.

26. Health and Public Policy Committee, American College of Physicians. The safety and efficacy of ambulatory cardiac catheterization in the hospital and free-standing setting. Ann Intern Med 1985;103:294–298.

27. ACC/AHA Joint Statement. The safety and efficacy of ambulatory cardiac catheterization in the Hospital and Free-standing Facility. Cardiol Newsletter 1985;15:2.

28. ACC/AHA Task Force on Ambulatory Cardiac Catheterization. Guidelines on Ambulatory Cardiac Catheterization. J Am Coll Cardiol in press, 1989.

5

Interventional Cardiac Catheterization for Myocardial Infarction: Logistics, Operation, and Results

Richard S. Stack, M.D.

INTRODUCTION

Coronary reperfusion within 6 hours of the onset of acute myocardial infarction partially salvages jeopardized myocardium and significantly improves both short- and long-term survival (1–6). Thrombolytic agents have become a standard therapeutic intervention in patients without contraindications. Despite the efficacy of these agents, all available thrombolytic drugs share at least two major limitations. First, even the best available agents fail to recanalize the infarction-related coronary artery in 20 to 30% of cases (7, 8). Second, even in those patients who have recanalization, there is a significant residual stenosis in many that often limits reperfusion and leads to reocclusion with or without either signs or symptoms of ischemia (9, 10). Unfortunately, noninvasive methods, such as chest pain, ST segment changes, or reperfusion arrhythmias, for identifying patients who have failed to recanalize have recently been shown to be unreliable (11, 12).

Because of the limitations of thrombolytic therapy and the inability to reliably identify patients who fail to reperfuse, urgent cardiac catheterization with percutaneous transluminal coronary angioplasty (PTCA) has been proposed. This approach permits patients with total coronary occlusion to be immediately identified and reperfusion can then be established directly with PTCA. Patients who have been reperfused by prior thrombolytic agents but have significant residual stenosis can also be identified and undergo PTCA to achieve wider patency, reducing the likelihood for reocclusion. Although several trials have shown excellent results using this approach, it is clear that PTCA in the setting of an unstable plaque may result in a lower acute success rate and a higher in-hospital reocclusion rate, as compared with elective PTCA (13, 14). This is particularly true if PTCA is applied in all instances regardless of the coronary anatomy (15).

Based on the above reasoning, a strategy was designed to attempt to maximize the efficacy, safety, and long-term outcome of coronary reperfusion. Thrombolytic therapy is administered immediately at local community hospitals within a 150-mile radius of the center, and the patient is transferred by helicopter or specialized ground transport emergency units. Emergency cardiac catheterization is performed, and infarction-related vessel patency status is documented angiographically. In patients found to be successfully recanalized with good antegrade flow, PTCA or bypass surgery is deferred until later when

50

the plaque may be more stabilized. However, patients who fail to reperfuse, those with poor antegrade flow, and patients in cardiogenic shock undergo emergency PTCA. This chapter reviews the logistics, operation, and results of this strategy as performed at the emergency Interventional Cardiac Catheterization (ICC) Program at Duke University Medical Center.

INTERVENTIONAL CARDIAC CATHETERIZATION PROGRAM

Emergency Transport

Emergency cardiac catheterization facilities staffed with highly trained personnel are expensive and beyond the means of many smaller community hospitals. Specialized emergency cardiac transportation facilities using helicopter and ground transport units offer a means of providing definitive myocardial infarction therapy to community hospitals within 150 to 200 miles of the interventional center. We use three helipads located adjacent to the emergency department and interventional laboratory facilities. Two of the crafts are large, specially equipped, twin turbo helicopters staffed on a 24-hr basis and occupy two of the helipads. The remaining helipad is used for aircraft from hospitals with their own helicopter services. A large specially equipped emergency ground transport unit is used for patients within a 25-mile radius of the interventional center or for longer distances during poor weather conditions when the helicopters are unable to fly. The ground transport unit is staffed by the same specially trained personnel that staff the helicopter.

When patients with acute myocardial infarction are identified by referring physicians at community hospitals, either the interventional cardiologist on call or the Life Flight control officer is notified to arrange transfer. Depending on distance and weather conditions, helicopter or ground transport units are dispatched with a crew consisting of an experienced pilot or emergency vehicle driver and two critical care Life Flight nurses. During our early experience, interventional cardiologists often accompanied the Life Flight crew during transport. At present, cardiologists rarely accompany the crew unless there are special needs such as balloon pump insertion at the local hospital. Both the helicopters and ground transport units are equipped with portable intraaortic balloon pumps. During transport, Life Flight crews are in continuous radio contact with the interventional cardiologists to receive medication orders and to report any changes in patient condition.

Recently, the safety and efficacy of air transport at our institution from March 1, 1985, through June 30, 1986, was reported (16). A total of 1,597 critically ill patients were transported. Within the group transported for cardiac reasons (n = 896 patients), 250 patients met criteria for acute myocardial infarction (AMI). These criteria included: a compatible history of chest pain of < 12 hr in duration; at least 1-mm ST segment elevation in two or more continuous ECG leads; no resolution of ST segment elevation with 0.4 mg sublingual nitroglycerin given in three consecutive doses. Once patients fulfilled these criteria, thrombolytic therapy was initiated unless there was contraindication due to risk of bleeding. Most patients (96%) were treated with thrombolytic therapy (intravenous streptokinase, 1.5 million/units, in 77% and intravenous tissue plasminogen activator (tPA) in 19%). No thrombolytic therapy was used in 4%. Time from onset of symptoms to administration of thrombolytic therapy ranged from 30 to 120 min (median 180 min); time of arrival at the Interventional Catheterization Laboratory ranged from 105 to 815 min after diagnosis (median 300 min). The actual flight time was 12 to 77 min (median 31 min). Transient hypotension, preflight (30 patients) and in-flight (21 patients), was the most common complication. Sustained hypotension (longer than 1 hr) occurred in 20 patients preflight and four patients in flight. Ventricular fibrillation or sustained ventricular tachycardia occurred before take-off in 38 patients (15%). No patients had ventricular fibrillation, asystole, or respiratory arrest during transport. Fluid boluses for hypotension were the most common intervention during flight. Five patients required cardiopulmonary resuscitation in flight (three prior to lift-off and two in-flight). Fourteen patients required vasopressors, antishock trousers, or both to maintain adequate blood pressure before and during flight. But cardioversion, defibrillation, and/or intubation were not required during flight.

Patient Selection

Selection criteria for interventional cardiac catheterization in patients with myocardial infarction have not yet been fully established. Presumably, some patients will not benefit or may be harmed. Available studies, however, suggest that most patients should benefit from early and complete restoration of coronary blood flow.

Although specific investigational protocols vary, our selection criteria for thrombolytic therapy are as follows:

1. Chest pain of ≤6 hr in duration or associated with ST segment elevation of >1 mm in two or more ECG leads.
2. Intermittent ("stuttering") chest pain of 6 to 24 hr in duration, provided that both persistent chest pain and ST segment elevation are present, indicating ischemic but viable residual myocardium.

Thrombolytic therapy is withheld if patients have any of the following: recent history of gastrointestinal bleeding, stroke, major surgery, or trauma (including prolonged cardiopulmonary resuscitation (CPR)); history of a bleeding diathesis; proliferative diabetic retinopathy; severe uncontrolled hypertension (diastolic pressure greater than or equal to 130, systolic greater than or equal to 200 mm Hg); or a history of allergic reaction to the thrombolytic agent. Patients over 75 years of age are individualized, based on their pre-infarction medical status. Patients with contraindications to thrombolytic therapy may be treated with PTCA alone, although the usual dosage of heparin used during the PTCA procedure (10,000 units) may be reduced.

Because time is critical when attempting to salvage jeopardized myocardium, treatment must often be based on a presumptive diagnosis of myocardial infarction before cardiac enzyme elevations can be detected. Several pitfalls in the presumptive diagnosis of acute myocardial infarction (AMI) are worth mentioning. One of the most common situations encountered is that of the patient with nonspecific chest discomfort associated with minor ECG changes later found to be of noncardiac etiology. To minimize treating such patients inappropriately, we require that ST segment elevation >1 mm be present in at least two ECG leads and that there be chest discomfort strongly suggestive of myocardial infarction. Despite these criteria, patients with early repolarization abnormalities or left ventricular hypertrophy may have ECG abnormalities that mimic acute infarction. Clues from the ST segment configuration, previous ECG tracings, and atypical features of the chest pain symptoms are all useful in making the correct diagnosis. Patients with acute pericarditis presenting with precordial chest pain and ST segment elevation are of particular concern. Administration of thrombolytic therapy to such patients is contraindicated because of the risk of pericardial tamponade. Diffuse ST segment elevation, extending beyond the ECG region usually influenced by a single coronary distribution, coupled with chest pain that changes with position or respiration, and a pericardial friction rub help to establish the diagnosis of pericarditis. Another important contraindication to thrombolytic therapy in patients with a syndrome masquerading as infarction is acute aortic dissection. This may be particularly confusing if the dissection compresses or involves a coronary artery, causing simultaneous myocardial ischemia or infarction. A tearing quality to the chest pain, often with radiation to the back, coupled with a history of hypertension or with unequal pulses, also favors the possibility of acute dissection.

Even in the presence of a definitive diagnosis of myocardial infarction, it is important to exclude other disorders that may cause an untoward result following administration of thrombolytic agents. Examples include retinal hemorrhage in diabetics, occult trauma which may occur during CPR, or head injuries that might have occurred during a syncopal episode associated with acute infarction.

We continually maintain a high index of suspicion for any contraindications to thrombolytic therapy. When we are in doubt about the diagnosis, we withhold thrombolytic therapy until after we have catheterized the patient. If the coronary angiogram and ventriculogram show definitive evidence of myocardial infarction, and the vessel is found to be occluded, we immediately proceed with PTCA.

Emergency Angioplasty Technique for Acute Reperfusion

On entering the ICC Laboratory, the patient is quickly evaluated with a brief and pertinent history and physical. The outside records are reviewed. The diagnosis of myocardial infarction is confirmed, and the precise time of onset of chest pain is recorded. A differential diagnosis including acute pericarditis and aortic dissection must always be considered. A consent form noting the potential need for pacemaker insertion, balloon flotation catheter insertion, balloon pump insertion, and general anesthesia and bypass surgery is signed prior to cardiac catheterization. The patient is transferred from the emergency stretcher directly to the fluoroscopy table, and a preprocedure, 12-lead ECG is obtained.

Radiolucent ECG monitoring leads and wires are placed on the patient so that 12-lead ECGs may be repeated during the procedure. A set of leads and wires are also placed to service the balloon pump console. A Foley catheter is inserted into the patient's bladder, and the right and left groins are shaved, prepped, and draped. A 6 Fr arterial sheath is inserted after carefully introducing the guidewire via a needle inserted through only the anterior wall of the femoral artery (not through the entire vessel), and arterial blood is immediately withdrawn for blood gas determination.

Standard 6 Fr coronary angiographic catheters are then used to first opacify the presumed noninfarction-related coronary artery if there is interest in documenting the degree of collateralization to the infarction-related vessel. The infarction-related coronary artery is then opacified in multiple views and biplane ventriculography is performed also with 6 Fr catheters. If the patient is found to have an occluded infarction-related artery, or a high-grade residual stenosis with either slow antegrade flow or hemodynamic compromise, emergency PTCA is performed (see selection protocol, Fig. 5.1). If emergency PTCA is to be performed, the 6 Fr sheath is exchanged for an 8 Fr sheath. Another 8 Fr sheath is inserted into the femoral vein. In patients presenting in cardiogenic shock, an intraaortic balloon pump is often inserted using the left groin prior to the diagnostic catheterization. Biplane

left ventriculography is performed during diagnostic catheterization unless severe hemodynamic compromise requires that PTCA be performed immediately. Ventriculography is then deferred until the end of the procedure.

An 8 Fr PTCA, thin-walled guiding catheter is inserted via the 8 Fr sheath and advanced to the coronary artery. A PTCA balloon dilation catheter is then advanced into the guiding catheter. The infarction-related lesion should always be approached cautiously with the tip of the guidewire. Although it is usually easy to readily cross acute total occlusions with the guidewire, one must guard against dissection with the wire in the presence of an ulcerated, unstable plaque. A slow, gentle spiral or augur-like motion of the wire tip, with frequent guiding catheter injections, will generally result in crossing the complete obstruction with ease. The guidewire should never be forced against a resistance. Acute total obstructions are considerably softer than chronic total occlusions, and when the wire is not subintimal, it should pass through the obstruction with minimal resistance.

After the balloon is localized at the center of the site of occlusion, it is inflated (see Fig. 5.2). Although no particular combination of rate, extent, or duration of inflation have proven to be superior, we generally begin with a low inflation pressure, gradually increasing pressure to 6 to 8 atm for 2 to 5 min. After balloon deflation, the results are assessed by guiding catheter injections with high resolution, large screen fluoroscopy, and digital subtraction angiography. Some laboratories use translesion pressure gradients, but we have found these gradients to be inaccurate and time consuming in the setting of acute infarction, so we no longer employ them. If the lesion appears to have been satisfactorily dilated on fluoroscopy with the deflated balloon across it, we withdraw the balloon catheter into the guiding catheter and perform multiple injections in the identical views obtained prior to PTCA using both cineangiography and digital subtraction angiography. Lesions dilated in the acute infarction setting are more likely to reclose abruptly than are those dilated in the elective setting. Thus, we generally repeat the dilation procedure until minimal residual stenosis

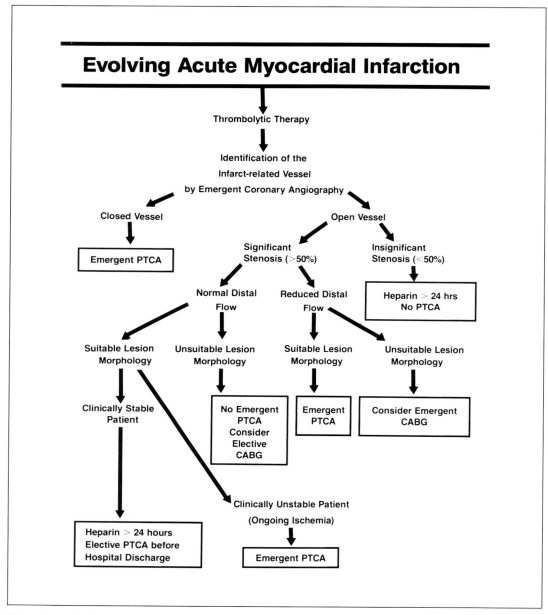

Figure 5.1. Selection protocol for evolving acute myocardial infarction resulting in emergency PTCA.

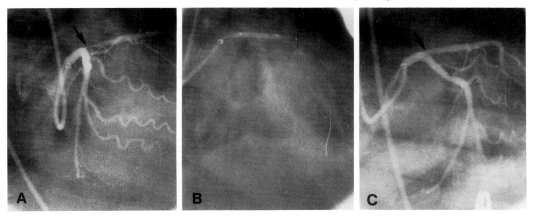

Figure 5.2. Inflated PTCA balloon (*B*) localized at the site of the occlusion (*A*) and final result (*C*).

(<25%) is obtained. We then wait 5 to 10 min following the last inflation to repeat the angiogram and confirm that vessel patency persists.

Management of Abrupt Reclosure after Emergency PTCA for Acute Infarction

Although the overall PTCA success rate (defined as ≤50% residual diameter narrowing) is high in the acute infarction setting, it is less than that for elective patients. In a recent study of 645 consecutive patients undergoing elective PTCA for angina or emergency PTCA for AMI, our success rates were 94% for elective patients and 87% ($p < 0.01$) for the emergency patients with acute infarction (13). The rate at which we were able to cross the lesion was 99% in both patient groups, despite a high percentage of total occlusions before PTCA in the acute infarction patients. The difference in success rates was due to a higher incidence of abrupt reclosure or early restenosis following an initially successful PTCA in the infarction patients.

If abrupt reocclusion occurs, the lesion should be gently recrossed with the guidewire, and further dilation performed using higher pressures for longer periods of time. When vessel size permits, a larger diameter balloon may be employed if repeat dilatations with the same balloon are not successful. Intracoronary nitroglycerin and sublingual nifedipine are administered to reduce any spastic component that may contribute to the reocclusion. Intracoronary streptokinase or

tPA may be utilized to lyse residual coronary thrombus. Recently, we have had some success with the use of very prolonged inflations (20 to 30 min) using either standard catheters or perfusion balloon catheters (17).

If a lesion continues to reclose, emergency surgery is indicated if reocclusion results in return of symptoms and/or ST segment elevation, indicating potentially salvageable myocardium, or if patients show hemodynamic compromise following reocclusion. Patients with reocclusion can be successfully managed by reperfusion catheter (18-20). The reperfusion catheter is a 4.5 Fr polyethylene conduit that tracks over a standard angioplasty exchange guidewire (Fig. 5.3). In patients with reocclusion, the original balloon catheter is advanced across the obstruction, and the original guidewire is replaced with an exchange wire. The balloon catheter is then exchanged for the reperfusion catheter, which is advanced across the lesion. The exchange guidewire is then removed. Blood enters proximal side holes from the aorta and proximal coronary artery, flows through the conduit to exit via the distal side holes beyond the occlusion to perfuse the jeopardized myocardial region (Fig. 5.4). Heparin solution (500 units/cc) is used to flush the reperfusion catheter every 5 min while transporting the patient to the operating room.

Adjunctive Medical Therapy

At the referring medical center prior to transport, each patient is prophylactically treated with lidocaine given as an IV bolus of 75 mg

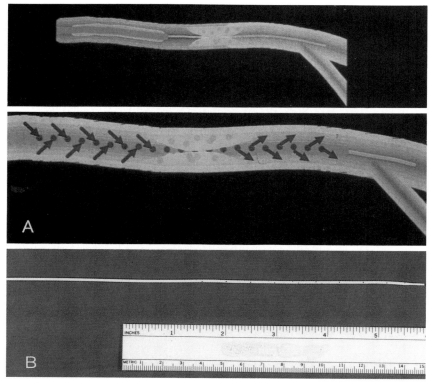

Figure 5.3.   Reperfusion catheter-4.5 Fr polyethylene conduit that tracks over a standard angioplasty exchange guidewire.

followed by 50 mg every 5 min for three doses for a total loading dose of 225 mg. Patients are also treated with diphenhydramine (25 mg IV) and cimetidine (300 mg IV) as prophylaxis against allergic reaction. Corticosteroids are not routinely administered. Morphine or demerol is given IV as needed for pain. Intramuscular injections are avoided because of hematoma formation in the presence of thrombolytic therapy. Thrombolytic therapy can now be selected from several agents, including streptokinase (1.5 million/units dissolved in 250 cc of 5% dextrose in water over 30 min); tissue plasminogen activator 100 mg (60 mg in the first hour with 10% given as a bolus, and 10 mg each hour for 4 hr); or urokinase (1.5 to 3 million units dissolved in 250 cc of 5% dextrose in water over 15 to 30 min). All patients are treated as soon as possible with one aspirin and 100 mg of dipyridamole p.o. One aspirin t.i.d and 75 mg t.i.d. of dipyridamole are continued for 6 months following the procedure.

Intravenous nitroglycerin is administered before, during, and after the procedure in order to maximize coronary blood flow and prevent spasm. Patients undergoing PTCA are treated with 10,000 units of heparin just prior to PTCA and are given 2,000 units/hr as a bolus during prolonged procedures. Patients are then maintained on a heparin infusion regulated by partial thromboplastin time determinations until the femoral sheath is removed approximately 24 hr later. Heparin is then restarted and continued for 3 to 7 days. Patients are generally discharged taking aspirin, dipyridamole, calcium channel antagonists, and long-acting nitrates. The use of β-blockers is individualized.

Postprocedural Management

Following PTCA, a balloon flotation catheter is inserted in patients with anterior myocardial infarction and in most patients with infe-

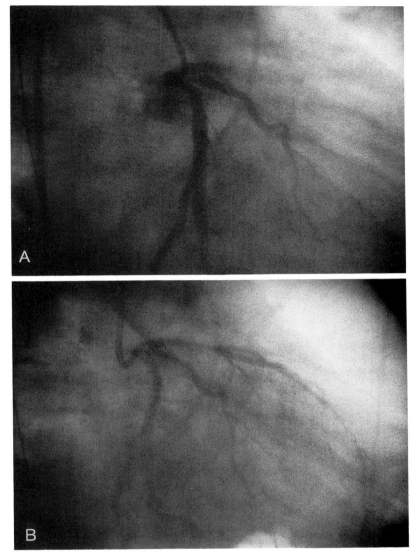

Figure 5.4. Blood enters proximal side holes from the aorta and proximal coronary artery, and flows through the conduit to exit via the distal side holes beyond the occlusion to perfuse the jeopardized myocardium.

rior infarction if there has been evidence of hemodynamic instability. Coronary care unit management includes bedside hemodynamic monitoring for 24 hr or until the patient is stable. Electrocardiographic monitoring is continued for 72 to 96 hr. The patient's hematocrit is frequently evaluated, and transfusion is indicated if the hematocrit falls below 30%. The patient is constantly monitored for signs or symptoms suggesting recurrent ischemia.

When present, emergency repeat PTCA is indicated. In patients with multivessel disease, only the infarction-related vessel is dilated during the acute infarction. Angioplasty of noninfarction-related vessels may be performed either prior to hospital discharge or after several months of convalescence, depending on the severity of the lesions and results of submaximal exercise testing done just prior to discharge.

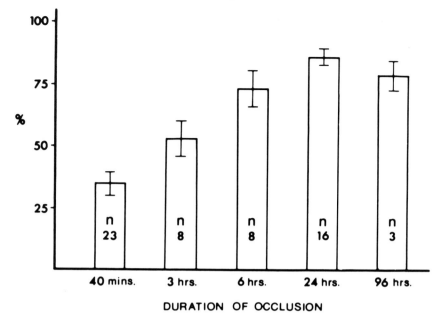

Figure 5.5. Histologic salvage of myocardium after various periods of temporary occlusion. Data show that the degree of histologic necrosis was essentially complete by 6 hours (75%). (From Reimer KA, Lowe JE, Rasmussen MM, Jennings RB. The wavefront phenomenon of ischemic cell death. 1. Myocardial infarct size vs. duration of coronary occlusion in dogs. Circulation 1977;56:786–794. By permission of the American Heart Association, Inc.)

RESULTS: IS EMERGENCY ICC WORTH THE COST AND EFFORT?

Importance of an Open Vessel

In an early animal study Reimer et al. (1) reported on the histologic salvage of myocardium after various periods of temporary occlusion (Fig. 5.5). These data show that the degree of histologic necrosis was essentially complete after 6 hr. This experimental study underscores the importance of reperfusion as soon as possible after the onset of myocardial infarction. Initial studies of thrombolytic therapy in man, using ejection fraction as a measure of global left ventricular function, showed little change between the initial and follow-up catheterizations (21). In an early clinical study we hypothesized that this could reflect the fact that global ejection fraction at the time of acute infarction represents a composite of depressed wall motion in the infarcted and jeopardized regions and hyperdynamic or compensatory increased wall motion in uninvolved regions of myocardium

(2). Thus, if there was significant return of function in the jeopardized region by the time of restudy, the hyperdynamic or compensatory wall motion of the uninvolved region may decrease, resulting in no overall change in global ejection fraction. We performed serial cardiac catheterization acutely, at 24 hr, and at 1 week after acute infarction. Figure 5.6 shows regional wall motion in patients who were successfully reperfused after intracoronary streptokinase. In patients whose global ejection fraction did not change or decreased after 1 week there was significant improvement in regional function of the infarction-related zone. The apparent decrease in global function was accounted for in each case by a reduction of the hyperdynamic compensatory wall motion observed in the uninvolved segments resulting between the acute study and 1-week study. In contrast, Figure 5.7 shows the regional wall motion changes in patients who were not successfully reperfused.

These results support the concept that a time-dependent salvage of jeopardized myocardium also occurs in humans like that docu-

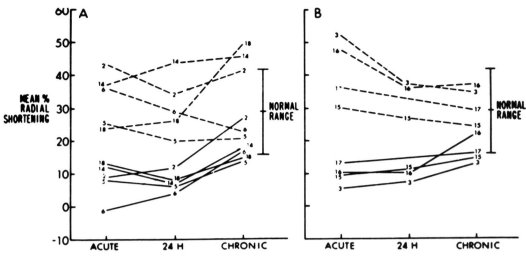

Figure 5.6. *A* illustrates those patients who had ≥5% increase in ejection fraction at 1 week. Their regional wall motion in the infarction-related zone (*solid lines*) improved dramatically, often into the low-to-normal range. Changes in the uninvolved compensatory region were mixed. Interestingly, each patient demonstrated a significant delay in return of function, indicating so–called "stunned myocardium". *B* shows the regional wall motion in patients whose global ejection fraction did not change or decreased after 1 week. (From Stack RS, Phillips HR, Grierson DS, et al. Functional improvement of jeopardized myocardium following intracoronary streptokinase infusion in acute myocardial infarction. J Clin Invest 1983;72:84–95. Used with permission from the American Society for Clinical Investigation.)

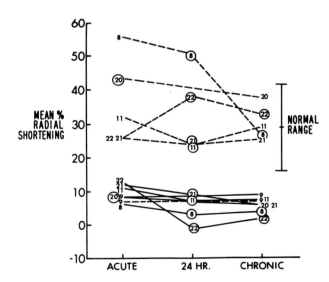

Figure 5.7. Regional wall motion changes in patients who were not successfully reperfused. There was no functional improvement in the infarction zone despite the fact that most patients (*open circles*) showed late reperfusion at the time of the 24 hour study. (From Stack RS, Phillips HR, Grierson DS, et al. Functional improvement of jeopardized myocardium following intracoronary streptokinase infusion in acute myocardial infarction. J Clin Invest 1983; 72:84–95. Used with permission of the American Society for Clinical Investigation.)

Table 5.1
GISSI Trial: 21-Day Mortality Overall and by Hours from Onset of Symptoms[a]

Hours		Mortality (%)		
	n[b]	Streptokinase	Control	p
Overall	13,861	10.7	13.0	0.0002
<1	1,277	8.2	15.4	0.0001
<3	6,094	9.2	12.0	0.0005
3–6	3,649	11.7	14.1	0.03
6–9	1,352	12.6	14.1	NS
9–12	594	15.8	13.6	NS

[a] Modified from GISSI. Effectiveness of intravenous thrombolytic treatment in acute myocardial infarction. Lancet 1986;1:397-401.

[b] n, number of patients; NS, not significant.

mented by Reimer et al. (1) in the dog model. Recent studies that have claimed high reperfusion rates with streptokinase or tPA based on elective cardiac catheterization studies at 24 to 72 hr should be interpreted with caution: since the rate of "spontaneous" reperfusion increases significantly with time, vessels that open late may simply deliver blood to a region of completed infarction (22).

Initial studies of survival following thrombolysis showed mixed results. In most of these studies, however, a survival benefit could not be detected because of an inadequate number of patients and cardiac events. Pooled data analysis from all randomized studies of intravenous streptokinase for myocardial infarction over a period of 25 years showed a significant survival benefit of 22% for patients treated with streptokinase, as compared with that of controls. The largest single study was the GISSI Trial, which reported on 11,806 randomized patients (4). This study again showed significant survival benefit in patients treated with streptokinase, as compared with that of controls (Table 5.1). Patients treated within 1 hr of the onset of chest pain showed a 47% improvement in survival, as compared with that of controls. However, patients treated after 6 hr showed no significant survival benefit.

In the recently reported ISIS-2 trial (6) 17,187 patients were given streptokinase (1.5 million units), aspirin (160 mg/day), or both up to 24 hr (median 5 hr) after the onset of suspected acute myocardial infarction. Streptokinase plus aspirin produced the greatest reduction (42%) in vascular deaths after 5 weeks (Fig. 5.8). Interestingly,

benefit was still observed in those receiving the treatment 13 to 24 hr after onset of infarction. In addition, aspirin seemed to reduce the reinfarctions and strokes. The difference in mortality rates of vascular and other causes with the use of streptokinase and aspirin remained significant after 15-month follow-up.

The Western Washington Trial showed a significant increase in survival at 30 days for patients treated with streptokinase, as compared with that of controls (23). Although a trend toward improved survival continued at 1 year, the difference was no longer statistically significant (23). However, review of initial cardiac catheterization findings showed that survival benefit was closely related to patency status of the infarction artery at time of acute infarction (24). Figure 5.9 shows 1-year survival in patients treated with streptokinase, as compared with that of controls. Among patients with anterior infarction (Fig. 5.9*A*), those treated with streptokinase showed a trend toward improvement in survival particularly at lower ejection fractions, as compared with that of controls. Because of a high incidence of failed thrombolytic therapy, with persistent occlusion of the infarction vessel, mean improvement of the overall population was not significantly different from that of controls. However, when Stadius and colleagues (24) separately plotted those patients who were successfully reperfused, a significant improvement in survival was evident. Importantly, the same relationship was found in patients with inferior myocardial infarction (Fig. 5.9*B*). Although several studies have shown less mortality risk with inferior infarc-

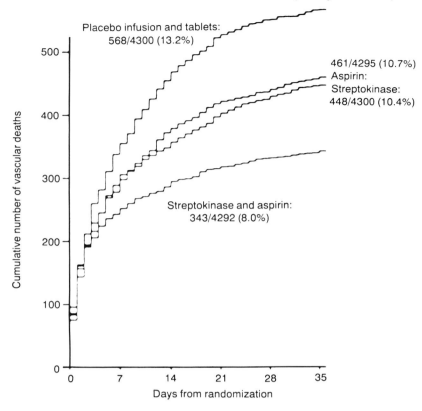

Figure 5.8. Cumulative vascular mortality in days 0–35. (From ISIS-2 (Second International Study of Infarct Survival) Collaborative Group. Randomized trial of intravenous streptokinase, oral aspirin, both, or neither among 17,187 cases of suspected acute myocardial infarction: ISIS-2. Lancet 1988; 2:349–360. Used with permission.)

tion, as compared with that with anterior infarction, it is clear from the Western Washington Trial that patients with inferior infarction and left ventricular dysfunction are at significant risk if treated conservatively. If the infarction vessel can be successfully reperfused, however, marked improvement in survival will result.

In an effort to overcome the limited reperfusion rate obtained with thrombolytic therapy alone, we studied a protocol involving combined therapy with immediate administration of thrombolytic agents in local emergency rooms followed by air transport for emergency PTCA (14). In this study 216 patients treated consecutively with immediate IV streptokinase (1.5 million units) followed by emergency PTCA were described. Median age of the population was 57 years, and 79% of patients were male. Community hospitals

were encouraged to send patients with hemodynamic compromise or other complications of infarction. Thus, 37% of the study group had one or more life-threatening complications related to infarction before arriving in the ICC Laboratory. Cardiogenic shock was present in 15%. Twenty percent had either sustained ventricular tachycardia or ventricular fibrillation prior to arrival. Median time from pain onset to streptokinase administration was 3.0 hr; median interval from pain onset to arrival in the ICC Laboratories was 4.5 hr. The results showed that 99% of infarction-related lesions were successfully crossed with the PTCA catheter. Ninety percent of patients left the laboratory with persistent reperfusion (Thrombolysis In Myocardial Infarction (TIMI) grade II or III flow). Successful complete dilation (defined as residual stenosis of ≤50%) was achieved in 87%, and

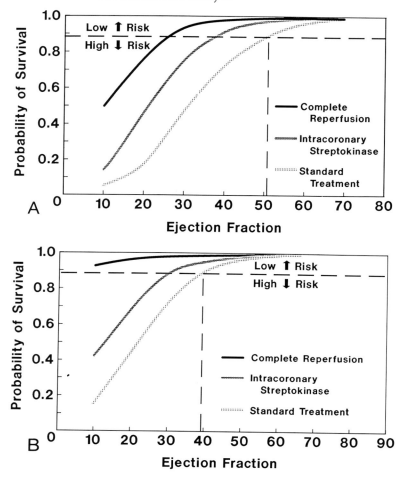

Figure 5.9. One-year survival in patients with anterior myocardial infarction treated with streptokinase, as compared with that of controls. (*A*) Patients with anterior infarction treated with streptokinase and showed a trend toward improvement in survival, particularly at lower ejection fractions, as compared with those of controls. Because of a high incidence of failed thrombolytic therapy, with persistent occlusion of the infarction vessel, mean improvement of the overall population was not significantly different from that of controls. (*B*) One-year survival for patients with inferior myocardial infarction treated with streptokinase. (From Stadius ML, Davis K, Maynard C, Ritchie JL, Kennedy JW. Risk stratification for one year survival based on characteristics identified in the early hours of acute myocardial infarction. The Western Washington Intracoronary Streptokinase Trial. Circulation 1986;74:703–711. By permission of the American Heart Association, Inc.)

partially successful dilation (stenosis of >50% but <100%) occurred in 3%.

Ten percent of patients had an unsuccessful procedure. Of these, one-third were referred for emergency coronary artery bypass grafting (CABG). All eight emergency CABG patients had a reperfusion catheter inserted to maintain myocardial blood flow prior to operation. The other two-thirds of the unsuccessful PTCA group were thought to

have completed their infarcts and were transferred to the coronary care unit for routine postinfarction care.

During PTCA, 6% of patients experienced ventricular tachycardia, and 5% had ventricular fibrillation. Ten percent of patients had severe bradycardia or asystole. Two percent required CPR. The procedural death rate was 0.5%. Stroke occurred during the procedure in 0.5% of patients.

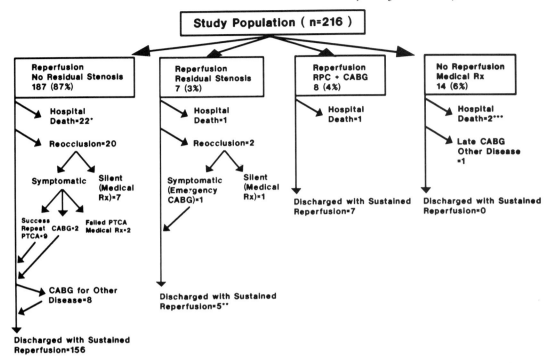

Figure 5.10. Final hospital outcome of the study population of 216 patients treated with streptokinase followed by emergency PTCA. (From Stack RS, O'Connor CM, Mark DB, et al. Coronary perfusion during acute myocardial infarction with a combined therapy of coronary angioplasty and high-dose intravenous streptokinase. Circulation 1988;77:151–161. By permission of the American Heart Association, Inc.)

The most common in-hospital complication (55% of patients) was development of groin hematoma at the site of catheterization. Forty-one percent of patients experienced a drop in hematocrit to <30%, and 40% received transfusions at some time during hospitalization. No deaths, however, were attributed to bleeding. Twenty-five patients (12%) died in-hospital, including during the initial procedure. Two of these patients had an intervening CABG. An additional 3% of patients had a cardiac arrest and were successfully resuscitated.

Of 158 eligible patients, 144 (91%) underwent follow-up cardiac catheterization. Of the 14 patients who were eligible but did not undergo a restudy, none had evidence of angina or new ECG changes at anytime prior to hospital discharge. Figure 5.10 shows the final hospital outcome of the study population (14). Silent reocclusion, diagnosed at the time of predischarge cardiac catheterization, occurred in 4% of patients

following an initially successful or partially successful PTCA. Symptomatic reocclusion prior to discharge occurred in 14 patients (7%) who were managed with repeat PTCA (11 patients; successful in 9) or CABG (3 patients). In patients with a fully successful initial PTCA, restenosis without reocclusion occurred in 12%. Conversely, in patients with only a partially successful initial PTCA (i.e., persistent reperfusion but >50% residual stenosis) reduction of the lesion to <50% stenosis at hospital discharge occurred in 28%.

A policy of aggressive management for producing sustained myocardial perfusion was maintained throughout hospitalization. Patients with reocclusion were managed with medical therapy alone only if occlusion of the infarction vessel was no longer associated with evidence of ischemia. Thus, 94% of all surviving patients who had sustained reperfusion after initial catheterization (with PTCA or reperfusion catheter plus CABG) were discharged with an open infarction-related vessel or bypass graft.

In a multicenter study, Thrombolysis and Angioplasty in Myocardial Infarction I (TAMI I), we compared the results of emergency PTCA with delayed angioplasty (8) (Fig. 5.11). In 386 patients with acute myocardial infarction, intravenous tPA was administered 2.95 ± 1.1 hr from symptom onset. Based on 90-min emergency coronary angiography, infarction vessel patency was achieved in 288 (75%) patients. To determine the role and timing of coronary angioplasty after emergency cardiac catheterization with documentation of successful thrombolysis, 197 patients with a patent vessel and high grade residual stenosis suitable for angioplasty were randomized to immediate (99 patients) or deferred (98 patients) angioplasty. Angioplasty success was high in both groups, but failure in nine immediate angioplasty patients necessitated emergency bypass surgery in seven. The incidence of reocclusion was similar in the two groups: immediate 11%, deferred 13%. There was regional infarction zone wall motion improvement from baseline to 7 days in both groups (immediate, −2.60 ± 1.1 to −2.24 ± 1.1 SD per chord, $p = 0.0001$; deferred, −2.26 ± 1.1 to −1.86 ± 1.3 SD per chord, $p = 0.002$) without differences in regional or global function between the groups. In the deferred group, the rate of crossover to emergency angioplasty for definite recurrent ischemia was 16% (vs. 5% in the immediate angioplasty group, $p = 0.01$) while 14% had an insignificant residual stenosis at 7-day follow-up catheterization.

On the basis of the TAMI I study, we concluded that patients who underwent emergency cardiac catheterization and were found to have successful thrombolysis and suitable coronary anatomy could undergo angioplasty or bypass surgery electively later during the hospitalization. In a subsequent study based on the TAMI I data, Califf et al. (12) attempted to use multiple noninvasive clinical factors for identifying the patency status of the infarction artery. Of 13 parameters and risk factors examined, only chest pain and ST segment elevation had any predictive value. Patients with complete resolution of ST segment elevation prior to coronary angiography had a 96% probability of reperfusion while patients with complete resolution of

chest pain had a 84% probability of an open vessel. However, these parameters were present in only 6 and 29% of the population, respectively. It appears from further analysis of these data that commonly used clinical indicators of reperfusion are not useful in the early hr following acute infarction in the great majority of patients presenting to the emergency room.

Long-Term Survival

Long-term outcome following thrombolytic therapy, as compared to that of a control group, was recently reported for the GISSI study (25). Results of this trial are shown in Table 5.2. Although there was a statistically significant difference in overall mortality when including in-hospital results, there was little difference in postdischarge mortality (approximately 7%) between patients treated with intravenous streptokinase, as compared with that of untreated controls.

In a recent study (5), we analyzed the 1-year and 1-year event-free survival in 342 patients with acute myocardial infarction who were consecutively enrolled in a treatment protocol of early intravenous thrombolytic therapy followed by emergency coronary angioplasty. Ninety-four percent of patients

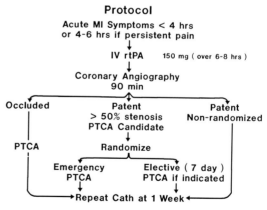

Figure 5.11. TAMI Trial. Results of emergency PTCA with delayed angioplasty in TAMI study (Modified from Topol EJ, Califf RM, George BS, et al., and the Thrombolysis and Angioplasty in Myocardial Infarction (TAMI) Study Group. A randomized trial of immediate versus delayed elective angioplasty after intravenous tissue plasminogen activator in acute myocardial infarction. N Engl J Med 1987;317:581–588.)

Table 5.2
GISSI Trial: One-Year Cumulative Percentage Mortality Overall and by Hours from Onset of Symptoms[a]

Hours		Mortality (%)		
	n[b]	Streptokinase	Control	p
Overall	11,697	17.2	19.0	0.008
≤1	1,275	12.9	21.2	0.00001
≤3	6,085	15.1	17.3	0.02
3-6	3,643	18.3	21.2	0.02
6-9	1,352	21.1	21.4	NS
9-12	594	21.9	18.5	NS

[a] Modified from GISSI. Long-term effects of intravenous thrombolysis in acute myocardial infarction: final report of the GISSI Study. Lancet 1987;2:871-874.
[b] n, number of patients; NS, not significant.

achieved successful reperfusion, including 3.5% with failed angioplasty whose perfusion was maintained by means of a reperfusion catheter prior to emergency bypass surgery. Procedural mortality was 1.2%, and total in-hospital mortality was 11%. Ninety-four percent of all 304 surviving patients were discharged from the hospital with an open infarction artery or bypass graft. Cumulative 1-year survival for all patients managed with this treatment strategy was 87%, and cardiac event-free survival was 84%. One-year survival for hospital survivors was 98%, and the infarction-free survival was 94% (Fig. 5.12). Multivariate analysis identified the following factors as independent predictors of subsequent cardiovascular death: cardiogenic shock, older age, lower ejection fraction, female sex, and a closed infarction vessel on the initial coronary angiogram. Among patients with cardiogenic shock, despite a 42% in-hospital mortality, only 4% died during the first year after hospital discharge. Similarly, in-hospital and 1-year postdischarge mortality was 19% and 4% for patients with an initial ejection fraction <40%, and 25% and 3%, respectively, for patients over 65 years. An aggressive treatment strategy including early thrombolytic therapy, emergency cardiac catheterization, coronary angioplasty, and bypass surgery, when necessary, results in a high rate of infarction vessel patency. Long-term mortality and reinfarction rates after hospital discharge are low even for patients in high-risk subgroups.

FUTURE STUDIES

Despite the large number of individual studies and clinical trials performed in recent years, major controversy continues over the proper role and timing of emergency cardiac catheterization and emergency PTCA. In addition, studies have shown conflicting results regarding the efficacy of tPA, particularly when used in conjunction with emergency angioplasty. For example, we have recently shown in a multicenter clinical trial (TAMI II) that the combination of urokinase plus tPA could markedly reduce the incidence of recurrent ischemic events, particularly in patients undergoing PTCA for failed thrombolytic therapy (26).

In an effort to prospectively compare the treatment strategy of thrombolytic therapy alone administered in a community hospital with an aggressive strategy of emergency transport to a tertiary center with cardiac catheterization, we have recently initiated the TAMI V trial. Patients with acute myocardial infarction are identified as candidates for thrombolytic therapy in a community hospital. Patients then undergo a three-way randomization at the community hospital to treatment with tPA, urokinase, or a combination of tPA and urokinase therapy. Each of the three groups are further randomized into a treatment strategy of emergency transport and cardiac catheterization at a tertiary center or to conservative management in the coronary care unit at the community hospital. All

Figure 5.12. One-year survival for hospital survivors after emergency coronary angioplasty was 98%, and infarction-free survival was 94%. (From Stack RS, Califf RM, Hinohara T, et al. Survival and cardiac event rates in the first year following emergency angioplasty for acute myocardial infarction. J Am Coll Cardiol 1988; 11:1141–1149. Used with permission.)

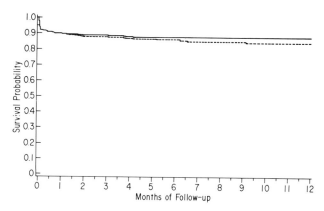

patients undergo angiography 7 to 10 days following infarction and left ventricular function will be compared using biplane ventriculography. In-hospital outcome and long-term outcome will be compared in all groups.

Further studies are needed to definitively identify patients who have failed to reperfuse using some method of noninvasive diagnosis. In addition, research must be directed towards improving thrombolytic regimens so that emergency catheterization and emergency PTCA can be reserved only for those who fail less invasive means of therapy. However, until such modalities are identified, emergency cardiac catheterization remains as the only method for accurate diagnosis of coronary reperfusion. It must also be shown that less aggressive methods of management can achieve the same long-term survival shown in patients with immediate PTCA, particularly for patients in high-risk subgroups such as cardiogenic shock.

References

1. Reimer KA, Lowe JE, Rasmussen MM, Jennings RB. The wavefront phenomenon of ischemic cell death. 1. Myocardial infarct size versus duration of coronary occlusion in dogs. Circulation 1977; 56:786–794.
2. Stack RS, Phillips HR, Grierson DS, et al. Functional improvement of jeopardized myocardium following intracoronary streptokinase infusion in acute myocardial infarction. J Clin Invest 1983; 72:84–95.
3. Yusuf S, Collins R, Peto R, et al. Intravenous and intracoronary fibrinolytic therapy in acute myocardial infarction: overview of results on mortality, reinfarction and side effects from 33 randomized controlled trials. Eur Heart J 1985;6:556–585.
4. Gruppo Italiano Per Lo Studio Della Streptochinasi Nell'Infarto Miocardico (GISSI). Effectiveness of intravenous thrombolytic treatment in acute myocardial infarction. Lancet 1986;1:397–401.
5. Stack RS, Califf RM, Hinohara T, et al. Survival and cardiac event rates in the first year following emergency angioplasty for acute myocardial infarction. J Am Coll Cardiol 1988; 11:1141–1149.
6. ISIS–2 (Second International Study of Infarct Survival) Collaborative Group. Randomized trial of intravenous streptokinase, oral aspirin, both, or neither among 17,187 cases of suspected acute myocardial infarction: ISIS–2. Lancet 1988;2:349–360.
7. TIMI Study Group. The Thrombolysis in Myocardial Infarction (TIMI) Trial. Phase I findings (special report). N Engl J Med 1985;312:932–936.
8. Topol EJ, Califf RM, George BS, et al., and the Thrombolysis and Angioplasty in Myocardial Infarction (TAMI) Study Group. A randomized trial of immediate versus delayed elective angioplasty after intravenous tissue plasminogen activator in acute myocardial infarction. N Engl J Med 1987; 317:581–588.
9. Harrison DG, Ferguson DW, Collins SM, et al. Rethrombosis after reperfusion with streptokinase: importance of geometry of residual lesions. Circulation 1984;69:991–999.
10. Fung AY, Lai P, Topol EJ, et al. Value of percutaneous transluminal coronary angioplasty after unsuccessful intravenous streptokinase therapy in acute myocardial infarction. Am J Cardiol 1986;58:686–691.
11. Kircher BJ, Topol EJ, O'Neill WW, Pitt B. Prediction of infarct coronary artery recanalization after intravenous thrombolytic therapy. Am J Cardiol 1987;59:513–515.
12. Califf RM, O'Neil WW, Stack RS, et al. Failure of simple clinical measurements to predict perfusion status after intravenous thrombolysis. Ann Intern Med 1988;108:658–662.
13. Ramirez N, Califf RM, O'Callaghan WG, et al. Does clinical indication for coronary angioplasty affect outcome? (abstr). J Am Coll Cardiol 1987; 9:182A.
14. Stack RS, O'Connor CM, Mark DB, et al. Coronary perfusion during acute myocardial infarction with a combined therapy of coronary angioplasty and

high–dose intravenous streptokinase. Circulation 1988;77:151–161.

15. Simoons ML, Betriu A, Col J, et al. The European Cooperative Study Group for Recombinant Tissue–type Plasminogen Activator (rTPA). Thrombolysis with tissue plasminogen activator in acute myocardial infarction: no additional benefit from immediate percutaneous coronary angioplasty. Lancet 1988;1:197–203.

16. Bellinger RL, Califf RM, Mark DB, et al. Helicopter transport of patients during acute myocardial infarction. Am J Cardiol 1988;61:718–722.

17. Stack RS, Quigley PJ, Collins G, Phillips HR. Perfusion balloon catheter. Am J Cardiol 1988;61:77–80.

18. Hinohara T, Simpson J, Phillips H, et al. Transluminal catheter reperfusion: a new technique to re-establish blood flow following coronary occlusion during percutaneous transluminal coronary angioplasty. Am J Cardiol 1986;57:684–686.

19. Ferguson TB, Hinohara T, Simpson J, Stack RS, Wechsler AS. Catheter reperfusion to allow optimal coronary bypass grafting following failed transluminal coronary angioplasty. Ann Thorac Surg 1986;42:399–405.

20. Kereiakes DJ, Topol EJ, George BS, et al. TAMI Study Group. Emergency coronary artery bypass surgery preserves global and regional left ventricular function after intravenous tissue plasminogen activator therapy for acute myocardial infarction. J Am Coll Cardiol 1988;11:899–907.

21. Rentrop P, Blancke H, Karsch KR, Kaiser H, Kostering H, Leitz K. Selective intracoronary thrombolysis in acute myocardial infarction and unstable angina pectoris. Circulation 1981;63:307–317.

22. Dewood MA, Spores J, Notske R, et al. Prevalence of total coronary occlusion during the early hours of transmural myocardial infarction. N Engl J Med 1980;303:897–902.

23. Kennedy JW, Ritchie JL, Davis KB, Stadius ML, Maynard C, Fritz JK. The Western Washington randomized trial of intracoronary streptokinase in acute myocardial infarction: a 12–month follow–up report. N Engl J Med 1985;312:1073–1078.

24. Stadius ML, Davis K, Maynard C, Ritchie JL, Kennedy JW. Risk stratification for 1 year survival based on characteristics identified in the early hours of acute myocardial infarction. The Western Washington Intracoronary Streptokinase Trial. Circulation 1986;74:703–711.

24. Gruppo Italiano Per Lo Studio Della Streptochinasi Nell'Infarto Miocardico (GISSI). Long–term effects of intravenous thrombolysis in acute myocardial infarction: final report of the GISSI study. Lancet 1987;2:871–874.

25. Topol EJ, Califf RM, George BS, et al. TAMI Study Group. Coronary arterial thrombolysis with combined infusion of recombinant tissue–type plasminogen activator and urokinase in patients with acute myocardial infarction. Circulation 1988;77:1100–1107.

Section

3

CATHETERIZATION AND RADIOGRAPHIC TECHNIQUES

6

Review of Techniques

James A. Hill, M.D.
Charles R. Lambert, M.D., Ph.D.
Carl J. Pepine, M.D.

INTRODUCTION

Performing cardiac catheterization involves a great deal of technical skill, sophisticated instrumentation, and mature judgment to choose the appropriate procedures from among the various techniques available. As the scope of cardiac catheterization has changed from primarily an elective diagnostic procedure in stable patients to a procedure often performed in combination with therapeutic interventions in critically ill patients, the operator needs to be very familiar with disease processes and therapeutic alternatives in order to select the best technique and its timing.

The purpose of this chapter is to describe the various techniques available for catheter introduction, summarize their advantages, disadvantages, and uses; and briefly discuss some of the associated procedures that may provide additional information and therapeutic benefit in a given patient. The following assumes that the patient has had a complete medical and cardiovascular evaluation, which also includes an ECG, chest x-ray, hemogram, BUN, and creatinine, prior to the procedure.

PREPARATION OF THE PATIENT

Prior to any catheterization procedure, the patients and, when appropriate, their relatives should be informed about the risks, benefits, and alternatives to the procedure. The patient should have a clear understanding of the indications and expected outcome for the procedure. The patient should know what to expect during and after the procedure, when results will be available, and their significance.

Patients should have an empty stomach to limit the nausea and emesis that occasionally occur with contrast administration or vagal reaction. For procedures done in the morning, this will generally mean fasting after midnight. When procedures are performed later in the day, a light liquid breakfast may be given. If the arm is to be used, intravenous lines should be moved away from the site. Patients should empty their bladders prior to catheterization procedures.

Anesthesia and Sedation

Generally, we feel that cardiac catheterization in adults is best performed using only local anesthesia. This ensures optimal patient cooperation, allows patients to report symptoms, and permits speedy recovery. In the extremely anxious patient, mild sedation with a benzodiazepine will be helpful. Routine administration of narcotics and sedatives prior to catheterization is not advocated since they inhibit the patient's ability to cooperate with coughing, deep breathing, and breath holding and may alter their reports of chest pain or other important symptoms. We administer diphenhydramine orally approximately 30 min prior to the procedure. This provides some mild sedation as well as anti-histamine effect to help in prophylaxis of possible contrast material allergy. There are special circumstances, however, wherein sedation or even general anesthesia may be necessary (e.g., an extremely agitated or uncooperative patient or a child) so that safety is not compromised.

Local Anesthesia

Lidocaine (1 or 2%) is used for local anesthesia given both superficially and near the vascular sheath. A 25-gauge needle is used in case a blood vessel or nerve is inadvertently punctured. Epinephrine is not added to the lidocaine because a substantial systemic effect or local vessel spasm may occur. Adding a small amount (approximately 10% of the total volume) of sodium bicarbonate solution to the lidocaine can limit the initial burning that some patients experience with the injection. The most important aspect is to administer enough anesthetic to render effective anesthesia before the cutdown or percutaneous puncture is started. If there is substantial pain locally, there is more chance for a vagal reaction or spasm to occur. The patient is less likely to be able to cooperate, and increases in heart rate and blood pressure may produce ischemia in patients with coronary artery disease. The local anesthetic effect lasts approximately 30 to 45 min with lidocaine, and supplementation should be anticipated when procedures last longer. Occasionally, a more potent or longer-acting local anesthetic such as mepivacaine hydrochloride (Carbocaine) may be necessary in patients who are rapid metabolizers of lidocaine.

METHODS USED TO INTRODUCE CATHETERS

There are two general methods currently in use for introduction of catheters into the central circulation regardless of the location of entry. These are (*a*) percutaneous introduction using needles and guidewires and (*b*) direct introduction after surgical isolation of the vessel. While either method may be utilized at any site, practical and anatomic considerations generally dictate which approach is used for any given vessel and in any given patient.

Percutaneous Introduction

The Seldinger technique or a modification of it is the method by which most percutaneous catheter insertion is accomplished (Fig. 6.1). Here, the operator locates the vessel to be cannulated using palpation and enters it with a needle inserted through the skin. An 18-gauge needle is generally appropriate in adults, but any size into which a guidewire will fit will work. One of two general types of needles is used: (*a*) a sharp, long-pointed beveled needle with a cutting edge, or (*b*) a blunt, short less-pointed beveled needle without a cutting edge containing an obturator (see Chapter 7). The techniques used for insertion of these differ somewhat in that the cutting needle ideally enters the vessel only on one side during advancement into the vessel. The bevel of the needle with an obturator is relatively blunt so the needle often must be advanced more forcefully and deeply to affect arterial puncture. Hence, this needle often enters both the front and back walls of the vessel. When the obturator is removed, the needle often must be withdrawn until blood flow results. This latter technique causes more trauma to the vessel, particularly if the vessel is diseased and calcified. Calcified or fibrotic arteries are difficult to puncture with a blunt needle. Some modified blunt needles contain obturators or stylets with small holes to permit a drop of blood to flow when the vessel is entered. We have not found these modifications to be advantageous, and their use often requires more time. We prefer to use a sharp, 18-gauge needle without an obturator for all arterial and venous punctures.

Once good blood return occurs either with or without aspiration, a guidewire is inserted through the needle into the vessel. We prefer an 0.035-inch, Teflon-coated, spring coil guidewire with a J-tip. If difficulty is encountered advancing this wire, an 0.025-inch wire is substituted. Pressure is applied proximally to the needle in arteries and both proximally and distally to the needle in veins as the needle is removed to leave only the guidewire in place. The guidewire is wiped with a sponge wetted with heparinized saline. As pressure is maintained, the skin puncture site is enlarged using a scalpel blade followed by dissection with a straight hemostat to create a percutaneous tunnel. This track must allow

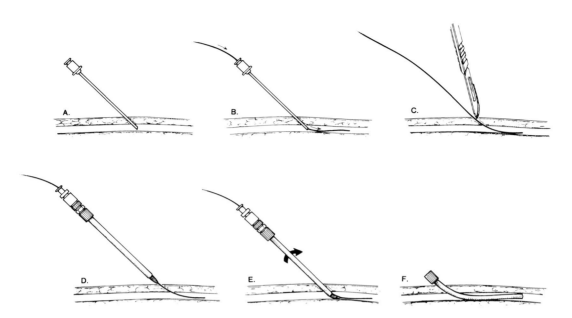

Figure 6.1. Modified Seldinger technique for percutaneous catheter sheath introduction. *A,* Vessel punctured by needle; *B,* Flexible guidewire placed into vessel via needle; *C,* Needle removed, guidewire left in place, and hole in skin around wire enlarged with scalpel; *D,* Sheath and dilator placed over guidewire; *E,* Sheath and dilator advanced over guidewire and into vessel; *F,* Dilator and guidewire removed while sheath remains in vessel.

the catheter to be inserted and move freely so that its tip is not damaged as it traverses the skin and subcutaneous tissue. A "burr" must not be created at the tip of the catheter, dilator, or sheath, as this can damage the vessel. Depending upon the type of catheter to be used, a stiff, short dilator may be useful for dilating the subcutaneous tissue and vessel. The dilator is advanced over the guidewire after the needle has been removed. After several passes into the vessel to make a tract, the dilator is removed as the wire is again wiped. The catheter is then advanced over the guidewire, and the guidewire is removed. In cases in which either scarring or calcification make entry difficult, a dilator several sizes smaller than the catheter to be used is first introduced. Serial dilations are made using successively larger dilators, with each introduced over the indwelling guidewire. Sometimes it is also helpful to use a larger guidewire (0.038-inch) when large dilators are needed in very scarred or calcified vessels. When only the guidewire is in place, the operator should maintain finger pressure over the vessel to limit bleeding. We routinely use a short

sheath, with a diaphragm to maintain hemostasis and facilitate catheter exchanges. Once the catheter or sheath is introduced into an artery, we administer 5000 units of heparin.

The advantages of the percutaneous technique make it the most popular method to introduce catheters into the vascular system. It is fast, requires minimal surgical skill, and is more easily taught and mastered than other techniques. Repeat procedures can be more readily performed with less trauma than a cutdown.

The primary disadvantage of the percutaneous technique is that blind introduction does not allow one to avoid diseased portions of vessels where excessive damage may occur. This may be a disadvantage when arterial cannulation is done in patients with peripheral vascular disease. Also, catheter control can be limited when there is a substantial amount of subcutaneous tissue, scar, or very tortuous vessel. Occasionally when catheters are removed, tamponade may be difficult in patients with clotting abnormalities, markedly widened pulse pressure, or severe hypertension.

Direct Surgical Cutdown

The cutdown is generally used only for the brachial approach. Cutdown in other sites is a more complex surgical procedure and offers no particular advantage, except in very select circumstances such as aortic valvuloplasty or in small children. Femoral cutdown technique will not be described, as it is generally not performed by physicians catheterizing adult patients.

The aim of brachial artery isolation is to mobilize about 1 to 2 cm of artery in an area of minimal branching prior to its bifurcation into radial and ulnar branches (Fig. 6.2). A transverse skin incision, 1.5 to 2 cm long, is made for isolation of a vein and brachial artery. The incision is smaller and more medial if only a vein is needed. With the elbow extended blunt dissection is done using standard surgical instruments. In some this may require a pad under the elbow. The cutdown is best done approximately 1 cm proximal to the medial epicondyle directly over the brachial artery pulse where the artery is becoming more superficial to cross the joint before it reaches the bicipital aponeurosis. This area is preferred because branches are limited, the artery is usually separated from the median nerve, and collateral flow is excellent, so that even with brachial artery obstruction in this area, ischemia of the arm is uncommon. A vein is usually isolated in the brachial sheath or by exploring more medially for the median cubital vein. The vein is controlled using a short length of 3-0 or 4-0 suture placed on both sides of the planned venotomy site.

The artery should be handled and controlled using either umbilical tapes or sterile rubber bands placed proximally and distally to the planned arteriotomy site. The isolated area should be mobilized to allow easy lifting of the segment to the level of the skin. This will allow for more parallel entry of the catheter into the artery, permitting easier catheter manipulation and less arterial trauma. Traction is applied on the distal tape to distend the artery proximally, and an incision is made large enough to allow introduction of the catheter tip. We use a pointed No. 11 blade and insert it slowly into the lumen. The hole is enlarged slightly as the blade is removed. A larger hole may permit substantial leakage around the catheter. We feel that a horizontal

incision is superior to a vertical one because the arteriotomy remains smaller, rather than enlarging longitudinally with catheter manipulation. Some prefer a vertical incision, reasoning that its extension by catheter manipulation will be in the longitudinal direction involving less of the circumference of the vessel. The vertical incision is then repaired in a horizontal direction. When the catheter is within the vessel, 5000 units of heparin are given.

When catheters are exchanged or the procedure is complete and catheters are removed, the operator should allow bleeding to occur from the vessel proximal and distal to the arteriotomy to establish adequacy of flow and to wash out debris. If flow is not brisk, balloon catheter thrombectomy should be performed. Additional heparin may be administered so that thrombus does not reform during the repair. Routine use of embolectomy catheters is not recommended since these catheters provide additional trauma to the intima. After adequate flow has been established, vascular clamps are placed on both sides of the arteriotomy to occlude flow. The arteriotomy is inspected for thrombus and intimal damage. After debris or damage is removed or repaired, the arteriotomy is closed using 6-0 or 7-0 vascular suture. The suturing technique should be either horizontal mattress, starting at either side and working toward the middle, or purse string. Some prefer a continuous running suture, usually with a nonbraided suture. The goal is to evert the edges and provide intima-to-intima approximation to lessen potential for thrombus formation without compromising the vessel diameter. Veins should be ligated, making sure to isolate the venotomy site between the proximal and distal ties.

Brachial artery cutdown offers some potential advantages over the percutaneous technique. It provides direct visualization of the vessel in case of difficulty in catheter introduction and allows most local vascular problems to be corrected by the operator without surgical assistance prior to finishing the procedure. If vascular surgical intervention is necessary, this can generally be performed under local anesthesia. Catheter control is generally better with direct exposure. Disadvantages of the technique include the greater surgical skills required, increased time of the

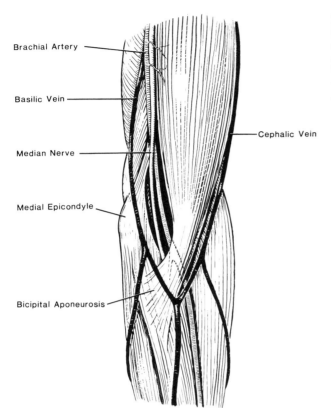

Brachial Artery

Basilic Vein

Median Nerve

Medial Epicondyle

Bicipital Aponeurosis

Cephalic Vein

Figure 6.2. Anatomy of the arm illustrating appropriate site for brachial artery cutdown. The ideal site is approximately 1 to 2 cm proximal to the bifurcation of the brachial artery in the triangle formed by the bicipital aponeurosis. This is generally less than 1 cm above the medial epicondyle of the elbow joint.

procedure, loss of venous access because of vein ligation, increased trauma required with repeat procedures and limited catheter sizes that can be used (usually no larger than 8 or 8.3 Fr in men and 7 or 7.5 Fr in women).

CATHETER-RELATED PERIPHERAL VESSEL SPASM

Occasionally, spasm of the artery or vein prevents the catheter from being easily removed or advanced, particularly when using the brachial approach and rarely with the femoral approach. Proper catheter sizing and not advancing catheters when they do not pass easily will limit this problem. However, if spasm occurs, the catheter should be replaced with a smaller size. If this is not possible, intravenous or arterial vasodilators, such as nitroglycerin or low dose tolazoline, and even mild sedation usually provide local vasodilation. Sometimes oral or buccal nifedipine is very effective for arterial spasm. If after several minutes the catheter cannot be removed, it is best to keep the patient anticoagulated

and try again about 30 min later after more vasodilator is given. Some have suggested light weight traction or even general anesthesia. In our experience, surgical removal has never been necessary, and major arterial damage has not occurred using this approach in our laboratories.

SITES FOR CATHETER INTRODUCTION

The two most commonly utilized sites used to enter the central arterial circulation and for performance of left-sided cardiac catheterization and angiography are the femoral and the brachial routes. While venous access can be achieved via multiple routes, if both arterial and venous catheterization are to be performed, one site is preferable for patient comfort and operator convenience. The well-equipped laboratory and skilled high-volume operator should be comfortable with both the femoral and brachial approaches, as well as with other methods used to insert catheters. There are circumstances when one approach is clearly advantageous or essential, such as with occlusion of the abdominal aorta, severe femoral-iliac disease, or an aberrant subclavian vessel. Certain procedures, such as bilateral internal mammary angiography, are more easily performed from one site over another. Other procedures can be performed from only one site, such as transseptal catheterization from the right femoral vein.

Femoral Site

The femoral site is probably the most commonly utilized approach for left heart catheterization. Percutaneous technique is generally used with the Seldinger technique, as previously described. The artery should be entered between the superficial femoral artery and inguinal ligament. Here, it is relatively straight without major branches and is large enough for passage of large catheters. If the superficial femoral artery is punctured, the guidewire will frequently not traverse the bifurcation because of the acute angle at the origin of the common femoral artery. Additionally, the superficial femoral artery may be too small for large catheters, and both spasm and trauma may result in occlusion. If venous catheterization is needed, the vein, which is directly medial to the artery, is punctured about 1 cm inferiorly or superiorly to the artery to help avoid the possibility of arteriovenous fistula formation.

In general, the femoral approach is faster to perform and easier to master. There are several other advantages, including larger vessels to allow for the introduction of larger catheters; ease of abdominal, renal, and bilateral internal mammary artery angiography; ready access to virtually the entire central arterial circulation with the appropriate catheter; and the multitude of catheters available for adapting the procedure to the patient. Disadvantages of this approach are few. However, the abdominal aorta and iliofemoral branches are generally more atherosclerotic and tortuous than upper extremity branches and can present problems for catheter passage. Coronary sinus cannulation can be difficult when needed for coronary sinus flow measurement, blood sampling, atrial pacing, or electrophysiologic study. In addition, if there is a local vascular complication, repair will

generally require surgical intervention in the operating room under general anesthesia.

Brachial Site

The brachial site may be utilized either percutaneously or by cutdown. Both techniques have their advantages and how the brachial approach is used will depend on operator experience and skill. If both arterial and venous catheterization are to be performed, a cutdown will generally be necessary. The location for brachial catheter introduction was described previously.

In general, catheterization via the brachial approach is performed through less diseased vessels and is preferable in patients with severe abdominoiliac disease. While some catheterization procedures such as cannulation of the coronary sinus are more easily performed from the arm, others, such as bilateral internal mammary artery angiography, are more difficult. In case of local vascular complications, many of the problems encountered can be dealt with in the catheterization laboratory by the person performing the procedure. Need for more extensive surgical intervention and general anesthesia is generally rare. Frequently, there are excellent collaterals so that surgical intervention may not be necessary, as limb ischemia is unusual, even with arterial occlusion. From the brachial approach, bleeding can be easily controlled in the patient receiving uninterrupted anticoagulation therapy, with a clotting disorder, or with widened pulse pressure. Finally, the brachial approach allows for more rapid ambulation, facilitating early patient release, as for outpatient catheterization.

Other Sites for Venous Access

Subclavian

The subclavian vein (Fig. 6.3) is an excellent access site to the central venous circulation and is currently used for a variety of different procedures (cardiac pacemaker insertion, both permanent and temporary; pulmonary artery catheterization; parenteral hyperalimentation; etc). Certain patient conditions make subclavian puncture somewhat more hazardous, and other approaches should

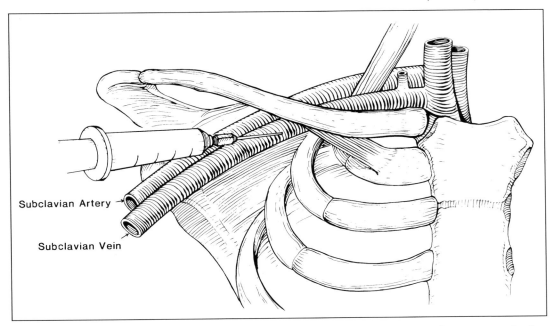

Subclavian Artery →

Subclavian Vein

Figure 6.3   Anatomic localization of the subclavian vein. The appropriate site for puncture (in the middle to distal third of the clavicle) and the direction of the needle (toward a point just above the suprasternal notch) are illustrated.

be used. These include patients in whom a pneumothorax would not be well tolerated, such as those who are receiving positive expiratory pressure for ventilatory support, with superior vena cava obstruction or with anatomic abnormalities that make the subclavian vein difficult to puncture.

The technique for subclavian catheterization is relatively simple but has some important hazards associated with it, primarily pneumothorax and hemothorax. Patients who do not have engorged neck veins should be in Trendelenburg (head-down) position to engorge the subclavian vein. It is helpful to place a small pillow or rolled sheet between the patient's shoulders to elevate the proximal and midclavicular area. The Seldinger technique, as previously described, should be utilized. After appropriate sterile preparation and local anesthesia, the needle is inserted perpendicularly to the skin in the area just inferior to and between the middle and distal third of the clavicle to a depth even with the bottom of the clavicle. The hub of the needle is then tilted, and the needle is aimed at a point 1 cm above the sternal notch. The needle is then advanced directly beneath the clavicle toward this point with constant

negative pressure. When the vein is entered, the needle should be grasped and immobilized, and the syringe should be removed. Just before and during the period when the hub of the needle is exposed, the patient should suspend breathing or perform a Valsalva maneuver to minimize the chance of air embolus. The guidewire is then placed, and the needle is removed. The procedure is then completed using whatever types of sheaths and catheters that are needed (see Chapter 7, General principles of central venous catheterization, regardless of route, are outlined in Table 6.1.)

Jugular

Internal. The internal jugular vein (Fig. 6.4) generally provides a straight pathway into the central venous circulation. Comparative data (1) suggest that using the external jugular vein approach is safer but less likely to be successful in reaching the superior vena cava than is the internal jugular. The internal jugular approach is, however, less likely to be associated with the pneumothorax and hemothorax complications of the subclavian approach. In patients with carotid artery abnormalities on the contralateral side, superior

Table 6.1.

General Principles of Central Venous Catheterization Technique

1. Choose the site for catheterization with which you are most familiar and which carries the least risk in the given clinical circumstance.
2. For cervical and subclavian punctures, place the patient in a head-down position to engorge the central veins, increase the central venous pressure, and decrease the chance of air embolism unless obvious venous engorgement is present.
3. Ensure free-flowing blood before advancing any catheter or guidewire.
4. Always keep the tips of catheters and needles sealed and perform catheter or guidewire exchanges during forced expiration or Valsalva maneuver to limit the possibility of air embolism.
5. If arterial puncture is possible or likely, use a relatively small bore needle (no larger than 18-gauge) and the Seldinger technique to minimize trauma.
6. Maintain aspiration (negative pressure) when withdrawing the needle, as the initial pass may have perforated the vein, and free flow of blood and venous access may occur with withdrawal.
7. If a sheath is left in place without a catheter in it, make sure the diaphragm or some other hemostatic device provides an appropriate seal to prevent air leakage.

vena cava obstruction, or in those with distorted or difficult landmarks on the side of the neck to be used for puncture, internal jugular puncture should probably be avoided.

Knowledge of the course of the internal jugular is essential to successful cannulation. After it enters the neck from the base of the skull, the internal jugular runs beneath and medial to the sternocleidomastoid muscle in its upper portion and medial to the lateral (clavicular) head of the sternocleidomastoid muscle in its lower portion. It joins the subclavian vein beneath the sternal end of the clavicle to form the innominate vein. The left internal jugular vein forms a much more acute angle with the subclavian than the right does, making it somewhat more difficult to use for catheter manipulations. In addition, the thoracic duct enters the subclavian vein near the same location, adding another structure that can be inadvertently punctured.

The best location for puncture of the internal jugular vein depends on operator preference and experience (2–6). There are at least three locations: **central**, **anterior**, and **posterior**. The technique and equipment are the same for all locations. For all locations, the patient's head should be turned approximately 45° off sagittal to the opposite side from where the puncture is to be performed. In a conscious patient, having him or her gently lift his or her head will allow better localization of the heads of the sternocleidomastoid muscle both visually and by palpation. The **central approach** utilizes a venipuncture near the apex of the triangle formed by the two heads

of the sternocleidomastoid muscle. After local anesthesia, the carotid artery is palpated beneath the sternal head of the muscle and gently retracted medially. The needle is advanced at an approximately 45° angle from the body's frontal plane and aimed laterally toward the ipsilateral nipple to the junction of the proximal and middle third of the clavicle. This approach should direct the needle

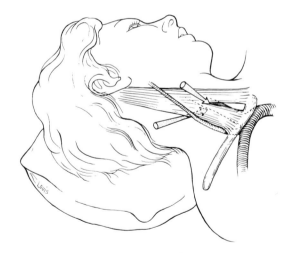

Figure 6.4. Anatomic localization of the internal and external jugular veins. *Arrows* illustrate the appropriate location for internal jugular puncture. The *top arrow* illustrates the anterior approach while the *lower arrow* illustrates the posterior approach (just above the external jugular vein and under the sternocleidomastoid muscle).

underneath the lateral (clavicular) head of the sternocleidomastoid muscle, and venipuncture should occur within 4 to 5 cm, or the needle should be withdrawn and redirected.

The **anterior approach** is similar, except that the needle is placed at the midpoint of the sternocleidomastoid muscle and directed at a slightly more acute angle with the skin. Again, the needle is aimed under the clavicular head of the sternocleidomastoid muscle toward the ipsilateral nipple. Some operators advocate an even lower approach just above the clavicle, using the notch on the medial clavicle as a landmark and a more medially directed puncture.

The **posterior approach** utilizes the lateral border of the clavicular head of the sternocleidomastoid muscle and the path of the external jugular vein as landmarks. The needle is introduced along the lateral border of the sternocleidomastoid muscle about 5 cm from the clavicle above the crossing point of the external jugular over the muscle. The needle is directed under the muscle caudally toward the suprasternal notch. Venipuncture should occur within approximately 5 cm, or the needle should be withdrawn and redirected. Introducing catheters is performed using standard techniques.

External. The external jugular vein provides a convenient location for central venous access as it courses posteriorly across the lateral belly of the sternocleidomastoid muscle. As with subclavian and internal jugular cannulation, the patient is placed in a slight head-down position, and the vein is entered as with any superficial vein. Methods for catheter introduction are identical to other percutaneous techniques. The major problem with this route is that occasionally the angle of entry of the external jugular into the subclavian is very acute and may not allow for easy entry into the superior vena cava without guidewires and fluoroscopy. For this reason, the external jugular is not frequently used for cardiac catheter introduction but only for fluid administration.

Direct Cardiac Puncture

Direct left ventricular puncture (7-10), still has application, particularly in patients with both mitral and aortic mechanical prosthetic valves (11). Direct left ventricular puncture may be performed via either the subxyphoid or intercostal route in the apical area. Chronic anticoagulation should be discontinued and heparin begun so that normal clotting studies can be achieved just prior to the anticipated catheterization and for several hours afterwards. It may help to place the patient in a shallow right anterior oblique (RAO) position. Ascending aortic and pulmonary artery catheters should be placed first by standard approaches in order to monitor pressures. We use the technique described by Brock et al. (8). After appropriate local anesthesia, an 18-gauge needle is inserted at the apical impulse and directed toward the right second costochondral junction with a posterior angulation of approximately 35°. It is advanced until the pulsating heart is felt, or ventricular ectopy is noted. We find it helpful to use fluoroscopy to note when ventricular contact is made. The needle is then advanced until blood flows freely. The pressure waveform should then be inspected and recorded to ensure that the needle is within the left ventricle.

Occasionally, in patients with right ventricular enlargement, the right ventricle may be inadvertently entered. If this occurs, the needle should be removed and reinserted 1 to 2 cm to the left and redirected more posteriorly. If angiography is to be performed, it is preferable to place a small (5 or 6 Fr, high-flow pigtail) catheter into the ventricle using a guidewire rather than inject contrast material in high volumes through the needle. After the catheter is removed, the patient is asked to remain quiet on his back or left side and is sent to the coronary care unit for observation. After 3 hr, heparin is restarted if needed. If any difficulty is suspected, an echocardiogram is done to evaluate for possible pericardial tamponade. In the authors' experience, this method has not resulted in major complications, but the possibility of trauma to coronary arteries and pericardial tamponade exists. The procedure should be done only in laboratories located in hospitals with cardiac surgery programs and in the presence of experienced operators.

Transseptal Puncture

The transseptal catheter apparatus consists of a tapered needle designed to puncture the atrial septum and a tapered catheter that passes over the needle to enter the left atrium (Fig. 6.5). In addition, a long, curved sheath (Mullins) can be utilized to facilitate catheter exchange. Use of the sheath will eliminate the need for a tip occluder and other equipment formerly necessary for good quality angiography with a Brockenbrough catheter. We prefer to use the sheath in our laboratories. Details of available transseptal equipment can be found in Chapter 7.

The most common indication for transseptal catheterization is when left atrial or left ventricular pressure is needed and cannot be obtained by means of retrograde technique. Another indication is the rare patient with severe aortic stenosis whose valve cannot be traversed in a retrograde fashion or with a mechanical (e.g., tilting disc) aortic valve prosthesis without a paravalvular leak that cannot be safely traversed as a route to the left ventricle. Also the rare patient with aortic stenosis who has no arterial access can be evaluated using the transseptal approach with a flow-directed CO_2-filled balloon catheter floated to the aorta from the left ventricle. In hypertrophic cardiomyopathy, to avoid catheter entrapment, left ventricular inflow and outflow pressures can be assessed by simultaneous transseptal left ventricular and retrograde aortic catheterization. Patients with severe pulmonary hypertension and mitral stenosis can be evaluated by means of transseptal technique when it is impossible to wedge the catheter. Diagnosis of cor triatriatum and pulmonary venoocclusive disease may require the transseptal approach. Mitral and antegrade aortic valvuloplasty can only be performed using the transseptal approach. Finally, the approach may be used for atrial septostomy in patients with complete transposition and atrioventricular valve atresia with an intact atrial septum.

There are several anatomic considerations that are important in patient selection for transseptal catheterization. Transseptal catheterization should not be done in patients with distortion of cardiac anatomy or cardiac position within the chest, including spinal deformities or abnormal heart position. An extremely large left atrium distorts the atrial septum and makes transseptal catheterization more difficult and more hazardous. In the presence of thrombi or masses in the left atrium, recent systemic embolism or suspicion of a left atrial myxoma or clot, the transseptal technique should not be utilized. If access to the right femoral vein and inferior vena cava is not available, the technique cannot be used. Finally, because of the stiff needle used, the patient must be cooperative and be able to lie still. General anesthesia may be necessary if transseptal catheterization is essential and the patient is unable to cooperate. Some other conditions may make the transseptal approach more hazardous but are not absolute contraindications. Giant right atria, markedly dilated aortic root with small left atrium, and complex congenital heart disease that distorts either the inferior vena cava or the atrial septum are some of these conditions.

For transseptal catheterization, biplane fluoroscopy should be used when available, and two-dimensional echocardiography may be useful to help determine catheter position in cases in which there is some question. Some prefer to have a pigtail catheter in the ascending aorta as a landmark. The right femoral vein is entered by percutaneous puncture. After the guidewire is in the inferior vena cava, the transseptal catheter and long sheath are passed as a unit over the wire, and the entire system is advanced into the superior vena cava. The sheath and dilator should move freely with good tactile perception. The guidewire is then removed, and the transseptal needle is advanced through the catheter with its stylet in place, to protect the dilator, to approximately 1 cm from the end of the catheter but remaining inside the catheter. The stylet is then removed from the needle, and the needle hub connected to a pressure transducer. The system is then withdrawn with the orientation of the needle and tip of the catheter rotated with clockwise torque to the "four o'clock" position, as gauged by the metal indicator arrow on the proximal end of the needle. The catheter tip is upward and to the right, as viewed by posteroanterior fluoroscopy. Because the atrial septum is oriented downward anteriorly and to the right, withdrawing the system with this orientation will cause the catheter to orient itself toward and "catch" in the fossa ovalis after it is pulled back across the "limbic ledge" or ridge in the right atrium formed by the indentation of the aorta. Here the lateral view should confirm a slight posterior orientation of the needle. Care

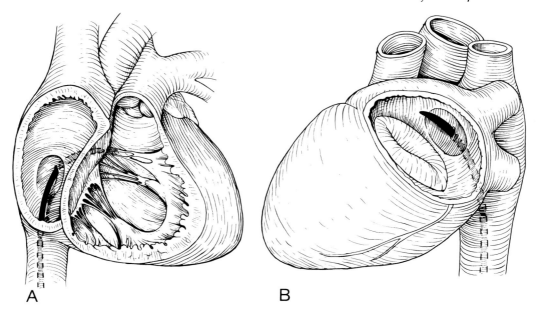

Figure 6.5. Anterior (*A*, front of the right atrium and right ventricle have been cut away) and posterior (*B*, back of the left atrium has been cut away) view of transseptal catheter in appropriate position across the atrial septum in the region of the foramen ovale.

must be taken not to let the needle advance beyond the tip of the catheter until it is in the appropriate position in the fossa ovalis. Once this position has been reached, the catheter should be advanced to maintain contact with the fossa ovalis and kept in this position with some pressure exerted. In approximately 20% or more of cases the catheter will cross a "catheter patent" foramen ovale to reach the left atrium without exposing the tip of the needle. If the catheter does not cross the foramen, the needle is then advanced out of the catheter to a position across the septum and into the left atrium. Generally, a "popping" sensation will occur with successful penetration of the atrial septum. Pressure measurement and oxygen saturation can be used to confirm that the needle is in the left atrium.

If the pressure tracing becomes damped and does not resemble left atrial pressure, contrast injection often reveals staining of the interatrial septum or posterior wall of the left atrium. If no other changes have occurred, the needle should be withdrawn and the system repositioned in the right atrium over a guidewire. The puncture approach is then started again.

When left atrial pressure is obtained, the needle position is fixed using the patient's right thigh. Without advancing the needle further into the left atrium, the catheter and sheath are then advanced over the needle, and the needle is removed. At this time heparin can be given. If the catheter does not go into the left ventricle as it assumes its preformed shape or with gentle advancing, the guidewire can be replaced and used to help guide the catheter into the desired location. In addition, the tapered catheter can be removed and replaced by another catheter through the sheath for either easier manipulation into the ventricle and aorta, or for angiography. A flow-directed balloon catheter may also be used through the sheath, but it should be filled with CO_2 as a safety precaution. Some use a transseptal pigtail catheter.

Complications of transseptal catheterization include aortic puncture, coronary sinus perforation, venous perforation, atrial puncture, and pericardial tamponade, as well as the other complications of left heart catheterization. The complication rate is determined by operator experience but is usually higher than with all other catheterization techniques. Because of the risk of vascular perforation, systemic anticoagulation should not be performed until the actual transseptal puncture has been successfully completed.

Other Sites for Arterial Access

Other sites have been utilized for arterial access for cardiac catheterization and angiography in very select circumstances. These include the translumbar (12) and axillary (13) approaches. The translumbar approach is appropriate in the rare case of occlusion of all peripheral arteries but obviously requires a change in routine patient preparation, positioning, and laboratory setup. With the advent of smaller catheters and the ease and safety of the percutaneous brachial technique, it is our opinion that the axillary approach offers no particular advantage, and the lack of collaterals may make it more risky.

Regardless of the site or method of catheter introduction used, arterial sites and distal pulses should be assessed when the patient leaves the laboratory, again within 4 to 6 hr of the procedure and 1 week postcatheterization. This should allow detection of both early and late arterial complications.

CATHETER MANIPULATION

There are a number of aspects of getting catheters into their desired locations that are not necessarily obvious to the beginner that become part of the skills of a catheterizing physician. Modern catheters have been designed to make the techniques easier, but control of the catheter tip is still the key to its manipulation. The first and most important principle of successful catheter manipulation is to choose the correct catheter for the purpose. Preformed catheters will assume their predetermined shape while in the patient, despite the manipulation and warming that occurs when placed at body temperature. The warming is generally not enough to alter the shape significantly but can make a small bore polyethylene catheter softer after a few minutes in the body, making it more difficult to control. With woven catheters, warming can change the shape of the catheter significantly. A good example of this is during coronary catheterization, when one is using a woven Dacron Sones catheter.

Catheters should never be forced to move in a vessel. If advancement is not smooth and effortless, something is generally wrong. It may be that the tip is impacted against the wall of a vessel; there is vasospasm; or the catheter has reached too small an area in the vessel to advance any further. In any case, the catheter must be withdrawn, redirected, or replaced. Generally when the tip of the catheter is against a vascular structure, it is difficult and sometimes dangerous to advance it further. With soft or balloon-tip catheters, or in certain cardiac chambers, such as the right atrium, forming a U-shaped loop in the catheter may be helpful or even necessary. This is true of coronary catheterization using the Sones technique or right heart catheterization from the arm using a non flow-directed catheter. It is important, however, not to force the tip against a vessel wall but to gently rotate the catheter as it is being advanced and to slide the tip up the vascular wall, not forcing it at a 90° angle.

Performing maneuvers to form loops at the end of a catheter will frequently create complex bends in the catheter in areas other than the end, particularly if the tip is not free to move. In catheters that are not preformed, this can be a problem because of the tendency of the catheter to "remember" these bends. Catheters generally are easiest to manipulate when all of their angles are in the same plane. In this way, coaxial pressure will be transmitted to the tip, not to other parts of the catheter. For example, with Sones coronary catheterization using a woven Dacron catheter, these extra bends will make the procedure much more difficult. An example of this with preformed catheters is an angled pigtail catheter being used in an angled sheath for right ventricular endomyocardial biopsy. If the bends in the sheath and the catheter are lined up to form one continuous bend in a single plane, maneuvering the system into the right ventricle is simple. Moreover, when advancing the sheath over the pigtail, it follows a natural gentle curve directly into the desired location. When using preformed catheters, the operator should take advantage of the curves that are present in them. For example, a pigtail catheter with a 30° or 45° angle at the tip is designed to cross the aortic valve, pointing directly along the long axis of the left ventricle.

Because catheters all must pass through the skin directly, a sheath, or the wall of a vessel to enter the circulation, there is some resistance to that movement. Whenever a catheter needs to be rotated, this will become a factor in maintaining control. Continuing to rotate a catheter without transmitting those turns to the tip will not allow for appropriate control of the catheter tip. Simple gentle movements of the catheter in and out, often only a very short distance, will enable torque to be transmitted to the tip as it is placed on the opposite end.

Finally, if a catheter is not doing what you want it to do because of shape, size, vascular abnormalities, or other factors, choose another one and start again. There is no advantage in trying to make a catheter do something it was not designed to do. This may be dangerous and frustrating. A well-equipped laboratory should have a wide selection of catheters so that the operator can choose the most appropriate catheter design.

Approach to Catheterization of the Right Heart

Right heart catheterization is always performed in antegrade fashion from a systemic vein. It can be performed from either an upper or lower extremity, as well as the subclavian or jugular veins. Catheter manipulation is somewhat different with each approach. In addition, the type of catheter chosen will also influence the type of manipulation performed.

Balloon flotation catheters (e.g., Swan-Ganz, Berman) are the most common types of catheters currently used for right heart catheterization, and only limited manipulation is possible. From the upper venous system, via the subclavian, jugular, or brachial vein, the catheter is advanced into the superior vena cava or right atrium, and the balloon is inflated. Generally, it will then float into the pulmonary artery as it is advanced. Occasionally, the catheter will loop in the atrium and not readily cross the tricuspid valve. In this circumstance, deflating the balloon and redirecting the catheter prior to reinflation will often allow it to pass. If this does not work, placing a guidewire into the central lumen will usually stiffen the catheter enough to allow better manipulation, either with or without the balloon inflated. This is particularly helpful when there is significant tricuspid regurgitation or a very large right atrium.

From the femoral vein, two techniques may be used with a balloon catheter. The first involves forming a loop in the right atrium. The loop should enlarge as the catheter tip is directed laterally. Advancing the catheter should allow the tip to be directed inferiorly along the lateral wall of the right atrium and then medially toward the tricuspid valve and into the pulmonary artery. Once the catheter is in the pulmonary artery, the redundant loop should be removed. Another technique used to enter the pulmonary artery involves passing the catheter directly across the tricuspid valve. The tip of the catheter is positioned directly across the valve, pointing up toward the outflow tract. This often requires rotating the catheter, generally in a counterclockwise direction, while the patient inspires. Otherwise, there is a tendency for the catheter to be directed toward the right ventricular apex, and from that position, floating into the pulmonary artery is most difficult. From the outflow tract, once the tip is directed toward the pulmonary artery, advancing the catheter will allow it to float into the desired pulmonary artery location.

With a stiffer, nonflotation catheter, such as a Cournand, Goodale-Lubin, or Zucker catheter, manipulation is very different. From the upper extremity, one should not generally attempt to pass these catheters directly into the pulmonary artery without first forming a loop in the right atrium. Without a loop, these catheters readily traverse the tricuspid valve to the right ventricular apex. The catheter is directed toward the lateral atrial wall until it is impeded by an irregular surface, usually the right atrium-inferior vena cava junction. From here it is advanced to form a large loop with the tip pointing up. Then it is rotated, generally about 180° counterclockwise, to turn the loop and direct the tip toward the pulmonary artery as the body of the catheter crosses the tricuspid valve first. Once this is accomplished and the catheter is not stuck on the right ventricular outflow region, advancing out into the pulmonary artery is straightforward. In general, more catheter should be fed into the vein to help the tip move to the pulmonary artery. If the catheter starts to buckle in the right ventricle, however, it should be withdrawn and redirected because perforation of the outflow tract may occur readily. From the lower extremity, a technique similar to that described for the direct passage of a balloon flotation catheter is performed. The tip of the catheter is placed across the tricuspid valve, with the tip turned up into the pulmonary valve as the catheter is advanced. Alternately, when the right atrium is large, a loop may be made as described with a balloon flotation catheter.

When a stiff catheter is directed toward the atrial septum, as with transseptal catheterization, it can often be advanced across a "probe patent" foramen ovale. Left atrial position can be verified by noting left atrial pressure, by measuring systemic arterial oxygen saturation, or by a small contrast injection. In this same manner, an atrial septal defect can be crossed often even with a balloon flotation catheter.

A brief note about **coronary sinus catheterization** is necessary. This is generally difficult from the inferior vena cava and should be performed from the upper extremity whenever possible. The ostium of the coronary sinus is inferior and medial to the tricuspid valve opening. When using a catheter with pressure monitoring capability, the catheter should be pointed toward the tricuspid valve and directly passed into the right ventricle. After ventricular pressure is noted, the catheter is pulled back until atrial pressure is noted. The tip of the catheter should be facing inferiorly and to the patient's left. Rotating the catheter counterclockwise approximately 90° and advancing it should place it in the coronary sinus. Atrial pressure will still be recorded, and the catheter appears as if it is going into the right ventricle. When pressure monitoring is not available, as with electrophysiology catheters, catheter position, recorded electrical signals and, when necessary, lateral fluoroscopy, will confirm catheter position. Absence of ventricular ectopy when the catheter looks like it is directed into the right ventricular outflow tract will also be a clue to the fact that the catheter is in the coronary sinus.

Obvious areas of venous obstruction should be avoided, as in the patient with deep vein thrombosis in a femoral vein or inferior vena cava obstruction. In this case, a different site should be used. In individuals with a persistent left superior vena cava, venous drainage from the left upper extremity is into the coronary sinus. Occasionally this can be identified on chest x-ray but often is first noted when a catheter takes an aberrant course from the left subclavian. Usually in this situation, manipulating a catheter into the right ventricle and pulmonary artery is quite difficult, and another site should be used.

What catheter is chosen for right heart catheterization depends on the function it is to perform. Out of the catheterization laboratory setting, the only catheter that will generally be used is the balloon flotation catheter. What specific model is chosen will be determined by what capabilities are necessary (pacing, cardiac output, etc.). In the catheterization laboratory, either a stiff or balloon catheter may be used. For pressure measurements, stiff catheters have a better frequency response and will give a phasic pressure without the "catheter whip" that often accompanies softer balloon catheters. This is important when measuring pulmonary-capillary wedge pressure, particularly in patients with pulmonary hypertension. For this application, an end-hole catheter, such as a Cournand, is most appropriate. Likewise, for determination of pressure gradients, as in the case with pulmonic stenosis, an end-hole catheter should be used. For angiography either of the right atrium, right ventricle, or pulmonary artery, a multiple side-hole catheter, such as a Berman angiographic, pigtail, or NIH, is necessary.

Approach to Catheterization of the Left Heart

Left ventricular catheterization is usually performed in retrograde fashion through the aortic valve. Here the left heart is approached by advancing a catheter to the descending aorta, removing the guidewire, and flushing the catheter. While usually performed with a pigtail catheter from the femoral approach, many other catheters can be used. Once the catheter has been flushed, it is advanced to the ascending aorta as pressure is monitored. Techniques utilized to cross the aortic valve include (*a*) the direct approach where the aortic valve is crossed with the tip of the catheter; (*b*) the indirect approach where a loop is formed so that the distal end of the catheter is "backed" across the valve and (*c*) either of these two techniques combined with a guidewire. Ventricular ectopy upon entering the cavity is a common occurrence, and the operator needs to be ready to position the catheter quickly to find a stable position.

The **direct approach** is most often accomplished with relatively rigid catheters. These include the NIH, Lehman ventriculography, multipurpose, and Gensini catheters. All of these catheters have multiple holes and handle high flow rates; therefore, they can be used for ventriculography. Single-hole catheters, such as the right Judkins coronary catheters, can also be advanced directly into the left ventricle, but they are not suitable for the high-volume power injection necessary for adequate ventricular filling with contrast material. This type of catheter must then be exchanged for an appropriate ventriculography catheter. With the direct approach the catheter is advanced into the area just above the aortic valve and turned so that the tip faces leftward toward the valve orifice. The catheter is then advanced gently until the valve is crossed or the left cusp stops forward motion of the catheter tip. If the cusp stops the catheter, it should be withdrawn slightly, redirected using either clockwise or counterclockwise rotation, and advanced again. Using this method, the valve is "explored" until the catheter tip advances easily into the left ventricle. In patients with aortic stenosis, identification of the jet of blood ejected through the valve by observing high-frequency vibrations of the catheter often can be used to help recognize the location of the orifice. In addition, moving the fluoroscope into the left anterior oblique position or use of biplane fluoroscopy may be helpful. With some catheters, such as a large (8 Fr or larger) NIH catheter, the direct approach is the only appropriate method for crossing the aortic valve because the catheter is too stiff to form a loop safely, and guidewires cannot be advanced beyond the tip.

The **indirect approach** is most commonly used with pigtail catheters but is also suitable for any catheter that will easily form a loop within the ascending aorta, such as a Sones or multipurpose catheter. The pigtail catheter is advanced to a position just above the aortic valve and rotated so that the "tail" is oriented toward the left coronary cusp. The catheter is then advanced so that the loop of the pigtail is pushed firmly against the cusp. When the aortic valve is normal, the catheter will generally enter the ventricle easily by simply advancing it and forming a larger loop. If this does not cause the catheter to spring into the left ventricle, having the patient breath as the catheter is withdrawn and rotated clockwise will allow it to easily cross the valve in most patients. The right anterior oblique view may help in some patients. In the case of Sones and multipurpose catheters, a loop is formed by rotating and advancing the catheter simultaneously from either the left or posterior cusp. Once the catheter is in the ventricle, the loop can be straightened by gentle retraction and rotation. Ventricular ectopy is usually controlled by these maneuvers.

Guidewires are often helpful for crossing the aortic valve and can be used in a number of ways, depending on the catheter. With an open-ended catheter, they can be advanced out of the end of the catheter, and a loop can be formed either with the guidewire alone or with the catheter. The valve can then be crossed indirectly with this loop. The catheter can also serve to steer the guidewire directly across the aortic valve. This method is particularly useful with a straight guidewire in the case of either a stenotic valve or dilated root. When aortic valve stenosis is suspected, it is often helpful to start with a pigtail catheter and reinsert the guidewire to begin the crossing procedure with the guidewire directed toward the center of the valve orifice. Many operators use a variety of different catheters for this purpose with different bends chosen to best reflect the specific anatomy of the aorta. These include pigtail catheters with and without preformed bends, right and left Judkins catheters, and Amplatz catheters. Guidewires can also be bent to reflect the specific anatomy to be negotiated. Again, if a single end-hole catheter is used, it must be exchanged for a more appropriate angiographic catheter prior to ventriculography using a 240- to 260-cm exchange wire of the largest diameter accepted by the catheter used. Creation of a large loop at the end of the exchange wire is helpful to keep the wire in a small left ventricular cavity with a minimum of ectopic beats. Guidewires can also be used to stiffen or straighten either an open- or closed-end catheter. Either the soft or hard end of the wire can be used for this purpose, but the hard end of the wire must never be advanced near or out of the end of the catheter tip. Crossing a stenotic valve can consume a considerable amount of time, so the amount of time that the wire is in the catheter should be closely monitored. The wire should be removed and wiped with heparinized saline and the catheter flushed every 2 min.

ASSOCIATED PROCEDURES

Catheterization of the heart and vascular system is performed in order to gain diagnostic information or perform therapeutic procedures. The diagnostic procedures performed include angiography, pressure and function measurements, blood sampling for shunt detection and metabolic parameter determination, electrophysiologic measurements and stimulation, as well as other techniques that are discussed in other chapters. Therapeutic techniques such as angioplasty and valvuloplasty are likewise discussed elsewhere in Chapters 15 and 17, respectively.

Endomyocardial Biopsy

Endomyocardial biopsy is unique among all catheterization procedures in that it is performed only to remove a piece of tissue from the heart. This technique has undergone marked improvement since it was first attempted. Older techniques have been largely abandoned since development of transvascular biotomes of the Konno, King, and Stanford types. These instruments vary somewhat, but all share the ability to be introduced via a sheath placed into the internal jugular, brachial, or femoral vein for repeated sampling from the right ventricle. The brachial or femoral artery can be utilized for left ventricular biopsy. The complication rate for transvascular myocardial biopsy is very low when performed by experienced operators. The complications include those related to the approach, such as vein thrombosis and hematoma, as well as air embolism. Arrhythmias are common with catheter manipulation, but it is rare to have a sustained arrhythmia. An occasional patient will develop transient right bundle branch or AV block, but permanent conduction abnormalities are rare. Cardiac perforation with tamponade has been reported in less than 0.05% in all series reported, and death is extremely rare, with only two deaths out of some 6,700 biopsies reported in a recent world survey. The overall complication rate in most series is reported to be between 1 and 2%. In addition, it is rare not to obtain adequate tissue for examination (14).

The technique for obtaining biopsy specimens from the heart is relatively simple (Fig. 6.6). The right ventricular approach will be described because it is the most commonly employed, but the technique is basically the same for the left ventricle. Either the internal jugular or femoral vein can be utilized. On occasion, we have used the brachial approach. The short Stanford biotome must be used only through the neck because of the length of the instrument, but other biotomes (Cordis™ and Mansfield™) come in lengths suitable for either the jugular or femoral approach. Regardless of the site or biotome to be utilized, a sheath designed for this purpose is placed in the vein. These sheaths are made with a 45° angle on the terminal portion to allow for more ready access to the right ventricle. After a long (145-cm) guidewire is placed in the vessel, a pigtail catheter inside the sheath is passed as a unit into the vessel. The guidewire is used to help place the pigtail in the apex of the right ventricle, and the guidewire is removed. The pigtail catheter is then fixed in this location as the sheath is advanced over it. When the sheath is in place, the catheter is removed, the sheath is flushed, and the side port is connected to a pressure transducer for monitoring. After right ventricular location is verified by pressure measurement, the biotome is advanced into the sheath to a distance approximately 2 cm from the tip. This should be done while flush solution is flowing through the sheath to prevent infusion of air and thrombus formation. The sheath can then be rotated toward the ventricular septum, keeping in mind that the biotome in the sheath will tend to straighten it. The handle controlling the biotome jaws should be moved to the open position so that the jaws will open immediately on exiting the sheath to limit the possibility of perforation. With the jaws opened, the biotome is pushed into the septal wall, and the jaws are closed and withdrawn with a jerking motion to remove a piece of the myocardium. Generally, there are several premature ventricular beats during this portion of the procedure but rarely are they sustained. This procedure can be repeated as often as necessary, and different locations in the septum can be sampled simply by moving the sheath. After each sample is taken, pressure should be checked to ensure that the sheath has not moved out of the ventricle. Generally three to five samples are adequate for most diagnostic purposes.

The technique for left ventricular biopsy is very similar, except that the approach is retrograde through the aortic valve. Extreme care must be used to avoid the introduction of air, when advancing the biotome into the sheath. Left ventricular biopsy should be avoided in patients with left ventricular thrombi and should not be considered in patients with right bundle branch block, because of the chance of inducing complete AV block. Since there does not appear to be a substantial difference in yield between left and right ventricular sites, it is not possible to justify routine use of left ventricular biopsy (15–17).

It is important to note that the person interpreting the specimen is at least as important as the proper performance of the biopsy. Biopsies taken from a beating heart are not the same as specimens taken from autopsy material. There are numerous artifacts related to the forceps, the size of the specimen, and the fact that the heart was actively contracting during the procedure, which can render accurate interpretation difficult.

Pericardiocentesis

Pericardiocentesis is a technique that is occasionally necessary for the diagnosis and/or management of acute and chronic pericardial disease. It is absolutely essential, how- ever, for those performing cardiac catheterization to be skilled in pericardiocentesis because it can be lifesaving in the event of tamponade due to cardiac perforation by a catheter or needle. Pericardiocentesis can be performed with fluoroscopic, two-dimensional echocardiographic, or electrocardiographic monitoring and guidance. Many use a combination of these monitoring techniques. Except under the most emergent circumstances, pericardiocentesis should not be performed without monitoring, as considerable cardiac damage can occur. Electrocardiographic guidance may be cumbersome and is occasionally misleading as the right ventricle or right atrium may be punctured without registering a change in the ECG. Direct fluoroscopic needle visualization is preferred by the authors. Pressure monitoring is not essential but is important in some cases to provide confirmatory evidence of tamponade (see Chapter 31).

The only instrumentation absolutely necessary for this procedure is a needle of adequate size for fluid aspiration and a syringe. A long 16- or 18-gauge needle is appropriate, as it will allow for the aspiration of even relatively viscous fluid and permit the introduction of a guidewire. The bevel on the needle should be relatively blunt. If catheters are to be placed for prolonged drainage or infusion, a soft, multiple side-hole catheter, such as a pigtail catheter, should be inserted over a guidewire.

We prefer the subxyphoid route, but many other sites can be used, depending on the location and volume of the effusion (Fig. 6.7). The advantage of the subxyphoid approach is that it is extrapleural and avoids coronary and mammary arteries. The patient should be recumbent at an angle of approximately 30 to 45° to allow for pooling of fluid. Under local anesthesia, the needle is inserted perpendicular to the skin in the subxyphoid region and advanced to just below the lower border of the ribs. This is usually approximately 5 to 8 mm, depending on the size of the patient. The hub of the needle is then angled inferiorly and the tip anteriorly by moving the barrel of the syringe toward the abdominal wall. If the patient is obese, considerable force may be necessary to force the syringe against the abdominal wall to direct the tip of the needle sufficiently anteriorly. The tip may be pointed toward either the left or right shoulder or in between, as long as it is directed cephalad and advanced while aspirating until fluid is withdrawn. Usually there is a distinct sensation of the needle "popping" through the parietal pericardium as the pericardial space is entered. Unless the fluid is under high pressure, it will usually only drip out unless negative pressure is applied. As more fluid is withdrawn, the needle will eventually come into contact with the heart, and the operator will be aware of the beating motion of the heart on the end of the needle. As a result, extensive cardiac trauma or perforation may occur, and it is prudent to replace the needle with a catheter prior to withdrawing large amounts of pericardial fluid.

If there is a question as to whether the fluid that is withdrawn is from an intracardiac site, the quickest method of determining this is to inject a small amount of radiographic contrast material. This may be either a radiographic agent, if the procedure is being

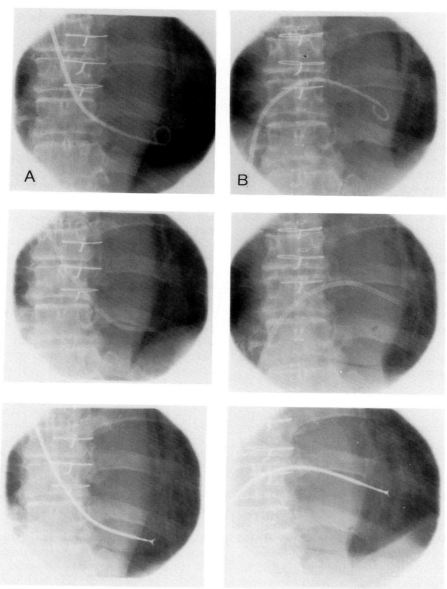

Figure 6.6. Radiographic appearance of the location of an endomyocardial biopsy apparatus in appropriate position. Notice that the sheath changes shape and position slightly with the catheter or biopsy forceps in it. *A*, Internal jugular approach. *Top*, Sheath and pigtail catheter in right ventricle. *Middle*, Sheath alone in right ventricle. *Bottom*, Biopsy forceps (open jaws) extended out of sheath and against the endocardium. *B*, Femoral vein approach. *Top*, Sheath and pigtail catheter in right ventricle. *Middle*, Sheath alone in right ventricle. *Bottom*, Biopsy forceps (open jaws) extended out of sheath and against the endocardium.

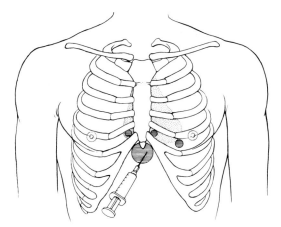

Figure 6.7. Schematic illustration of proper location and direction of needle entry for pericardiocentesis from the subxiphoid area (*large stippled circle*). The needle is placed immediately under the xiphoid process and directed toward the left shoulder. Alternate sites are noted in the apical and left and right parasternal regions (*smaller stippled circles*).

performed with fluoroscopic guidance, or saline, to detect microbubbles by two-dimensional echocardiography. Contrast material will either pool in the de-pendent part of the pericardial space or rapidly wash out into the vascular space if a cardiac chamber has been entered. In addition, performing a hematocrit on the fluid may be helpful but takes longer. Bloody pericardial fluid will generally be of a lower hematocrit than peripheral blood and will not clot because of defibrination that occurs when fluid has been in the pericardial space for a prolonged period.

Processing, analyzing, and interpreting pericardial fluid data are important. However, analysis of pericardial fluid generally does not yield a great deal of diagnostic information. While certain diseases, such as cholesterol pericarditis, rheumatoid arthritis, and hypothyroidism, may yield characteristic pericardial fluid profiles, most do not.

Retrieval of Intravascular Foreign Bodies

Cardiologists and radiologists who perform invasive procedures are occasionally called upon to remove intravascular foreign bodies. Major differences have developed in the type of foreign bodies that get marooned in the vascular system, as catheter and guidewire systems have changed, but usually it is a catheter or guidewire or some portion of them that necessitates retrieval. Because of the type of catheter fragment concerned, most lay with their proximal end in the inflow area of the right atrium or completely in the pulmonary artery (18). Migratory patterns are variable, but the distal ends of these right-sided catheters may be distributed in the right atrium, right ventricle, or pulmonary artery with a similar frequency, depending on length. A discussion of the different retrieval methods is beyond the scope of this chapter, but a brief description of some of the more commonly used techniques will be provided.

There are at least three basic methods for retrieval of intravascular foreign bodies: entangling, snaring, and grabbing. Often modifications of the position of the foreign body within the circulation are necessary before any of these techniques are possible. Moving the foreign body may be necessary to dislodge the end in order to snare it or to get it into a position that is more easily approached. This can frequently be done with soft, standard catheters, such as a preformed coronary or pigtail catheter. Simply by hooking the end of these catheters around some portion of the foreign body, it can frequently be dislodged or reoriented. The entangling technique is performed by carrying this one step further. A pigtail catheter can be turned in such a way as to tangle the foreign body around it. Once the catheter to be removed is securely around the pigtail catheter, the entire system is gently pulled back and removed. The difficulty with this technique is that the foreign body may become dislodged and embolize during removal, as there is no way to secure it.

The snare technique is the most commonly used and entails passing a loop of exchange length guidewire into a catheter which generally will be of large enough bore to accommodate the two wires without kinking. We usually use a 240-cm, 0.025-inch guidewire in a 7 or 8 Fr open-ended catheter. Removal of the movable core of standard guidewires will soften the wire and limit kinking, but this is not essential. Systems are commercially available that are variably elaborate but basically perform the same function. A catheter-snare system similar to a urologic stone basket retrieval system is also available and provides several loops for snaring purposes. Basically, the snare is advanced with an open loop adjacent to the tip of the catheter to be removed. When the piece to be removed is in the loop, the snare is closed by retracting the guidewire ends. Tension is maintained on these ends, and the catheter snare is slowly removed with the foreign body.

Another technique is to directly grasp the foreign body with a biopsy instrument like that used for endomyocardial biopsy. This allows retrieval of a foreign body that does not have a readily free end by grasping it at any point. Once the foreign body is grasped, the biopsy forceps should be removed with any sheath that has been used for its introduction while the grasp is maintained. Occasionally, it is possible to use the biopsy forceps to free a catheter, particularly one that has been in place for a prolonged period, such as a permanent pacemaker lead. Forceps can be used to remove small pieces of tissue near the lead to free it, allowing removal. Obviously, this should be done with great care, preferably in the ventricle only after more conventional methods have failed. These biopsy instruments are relatively rigid and difficult to maneuver, and perforation of a vascular structure is possible.

Several general rules should be kept in mind when planning removal of an intravascular foreign body. It is best to move the piece to be removed to a large chamber or vessel. The pulmonary artery and small peripheral vessels are the most difficult sites from which to retrieve a foreign body. A large venous sheath will allow removal of the foreign body and retrieval device, occasionally without removing the sheath, thus maintaining venous access. If the body to be removed is in the arterial system, a cutdown and use of a large vessel such as the femoral artery will lessen the chance of peripheral arterial injury on exit.

In our experience, retrieval of intravascular foreign bodies has been fairly safe, and this has been confirmed by others (18). Each situation is different, however, and few general rules can be established as to the proper approach. This type of manipulation should be performed only by very experienced operators with a full array of catheters at their disposal and the ability to view the heart from a variety of vantage points fluoroscopically and echocardiographically, as serious adverse effects are possible.

SUMMARY

The various techniques of cardiac catheterization offer the physician a large number of options in terms of approach, site, procedures, and methods to aid in the diagnosis and treatment of a variety of conditions. The procedures are very safe when appropriately adapted to various circumstances and performed by trained individuals. Further improvements can be expected in both the techniques and the hardware available. However, as catheterization techniques and their indications expand, it is important to apply them with the knowledge that they are not without some degree of risk.

References

1. Belani KG, Buckley JJ, Gordon JR, Castaneda W. Percutaneous cervical central venous line placement: a comparison of the internal and external jugular vein routes. Anesthesiology 1980; 59: 40-44.
2. English ICW, Frew RM, Pigott JF, Zaki M. Percutaneous catheterization of the internal jugular vein. Anaesthesia 1969; 24:521-531.
3. Defalque RJ. Percutaneous catheterization of the internal jugular vein. Anesthesia Analgesia 1974; 53:116-121.
4. Seneff MG. Central venous catheterization: a comprehensive review. Part I. J Intens Care Med 1987; 2:163-175.
5. Seneff MG. Central venous catheterization: a comprehensive review. Part II. J Intens Care Med 1987; 2:218-231.
6. Rao TLK, Wong AY, Salem MR. A new approach to percutaneous catheterization of the internal jugular vein. Anesthesiology 1977; 46:362-364.
7. Bjork VO, Cullhed I, Hallen A, Lodin H, Malers E. Sequelae of left ventricular puncture with angiocardiography. Circulation 1961; 24:204-212.
8. Brock R, Milstein BB, Ross DN. Percutaneous left ventricular puncture in the assessment of aortic stenosis. Thorax 1956; 2:163-171.
9. Greene DG, Sharp JT, Griffith GT, Bunnell IL, Macmanus JE. Surgical application of anterior percutaneous left heart puncture. Surgery 1958; 43:1-5.
10. Yu PN, Lovejoy FW, Schreiner BF, Leahy RH, Stanfield CA, Walther H. Direct left ventricular puncture in the evaluation of aortic and mitral stenosis. Am Heart J 1958; 55:926-941.
11. Baxley SW, Soto B. Hemodynamic evaluation of patients with combined mitral and aortic prostheses. Am J Cardiol 1980; 45:42-47.
12. Marcus R, Grollman JH Jr. Translumbar coronary and brachiocephalic arteriography using a modified Desilets-Hoffman sheath. Diagnosis 1987; 13:288-290.

13. Valeix B, Labrunie P, Jahjah F, et al. Selective coronary arteriography by percutaneous transaxillary approach. Cathet Cardiovasc Diagn 1987; 10: 403-409.

14. Fowles RE, Mason JW. Role of cardiac biopsy in the diagnosis and management of cardiac disease. Prog Cardiovasc Dis 1984; 27:153-172.

15. Brooksby IAB, Jenkins S, Davies MJ, Swanton MB, Coltart DJ, Webb-Peploe MM. Left ventricular endomyocardial biopsy. I. Description and evaluation of the technique. Cathet Cardiovasc Diagn 1977; 3:115-121.

16. Davies MJ, Brooksby IAB, Jenkins S, et al. Left ventricular endomyocardial biopsy. II. The value of light microscopy. Cathet Cardiovasc Diagn 1977; 3:123-130.

17. Davies MJ, Kennedy S, Brooksby IAB, et al. Left ventricular endomyocardial biopsy. III. Ultrastructural characteristic of cardiomyopathy and cardiac hypertrophy with good or poor ventricular function. Cathet Cardiovasc Diagn 1977; 3:131-137.

18. Bloomfield DA. The nonsurgical retrieval of intracardiac foreign bodies—an international survey. Cathet Cardiovasc Diagn 1978; 4:1-14.

7

Catheters, Sheaths, Guidewires, and Needles

Robert G. Macdonald, M.D.

INTRODUCTION

Performance of a hemodynamic or angiographic study should meet two important requirements. First, the procedure must be completed in such a way that all necessary information has been obtained. Second, this must be done quickly and efficiently with a minimum of risk and discomfort to the patient. In meeting these requirements, the catheterizing physician draws not only upon his experience in performing a large volume of varied procedures, but also upon a knowledge of the "tools of his trade." Development and marketing of equipment for cardiac catheterization is a major industry, even more so with recent advances in interventional catheterization procedures. The invasive or interventional cardiologist must be familiar with the relative merits of particular equipment designs and must keep abreast of new developments by various manufacturers as these become available.

This chapter will provide an overview of the "tools" currently available for cardiac catheterization, with a brief discussion of the technical considerations leading to selection of items for specific purposes. This review will be limited to those items necessary for diagnostic catheterization and will, in general, focus on items common to most types of catheterization procedures. Highly specialized catheters and guidewires used for percutaneous transluminal coronary angioplasty (PTCA) and valvuloplasty will be discussed in

Chapters 15 and 17, respectively. An understanding of the basic construction of these tools is very important relative to selection of equipment for specific cases, optimal manipulation of equipment, and avoidance of complications. This is further emphasized in selection of equipment when the first choice fails during a procedure.

Discussion of equipment available for catheterization will follow in order of use during the procedure: first, needles for percutaneous vascular access; second, the varied guidewires available; third, sheaths and dilators for establishment and maintenance of a route for catheter insertion; and finally, catheters for hemodynamic assessment and ventricular and selective coronary angiography.

NEEDLES FOR PERCUTANEOUS VASCULAR ACCESS

Choice of a specific needle for vascular access may seem to require little consideration. There are, however, two major differences in needle design which result in different insertion techniques (Seldinger vs. direct) and considerable variations in needle size and shape. A description of the components of a needle is necessary before further discussion can ensue. Figure 7.1 shows an example of standard disposable Seldinger and direct front-wall-type needles. In Figure 7.2, a Seldinger needle is illustrated with labeled components. Needles of this type are modifications of the older Riley and Cournand needles and have a

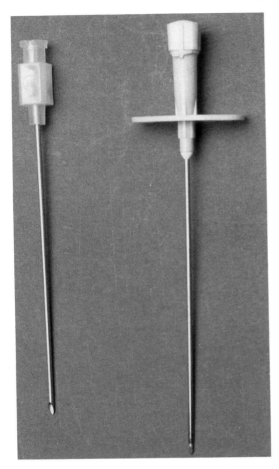

Figure 7.1. The two most commonly used needle types for vascular access. On the *left*, a single-piece, thin-walled "front wall needle"; on the *right*, a two-component, thin-walled Seldinger needle.

blunted needle bevel and one or two stylets. The innermost stylet is solid and is designed to prevent the lumen from becoming blocked with skin and subcutaneous tissue and blood as the needle is inserted into the artery. Most contemporary designs have a single stylet or use the direct method with no stylet at all.

The hub of the needle must incorporate several features. It must fit firmly on the body of the needle and internally have a smooth funnel into the body to facilitate wire insertion. Most hubs have a female luer lock connector, allowing attachment to the male luer connector on a syringe with an airtight seal. This is important for maintenance of negative pressure when withdrawing a needle into the

lumen of a low pressure vessel and observing blood return, as in the Seldinger technique. The hub section may have a "winged" baseplate or flange to allow gripping between the first two fingers and thumb, as used in the Seldinger technique, so that the needle can be controlled with one hand. During insertion, the needle should always be controlled by the hand-held wing rather than an attached syringe. Numerous arterial needles are available and some examples are shown in Figure 7.3. One design (Argon Inc.) incorporates a detachable plastic baseplate allowing for variations in personal preference among different operators in the same laboratory (Fig. 7.4).

Needles are sized according to their external diameter and an arbitrary gauging system (Table 7.1). With increasing gauge number, the diameter decreases.

Needles may be standard or thin-walled, allowing greater internal to external diameter ratios. Most 18-gauge needles will allow passage of a 0.035- or 0.038-inch standard guidewire, and these sizes are commonly stocked in most laboratories. A needle must be long enough to pass through a considerable depth of subcutaneous tissue in obese patients and short enough to be manipulated skillfully in

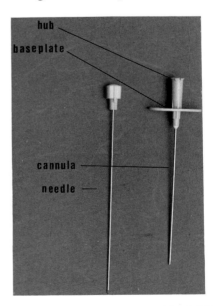

Figure 7.2. A two-piece disposable Seldinger needle with labeled components.

Table 7.1
Conventional Needle Sizing System

Stubs Needle Gauge No.	Outer Diameter (inches)
13	0.095
14	0.083
15	0.072
16	0.065
17	0.058
18	0.049
19	0.042
20	0.035

puncturing the artery or vein. A standard length of 2.75 to 3.0 inches for arterial needles is acceptable in all but rare cases. The tip of the needle has a bevel that forms an angle less acute than that of standard injection needles. The needle must, of course, be sharp enough to avoid tearing the arterial wall on vessel entry and strong enough to pass through calcified arterial walls or subcutaneous fibrous tissue resulting from previous catheterizations or operations. Needles for other uses such as pericardiocentesis and direct percutaneous left ventricular puncture come in various designs and lengths up to 22 cm, as shown in Figure 7.5. The bevels on these needles should be about 45° and the point must be kept sharp, as many special types are sterilized and reused.

The cost of standard arterial needles can vary as much as fivefold, depending on design and manufacturer. Since this amount is very small relative to the total cost of all equipment used during a procedure, the quality and design of the needle, rather than cost, should dictate its selection. Needles designed for resterilization and multiple uses are no longer desirable from a technical or financial point of view.

GUIDEWIRES
Construction

Discussion of guidewires may be divided into a description of the basic components and differences in length, size, and shape that are suited to specific uses.

Basic wire construction is illustrated in Figure 7.6. The coil is made by spinning a thin strand of wire around a metal tube or rod. The coil is then advanced over a core or mandrel and fixed at the ends by a soldered bond. At the flexible end or tip a safety ribbon is soldered and runs the length of the guidewire adjacent to the core.

From Figure 7.6 it can be appreciated that the length of the tip segment without a core

Figure 7.3. A selection of disposable arterial needles illustrating some of the different designs available.

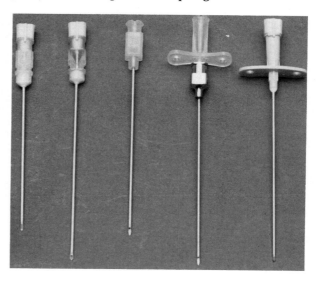

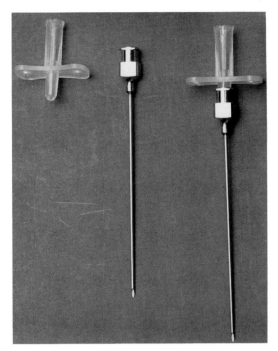

Figure 7.4. A single-use, front wall needle made by Argon Inc. Note the detachable winged baseplate.

will determine how much wire can be advanced through a tortuous segment before the core meets a sudden bend. A gradually tapered core allows for a smoother transition from the very flexible end or tip to the stiffer body of the wire. One of the disadvantages of some movable core wire designs is that with the core retracted a very flimsy wire tip may be advanced around a sharp bend or complex atherosclerotic plaque, but then the stiff core will not follow. Gradual tapering of the core wire in both "fixed" and movable designs can overcome this problem.

Another feature of certain wire designs is an external Teflon coating. This may be applied as a bath or spray to the assembled wire and then bake-dried in an oven to ensure adequate bonding. This provides for "lubricity" (i.e., a reduction in friction between wire and catheter lumen) and reduced thrombogenicity. Despite this feature, the irregular surface of coiled guidewires continues to predispose to thrombus formation. All wires must, therefore, be left in the vessel for only the minimum time necessary for catheter positioning. Stainless steel wires are currently

used predominately for venous access and not for catheter guidance or manipulation in the arterial system.

Recently, a newer design has been marketed. The Radifocus Guidewire "M" made by Terumo Corporation consists of an elastic alloy core coated with a hydrophilic plastic polymer. This provides for a pliable tip, a smooth outer coating, and excellent torque control.

Length

Guidewires are available in lengths from 35 to 260 cm and may be cut to any length. In general, a guidewire should be at least 20 cm longer than the catheter for which it is to be used. The shorter length is used for the introduction of vascular sheaths predominantly into the venous system. A 145-cm wire is usually adequate for insertion or removal of

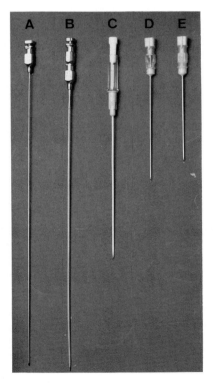

Figure 7.5. Variations in needle length. *A* and *B*, A reusable needle for pericardiocentesis or percutaneous left ventricular puncture. *C*, An intermediate length needle. *D* and *E*, Two shorter arterial needles.

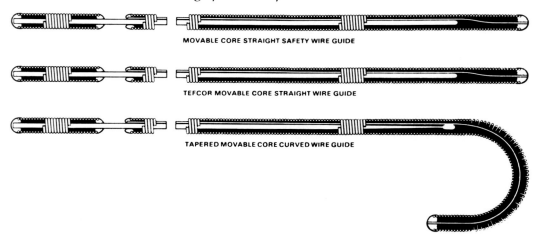

MOVABLE CORE STRAIGHT SAFETY WIRE GUIDE

TEFCOR MOVABLE CORE STRAIGHT WIRE GUIDE

TAPERED MOVABLE CORE CURVED WIRE GUIDE

Figure 7.6. Movable core wire guide construction. Diagram of basic construction of guidewires. (From Cook Product Literature, "Diagnostic and Interventional products for radiology, cardiology and surgery." 1986:4.).

Figure 7.7. Safety guidewires. On the left is a 35-cm stainless steel "J-tipped" wire for venous sheath insertion. On the right is a 135-cm Teflon- coated "J-tipped" wire in its packaging ring.

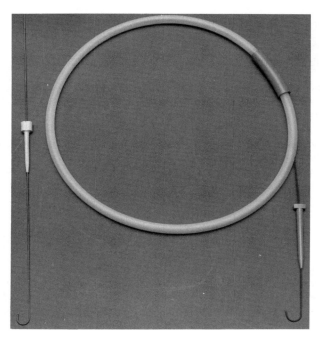

catheters where only a short length of wire needs to remain in the artery. In cases where difficulty has been encountered crossing a tortuous arterial segment from either the leg or arm approach, an exchange wire of approximately 240 to 260 cm in length may be used. When changing catheters, this avoids withdrawing the tip of the wire back through the tortuous segment already negotiated and, thus, minimizes trauma to the vessel at this region. An example of stainless steel wire for venous access and coiled Teflon-coated wire are shown in Figure 7.7.

Diameter

Guidewires most frequently used during diagnostic angiography are either 0.035-inch or 0.038-inch external diameter. Both will pass through an 18-gauge or larger needle and will accommodate most angiographic catheters

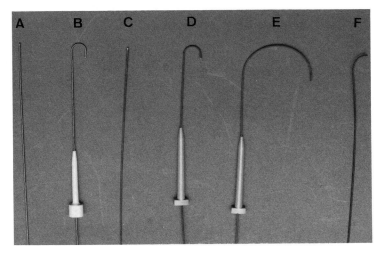

Figure 7.8. A selection of spring tip guidewires. *A*, Stainless steel straight tip. *B*, Stainless steel 3-mm J-tipped wire. *C* and *D*, Teflon-coated straight and 3-mm J-tipped wires. *E*, Teflon-coated 16-mm J-tipped wire. *F*, Terumo "m" wire.

used in adults. The 0.035-inch wire, being slightly smaller in diameter than a 0.038-inch wire, allows advancement of a catheter over it with less internal friction and, hence, greater ability to feel resistance when vascular obstruction or tortuosity are encountered. The wire itself is somewhat more flexible, softer, and potentially less traumatic and more easily manipulated through tortuous arterial segments. The stiffer 0.038-inch wire, however, is less likely to bend when one is trying to advance a dilator through fibrotic subcutaneous tissue or a calcified arterial wall and when one is inserting a pigtail catheter over the wire through a distorted stenotic aortic valve via the retrograde approach. The 0.035-inch wire is perhaps a better wire for routine use, and the 0.038-inch wire is best reserved for specific indications, such as those described above. The 0.025-inch wire is usually reserved for smaller diameter catheters (e.g., 4 Fr or less) or used when there is difficulty advancing a 0.035-inch wire. In the latter case, the smaller wire will be less traumatic to the vessel wall.

Shape

Current wire selection involves not only a straight tip with a flexible or movable core but also J tips of several sizes (Fig. 7.8). J wires are described by the radius of curvature in the tip (e.g., 3-mm "J").

The 3-mm J is indicated for routine use and has advantages over straight wires in its tendency to avoid entering side branches and to curve or "glance off" of atherosclerotic plaques rather than dissect beneath them. With larger plaques in highly tortuous vessels a larger J is sometimes helpful for atraumatic guidewire advancement. The only significant disadvantage of the J wire is that some physicians may have difficulty introducing the tip through a needle or catheter hub. This is facilitated by a plastic tip introducer that is packaged with all J-tipped guidewires. There is also a technique whereby the operator can pinch the wire between the thumb and index finger and retract a more proximal segment of wire between the palm and remaining fingers to straighten the spring tip. In rare cases a J-tipped wire with a movable core may be advanced through an arterial segment where a standard J tip has been unsuccessful. Larger J's and other configurations are sometimes helpful for exchange purposes, particularly within the left ventricular cavity. Different tip configurations can be added by pulling the region to be curved between the thumb and the rounded edge of a hemostat.

Use of a straight-tipped wire is indicated when attempting to cross a stenotic aortic valve in retrograde fashion. In this situation the J tip has too large a diameter to negotiate a narrow orifice, and the straight tip more readily penetrates the jet of blood exiting the valve and can better probe the valve orifice. Wires with a flexible J tip on one end and a flexible straight tip on the other are available from most manufacturers at slightly higher cost. A straight-tipped wire can also be shaped using the technique described above.

In summary, catheter guidewires are available in various lengths, diameters, and tip configurations. Knowledge of different wires allows a selection matched to particular needs, thus enhancing the success and safety of a procedure.

VASCULAR SHEATHS AND DILATORS

With advances in angiographic equipment, techniques used to achieve and maintain vascular access have seen considerable refinement. Previously, most arterial catheterization was done via the Seldinger technique, with catheter insertion directly over a guidewire or by cutdown technique. With this technique, an arterial dilator was advanced over the wire to provide a tract through the subcutaneous tissue and vessel wall for subsequent catheter insertion. The dilator used was generally of at least one French size smaller than the body of the catheter to be inserted to reduce the possibility of leakage of blood around the catheter once in place. The development of thin-walled vascular sheaths offers a different approach and in many laboratories their use has become common practice.

Current sheath designs incorporate a side port to allow for flushing of sheaths and pressure monitoring from the sheath itself. Increasingly efficient backbleed valves provide a tight seal around the catheter, and even with the catheter removed or with only a guidewire inserted, there is little backbleeding. Yet, they cause little resistance to catheter insertion and manipulation.

These features make catheterization easier for both the physician and patient. Catheter changes are rapid, and there is reduction of both arterial trauma and the possibility of bleeding into the subcutaneous tissues during the catheterization procedure. Following use of thrombolytic and anticoagulant agents, the sheath may be left in place until coagulation status has returned to baseline or has been reversed by protamine. A sheath may be left in place to allow for rapid vascular access, as in

unstable cases or following PTCA, wherein reocclusion is a possibility and an emergency repeat dilation may be necessary. Detailed below are some of the features of different sheath and dilator designs. In Figure 7.9, several vascular sheaths and introducers are illustrated.

Dilators

A vascular dilator can be of various lengths and French sizes but must meet certain requirements. The dilator must be of hard plastic, usually Teflon or polyethylene, to allow passage through fibrous tissue or atherosclerotic or calcified arterial walls. The tip must be tapered smoothly to minimize the possibility of tearing the arterial wall.

The final tip taper and internal diameter of the dilator should closely fit the guidewire diameter to allow smooth advancement of the dilator over the wire with little blood between the wire and dilator lumen and minimal trauma to the vascular wall. In certain cases where considerable resistance to dilator insertion occurs, serial dilation with progressively

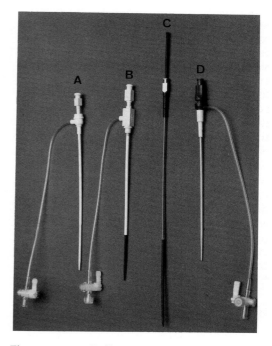

Figure 7.9. Different introducer-sheath designs. *A*, Cordis 8 Fr. *B*, USCI 8 Fr. *C*, USCI Desilets-Hoffman sheath for venous access. *D*, Terumo radifocus 8 Fr.

larger dilators may be beneficial. Most dilators have a female luer lock hub to allow secure attachment with the male luer connector of a syringe. Ideally, the French size of the dilator should be imprinted on the hub, or different dilators may be color coded according to size to permit rapid identification.

Sheaths

Vascular sheaths come in a variety of lengths and sizes, as illustrated in Figure 7.10. Size ranges from 5 Fr through 14 Fr are available, with the larger sizes used for insertion of intraaortic balloons or valvuloplasty balloon catheters. Lengths as short as 6 cm may be used for percutaneous brachial entry and longer sheaths (23 cm) for PTCA via tortuous iliac arteries with the femoral approach. In sheaths with side extensions the tubing is polyethylene and extends to a three-way stopcock, providing separate ports for pressure monitoring and flushing or administering medications. The sheath itself is made of a nonthrombogenic material, usually Teflon or polyethylene, which is extremely strong, thin, pliable, and radiolucent. The tip of the sheath is tapered by "pulling" while it is hot during manufacture. This minimizes trauma as the sheath is advanced over the dilator into the vessel. There are various hub designs as shown in Figure 7.11. One design, made by Arrow Inc., incorporates an accordion-like neck on the proximal end of the sheath to allow angulation of the hub without kinking the sheath itself. Others have a sleeve-like support at the neck region. If a backbleed valve is not incorporated, a luer lock hub should be present to allow attachment of a syringe or stopcock for aspiration or flushing. Separate backbleed valves are available for attachment to valveless sheaths when control of bleeding is necessary.

The hemostasis valves may be of several designs. Cordis has a "Unistasis valve" that is a one-piece valve that will not backbleed even with a thin wire through it. USCI has a hemaquet valve that consists of a rubber "0" ring, and other companies have recently introduced valves with a diaphragm consisting of multilayered overlapping sheets of rubber. The Terumo Radifocus Sheath has a valve consisting of a silicone plug with a crosscut for a tight seal with excellent lubricity.

Selection of a particular sheath is most

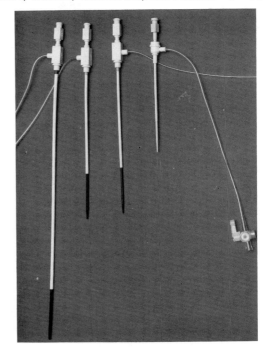

Figure 7.10. Variable sheath lengths and diameters, ranging from a USCI 9 Fr PTCA sheath on the left to a Cordis 7 Fr short percutaneous brachial sheath on the far right.

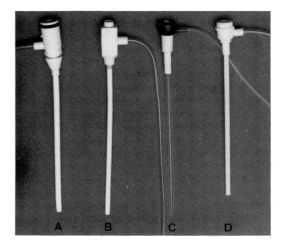

Figure 7.11. Different hub designs. *A*, Arrow 8.5 Fr. *B*, USCI 8 Fr. *C*, Terumo 8 Fr. *D*, Cordis 8 Fr.

often based on the quality of the hemostasis valve. Valves which are too tight or do not maintain lubricity tend to "grab" the catheter, interfering with insertion, withdrawal, and rotation. This may significantly impair the operator's ability to safely position an angiographic catheter. It is also important that the valve not be too loose such that bleeding occurs through the insertion port after catheter removal or when only an exchange wire as small as 0.035-inch in external diameter remains in the sheath. Regardless of the design, it is important to moisten the catheter frequently to keep the hemostasis valve lubricated during catheter insertion and manipulation. Selection of a catheter at least one size smaller than the sheath (e.g., 7 Fr catheter with an 8 Fr sheath) will also permit blood sampling and pressure recording from the sheath sidearm (e.g., during dye dilution studies or for simultaneous pressure recording).

Obturators

The Arrow Sheath System (Fig. 7.12) also incorporates an obturator and cap to be inserted for stabilization of the sheath when left in place for continued anticoagulation or pressure monitoring after the catheterization procedure. Presence of the obturator reduces compression and kinking of the sheath and the tendency for bleeding into the subcutaneous tissues around the sheath at the arterial puncture site. The obturator is 1.5 Fr size smaller in diameter than the sheath to allow side port pressure monitoring with the obturator inserted.

In summary, although a vascular sheath may, at first, seem like a very simple equipment item, there are certain features leading to selection of a product from a particular manufacturer. A well-designed sheath markedly facilitates the catheterization procedure, while a poor design may not only make the procedure more difficult but also may significantly increase the duration of the procedure and risk of complications.

CATHETERS

More than any other type of catheterization equipment, catheters are extremely diverse in shape, design, and specific features. This section will review some of the terminology used to describe catheters, basic principles of catheter construction, and the wide selection of catheter configuration and size currently available for cardiac angiography.

In describing the merits or demerits of a specific catheter, the catheterizing physician

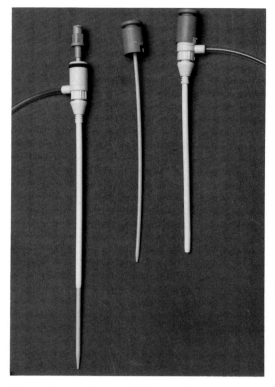

Figure 7.12.   Arrow 8.5 Fr sheath with 7 Fr obturator shown separately and inserted into the sheath. (Note: It has a twist lock cap).

or manufacturer relies on specific terminology applied to catheter performance. Listed below is a short glossary of terms that are frequently encountered in product literature and may be used in discussions in the remainder of this chapter.

Axial control—Ability to directly transmit forces from the end of the catheter to the tip.

Body—Segment of catheter between the tip and hub.

Contrast medium delivery or maximum flow rate—Ability to deliver high contrast material flow rates within a specified injection pressure range.

Flexibility—Ability of a section of catheter to bend on contact with a resistant surface.

Hub—Fitting on the proximal end of the catheter.

Internal diameter—Diameter of the internal lumen of the catheter; determines which guidewires can be accommodated and expected contrast medium delivery.

Maneuverability—Ability to advance a catheter around sharp bends or through tortuous vascular segments. Implies flexibility and torque control.

Memory—Ability to recover and maintain a specific configuration after insertion and guidewire removal.

Pliability—Ability to bend and to be shaped.

Pressure monitoring characteristics—Capacity to accurately transmit pressure from catheter tip to pressure transducer, a function of length, internal diameter, and catheter stiffness.

"Pushability" or power—Ability to directly transmit force applied to the hub of the catheter longitudinally to the tip. (Of considerable importance in balloon angioplasty catheters).

Radiopacity—Ability to visualize the catheter under x-ray fluoroscopic control.

Softness—Ability to easily bend. Incorporates flexibility and implies poor stiffness and poor memory.

Stability—Ability of a catheter to remain in position, a function of stiffness, memory, and matching of catheter configuration to anatomy.

Stiffness—Ability to resist bending, a lack of flexibility.

Strength—Ability to withstand high pressure injections. A term generally used in reference to angiographic catheters, which need to withstand high injection pressures associated with high contrast flow rates.

Support or backup—Ability to remain in position despite resistance, used in reference to angioplasty guide catheters when advancing a balloon catheter against resistance. A function of stiffness and configuration.

Tip—The final taper or distal end of the catheter. The part inserted into the patient first.

Torque control—Ability to directly transmit rotational forces from the end of the catheter to the tip. Synonymous with axial control.

Trackability—Ability of a catheter to follow a guidewire along its course through the vascular anatomy. A function of the proper combination of flexibility and pushability.

Catheter Components

A cardiac catheter is composed of several segments and parts, as illustrated in Figure 7.13. The body of the catheter is generally straight over most of its length and may have different configurations toward the tip. The bends in a catheter are called curves, and the terms primary, secondary etc. are applied to each additional curve away from the tip, as in Figure 7.13. The catheter tip is its most distal segment. Catheter tips may have any combination of a single end hole or closed end and any number of side holes. The presence of side holes allows for increased contrast delivery

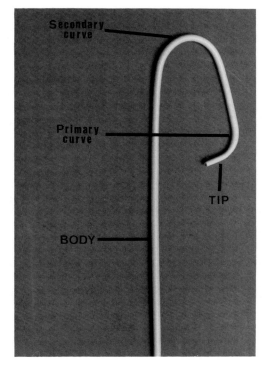

Figure 7.13. Sections of a catheter. The different sections on a Judkins left 4-cm (JL4) catheter are indicated.

with less tendency for catheter recoil. In the case of many end-hole catheters there is a taper over a short segment to allow catheter insertion over a guidewire directly through the skin. Catheters designed for insertion through an arteriotomy or sheath may not necessarily have a tapered tip. Newer catheter tip designs may incorporate grooved tips or a "soft tip" to be discussed in more detail later.

The hub of the catheter is bonded to the body and must have a strong, airtight seal. Specific design features include a female luer lock for syringe or manifold attachment, winged tips or squared hubs for easier rotation and handling, and imprinting of catheter specifications on the hub for easy identification (Fig. 7.14). The internal portion of the hub must have a smooth taper to facilitate guidewire insertion. In many designs the hub connection to the body of the catheter is reinforced by shrink tubing or a sleeve to decrease the chance of kinking or bending. Catheter specifications may also be imprinted on the sleeve.

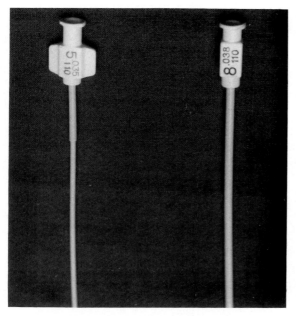

Figure 7.14. Catheter hubs. The hubs from a Cordis 5 Fr and 8 Fr pigtail catheter are shown to demonstrate the winged hub design and reinforcing sleeve on the 5 Fr catheter and the specifications imprinted on the hub of both catheters.

Principles of Catheter Construction

Cardiac catheters may be composed of one or several layers. In most multilayered designs one tube is stretched or "extruded" over another to form a bond. In catheters composed of several layers, the components determine performance characteristics (Fig. 7.15).

Most multilayered catheters consist of an inner tube of Teflon, over which is a layer of nylon, woven Dacron, or stainless steel braiding. A tube of polyethylene or polyurethane is then heated and extruded over the two inner layers to bond firmly as a third or external layer of the catheter. Others might consist of a polyurethane core covered by stainless steel braiding and an external polyurethane "jacket."

The inner layer provides a smooth surface through which guidewires and contrast agents may pass and should be nonthrombogenic. The thickness of the filaments and density of wire or nylon braiding in the middle layer and the type of plastic used determine the stiffness and torque control of the catheter. Some newer catheter designs involve a much thinner wall, allowing high flow characteris

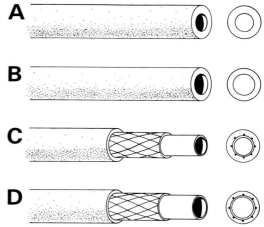

Figure 7.15. Basic catheter construction. Standard (*A*) and thin-walled (*B*) designs are shown above for a single-layer extruded catheter. Below are standard (*C*) and thin-walled (*D*) designs for a multilayered catheter with a braided stainless steel middle layer.

tics but less torque control and strength. This may be accomplished by incorporating the braiding into the inner layer and reducing the number or thickness of layers in the catheter wall. Use of a nylon layer or core imparts a stiffness to the catheter that is heat resistant, as in the Edwards "Uniweave" 6 Fr design and in some right heart and ventriculographic catheters.

Components of the external layer are also important determinants of catheter performance. The external layer must be impregnated with a radiopaque material such as barium or bismuth to provide the catheter with radiopacity for easy fluoroscopic visualization. This process may soften the catheter material and may produce fine pitting of the surface of the catheter, leading to increased thrombogenicity. To overcome this, materials may be incorporated into the middle layers of the catheter, or a coating of silicone or other nonthrombogenic material may be applied to the outer catheter surface.

Polyethylene and polyurethane impart very different characteristics to a catheter. Both are thermoplastic materials. Polyethylene is relatively resistant to the softening effect of radiopaque materials but can be softened by heating to allow reshaping for special tip configurations. Polyethylene is more easily extruded over the inner two catheter layers.

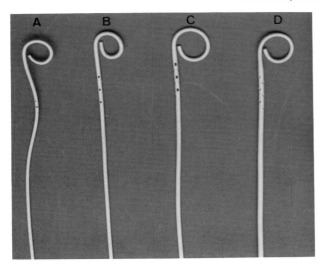

Figure 7.16. Catheter sizes. Four pigtail catheters are illustrated in order of increasing French size. *A*, 5 Fr. *B*, 6 Fr. *C*, 7 Fr. *D*, 8 Fr.

Due to its heat instability polyethylene must be gas sterilized. Polyurethane, being less resistant to heating, is claimed to provide a catheter with better memory and yet is a softer material due to more random molecular alignment. This softness is particularly desirable at the catheter tip to reduce risk of arterial trauma during selective positioning. Now that most catheters are preformed in a large variety of configurations and intended for one-time use, reshaping by heating is rarely needed, and polyurethane is the more common material used in catheters for selective angiography.

Catheter Sizes

Diameter

Catheters for angiographic use are sized by external and internal diameter and length. The internal diameter is specified either by actual diameter in thousandths of an inch or by the maximum diameter guidewire in millimeters which can be passed through the catheter. With newer thin-walled catheter designs, a much larger internal lumen to external diameter ratio can be achieved. This has resulted in catheters which can accommodate much more rapid contrast agent flow rates and has led to the use of smaller diameter catheters for angiography.

External diameter is expressed in French sizes which are obtained by multiplying the actual diameter in millimeters by 3.0. Conversely, the actual size of any catheter in millimeters may be calculated by dividing its French size by 3.0 (e.g., 9 Fr is 3.0 mm in diameter). French sizes from 5 through 8 are currently used for diagnostic angiography. The relative differences in size are illustrated in Figure 7.16. In Table 7.2 the internal and external diameters of conventional and thin-walled designs in various French sizes are compared. From the table it is obvious that the thin-walled design allows for potentially greater contrast flow rates, enhancing opacification and improving potential for diagnostic quality angiograms. It has also allowed for routine use of smaller diameter catheters that theoretically result in smaller arterial punctures, less time to achieve hemostasis after catheter removal, and less trauma to the vessel wall. Smaller catheters have been advocated for use in outpatient catheterization, but their potential advantages have not been substantiated in controlled clinical trials (1, 2).

In order to maintain catheter control, as noted previously, the thin-walled designs incorporate much stiffer plastics and, hence, reduce the pliability of the catheter tip. This decreases the ability to position the catheters in anatomical orientations not perfectly matched to the catheter configuration. Secondly, there is some concern that these stiffer catheter tips may increase the chance of arterial injury during selective coronary intubation. Some manufacturers have, therefore, included a soft tip design in an attempt to overcome this problem while maintaining stiffness in the body and curvatures necessary for catheter tip placement. Although conceptually attractive, this modification has yet

Table 7.2
External and Lumen Diameter Measurements in Standard and Thin-Walled Catheters

French	External Diameter		Internal Diameter			
Size	(inches)	(mm)	Standard		Thin-Walled	
			inches	mm	inches	mm
5	0.065	1.67	0.026	0.66	0.034	0.86
6	0.078	2.00	0.036	0.91	0.046	1.17
7	0.091	2.33	0.046	1.17	0.058	1.47
8	0.104	2.67	0.056	1.42	0.068	1.73
9	0.118	3.00	0.064	1.63	0.078	1.98

to be proven advantageous in controlled clinical trials (3).

Length

Catheters vary in length, depending on configuration and purpose and on the route of insertion (brachial vs. femoral). Most frequently used pigtail catheters are 110 cm in length whereas Judkins catheters are 100 cm in length. Most frequently used brachial catheters are 80 or 100 cm in length. Variations in length occur with catheters for other specific designs or purposes.

Configuration

Numerous catheter configurations are available for ventriculography, large vessel angiography, and selective coronary angiography. A detailed discussion of all of the many catheters used is not possible, but an overview of available catheter selections from the brachial and femoral approach will be provided.

Specific Types
Central Venous Catheters

Catheters for central venous access are often not routinely stocked in catheterization laboratories, but rather in critical care areas, where they are frequently used. These are short (usually 20 to 30 cm) catheters designed for insertion into the internal jugular, subclavian, or brachial antecubital vein. They are intended for longer-term access to the central venous system for measurement of central venous pressure and administration of nutrients or medications.

Currently used catheters are made of soft material, such as polyurethane, Teflon, or Silastic and, hence, will soften with body temperature in situ. Newer versions of central venous catheters incorporate more than one lumen. Triple-lumen catheters (Fig. 7.17) are now frequently used in critical care units, where a 16-gauge lumen should be available for administration of blood products and two 18-gauge lumens should be available for administration of crystalloids or medications. External sizing ranges from pediatric 4 Fr to adult 7 Fr. These catheters are very useful items in intensive care unit settings but do carry a small risk of central venous or right heart perforation. Although new designs involve softer materials, the importance of proper positioning and maintaining the tip at the superior vena cava right atrial junction should be emphasized.

Balloon Flotation Catheters

Since the introduction of the balloon flotation catheter by Swan and Ganz in 1970, numerous developments have occurred. The use of a flow-directed catheter for right heart catheterization without fluoroscopic control has significantly advanced management of patients in intensive care units.

In addition, when conventional right heart catheters cannot be directed into the pulmonary artery, a balloon flotation catheter will often be successful. This factor and the ease of obtaining a pulmonary-capillary wedge pressure have led to use of the flotation catheter as the first choice for right heart catheterization in many laboratories.

Most balloon flotation catheters are made from polyvinyl chloride (PVC) in a multiple extrusion, multilumen construction. The PVC is soft and becomes softer in situ when warmed by body temperature. The balloon is usually composed of latex and has inflated volumes ranging from 0.8 to 2.2 cc. The balloon is positioned within several millimeters

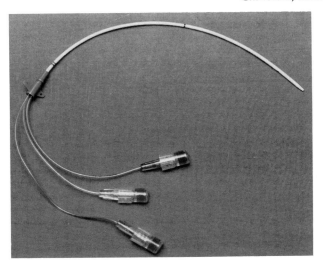

Figure 7.17. A 7 Fr triple-lumen central venous catheter 30 cm long (Cardiomed).

of the tip to reduce contact of the tip with the myocardium during advancement. Catheters vary in length and diameter from 60 cm 5 Fr for pediatric use to 110 cm 7 Fr for use in adults.

The catheter has a minimum of one lumen for balloon inflation and additional lumens according to intended use. A Berman angiographic catheter (Fig. 7.18) has its second lumen for injection of radiographic contrast and has no end hole but has multiple side holes to help prevent catheter recoil during rapid injection of contrast material.

Balloon flotation pacing catheters may have a second channel for wires leading to the two electrodes at the catheter tip (Fig. 7.19). Balloon catheters for cardiac output determination by thermodilution technique (Fig. 7.20) have a lumen for pressure measurement from the tip, a thermistor placed about 4 cm from the tip, and a proximal port (20 to 30 cm from tip) for measurement of pressure in proximal chambers (right atrium) and injection of indicator. In some models, incorporation of two additional lumens and side ports allows for transcatheter placement of right ventricular and right atrial pacing wires for ventricular or A-V sequential pacing. A comparison of three balloon catheter tips is illustrated in Figure 7.21.

Right Heart Catheters

Several right heart catheters are shown in Figure 7.22. The Cournand catheter is a thin-walled, woven Dacron, polyethylene or poly-urethane, single end-hole catheter designed specifically for right heart catheterization. It can be used for selective blood sampling, and with its single end hole can be used for obtaining pulmonary-capillary wedge pressure measurements with excellent pressure-monitoring characteristics.

Gorlin and Zucker catheters have configurations similar to that of the Cournand catheter but incorporate electrodes near the tip for optional cardiac pacing or simultaneous measurement of intracardiac pressures and electrograms. The Goodale-Lubin catheter is very similar to the Cournand catheter, except that it has two side holes close to the tip in addition to its end hole.

Transseptal Catheters

The transseptal catheter was developed specifically for crossing from right to left atrium through the interatrial septum at the fossa ovalis. The transseptal, or Brocken-brough, catheter is advanced over a Brocken-brough needle for left atrial catheterization. The catheter must then be manipulated from left atrium to left ventricle directly, or assisted by a 0.035-inch guidewire. The Brocken-brough needle (Fig. 7.23) is 18-gauge in its shaft and tapers to 21-gauge at its tip. It has a central lumen for blood sampling and pressure measurement and at its proximal end has a flange with a pointer to indicate tip direction.

The Brockenbrough catheter is constructed from Teflon and is more rigid than

Figure 7.18. A 7 Fr Berman
angiographic catheter (*arrow*).

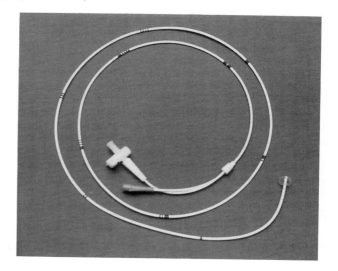

Figure 7.19. A 5 Fr Swan-Ganz bipolar
pacing catheter (Edwards).

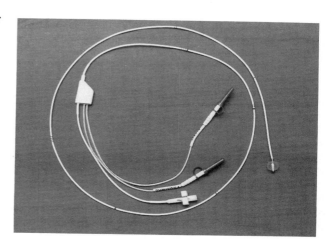

Figure 7.20. A 7 Fr Sorenson
thermodilution catheter (Abbof).

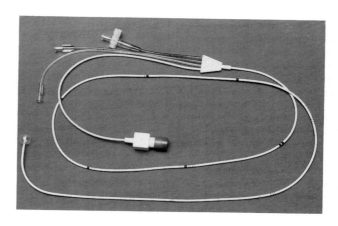

conventional catheters. It has a tapered tip with an end hole and from two to six side holes for angiography. The catheter tip is curved to facilitate advancement from left atrium to ventricle. Catheters are available with different curves to accommodate variations in left atrial size. Standard radii of curvature of 2.0, 2.5, and 3.0 cm are available. Comparative sizing is illustrated in Figure 7.24.

The transseptal catheter concept has been modified to a sheath design to facilitate insertion of different catheters into the left atrium or ventricle. The Mullins sheath and introducer, along with the Brockenbrough needle, are shown in Figure 7.23. The introducer is advanced over the needle in a fashion similar to that of the transseptal catheter. The sheath is then advanced, along with the introducer, across the septum. Sheath sizes range from 6 Fr to 8 Fr with internal diameters of 0.078 inch to 0.104 inch, respectively. The 8 Fr sheath will accommodate a 7 Fr catheter of conventional or balloon flotation type.

Angiographic Catheters

Numerous ventricular catheters are illustrated in Figure 7.25. The NIH catheter is a thick-walled, closed-end, rounded-tip catheter with four to six side holes at the tip. This catheter can be easily maneuvered and positioned directly through a sheath or cutdown. It is useful for crossing stenotic valves, and with a closed end, is stable during high flow injections. It is frequently used from the brachial approach for right or left ventriculography and angiography in any of the major vessels. It has excellent pressure-monitoring and angiographic characteristics.

The Gensini catheter is a thin-walled woven Dacron catheter with an open end and six side holes. It is useful in crossing the aortic valve from the brachial approach, where guidewire assistance is necessary, and it is well suited to high-flow contrast studies. The Lehman ventriculography catheter consists of a woven Dacron core and has a flexible, tapered, closed-end tip with four side holes. Its primary use is in crossing the aortic valve from the brachial approach and can be used for left ventriculography and ascending aortography.

Pigtail catheters are primarily used for high-flow contrast studies and achieve

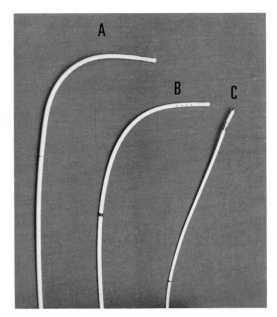

Figure 7.21. Comparison of catheter tips from: *A*, Sorenson thermodilution. *B*, Berman angiographic. *C*, Swan-Ganz pacing.

stability through their curled-tip design and multiple side holes. The curled end may be in a normal or tight radius configuration. The distal catheter segment can be straight or angled to allow easier entry into the left ventricle from the aorta, particularly in cases of aortic stenosis in which the left ventricle assumes a horizontal orientation. These angles are generally 145 or 155°. The number of side holes varies considerably with different designs and influences the contrast flow rates that can be achieved at a given injection pressure. Addition of more than eight side holes provides little advantage and increases the chance of thrombus formation on the catheter. This catheter has to be flushed forcefully to ensure that the flush will include the end hole and not just the side holes.

Coronary Angiographic Catheters

Coronary angiographic catheters can be grouped into numerous series: Sones, Judkins, Amplatz, multipurpose, and bypass graft. The general features are reviewed below.

Sones catheters (Fig. 7.26) were initially designed for insertion via brachial artery cutdown, as described in Chapter 6, and more recently have been modified for percutaneous

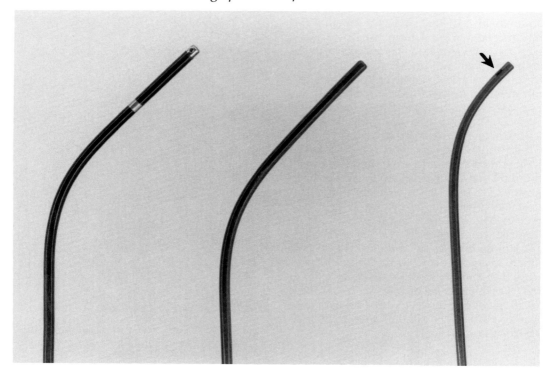

Figure 7.22. Right heart catheters. *A*, Zucker. *B*, Cournand. *C*, Goodale-Lubin.

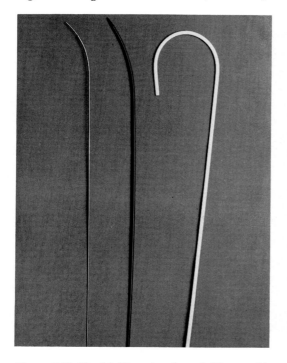

Figure 7.23. The Mullins sheath and dilator with Brockenbrough transseptal needle.

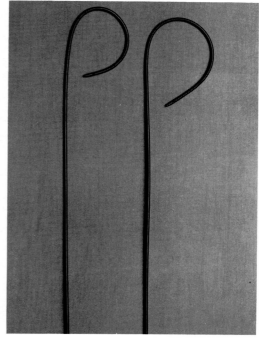

Figure 7.24. Brockenbrough transseptal catheters showing different tip curvatures.

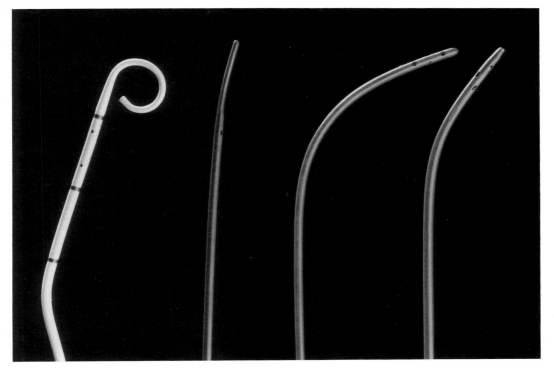

Figure 7.25.   Ventriculographic catheters: *A*, Pigtail. *B*, Lehman ventricular. *C*, NIH. *D*, Gensini.

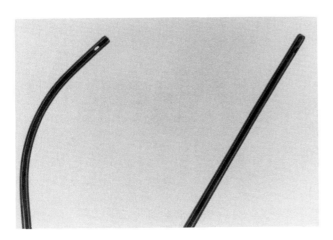

Figure 7.26.   Sones catheters.

Figure 7.27. Judkins left coronary
catheters: *A*, JL3.5. *B*, JL4. *C*, JL5.

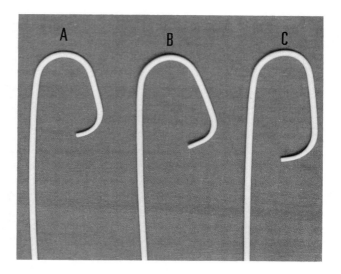

brachial insertion via a sheath system. Original construction was based on a woven
Dacron design, but polyurethane and
polyethylene may also be used. The percutaneous systems are frequently layered with
external polyethylene or polyurethane coats
(see Chapter 13).

The Judkins catheters (Figs. 7.27 and 7.28)
are intended for insertion over a wire from a
femoral percutaneous approach. The principal
advantage of Judkins catheters lies in their
ability to naturally seek the coronary orifice
when advanced into the respective sinus of
Valsalva. The specifics of the Judkins technique are discussed in Chapter 13.

The Amplatz configurations and sizes for
left and right coronaries are shown in Figure
7.29 and 7.30, respectively. The Amplatz
catheters are particularly useful in situations
in which Judkins catheters are not suited to a
given anatomical variation, particularly when
the coronary artery originates from high in
the sinus of Valsalva. The Amplatz configurations have also been adapted for use from the
brachial approach in situations in which the
Sones catheter cannot be manipulated into the
coronary orifice.

The multipurpose catheter (Schoonmaker
and King, single catheter technique) (Fig.
7.31) is relatively unique from the femoral
approach in its use for both ventriculography
and selective coronary angiography. It can also
be used for aortography, although the jet of
contrast from the end hole may artificially

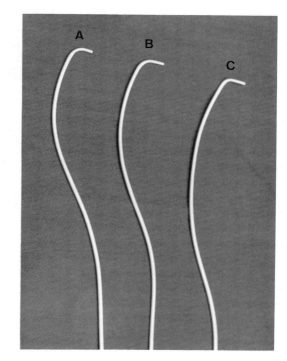

Figure 7.28. Judkins right coronary catheters: *A*,
JR4. *B*, JR5. *C*, JR6.

magnify the severity of aortic insufficiency as
assessed angiographically. As can been seen
in Figure 7.31, the multipurpose catheter is
comparable with the Sones catheter in configuration and is manipulated in similar fashion.

Saphenous vein bypass graft and internal

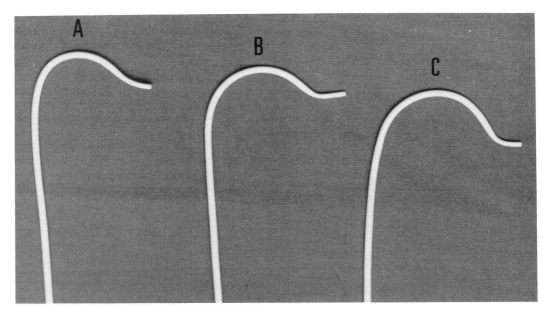

Figure 7.29. Amplatz left coronary catheters: *A*, ALI. *B*, ALII. *C*, ALIII.

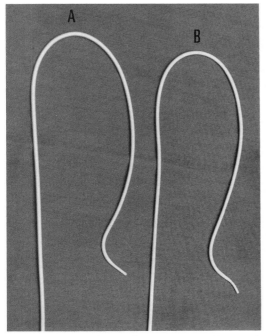

Figure 7.30. Amplatz right coronary catheters: *A*, ARI. *B*, ARII.

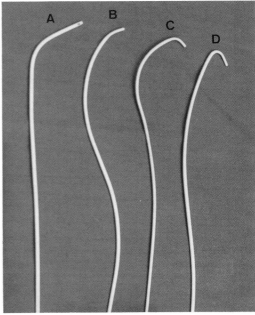

Figure 7.31. Multipurpose and bypass graft catheters. *A*, Multipurpose. *B*, Right bypass. *C*, Left bypass. *D*, Internal mammary artery.

mammary artery catheters are available in several designs (Fig. 7.31). Separate configurations are available for venous bypass grafts to the right and left coronary arteries and for selective internal mammary angiography. Use of these catheters requires considerable expertise for proper manipulation.

SUMMARY

In summary, there is an extensive selection of catheters available for use from both the brachial and femoral approach. A thorough knowledge of the specific indications for the different configurations enhances the operator's ability to consistently position a catheter where desired and obtain a high quality angiographic study. Many of these technical considerations will be detailed in other chapters.

References

1. Molajo AO, Ward C, Bray CL, Dobson D. Comparison of the performance of superflow (5F) and conventional 8F catheter for cardiac catheterization by the femoral route. Cathet Cardiovasc Diagn 1987;13:275–276.

2. Brown RIG, MacDonald AC. Use of 5 French catheters for cardiac catheterization and coronary angiography. Cathet Cardiovasc Diagn 1987;13:214–217.

3. Finci L, Meier B, Steffenino G, Rutishauser W. Clinical evaluation of soft–tipped catheters for coronary angiography. Cathet Cardiovasc Diagn 1986;12:347–351

8

Radiographic Techniques Used in Cardiac Catheterization

David Holmes, M.D.
Merrill A. Wondrow[a]
Paul R. Julsrud, M.D.

Cardiac catheterization has changed rapidly over the past 10 years (1–3). With the introduction of interventional techniques, such as percutaneous transluminal coronary angioplasty (PTCA), the demands on radiographic equipment have become more stringent (4, 5). These demands are being met by advances in both video and cine imaging capabilities (6-9). The invasive cardiologist must be familiar with radiographic techniques and principles to be able to understand the benefits and limitations of the imaging chain, to relate to support personnel, and to maximize equipment performance.

ANGIOGRAPHIC EQUIPMENT

Angiographic equipment has changed substantially. In the past, floating tabletop/rotational cradle combinations were used exclusively. These systems had the advantage of improved protection from radiation and short source-to-image distance (Fig. 8.1). This type of system subsequently was modified by mechanically coupling the image intensifier and x-ray tube. This modification allowed for cranial and caudal angulation in the sagittal plane. Such angulation is essential for optimal assessment of different segments of the coronary anatomy (10, 11).

These modified systems have had significant advantages. The proximal left anterior descending coronary artery could be seen very well, particularly in a cranial left anterior oblique (LAO) view. When the patient was rotated, rather than the equipment rotated, into a LAO view, the heart shifted off of the spine. This counterclockwise rotation of the heart allowed the proximal left anterior descending artery to be seen well, with improved visualization of fine details. Another major advantage was easy access for a brachial artery approach. Other advantages were that the cradle could be rotated and the tabletop moved faster than the imaging equipment itself. Finally, access to the patient's head and airway was easier.

However, these systems had disadvantages. For some patients, rotation was uncomfortable and disturbing, particularly the tight straps required to permit rotation without patient movement within the cradle. During rotation of the patient, catheter position, particularly with a Sones catheter, could be lost. In addition, to change cranial and caudal angulation required manual manipulation of the tower itself. Finally, the degree of sagittal plane angulation was limited to approximately 30° cranial and 10° to 15° caudal.

Most newer cardiac laboratories have x-ray equipment that rotates around the patient. Various configurations are available including, among others, an L-U arm combination, a U arm with a parallelogram, and a C arm with rotation around two axes (Fig. 8.2). These

[a]Associate, Mayo Clinic and Mayo Foundation.

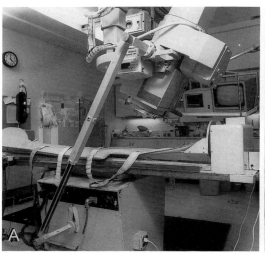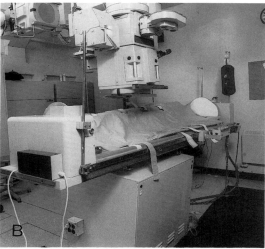

Figure 8.1. (*A*, Floating tabletop with rotational cradle. This system had the advantage of a short source-to-image distance. Sagittal plane angulation was not possible without the use of a wedge. *B*, To obtain cranial or caudal sagittal plane angulation, the image intensifier and the x-ray tube were mechanically coupled.

systems allow for maximal angulated views and excellent catheter stability because the patient is not moved. For some patients, the flat table is also more comfortable than the rotating cradle with its straps. In addition, the operator can adjust the cranial and caudal angulations from the table itself.

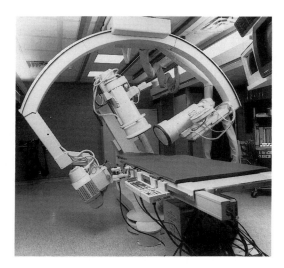

Figure 8.2. Current laboratory equipment that rotates around the patient. Various configurations are available, including a biplane L-U-C arm system, as shown here.

The disadvantages are a longer source-to-image distance and increased radiation exposure (12). It is more difficult to perform brachial artery procedures, particularly if biplane angiography is used. Other disadvantages include less than optimal access to the patient's head and airway. This is a substantial problem in critically ill patients who require ventilator support. Another problem is the fact that, even though multiple angulated views can be achieved, the proximal left anterior descending coronary artery may not be seen as well because the heart does not move relative to the spine (as it does when the patient is rotated to the LAO position with a cradle). Because of the importance of this view, particularly with PTCA, we have combined a rotational equipment support system with a rotational cradle (Fig. 8.3). This cradle allows for table rotation up to 30°. This combination provides excellent visualization of all aspects of the coronary arterial tree, particularly the proximal left anterior descending coronary artery in the LAO view.

The choice between **biplane** and **monoplane** equipment depends on the purpose of the laboratory as well as on operator preference. All of our rooms have biplane capability. This allows simultaneous orthogonal biplane angiography of the left ventricle, ascending aorta, and other cardiac structures. All left ventriculograms are recorded by using 30° right anterior oblique (RAO) and 60° LAO views. This allows assessment of more segments of the left ventricle than would be possible with a single-plane RAO view alone. Because coronary artery disease produces heterogeneous effects on regional left ventricular function, biplane views are important (13, 14). This is particularly the case in assessing the effect of reperfusion on ventricular function (13). In these patients, improvements may be seen in either the RAO or LAO views. The two projections are complementary, providing information about regional function not obtained from either view alone. Septal and posterolateral walls are not seen in the RAO view. If a biplane system is not available, the left ventricular angiogram may be repeated, once in the RAO view and once in the LAO view. This has the disadvantages of increasing the amounts of contrast agent, radiation, and time required.

For biplane left ventricular angiography, we **view both images on a single monitor** (15). The images from the anteroposterior and lateral video cameras are transmitted to a biplane video switcher. This allows them to be synchronized temporally for display on a single monitor. A common video-synchronizing generator drives a timing and control device to achieve synchronization (Fig. 8.4). Biplane imaging is being used with increasing frequency during other procedures. In transseptal catheterization, it facilitates safer entry into the left atrium. It is also used with increasing frequency in PTCA, although it is not essential. Optimal views in each plane are "frozen" for review. Recording of the angles used to obtain the diagnostic shots is helpful in setting up these optimal views. During dilation it may not be necessary to move the imaging equipment at all, except to switch from one video projection to the other. Biplane recordings cannot be used during dilation performed from the arm because the lateral tube interferes with operator position.

IMAGE SYSTEM

During imaging, radiation produced by the x-ray tube is attenuated as it passes through the patient (Fig. 8.4). This attenuated radiation is then detected by the image intensifier tube, which converts the x-ray energy (photons) to a

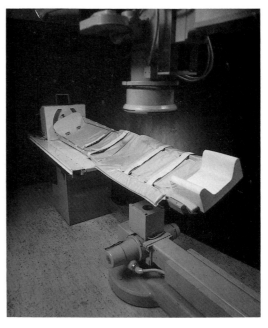

Figure 8.3. To improve cranial angulation images of the proximal left anterior descending artery, a modified cradle may be added to the system.

light image that is coupled optically to the detector. An automatic brightness control that senses directly from the image intensifier output is used to maintain video output and cine-film darkening over a wide range. In addition to the automatic brightness control, we use a manual iris to optimize the video image (15).

Cardiac imaging places unique demands on the imaging system. Because the structures to be visualized are moving rapidly, for example, the coronary arteries, exposure times should be short to avoid blurring caused by motion. If the catheterization suite is used for pediatric as well as adult patients, the demands are even greater. In pediatric patients with rapid heart rates, an exposure time of 2 to 3 msec is required; in adults, an exposure time of 5 msec or less is usually satisfactory.

X-Ray Generation
X-Ray Generator

The x-ray generator produces the power that accelerates electrons in the x-ray tube. Various generators are available for cardiovascular applications. There are advantages and

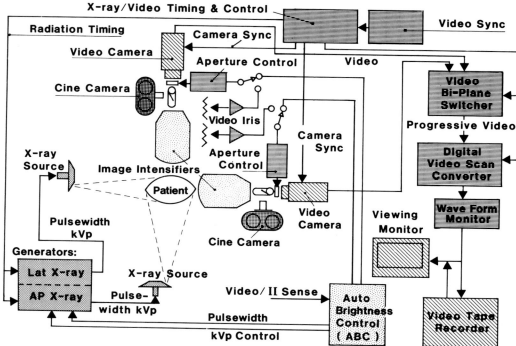

Figure 8.4. Block diagram of a cardiac biplane video/cine imaging system. A common video-synchronizing generator drives a timing-and-control device. This is necessary to achieve synchronization and also is essential for progressive scanning. (From Julsrud PR, Wondrow MA, Stears JG, Gray JE, Zahasky PE. X-ray equipment. In: Holmes DR Jr, Vlietstra RE, eds. Interventional cardiology. Philadelphia: FA Davis Company, Chap. 3, 1988. By permission of Mayo Foundation.)

disadvantages to each type. Selection of the appropriate one depends on the equipment design, x-ray tube selected, and intended use of the room. Constant-potential and pulsed generators are both suitable. Important considerations include kVp, mA, and kW ratings and characteristics of timing. These specifications can be obtained from the manufacturers. Recommended minimal requirements are given in Table 8.1.

X-Ray Tube

There also is wide variability in x-ray tubes among different manufacturers and in types by the same manufacturer. Selection of the appropriate tube depends on the generator and on the major purpose of the room. Rooms designed for interventional procedures have somewhat different requirements than rooms designed only for diagnostic purposes. This has led some authors to suggest that there should be designated interventional rooms and other designated diagnostic rooms (16).

However, few laboratories can afford the luxury of a designated interventional room. In addition, there is increased emphasis on combined diagnostic and therapeutic procedures, such as PTCA at the same time as initial diagnostic angiography (17). Therefore, given the

Table 8.1
Generators

Feature	Value
kVp	
Minimum	40
Maximum	150
mA	
Maximum	200 rms
Timing	
Maximum exposure time (pulsed, msec)	5 (grid base)
kW rating	
At 80 kVp	100
Automatic exposure control	mA-kVp combined

ᵃ rms, root mean square.

expanding scope of interventional catheterization practice, at our institution all new angiographic suites are suitable for both diagnostic and therapeutic procedures.

Various tubes are available. New advances include ceramic and graphite tubes and modified support structures. These tubes are significantly more expensive than conventional tubes but have the advantage of longer tube life and higher heat load capacity. The importance of sufficient heat load capacity and cooling capacity must be emphasized. If these are not sufficient, procedures will be prolonged in order to allow the units to return to normal temperatures during the procedure, and tube life probably will be shortened. Current tubes should be selected with a heat load capacity of 1.0 to 1.5 million heat units.

Focal spot sizes also vary. They should be between 0.5 and 1.0 mm for fluoroscopy and cineangiography. Smaller focal spots, 0.2 or 0.3 mm, may enhance resolution. Operating at smaller focal spot sizes increases the demand for adequate cooling because of increased heat production. Heat capacity should be monitored during procedures. If it decreases substantially, extra time between angiographic filming sessions may be required. Off-focal spot radiation may be a significant problem. During acceptance evaluation, we test each tube to ensure that off-focal spot radiation is absent. Our recommended specification minima for x-ray tubes are shown in Table 8.2. These specifications should be obtained from the manufacturers prior to purchase of new x-ray tubes.

The interface between x-ray generator and tube is undergoing considerable change (6, 8). In the past, video images and pulsed cine images have been achieved by secondary electronic switching. The x-ray pulse produced by secondary electronic switching has a prolonged decay (Fig. 8.5). This is the result of the capacitive characteristics of the high-voltage cables between the generator and x-ray tube that must be charged and discharged during each exposure. Secondary electronic switching does not suffice for pulsed fluoroscopy or for cineangiography when the x-ray output per exposure is relatively small. To solve these problems, a preferred alternative design is grid control of x-ray production (Fig. 8.6). With this system, the grid of the x-ray tube controls the length of the exposure. This

Table 8.2
Minimum Specifications of X-ray Tubes

Feature	Value
Focal spot size, mm	
Small	0.5
Large	1.0
Star measurements for testing	Yes
Rating, kW	
Small focal spot	40–60
Large focal spot	80–100
Anode characteristics	
Angles	
Small focal spot	7°
Large focal spot	7°
Heat capacity	700,000 heat units
Cooling rate (maximum)	150,000 heat units/min
Housing characteristics	
Heat capacity	1,750,000 heat units
Cooling capacity with liquid circulation system maximum	150,000 heat units/min

eliminates prolongation of the x-ray rise and fall times at all exposure rates and pulse widths.

Image Intensifier

The image intensifier converts an x-ray image into a visible light image. It is an evacuated bell-shaped glass tube or envelope that contains an input and an output phosphor. X-ray photons passing through the patient interact with the input phosphor, which produces light photons. These light photons are then converted to electrons by the photocathode in the image intensifier to produce an electronic image. This image is focused by high-voltage potentials onto the output phosphor.

There have been major improvements in image intensifier technology (4, 7). Modern cesium iodide input phosphors and improved conversion factors have allowed lower cine exposure rates. The x-ray tube should deliver 20 to 40 mr per cineframe to the image intensifier in the 5- to 7-inch field of view ideally at 75 to 85 kVp and 2 to 6 mr per video frame. Improved resolution has been achieved by use of columnar separation of phosphor crystals and low-absorption metallic input windows.

Veiling glare and **detective quantum** efficiency are important considerations that affect image intensifier performance. Veiling glare is

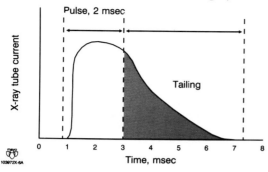

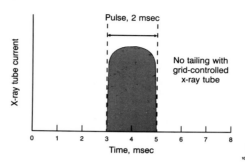

Figure 8.5. Secondary high-voltage electronic switching is often used to generate pulsed x-rays. The x-ray pulse produced in this manner has a prolonged decay that is the result of cable capacitance and varying x-ray tube current. (From Julsrud PR, Wondrow MA, Stears JG, Gray JE, Zahasky PE. X-ray equipment. In: Holmes DR Jr, Vlietstra RE, eds. Interventional cardiology. Philadelphia: FA Davis Company, Chapter 3, 1988. By permission of Mayo Foundation.)

Figure 8.6. Grid-controlled system can be used to produce x-rays. Since a grid in the x-ray tube performs the switching, the high-voltage cables remain constantly charged. X-rays produced in this fashion are of short duration and do not have the "tailing" seen in Figure 8.5. With this system and progressive scanning, a snapshot picture can be obtained. (From Julsrud PR, Wondrow MA, Stears JG, Gray JE, Zahasky PE. X-ray equipment. In: Holmes DR Jr, Vlietstra RE, eds. Interventional cardiology. Philadelphia: FA Davis Company, Chapter 3, 1988. By permission of Mayo Foundation.)

caused by extraneous light from internal image intensifier light scatter; this extraneous light degrades the image. Use of gray glass at the output phosphor and fiber optic coupling decreases veiling glare (16). Detective quantum efficiency is the efficiency with which the input phosphor absorbs x-ray photons. Improved detective quantum efficiency is characterized by a decrease in image noise at constant entrance exposure. Because keeping entrance x-ray exposure constant and low is important, improved detective quantum efficiency has been achieved by finding an optimal cesium iodide input phosphor thickness. Although increasing the thickness of the input phosphor will increase the absorption of x-rays, lateral light scatter is inversely proportional to input phosphor thickness. Therefore, there must be a balance between increasing thickness to improve x-ray absorption and decreasing thickness to minimize lateral light scatter.

Contrast ratio is an important factor in assessing image quality. This ratio is measured by placing a lead disc in the x-ray field to completely block a portion of the field from radiation. The light level is measured in the blocked area. The ratio of the intensities measured without the lead disc and with the

lead disc in place is the contrast ratio. Both large area and small area contrast ratios are measured by using either a disc that covers 10% of the input screen or a smaller disc (10 mm). The contrast ratio should be at least 20:1.

As was true for pulse generators and x-ray tubes, image intensifiers can be rated with the information obtained from the manufacturers. The minimal specifications are shown in Table 8.3.

Table 8.3
Minimal Specifications
for Image Intensifiers

Feature	Value
Input field size, inches (cm)	
Small	4.5 (11.4)
Medium	6.0 (15.2)
Large	9.0 (22.9)
Resolution cycles/min	
Small field center	5.3
Medium field center	4.6
Large field center	4.0
Conversion factor	
Medium field	100
Contrast ratio	
Small area	20:1

Optical Systems

The basic optical subsystem in an image chain consists of an objective lens and a camera lens. These lenses gather light generated in the image intensifier and focus it onto an image detector. To accomplish this, the output screen of the image intensifier tube is located at the focal point of the objective lens. Therefore, all light rays emerging from the objective lens are parallel. The camera lens then collects the parallel light rays and forms an image at its focal plane.

Camera lenses of different focal lengths are available. The selection of the focal length depends on the degree of overframing used. Horizontal overframing is usually used to increase magnification and to eliminate marginal image area.

Optical systems are rated by their relative aperture size. Optical systems for cardiac imaging have apertures ranging from f-20 to f-75. The smaller the f-stop, the faster the lens. A fast lens has a large effective diameter and allows more light to pass through it. However, the lens aperture size determines the depth of the field, and if the aperture is large, the depth of the field in sharp focus is limited. As the aperture size decreases, the range of image sharpness increases. If the aperture size is too small (i.e., high f-stop), however, more radiation will be required to produce diagnostic images. Decreased contrast and resolution can also result from veiling glare in the optical subsystem. Use of an antireflective coating may minimize this.

Video Systems

The video system consists of a video camera, a monitor, and a recording system. These systems have become more important as use of interventional procedures has increased (8, 9). Being able to visualize fine details of complex coronary anatomy is essential. This is particularly true in laboratories in which PTCA is performed at the same time as diagnostic coronary angiography. As video technology advances, it is likely that it will replace cinefilm.

Video Camera

The television camera pickup tube is one of the most important components in the video chain. It consists of a target and an electron gun. The target itself has two layers, a photoconductive layer and a signal plate. The metallic signal plate is applied to the inner surface of the faceplate. This layer must be thin enough to allow light photons to penetrate it but must be thick enough to hold an electrical charge. The photoconductive layer is applied to the signal plate. The electrical resistance of this layer changes in proportion to the intensity of the light transmitted through the signal plate. During operation, the image from the output phosphor of the image intensifier is projected through the faceplate onto the target. The intensity of the light photons changes the resistance in the photoconductive layer. The electron gun beam scans the photoconductive layer, recharging the target to near equilibrium. The final video signal is proportional to the recharge current on the photoconductive layer.

Target material and design, faceplate, and gun structure determine the performance characteristics of the pickup tube. Important considerations include lag or image retention time, signal dynamic range, contrast, and sensitivity. Lag or image retention is the result of failure of the initial scan to neutralize the charge on the photoconductive layer completely. Minimal lag will give the sharpest image for viewing rapidly moving cardiac structures. Conventional Vidicon tubes are less efficient in neutralizing the charge on the photoconductive layer and thus have inherently more lag than Plumbicon tubes or tubes with newer target materials such as selenium arsenic tellurium (Saticon) and selenium tellurium arsenic (Primicon). These newer targets have the best lag characteristics, i.e., not more than 10% of the peak video signal in the third video field.

The signal dynamic range is a measure of image brightness and is expressed as the ratio of the logarithms of maximum brightness and minimum brightness. Contrast sensitivity also depends on target and faceplate design. Newer tubes have excellent contrast sensitivity in addition to good dynamic range and lag specifications.

Image stabilization is as important during video imaging as during cine recording. Various approaches to this are available. Burnout, saturation, and blooming are specific problems, particularly during "panning," when portions of the lung field are included in the

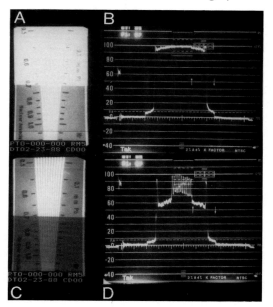

Figure 8.7. Adjustment of the video waveform is performed by an x-ray technician. Video image (*A*) and waveform (*B*) have improper manual iris settings and show saturation. The proper waveform and image are seen with optimal settings (*C* and *D*).

field of view. During panning, careful attention to minimizing the amount of lung in the field of view is essential. Use of radiation-absorbing filters also can help, particularly during digital image processing when panning is not used but when there is overlap with the lung field. Automatic exposure and gain controls are also useful. In addition, recent changes in amplifier design which prevent saturation may be helpful (6). These designs require adequate overrange capability in the pickup tube and preamplifier. An electron-processing stage is then used to compress the highlighted signals. In our system, the video waveform is monitored and adjusted with a manual iris to give optimal images (Fig. 8.7) (15). Expert in-house technical assistance is required for this approach to optimize the image.

A major factor affecting the optimal design of the video imaging system is selection of the video line scan rate. High-line rate (1023-line) systems have been given increasing attention, although there are few data comparing high-line rate and 525-line systems (16, 18, 19). Some of the differences between these are subjective, and some are related to failure to optimize whichever system is in use (18). If a 1023-line system is used, the video band width must be increased to keep vertical and horizontal resolutions equal. The video bandwidth must be 20 to 25 mHz, as compared with 10 to 15 mHz for a 525-line system. With this increase in video amplifier bandwidth, the signal-to-noise ratio decreases significantly to below the 45 to 50 dB recommended for cardiac imaging. In addition to a decrease in signal-to-noise ratio, quantum noise is more clearly seen and results in further image degradation. Some of this degradation is clearly subjective. Because important decisions in invasive cardiology are based increasingly on video images, these are important considerations. It is possible to obtain excellent images with a high-definition 525-line unit that achieves a signal-to-noise ratio of at least 45 dB (18). Newer video systems have the capability of both 525 and 1,023 lines.

The optimal configuration will depend on the entire video image system. Our video system provides a 525-line EIA RS-1702 signal with progressive scanning and a video bandwidth of 10 to 15 mHz (6, 15, 18, 20).

Progressive vs. Interlaced Scanning

Video fluoroscopy used interlaced scanning in the past (8, 9). For this, radiation exposure at 60 x-ray pps was required. Each video frame was scanned from top to bottom in 1/30 sec. However, each frame was composed of two fields, each of which contained 262.5 horizontal lines. Alternate horizontal lines were scanned, starting with line 1 of the first field (Fig. 8.8). There was motion blurring because each frame was scanned twice. In the past, attempts were made to decrease the x-ray exposure by decreasing the x-ray pulses from 60 to 30 pps. This resulted in image degradation and increased flicker. During cine recording, video flicker is also an annoyance when rates of 30 frames/sec are used.

One of the most important developments in cardiac imaging has been the introduction of pulsed progressive scanning (Fig. 8.9) (8, 9). This system is based on a different principle. A special video circuit sweeps the entire 525-line target once every 33.3 msec. While the x-ray source is pulsed for 3 to 5 msec, the image is written on the target. This

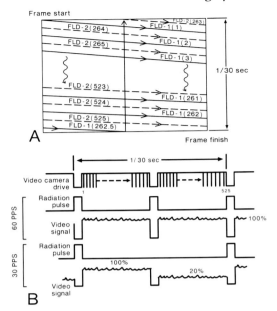

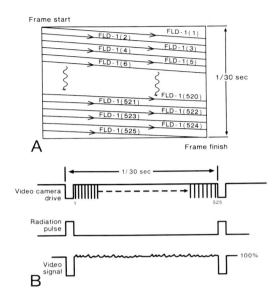

Figure 8.8. Conventional interlaced scanning. *A*, A 525-line video frame is scanned from top to bottom in 1/30 sec. Each frame is composed of two fields, each containing 262.5 horizontal lines. The starting point for scanning is line 1 of field 1 *(FLD-1(1))*. The line scans from left to right on alternate lines until it reaches the middle of the image at the bottom *(FLD-1(262.5))*. The scan then shifts back to the middle of the image at the top *(FLD-2(263))*. For field 2, the remaining lines are scanned *(dashed lines)* to complete the frame. *B*, The radiation and video timing for interlaced scanning at 60 pps are shown in the second and third waveforms. If the radiation is pulsed at 30 pps (fourth waveform), image brightness is decreased. (From Holmes DR Jr, Bove AA, Wondrow MA, Gray JE. Video x-ray progressive scanning: new technique for decreasing x-ray exposure without decreasing image quality during cardiac catheterization. Mayo Clin Proc 1986;61:321–326. By permission of Mayo Foundation.)

Figure 8.9. Progressive video scanning. The entire field is scanned in 1/30 sec. *A*, Each frame is composed of a single scan (field). *B*, Radiation can be pulsed at 30 pps with no degradation in image quality. (From Holmes DR Jr, Bove AA, Wondrow MA, Gray JE. Video x-ray progressive scanning: new technique for decreasing x-ray exposure without decreasing image quality during cardiac catheterization. Mayo Clin Proc 1986;61:321–326. By permission of Mayo Foundation.)

specialized video signal is converted into standard video format by a real-time digital scan converter to produce a digital image (768 × 512 pixels with 256 (8-bit) gray level resolution). This image is then converted in real time to a composite standard EIA RS-170 video signal. Progressive scanning has the advantages of improved image quality because it uses the short (3 to 5 msec) snapshot mode, improved resolution because of the lack of interfield blurring that is inherent in interlaced scanning,

and improved signal-to-noise ratio, as compared with that of conventional interlaced scanning (Fig. 8.10). A major clinical advantage is that because 30 pps can be used, the radiation exposure is decreased by 50% (Table 8.4). Progressive scanning can be used to enhance image quality for both cine and video recording. Optimal decrease in radiation exposure and improvement in image quality are achieved with grid-biased x-ray generation because of the short rectangular pulse

Figure 8.10. Right anterior oblique images from a 74-kg patient undergoing dilation of the right coronary artery. The images were recorded at identical angles with interlaced scanning (*left*) and progressive scanning (*right*). Two distinct guidewires are seen with conventional recording. Because of the snapshot effect in progressive scanning, only a single wire is seen, and image quality is improved. (From Holmes DR Jr, Bove AA, Wondrow MA, Gray JE. Video x-ray progressive scanning: new technique for decreasing x-ray exposure without decreasing image quality during cardiac catheterization. Mayo Clin Proc 1986;61:321–326. By permission of Mayo Foundation.)

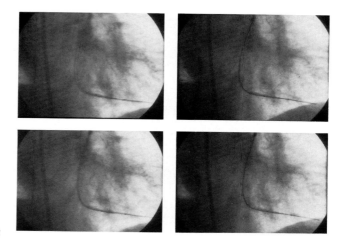

waveform, as compared with the continuous wave from x-ray generators (Fig. 8.5 and 8.6). Various similar scanning systems have now come into common use.

Video Monitor

The video image is becoming more important in the catheterization laboratory because it permits one to be certain that a diagnostic study has been performed and it facilitates decisions made during interventional procedures. The configuration of the video monitor depends on the details of the laboratory suite and on personal preference. The monitors should be as close as possible to the operator but not closer than four times the diagonal length of the monitor for optimal analysis and viewing. The stored freeze-frame video images should be displayed side by side with the live television images. In laboratories that use biplane video, a ceiling boom with four mounted video monitors may be optimal. The ability to move this along a ceiling support improves visualization.

The video monitor displays the radiographic image in a visible form. It should be able to display all of the information acquired by the imaging chain and therefore should allow the operator to assess fine details of cardiac anatomy accurately. This is particularly true for coronary dilation, during which decisions are made based on the video images. The spatial resolution should match that of the imaging system and have a similar bandwidth

(Table 8.5). The dynamic range should allow for reproduction of ten levels of video gray scale. The monitor also should have circuitry that allows clamping of the black portion of the image to a reference level. The output phosphor used varies. We have found that a P-4 phosphor most closely matches the film color most physicians are used to and is the accepted standard.

Videotape Recorder

Videodisc, video cassette, and videotape recorders all are used. Videotape recorders range in format from 8 mm to 1-inch broadcast type. Minimal specifications for recording a 525-line video image include a bandwidth of 5 to 10 mHz and signal-to-noise ratio of 45 dB. For optimal image recording, several factors must be kept in mind: (*a*) sufficient bandwidth to reproduce the original image; (*b*) signal-to-noise ratio similar to that of the rest of the system; (*c*) precision tracking during replay without misrepresentation; and (*d*) time base correction (15, 21, 22). This last feature allows absolute video registration. The ability to provide slow motion and freeze-frame without flicker or noise bars is also essential.

A broadcast standard, helical scan, 1-inch type C recorder is optimal. These have the bandwidth and signal-to-noise ratio sufficient to preserve the quality of the image. The image obtained with these recorders are similar to that with cinefilm.

Table 8.4
Radiation Entrance Exposure Rates at a Standard Vascular Phantom with Various Fluoroscopic X-ray Systems [a]

Mode[b]	15-cm (6-inch) image		23-cm (9-inch) image	
	Rate (r/min[c])	Difference	Rate (r/min[c])	Difference
Conventional cineangiography at 60 pps	50.1		26.0	
Cineangiography progressive scanning at 30 pps	24.1	-52%	12.1	-53%
Conventional fluoroscopy at 60 pps (30 fps)	3.7		1.3	
Fluoroscopy, progressive scanning at 30 pps (30 fps)	1.78	-52%	0.88	-32%

[a] From Holmes DR, Bove AA, Wondrow MA, Gray JE. Video x-ray progressive scanning: new technique for decreasing x-ray exposure without decreasing image quality during cardiac catheterization. Mayo Clin Proc 1986;61:321-326. By permission of Mayo Foundation.
[b] fps, frames/sec.
[c] 1 r = 0.258 mCi/kg.

Table 8.5
Video Systems

Feature	Preferred Optimal
Video tube	
Type (e.g., Vidicon, lead oxide, Vidicon, Plumbicon)	Plumbicon
Target voltage, V	45
Camera-video tube-amplifier chain	
Bandwidth (MHz at −3 dB)	15
Signal-to-noise ratio (minimum, dB)	50
Scan lines per frame	525
Shading correction	Yes
Gamma correction	No
Other signal processing (e.g., white clip or crush)	Extended dynamic range
Composite video signal (V)	1.0
Sync pulse (V)	0.3
RS-170 standard signal	Yes
Does video signal contain serrations and equalizing pulse?	Yes
AGC or ATC	AGC
Aspect ratio (4:3, 1:1, etc.)	4.3
Pulsed progressive scanning	
X-ray pulsing (type)	Grid-bias
Pulse width (msec)	3–5
Frame rate, no./sec	30
Monitor	
Size (diagonal, inches)	17–20
Bandwidth (MHz at −3dB)	15
Signal-to-noise ratio (dB)	45
Black level clamping	Yes
Videotape recorder	
Format	1-inch type C (R-170 525 lines)
Bandwidth (MHz at −3 dB)	5
Signal-to-noise ratio (dB)	45

Table 8.6
Quality Control Testing

Component Tested	Testing Frequency	Testing Equipment Used
Cinefilm processor	Daily	Sensitometer; densitometer
Cinefilm resolution	Daily	Visual assessment of resolution pattern
X-ray generator	Quarterly	kVp test device: high-voltage divider and oscilloscope
X-ray tube	Quarterly	Star resolution test pattern
Image intensifier	Quarterly	Assessed by observation of cine and video specification and recordings
Video system	Quarterly	Video signal generator; waveform monitor
Exposure rates	Quarterly	Dosimeter; half-value layer attenuator; patient-equivalent phantom
Cineprojectors	Quarterly	Projection test film

Videodisc recorders also can be used, particularly in combination with videotape recorders during PTCA. These devices can be used with either standard or high-line rate systems and operate with a signal-to-noise ratio of 40 to 45 dB and a bandwidth of 6 or 10 mHz.

QUALITY CONTROL

Quality control is an essential part of the operation of every cardiac catheterization laboratory and the responsibility of the laboratory director (5). This includes preventive maintenance of the system, evaluation of proposed equipment additions, continuing in-service education, and a constant review of the system's performance.

The aim of quality control is to obtain optimal fluoroscopy and cineangiography at all times with the least possible amount of radiation exposure. All parts of the system can be checked (Table 8.6). The effective kVp, pulse width, and pulse waveform of the x-ray generator can change with time; all of these can be monitored with a kVp test device. The x-ray tube should be checked either at the factory (this is preferable) or after installation. The measured focal spot size should be compared with the manufacturer's specifications; a star resolution test pattern is used most frequently. In addition to the x-ray generator and tube, the x-ray beam collimation and filtration should be assessed. The collimator blades should be checked to see that they are just visible on the edge of the image.

An important area of quality control is the exposure rate. This needs to be measured periodically in all modes (Table 8.7). It should be measured under different conditions, including direct readout with a dosimeter, with attenuators, and with a patient-equivalent phantom. Use of the phantom simulates clinical conditions and is helpful in evaluating patient entrance exposure rates.

The video imaging chain can be tested by viewing a resolution test target on the video display monitor (Fig. 8.11). In addition to resolution, the contrast and characteristics of the video signal are checked by using either a waveform monitor or an oscilloscope. The waveform monitor is also used to measure the noise in the video image. The video viewing monitor also should be checked. For this, the video signal generator is used. This has standard outputs so that the characteristics of the monitor, for example, flat field resolution and gray scale, can be tested independently of the rest of the video imaging chain.

Table 8.7
Entrance Image Intensifier Exposure Rates

Modality	Exposure rate (mr/frame)
Fluoroscopy	
6-inch	1–6
9-inch	0.5–3
Cine	
6-inch	25–35
9-inch	12–15
Video recording	
6-inch	16–30
9-inch	8–14

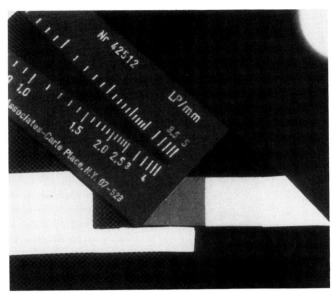

Figure 8.11. Cine resolution and density test pattern. (From Julsrud PR, Wondrow MA, Stears JG, Gray JE, Zahasky PE. X-ray equipment. In: Holmes DR Jr, Vlietstra RE, eds. Interventional cardiology. Philadelphia: FA Davis Company, Chapter 3, 1988. By permission of Mayo Foundation.)

A final area of quality control is periodic testing of the cinefilm images. The focus characteristics of the image intensifier and optical lenses determine the sharpness of the cine images. This can be assessed by using a step-wedge and resolution pattern filmed as part of the identification marker at the start of each case. Other aspects of the cinefilm images deal with the cinefilm processor and cineprojector, both of which need ongoing quality control assessment (Chapter 11).

In addition to quality control, preventive maintenance with both mechanical and electrical inspection is essential for providing high-quality radiographic images, reducing the number of equipment failures, early detection of failing equipment, and improved patient and operator safety.

IMAGE RECORDING AND STORAGE

Thirty-five millimeter cinefilm remains the standard for recording and storage of coronary angiographic images. Depending on the specific circumstances, other modalities may be used. For some pediatric cardiology applications, large cut film angiography is used in addition to cineangiography. For visualization of the details of the pulmonary arterial tree

and thoracic aorta, cut film may be useful. In addition, for peripheral vascular angiography, cut film is most commonly used. Some coronary angiographic laboratories use 105-mm film in addition to 35-mm film. The 105-mm spot film images may be used as a permanent record to be placed within the patient's chart or may be used to send to the referring physicians for their records. In addition, the 105-mm spot film images may be useful in the operating room to remind the surgeons of the specific anatomy. In the future, image recording and storage modalities are expected to change dramatically. Continued development of optical disks or digital tape probably will eventually lead to replacement of cinefilm.

RADIATION SAFETY

Radiation safety has become an increasingly important issue as the catheterization laboratory has become more therapeutic. Procedures such as PTCA are associated with increased radiation exposure because of longer fluoroscopy times. These longer fluoroscopy times reflect the need to position guidewires and dilation balloons within the coronary arterial tree. Dash and Leaman (23) found that mean cineangiographic times are similar for PTCA and diagnostic coronary angiography. However, fluoroscopy time is substantially longer. This prolonged fluoroscopy time resulted in a mean radiation exposure for PTCA procedures of 17 mrad/case/operator, compared with 9 mrad/case for routine coronary angiography. Overall, there was a 93% increase in operator radiation exposure during PTCA. There is obviously also increased radiation exposure to patients during PTCA. Cascade et al. (24), using patient dosimeter probes, found that the average radiation exposure was 20 ± 16 rads for coronary angiography and 69 ± 61 rads for PTCA procedures. When dilations were attempted on two lesions, radiation exposure was significantly greater than when attempted on one (100 rads, as compared with 47 rads). As increased numbers of multivessel dilation procedures are performed, this increased exposure may become more pronounced. These higher radiation exposure procedures have very important implications, affecting not only physicians but also paramedical persons and patients.

The issue of radiation safety and protection is multifaceted. The radiographic equipment must be checked according to the preventive maintenance specifications to see if it is operating within accepted limits. The goal should always be to deliver optimal images with the least amount of radiation. The operators and room personnel should wear adequate shielding aprons, thyroid collars, and leaded glasses. For personnel who are exposed to radiation to the back, for example, technicians who are turned away from the imaging equipment, wrap-around aprons are essential. Many kinds of equipment shields are available, ranging from movable freewheeling full-length shields to ceiling-mounted clear shields and a variety of lead beads (25). All of these can significantly decrease radiation exposure but only if they are used routinely and properly. Careful avoidance of unneeded x-ray exposure is also essential. If the x-ray foot switch is turned on only when necessary, radiation exposure can be minimized. Monitoring radiation exposure is essential and must be enforced. Overexposure must evoke a review of physician and laboratory techniques. Finally, improvements in video techniques, for example, progressive scanning, can also significantly reduce x-ray exposure by changing x-ray pulsing from 60 to 30 pulses/sec.

THE FUTURE

Cardiovascular imaging is changing rapidly. Video recording techniques have improved markedly over the past few years. Digital image processing and, eventually, digital acquisition are expected to enhance image quality further (see Chapter 9). It can be anticipated that cinefilm will be replaced by digital storage of images within 5 years. Questions remain about the development of an industry standard for recording, storage, and postprocessing. The probable end product will be digital acquisition of data, a standard piece of recording equipment, and unit record storage for easy access. Whether this storage will be an optical disc or an individual cassette remains to be determined. These developments should yield improved images and decreased cost (by virtue of elimination of cinefilm and processing) with less radiation exposure.

References

1. Vlietstra RE, Holmes DR Jr. PTCA: percutaneous transluminal coronary angioplasty. Philadelphia: FA Davis Company, 1987.
2. Ischinger T, ed. Practice of coronary angioplasty. Berlin: Springer–Verlag, 1986.
3. Grossman W, ed. Cardiac catheterization and angiography. 3rd ed. Philadelphia: Lea & Febiger, 1986.
4. Thompson TT. A practical approach to modern imaging equipment. 2nd ed. Boston: Little, Brown and Company, 1985.
5. Gray JE, Winkler NT, Stears J, Frank ED. Quality control in diagnostic imaging: a quality control cookbook. Baltimore: University Park Press, 1983.
6. Julsrud PR, Wondrow MA, Stears JG, Gray JE, Zahasky PE. X–ray equipment. In: Holmes DR Jr, Vlietstra RE, eds. Interventional cardiology. Philadelphia: FA Davis Company, Chapter 3, 1988.
7. Friesinger GC, Adams DF, Bourassa MG, et al. Optimal resources for examination of the heart and lungs: cardiac catheterization and radiographic facilities: examination of the chest and cardiovascular system study group. Circulation 1983; 68: 893A–930A.
8. Holmes DR Jr, Bove AA, Wondrow MA, Gray JE. Video x–ray progressive scanning: new technique for decreasing x–ray exposure without decreasing image quality during cardiac catheterization. Mayo Clin Proc 1986;61:321–326.
9. Wondrow MA, Bove AA, Holmes DR Jr, Gray JE, Julsrud PR. Technical consideration for a new x–ray video progressive scanning system for cardiac catheterization. Cathet Cardiovasc Diagn 1988;14:126–134.

10. Aldridge HE. A decade or more of cranial and caudal angled projections in coronary arteriography—another look (editorial). Cathet Cardiovasc Diagn 1984;10:539–542.

11. Lesperance J, Saltiel J, Petitclerc R, Bourassa MG. Angulated views in the sagittal plane for improved accuracy of cinecoronary angiography. Am J Roentgenol 1974;121:565–574.

12. Balter S, Sones FM Jr, Brancato R. Radiation exposure to the operator performing cardiac angiography with U–arm systems. Circulation 1978;58:925–932.

13. Holmes DR Jr, Bove AA, Nishimura RA, et al. Comparison of monoplane and biplane assessment of regional left ventricular wall motion after thrombolytic therapy for acute myocardial infarction. Am J Cardiol 1987;59:793–797.

14. Cohn PF, Gorlin R, Adams DF, Chahine RA, Vokonas PS, Herman MV. Comparison of biplane and single plane left ventriculograms in patients with coronary artery disease. Am J Cardiol 1974;33:1–6.

15. Gray JE, Wondrow MA, Smith HC, Holmes DR Jr. Technical considerations for cardiac laboratory high–definition video systems. Cathet Cardiovasc Diagn 1984;10:73–86.

16. Aker UT, Ischinger T. The cardiac catheterization laboratory for coronary angioplasty. In: Ischinger T, ed. Practice of coronary angioplasty. Berlin: Springer–Verlag, 1986:61–92.

17. O'Keefe JH Jr, Miller GA, Holmes DR Jr. Coronary angioplasty performed at the time of diagnostic catheterization: safety and efficacy (abstr). J Am Coll Cardiol 1988;11:129A.

18. Holmes DR Jr, Smith HC, Gray JE, Wondrow MA. Clinical evaluation and application of cardiac laboratory high–definition video systems. Cathet Cardiovasc Diagn 1984;10:63–71.

19. Haendle J, Horbaschek HH, Alexandrescu M. High resolution x–ray television and the high–resolution video recorder. Electromedica 1977;3:83–91.

20. EIA Standard RS–170: Electrical performance standards–evision studio facilities. Washington, DC: Electronics Industries Association, 1957.

21. Hathaway RA, Ravizza R. Development and design of the Ampex auto scan tracking (AST) system. J Soc Motion Picture Television Eng 1980;89:931–934.

22. Fibush D. SMPTE type C helical scan recording format. J Soc Motion Picture Television Eng 1978;87:775–780.

23. Dash H, Leaman DM. Operator radiation exposure during percutaneous transluminal coronary angioplasty. J Am Coll Cardiol 1984;4:725–728.

24. Cascade PN, Peterson LE, Wajszczuk WJ, Mantel J. Radiation exposure to patients undergoing percutaneous transluminal coronary angioplasty. Am J Cardiol 1987;59:996–997.

25. Gertz EW, Wisneski JA, Gould RG, Akin JR. Improved radiation protection for physicians performing cardiac catheterization. Am J Cardiol 1982;50:1283–1286.

9

Clinical Application of Digital Angiography in the Cardiac Catheterization Laboratory

Alan G. Wasserman, M.D.
Allan M. Ross, M.D.

INTRODUCTION

Digital subtraction angiography is the result of synergistic application of two related technologies to create enhanced images and processing options not available with conventional diagnostic radiographic imaging. The applicability of digital subtraction angiography for the diagnosis and evaluation of patients with cardiovascular disease is expanding. This technique has become feasible with the development and application of microprocessor technology that allows for rapid data acquisition and storage. Speed is essential since angiocardiographic images must be generated at the rate of at least 30 / sec in order to prevent distortion due to the heart's motion.

TECHNIQUE

Basically, in order to obtain a digital image (necessary for computer processing), the x-ray image is amplified and then subdivided into a matrix of small picture elements, or pixels. The brightness of the image in each pixel is represented by a value that ranges from 1 to 256 shades of gray. Most current digital subtraction systems use a matrix of 512×512 pixels. A computer stores the digital information, manipulates it, and reconverts the data to analog format for display.

The original and most frequently used processing method for enhancing images obtained in this fashion is "mask mode subtraction." A "background" digitized image is collected and stored from the region of interest prior to contrast administration. This background image is termed the "mask." After the mask is stored, radiographic contrast material is then injected, and a digitized image of the angiogram is obtained. From each frame of the angiogram the previously stored mask is subtracted, pixel by pixel. This can be done rapidly on-line, with the resultant image displayed immediately in the catheterization laboratory. The resulting image is in essence a "background-suppressed", enhanced study of contrast flow through the structure under investigation. This technique has the added advantage of requiring smaller amounts of contrast material and rapid digital processing for further quantitation analysis (e.g., ejection fraction, regional wall motion, percent stenosis) and digital storage or transmission. Thus, labor-intensive efforts required for quantitative angiography are reduced to a minimum. Large cinefilm libraries and time-consuming handling (mailing, etc.) are reduced or eliminated.

The major disadvantage of mask mode subtraction is misregistration artifact resulting from respiratory or cardiac-related motion. Motion can be minimized by increasing the sampling rate, summing masks, using multiple-image subtraction, or continuously updating the mask over time. Since data are stored in solid state memory or disk, artifacts can also be smoothed by postprocessing. Manipulation of the mask to achieve better alignment can be done, and if necessary, a new mask that achieves a better fit can be chosen.

Reduction of background structures, obscuring vascular or cardiac structures under investigation, allows for reduction in the volume of contrast material needed for visualization. With conventional angiography, an intravenous contrast injection often becomes so rapidly diluted that many right-sided and most left-sided cardiac structures cannot be adequately visualized. The image enhancement provided by digital angiography results in excellent quality images of many cardiac chamber and great vessel structures with only intravenous injections. Alternatively, small-volume arterial contrast injections can be used. This advantage, of course, has the potential to reduce the risks associated with radiographic contrast material administration (see Chapters 3 and 10).

LEFT VENTRICULOGRAPHY

Direct Angiography

Direct injection of contrast material into the left ventricular cavity with background subtraction produces high-quality images with doses of contrast agent approximately one-third of that necessary for conventional angiography. This allows for a lower osmotic and volume load in patients who may be at high risk for contrast-related toxicity, such as those with aortic stenosis, congestive heart failure, diabetes, or renal insufficiency. In addition, the radiation exposure to the patient and operator can be markedly reduced because fluoroscopic energies may be used with digital subtraction angiography rather than the high energies required for cineangiography. (see chapter 8)

The actual technique is very similar to that used for conventional cineangiography. After the patient and image tube are optimally positioned, the patient is asked to hold his breath, and the mask image is obtained over one to three cardiac cycles. Image acquisition is continued while contrast material is injected and is terminated two to three cycles after the contrast has cleared. The digital angiogram may be viewed immediately, or postprocessing may be done for further image enhancement. It has been our experience that better quality images are achieved when the reduced volume of contrast material is diluted by adding one or two equal volumes of saline to a total volume of 40 cc to be injected over 2 to 3 sec. Obviously, "panning" or movement of the table top or image tube will not be possible

during digital angiography. So, it is wise to use a somewhat larger field size than one uses when panning is available.

Intravenous Angiography

Following an intravenous injection of contrast material through the lungs to film its levophase with conventional cineangiography often does not allow for diagnostic left ventriculograms. Dilution of the contrast material bolus, as it mixes with large volumes of blood during its movement through the right heart and pulmonary vessels, results in reduced visualization of the left ventricle. Even when relatively large volumes of contrast material (≥ 60 cc) are injected rapidly, less than optimal visualization results. However, image enhancement by digitization with background subtraction permits diagnostic studies from intravenous injections that are often comparable to ventriculograms made by direct injection (1–7). Although studies may be performed with peripheral venous injections of contrast material, we have found that either central venous or right atrial administration is often more comfortable for the patient and adds to the image quality because higher injection rates can be used. A high-flow 5 Fr pigtail catheter may be inserted into the superior or inferior vena cava under fluoroscopic guidance. Contrast material may be injected close to or even in the right atrium.

Patient instruction and cooperation are very important since even slight motion may render a study uninterpretable. Patients must learn to hold a breath in end inspiration for up to 15 sec in order to eliminate excursion of the diaphragm and heart movement with respiration. Just prior to contrast injection, one to two seconds of imaging are recorded to provide a contrast-free background mask for subtraction. Thirty-five to forty cc of contrast material are then injected at a rate of 20 cc/sec into the inferior or superior vena cava with continuous imaging as the bolus traverses the right heart and lungs and then returns to the left atrium and ventricle (Fig. 9.1). Since there is considerable mixing and dilution of the contrast bolus as it travels towards the left ventricle, reduced contrast material flow rates and volumes are usually not adequate for diagnostic images.

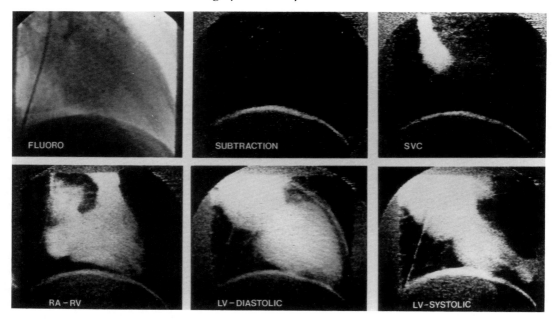

Figure 9.1. Stages in performing a first–pass digital subtraction ventriculographic study. From top left to right a mask is created and subtracted from the fluoroscopic (*fluoro*) image. The bolus of contrast is visualized as it passes through superior vena cava (*SVC*) and right– and left–sided cardiac chambers. *LV*, left ventricle; *RA*, right atrium; *RV*, right ventricle. (From Nissen SE, Booth D, Waters J, Fassas T, DeMaria AN. Evaluation of left ventricular contractile pattern by intravenous digital subtraction ventriculography: comparison with cineangiography and assessment of interobserver variability. Am J Cardiol 1983; 52:1293–1298. Reprinted with permission of American Journal of Cardiology.)

Imaging, subtraction, and storage can all occur in "realtime," allowing for continuous observation of the image on a video monitor. However, one retains the option of postprocessing the image. For example, if the patient has moved or breathed slightly during the procedure, an alternative mask, chosen from the end of the study after contrast has cleared the left ventricle, may result in significant improvement of image quality.

A good quality left ventricular study can be obtained in the majority of patients as long as they can effectively cooperate (Fig. 9.2). Patients in whom the bolus may become excessively diluted, such as those with significant tricuspid regurgitation, may not be good candidates for intravenous studies. Patients with severe pulmonary hypertension should not receive large-volume intravenous or right heart injections to visualize their left ventricle. They may be examined more safely using direct left-sided injections.

Comparison with Conventional Left Ventriculography

Comparison of digital subtraction ventriculography with conventional cineangiography has been made by multiple investigators (Fig. 9.3) (1-7). We evaluated wall motion in 40 consecutive patients who had both conventional left ventricular cineangiograms and intravenous digital left ventriculograms (4). Both studies were performed in the 30° right anterior oblique (RAO) projection. Separate readers evaluated the two types of studies for either a normal or abnormal contractile pattern in each of three ventricular segments (anterior, apical, and inferior). Complete concordance was found in 39 (97%) of the 40 comparisons.

Nissen et al. compared volume determinations made using these two methods (6). Close correlation was found for end-diastolic volume, end-systolic volume, and ejection

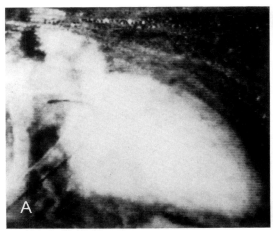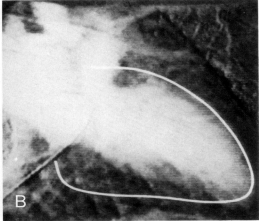

Figure 9.2. Abnormal rest intravenous digital ventriculogram at end diastole (*A*) and end systole (*B*) with the end–diastolic edge superimposed. A large area of anterior wall akinesis is detected. (From Johnson RA, Wasserman AG, Leiboff RH, et al. Intravenous digital left ventriculography at rest and with atrial pacing as a screening procedure for coronary artery disease. J Am Coll Cardiol 1983;2:905–910. Reprinted with permission of Journal of American College of Cardiology.)

fraction using the Sandler-Dodge method ($r = 0.88$, $r = 0.92$, and $r = 0.93$, respectively).

Another potential advantage of digital angiography for left ventricular study is the ability to quantify the density of the contrast agent in the left ventricular cavity. A logarithmic equation (programmed into the computer) can be used to produce a linear relationship between radiographic density and the numerical value for each pixel in the image. Densitometric determination of ejection fraction, similar to that used for radionuclide determination of ejection fraction, is then made. The densitometrically derived ejection fraction is independent of geometric assumptions inherent in the either the area-length or center line methods (8-10). Calculations for ejection fraction are similar to those used for nuclear methods. End-diastolic and end-systolic regions of interest are identified, and an area of background, chosen at end systole, is subtracted. Tobis et al. found a close correlation comparing ejection fractions ($r = 0.94$) obtained in 25 patients, using the area-length method with those obtained using videodensitometric analysis (8).

Interventional Studies

Use of the intravenous route allows for multiple ventricular function studies to be performed while minimizing both contrast and

radiation doses. For example, stress-induced changes in regional or global left ventricular function may be elicited at the time of coronary angiography to assess the functional significance of a coronary artery stenosis. Supine bicycle exercise and atrial pacing have been employed for stress tests with digital ventriculography (11-15). Since wall motion abnormalities are an earlier and a more frequent finding in the course of transient ischemic episodes than electrocardiographic changes, this approach has some theoretical advantages in the assessment of the functional significance of coronary stenosis.

EXERCISE STUDIES

Intravenous digital ventriculography combined with supine bicycle exercise stress has provided left ventricular function data comparable to that obtained by means of exercise radionuclide ventriculography. Exercise stress, however, may cause particular difficulties when combined with digital subtraction imaging. Since maximal exercise limits the ability of the patients to hold their breath, misregistration artifact produced by diaphragmatic motion may be an important problem. To avoid this problem, patients are allowed to breath normally while the intravenous bolus traverses the right heart and are required to

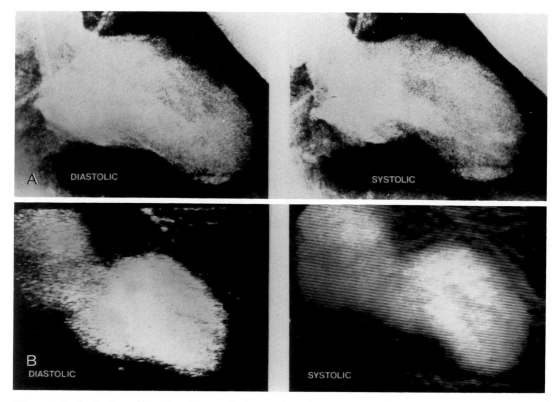

Figure 9.3. End–diastolic and end–systolic frames for cineangiography (*A*) and digital subtraction ventriculography (*B*) in the same patient. A large anteroapical aneurysm is detected with both techniques. (From Nissen SE, Booth D, Waters J, Fassas T, DeMaria AN. Evaluation of left ventricular contractile pattern by intravenous digital subtraction ventriculography: comparison with cineangiography and assessment of interobserver variability. Am J Cardiol 1983;52:1293–1298. Reprinted with permission of American Journal of Cardiology.)

hold respirations for only 2 to 3 sec when the bolus reaches the left ventricle.

Yiannikas et al. studied 79 patients referred for cardiac catheterization using exercise digital subtraction ventriculography (15). Significant coronary artery disease (CAD) was defined as at least one major coronary artery with ≥75% diameter stenosis. Development of a new left ventricular wall motion abnormality with exercise had a 94% sensitivity and 88% specificity for detection of significant CAD. Using failure of ejection fraction to increase by 5%, they found that the high sensitivity was retained (89%) but that specificity declined (56%). Detrano et al. compared stress thallium-201 scintigraphy with stress digital subtraction ventriculography in 97 consecutive patients (16). They chose a 50% diameter stenosis to represent significant CAD. Digital ventriculography was found to yield a higher sensitivity (79%) but lower specificity (72%) than stress thallium (62% and 82%, respectively) for identification of significant CAD. External body motion related to exercise can be an important limitation.

ATRIAL PACING STUDIES

Other investigators utilized atrial pacing to induce tachycardia stress combined with digital subtraction ventriculography (4, 13, 14). The major advantages of pacing are that it increases myocardial oxygen demand but does not limit the patient's ability to hold his or her breath and external body motion related to exercise is absent.

We used atrial pacing and digital subtraction ventriculographic studies to evaluate 61 consecutive patients undergoing cardiac catheterization further evaluates the basis for chest pain (4). A special dual pacing-angiographic 6 Fr catheter was made so that with only one venous puncture we were able to pace the right atrium and deliver contrast through its six spiral side holes. A digital angiogram was done with the patient at rest. Incremented atrial pacing was then performed at 2-min intervals after starting at a heart rate of 105 bpm. Heart rate was increased until either chest pain occurred or a maximal rate of 150 bpm was reached. Pacing stress was terminated as the contrast bolus traversed the right ventricle. Therefore, the left ventriculogram was obtained several beats after cessation of tachycardia stress, with the patient again in sinus rhythm. The postpacing ventriculogram was compared with that obtained at rest for development of new wall motion abnormalities. New wall motion abnormalities identified 38 of 44 patients with significant CAD (>70% diameter narrowing). There were six false-negative results (82% sensitivity) and one false-positive result (94% specificity). Studies by Mancini et al. (13), using intravenous ventriculography, and Tobis et al. (14), using direct low contrast ventriculography combined with atrial pacing, produced similar results.

We also compared intravenous digital ventriculography, using atrial pacing stress and exercise radionuclide ventriculography, for detection of wall motion abnormalities in 40 patients referred for cardiac catheterization (12). Neither technique produced a new wall motion abnormality in the 12 patients with normal coronary arteries. Six patients with coronary artery disease had a history of a myocardial infarction, and a resting wall motion abnormality was present in all six, as demonstrated by both techniques (Fig. 9.4). Of the remaining 22 patients with coronary artery disease, a new wall motion abnormality was detected by means of digital subtraction ventriculography after atrial pacing in 18 patients, as compared with that found in 15 patients after exercise radionuclide ventriculography. Thus, it seems appropriate to conclude that intravenous digital subtraction ventriculography using atrial pacing stress and exercise radionuclide ventriculography are substantially equivalent for detection of

stress-induced wall motion abnormalities in patients with CAD.

CORONARY ARTERIOGRAPHY

Use of digital angiography offers multiple advantages when visualizing the coronary arteries. The digitally obtained images are available for immediate review during the cardiac catheterization procedure, as they do not require film development. The ability to enhance images following acquisition can minimize the effect of background structures on stenosis recognition (7) (Fig. 9.5). Because the image is in a digital format, computerized edge detection algorithms and videodensitometry may be used, and these techniques should improve quantification of coronary artery stenosis (see Chapter 23). However, the major role for digital coronary angiography may be in providing a means by which we may actually assess coronary blood flow and coronary flow reserve.

Vogel et al. used digital imaging to quantify the time between contrast injection and its appearance within the myocardium (17, 18). Classical indicator dilution principles define an inverse relationship between indicator appearance time and blood flow. The myocardial contrast appearance time measured by digital techniques was found to correlate closely with regional blood flow. By combining regional appearance time of contrast material under basal and hyperemic conditions, with a densitometric estimate of the relative change in intravascular volume induced by the hyperemic state, an index of coronary flow reserve is obtained.

LeGrand et al., applying this technique, found reduced coronary flow reserves in an interesting group of patients with angiographically defined normal epicardial coronary arteries (19). These patients, however, also had other abnormal findings on either exercise thallium-201 scintigraphy or radionuclide ventriculograms. These abnormal findings suggest that this apparent reduced coronary flow reserve was probably secondary to true coronary vascular flow abnormalities, perhaps at the small vessel level. The technique of measuring coronary flow reserve by digital imaging has also been used to assess results of both coronary bypass surgery and coronary angioplasty (20, 21).

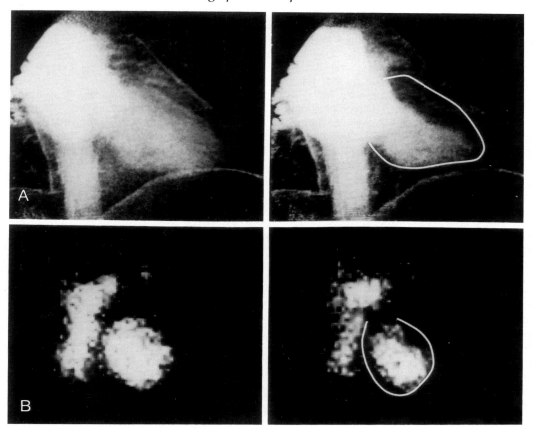

Figure 9.4. Intravenous digital ventriculogram (*A*) and radionuclide ventriculogram (*B*) from a patient with an inferior wall myocardial infarction. There is inferior akinesis. (From Wasserman AG, Johnson RA, Katz RJ, et al. Detection of left ventricular wall motion abnormalities for diagnosis of coronary artery disease: a comparison of exercise radionuclide and pacing intravenous digital ventriculography. Am J Cardiol 1984;54:497–501. Reprinted with permission of American Journal of Cardiology.)

Nissen et al. developed an alternative method of evaluating coronary flow reserve (22). They used contrast intensity-time curves generated from a region of interest over a coronary artery during successive end-diastolic frames. Time intensity curves are generated both under basal conditions and then under presumed maximal hyperemia conditions. The ratio of hyperemic flow to basal flow (flow reserve) may be estimated from the ratio of the area under the basal curve to the area under the hyperemic curve. Flow reserve estimated from digital angiograms was compared using an animal model with flow reserve measured by direct electromagnetic flow probe recordings. Coronary flow limitations were imposed by creating various degrees of stenoses, and a good correlation ($r = 0.86$)

between flow reserve estimated from digital angiograms and flow reserve measured by flow probe was found.

DIGITAL CORONARY ROADMAPPING

In order to facilitate positioning of guidewires and balloons during transluminal coronary angioplasty, Tobis et al. introduced a method called "coronary roadmapping" (23). A previously obtained digital subtraction image of the coronary artery is superimposed onto a "live" fluoroscopic image of the guide or balloon catheter. Thus, the operator can position the guidewire and balloon without the need for repeated injections of contrast agent to help

CINEANGIOGRAM

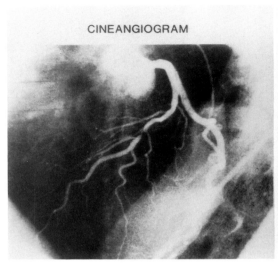

DIGITAL ACQUISITION
MASK MODE SUBTRACTION

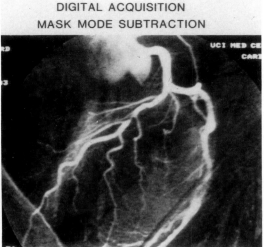

Figure 9.5.   Standard film–based cineangiogram in 60° left anterior oblique projection with 45° of cranial angulation. There is a significant lesion in the mid–left anterior descending coronary artery. A digitally acquired angiogram of the same patient in the same projection. A single–frame mask mode subtraction process was applied. Density from bones and soft tissue have been subtracted so that contrast resolution is improved. (From Tobis J, Nalcioglu O, Iseri L, et al. Detection and quantitation of coronary stenoses from digital subtraction angiograms compared with 35–millimeter film cineangiograms. Am J Cardiol 1984;54:489–496. Reprinted with permission of American Journal of Cardiology.)

localize the artery and stenosis. Digital techniques further aid the angioplasty procedure by allowing for rapid presentation of multiple stored images to help better define complex anatomy in various obliquities. The ease of operation and better image quality suggest that this application may supplant videotape recorded images for these purposes.

NONSELECTIVE CORONARY ANGIOGRAPHY

With the advent of digital angiography some have advocated that coronary angiography can be accomplished by nonselective means (Fig. 9.6). Various reasons have been proposed for performing digital coronary angiography by aortic root injection, including: (*a*) A total coronary evaluation could be performed using a smaller total dose of contrast agent. (*b*) There are obvious risk advantages in not directly engaging the coronary arteries. (*c*) Advances in catheter technology and power injectors allow the needed contrast to be delivered through a smaller catheter (5 Fr) and, hence, a smaller-sized arterial puncture. (*d*) The patient would receive a lower cumulative radiation dose. and

(*e*) With the use of fluoroscopic energies and already existing portable digital units, potentially a study would not require a conventional angiographic suite capable of generating high-dose cinetechnique. The latter raises the possibility of nonselective digital coronary angiography being done in critical care settings.

We investigated the potential for nonselective digital coronary angiography by studying a series of 23 consecutive patients who were undergoing conventional selective coronary cineangiography for evaluation of chest pain (24). Following selective coronary angiography, a pigtail catheter was positioned just above the aortic valve. Contrast agent (20 cc) was injected at 20 cc/sec. Two views were obtained: a 30 to 50° RAO and a 40 to 50° left anterior oblique (LAO) with a small degree of cranial angulation.

We evaluated the proximal third of each major coronary artery with both techniques, using conventional selective cineangiography as the reference standard. Of the 23 patients, 10 were found to have no stenoses, and 13 had at least one proximal coronary stenosis. Seventeen of the 22 (77%) proximal stenotic lesions found in these 13 patients were correctly identified by nonselective digital techniques.

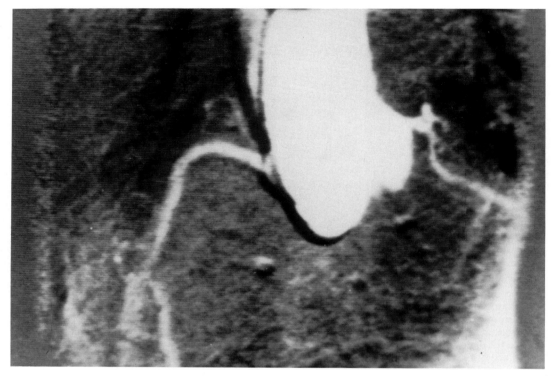

Figure 9.6. A 10–cc aortic root injection of contrast in the LAO projection. Digital angiography shows a total proximal occlusion of the left anterior descending artery. A mid–right coronary artery lesion is also seen.

Twelve of these 13 patients with coronary disease had digital studies adequate for complete analysis, and in 9 at least one diseased artery was identified. Of the 10 patients without proximal stenoses, 9 had adequate digital studies, and all were correctly identified.

Based upon our study, the **specificity** of nonselective coronary visualization with the use of digital techniques and aortic root injection appears to be excellent. However, the **sensitivity** for detecting only significant proximal disease is not adequate at present to propose that this method be used for coronary disease screening. Of course, advances in technique may change these results in the near future.

Similar problems exist in the evaluation of aortocoronary bypass grafts. However, Wholey, using digital intraaortic angiography, found a sensitivity of 93% with a specificity of 96% (25). It is necessary in evaluating graft patency to visualize both proximal and distal graft sites. Therefore, any misregistration arti-

fact may seriously limit the digital study. In our experience this approach for graft evaluation is not yet sufficiently accurate and comprehensive to supplant conventional selective angiography.

CONGENITAL HEART DISEASE

Digital subtraction angiography has been used in a wide range of patients with congenital heart disease (26-30). It has been particularly useful in assessing shunts and the adequacy of their repair. Yiannikas et al. found an excellent correlation between the calculated pulmonary to systemic flow ratios (Qp/Qs) obtained by nuclear technique and those obtained by densitometric techniques from digital angiography ($r = 0.89$) (28). Other congenital abnormalities in which digital angiography has been helpful include tricuspid atresia, Ebstein's anomaly, tetralogy of Fallot, pulmonary valve stenosis, and abnormalities of the aorta and aortic arch (29, 30). The contrast volume load and radiation limitation advantages may be of even more importance in the pediatric, as compared with the adult, population.

NONCARDIAC APPLICATION

The advantages of digital angiography in allowing for reduced contrast material concentrations, as well as "on-line" angiographic assessment, have renewed an interest in performance of digital angiography of noncardiac structures during diagnostic cardiac catheterization. However, the decreased resolution with digital angiography, as compared with that of standard film angiography and the occasional need for selective catheterization of the vessel under study (Fig. 9.7), limit this use for the practicing cardiologist.

Carotid arteries in patients with bruits and the renal arteries in those with hypertension may be the two most common noncardiac structures requiring angiographic evaluation during cardiac catheterization.

The cervical portion of the carotid arteries can be evaluated by means of digital technique from injections made with a pigtail catheter located in the aortic arch (31, 32). Multiple oblique views are required for complete visualization. Assessment of the renal arteries may be performed using digital technique from an injection made in the descending aorta in patients with a history of hypertension (33). Difficulty can arise with image degradation secondary to motion artifact from bowel peristalsis. Other areas that may be satisfactorily studied using digital technique at the time of cardiac catheterization include the aortic arch, abdominal aorta, pulmonary arteries, and peripheral vessels (34–36).

CONCLUSIONS

In view of the significant advantages discussed above, one might have expected a more widespread acceptance and utilization of digital subtraction angiography in cardiac catheterization laboratories. In fact, this technology has been slow to find its way into these traditional film-based laboratories. There are, no doubt, multiple explanations for this, perhaps including fiscal constraints. It is the authors' opinion, however, that industry decisions have retarded the acceptance and development of those advances. Manufacturers

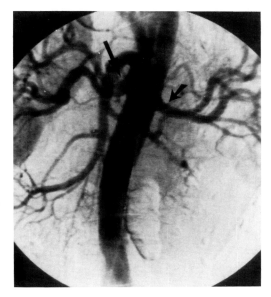

Figure 9.7. Intraarterial abdominal aortic injection, in a 5 to 10° right posterior oblique projection, demonstrates both renal arteries (*arrows*), by means of the digital subtraction technique. This selective injection into the abdominal aorta was required to provide adequate visualization of the proximal renal arteries. (From Van Breda A. Noncardiac application of digital angiography. In: Wasserman AG, Ross AM, eds. Cardiac application of digital angiography. Mount Kisco, NY: Futura, 1988. Reprinted with permission of Futura Publishing.)

have concentrated on image enhancement for conventional radiologic applications and spent relatively little effort in developing improved "user friendliness" for cardiac studies. Development and production of effective quantitative software for integration into the imaging apparatus has lagged behind software development for most other applications. One major problem is that radiographic equipment manufacturers have not readily accepted and interfaced hardware designed by digital equipment manufacturers. It is unlikely that a company focused in conventional radiographic equipment will have the depth and expertise possessed by digital equipment manufacturers. When these aspects are addressed, the full potential of digital subtraction technology in the catheterization laboratory may be better appreciated.

For the future, potential clinical applications for the combination of digital processing and subtraction angiography seem almost endless. Foremost among these are techniques to provide angiographic data not previously attainable in conventional clinical angiographic settings. Generation of data to quantify regional myocardial flow and coronary arterial phase flow dynamics and flow reserve are just a few examples. These techniques have the potential to widely expand the use of angiography from the anatomic to the physiologic or even pathophysiologic level. Other emerging applications should allow enhancement of conventional angiography in a manner not previously possible. Electronic acquisition, storage, and transmission of data in this modern era of telecommunications will become realities or spinoffs of the transition from film-based to digital-based handling of angiographic information.

References

1. Tobis JM, Nalcioglu O, Johnston WD, et al. Left ventricular imaging with digital subtraction angio-graphy using intravenous contrast injection and fluoroscopic exposure levels. Am Heart J 1982;104:20–27.
2. Goldberg HL, Borer JS, Moses JW, Fisher J, Cohen B, Skelly NT. Digital subtraction intravenous left ventricular angiography: comparison with conventional intraventricular angiography. J Am Coll Cardiol 1983;1:858–862.
3. Norris SL, Slutsky RA, Mancini GHJ, et al. A comparison of intravenous ventriculography with direct left ventriculography for quantitation of left ventricular volumes and ejection fractions. Am J Cardiol 1983;51:1399–1403.
4. Johnson RA, Wasserman AG, Leiboff RH, et al. Intravenous digital left ventriculography at rest and with atrial pacing as a screening procedure for coronary artery disease. J Am Coll Cardiol 1983;2:905–910.
5. Vas R, Diamond GA, Forrester JS, et al. Computer–enhanced digital angiography: correlation of clinical assessment of left ventricular ejection fraction and regional wall motion. Am Heart J 1982;104:730–732.
6. Nissen SE, Booth D, Waters J, Fassas T, DeMaria AN. Evaluation of left ventricular contractile pattern by intravenous digital subtraction ventriculography: comparison with cineangiography and assessment of interobserver variability. Am J Cardiol 1983;52:1293–1298.
7. Tobis J, Nalcioglu O, Iseri L, et al. Detection and quantitation of coronary artery stenoses from digital subtraction angiograms compared with 35–millimeter film cineangiograms. Am J Cardiol 1984;54:489–496.
8. Tobis JM, Nalcioglu O, Seibert JA, Johnston WD, Henry WL. Measurement of left ventricular ejec-

9. Nissen SE, Elion JL, Grayburn P, Booth DC, Wisenbaugh TW, DeMaria AN. Determination of left ventricular ejection fraction by computer densitometric analysis of digital subtraction angiography: experimental validation and correlation with area–length methods. Am J Cardiol 1987;59:675–680.
10. Detrano R, MacIntyre WJ, Salcedo EE, et al. Videodensitometric ejection fractions from intravenous digital subtraction left ventriculograms: correlation with conventional direct contrast and radionuclide ventriculography. Radiology 1985;155:19–23.
11. Goldberg HL, Moses JW, Borer JS, et al. Exercise left ventriculography utilizing intravenous digital angiography. J Am Coll Cardiol 1983;2:1092–1098.
12. Wasserman AG, Johnson RA, Katz RJ, et al. Detection of left ventricular wall motion abnormalities for diagnosis of coronary artery disease: a comparison of exercise radionuclide and pacing intravenous digital ventriculography. Am J Cardiol 1984;54:497–501.
13. Mancini GBJ, Peterson KL, Gregoratos G, Higgins CB, Einsidler E. Effects of atrial pacing on global and regional left ventricular function in coronary heart disease assessed by digital intravenous ventriculography. Am J Cardiol 1984;53:456–461.
14. Tobis J, Nalcioglu O, Johnston WD, et al. Digital angiography in assessment of ventricular function and wall motion during pacing in patients with coronary artery disease. Am J Cardiol 1983;51:668–675.
15. Yiannikas J, Simpfendorfer C, Detrano R, Salcedo EE, Sheldon WC. Stress digital subtraction angiography to assess presence of coronary artery disease in patients without myocardial infarction (abstr). Circulation 1963;68:III–41.
16. Detrano R, Simpfendorfer C, Day K, et al. Comparison of stress digital ventriculography, stress thallium scintigraphy, and digital fluoroscopy in the diagnosis of coronary artery disease in subjects without prior myocardial infarction. Am J Cardiol 1985;56:434–440.
17. Vogel R, LeFree M, Bates E, et al. Application of digital techniques to arteriography: use of myocardial contrast appearance time to measure coronary flow reserve. Am Heart J 1984;107:153–164.
18. Vogel RA, Bates ER, O'Neill WW, Aueron FM, Meier B, Gruentzig A. Coronary flow reserve measured during cardiac catheterization. Arch Intern Med 1984;144:1773–1776.
19. LeGrand V, Hodgson JM, Bates ER, et al. Abnormal coronary flow reserve and abnormal radionuclide exercise test results in patients with normal coronary angiograms. J Am Coll Cardiol 1985;6:1245–1253.
20. Bates ER, Aueron FM, LeGrand V, et al. Comparative effects of coronary artery bypass graft surgery and percutaneous transluminal coronary angioplasty on chronic regional coronary flow reserve. Circulation 1985;72:833–839.
21. Bates E, Vogel RA, LeFree MT, et al. The chronic coronary flow reserve provided by saphenous vein

bypass grafts as determined by digital radiography. Am Heart J 1984;108:462–468.

22. Nissen SE, Elion JL, Booth DC, Evans J, DeMaria AN. Value and limitations of computer analysis of digital subtraction angiography in the assessment of coronary flow reserve. Circulation 1986;73:562–571.

23. Tobis J, Johnston WD, Montelli S, et al. Digital coronary roadmapping as an aid for performing coronary angioplasty. Am J Cardiol 1985;56:237–241.

24. Ross AM, Johnson RA, Katz RJ, et al. Diagnosis of coronary disease by aortic digital subtraction angiography (abstr). Circulation 1983;68:III–43.

25. Wholey MH. Digital subtraction angiography in the evaluation of the ascending aortic and the pulmonary circulation. In: Wasserman AG, Ross AM, eds. Cardiac application of digital angiography. Mount Kisco, NY: Futura, 1988.

26. Moodie DS, Buonocore E, Yiannikas J, Gill CC, Pavlicek WA. Digital subtraction angiography in congenital heart disease in pediatric patients. Cleve Clin Q 1982;49:159–171.

27. Buonocore E, Pavlicek WA, Modic MT, et al. Anatomic and functional imaging of congenital heart disease with digital subtraction angiography. Radiology 1983;47:647–654.

28. Yiannikas J, Moodie DS, Gill CC, Sterba R, MacIntyre R, Buonocore E. Intravenous digital subtraction angiography in the assessment of patients with left–to–right shunts before and after surgical correction. J Am Coll Cardiol 1984;3:1507–1514.

29. Gordon T, Keyser PH, Moodie DS, Sterba R, Gill CC, Yiannikas J. The use of intravenous digital subtraction angiography in the evaluation of tetralogy of Fallot. Am Heart J, in press, 1989.

30. Moodie DS, Yiannikas J, Gill CC, Buonocore E, Pavlicek WA. Intravenous digital subtraction angiography in the evaluation of congenital abnormalities of the aorta and aortic arch. Am Heart J 1982;104:628–634.

31. Strother CM, Sackett JF, Crummy AB, et al. Clinical application of computerized fluroscopy, the extracranial carotid arteries. Radiology 1980; 136: 781–783.

32. Francis DA, Sheldon JJ, Soila K, Tobias J. Carotid artery and aortic arch imaging with ECG gating in DSA. Radiology 1985;155:827.

33. Gomes AS, Pais SO, Barbaric ZL. Digital subtraction angiography in the evolution of hypertension. Am J Radiol 1983;140:779–783.

34. Grossman LB, Buonocore E, Modic MT, Meaney TF. Digital subtraction angiography of the thoracic aorta. Radiology 1985;150:323–325.

35. Reilly RF, Smith CW, Price RR, et al. Digital subtraction pulmonary angiography. Am J Radiol 1982; 139:305–309.

36. Guthaner DF, Wexler L, Enzmann DR, et al. Evolution of peripheral vascular disease using digital subtraction angiography. Radiology 1983;147:393–398.

10

Radiographic Contrast Agents

James A. Hill, M.D.
Charles R. Lambert, M.D., Ph.D.
Carl J. Pepine, M.D.

INTRODUCTION

Essential to the generation of any image is a difference in contrast. Radiographic examination of the cardiovascular system primarily involves imaging structures of similar radiodensity, that of tissue. In general, there is not enough difference between such densities to generate an image when using conventional x-ray imaging techniques. Therefore, it is often necessary to enhance the minor degrees of contrast present through the use of various contrast agents, which absorb the transmission beam of x-rays to a greater extent than the surrounding tissue. Contrast agents are used in three basic ways in diagnostic imaging: by means of direct injection into a vascular lumen to outline the lumen, intravenous administration to evaluate distribution in various compartments, as is used in contrast enhanced CT scanning; and intravenous or oral administration to visualize their excretion from the body, such as in diagnostic urography or biliary imaging. At the current time, for cardiovascular imaging using x-rays, direct visualization after intravenous or intraarterial injection is the only way these agents are utilized.

As with any drug, these contrast agents should perform their function (i.e., provide for effective tissue contrast), without causing any untoward effects or altering physiologic function. However, the ideal agent that meets these criteria does not exist. The purpose of this chapter is to provide an overview of intravascular radiographic contrast agents and their properties, to discuss adverse effects that occur as a result of contrast media administration and how to manage them, and to specifi- cally discuss existing agents that are appropriate for cardiac angiography.

PHYSICAL PROPERTIES

All currently available contrast agents contain iodine, which in an appropriate concentration is an effective absorber of x-rays in the energy range of clinical imaging systems. While they differ structurally, they are all derivatives of triiodinated benzoic acids. There are a number of other compounds that will absorb x-rays and could therefore be utilized as contrast agents but they are too toxic. Toxicology data suggest that all iodine-containing agents are relatively biologically inert, but that they differ greatly in osmolality, viscosity, and other properties (Table 10.1). The amount of elemental iodine necessary to provide diagnostic imaging often is as much as 50 to 80 gm, which is approximately 1 million times the body's average daily turnover of iodine. The molecular weights of the available agents range from 600 to 1700.

Available agents used for vascular imaging may be divided into those that ionize in solution (ionic agents) and those that do not (nonionic agents). The conventional ionic contrast agents are all monomeric with either diatrizoate or iothalamate as the iodine carrier. These anions are combined with some combination of sodium and methylglucamine as cations. The ideal sodium-methylglucamine ratio, at least for coronary angiography, appears to be 1:6.6. The fact that these agents ionize in solution is relevant as to how they affect osmolality and electrophysiologic properties of tissue.

Table 10.1.
Contrast Agents Currently Utilized[a]

Generic Name	Trade Name (Manufacturer)	Iodine (mg/ml)	Osmolality (mOsm/kg)	Viscosity (25°C 37°C)		Na Content (mEq/liter)	Additives
Ionic							
Diatrizoate	Renografin-76	370	1940	13.8	8.4	190	Sodium citrate, 0.32%
sodium 100 mg/ml	(Squibb Diagnostics)						Disodium EDTA, 0.04%
meglumine 660 mg/ml							
Diatrizoate	Hypaque-76	370	2016	13.34	8.32	160	Calcium disodium EDTA, 0.01%
sodium 100 mg/ml	(Winthrop-Breon)						
meglumine 660 mg/ml							
Diatrizoate	Angiovist	370	2100	13.8	8.4	150	Calcium disodium EDTA, 0.01%
sodium 100 mg/ml meglumine 660 mg/ml	(Berlex)						
Ioxaglate sodium 19.6% meglumine 39.3%	Hexabrix (Mallinckrodt)	320	600	15.7	7.5	157	
Nonionic							
Iohexol	Omnipaque (Winthrop-Breon)	180 240 300 350	411 504 709 862	2.81 4.43 10.35 18.5	2.05 3.08 6.77 11.15		Calcium disodium EDTA, 10 mg/dl Tromethamine, 121 mg/dl
Iopamidol	Isovue Isovue (Squibb-Diagnostics)	300 370	616 796	8.8[b] 20.9[b]	4.7 9.4	200 200	Calcium disodium EDTA, 39 mg/dl (I–300) 48 mg/dl (I–370) Tromethamine, 100 mg/dl

[a]Modified from Fischer HW. Special report. Catalog of intravascular contrast media. Radiology 1986; 59:561–563 and Manufacturer Package Inserts (Berlex Laboratories, Inc., Wayne, NJ; Mallinckrodt, St. Louis, MO; Squibb Diagnostics, Princeton, NJ; Winthrop-Breon, New York, NY).
[b]Measured as meant: 20° C.

Osmolality is related to the number of particles in solution. The cations are radiologically inactive and only serve to increase the number of particles in solution. Osmolality can be reduced by either providing a compound that does not ionize, creating relatively more particles in solution that contain iodine, or providing more iodine molecules per particle in solution. A newer ionic agent, sodium methylglucamine ioxaglate (Hexabrix™), is a dimer and as a result contains twice as much iodine per molecule. This allows for major reduction of osmolality with equivalent iodine concentrations, as compared with conventional high osmolality ionic agents. Osmolality seems to be related to many physiologic and adverse effects caused by intravascular contrast agents. Considering that the osmolality of a widely used ionic contrast agent, meglumine sodium diatrizoate (Renografin-76™), is approximately seven times the serum osmolality, the potential implications for adverse physiologic effects are obvious, and reducing osmolality is a desirable goal.

Newer nonionic contrast agents do not ionize in solution and thus provide more particles that contain iodine in a given volume. Iopamidol (Isovue™) and iohexol (Omnipaque™) are two examples of these agents that are applicable to cardiac angiography. They are structurally different from ionic agents and can have an equivalent iodine content with a lower osmolality, as compared with conventional ionic agents. In addition, these newer nonionic agents tend to associate in solution, thereby further reducing the number of particles in solution and lowering the osmolality more than might be expected on a molecular basis alone.

PHARMACOLOGY

Available intravascular radiographic contrast agents have low lipid solubility and minimal plasma protein binding. They rapidly distribute in the body's extracellular space. Their molecular size and low lipid solubility effectively prevent passage across cell membranes in any significant amount, and thus, very little is absorbed. This size also allows them to be effectively filtered by glomeruli, and they are almost entirely excreted by the kidney.

The half-life for excretion in patients with normal renal function is 30 to 60 min. Other routes of excretion include the liver and bile, as well as other body secretions, such as sweat, tears, and saliva. These agents are freely filtered by the kidney but are neither secreted nor absorbed. The amount of contrast agent entering tubules is determined by the glomerular filtration rate and plasma concentration. As water and sodium are reabsorbed, the contrast agent is concentrated to a level markedly higher than that entering the tubule. Contrast agents also enhance urinary excretion of oxalate and uric acid with diatrizoate, having been shown to increase oxalate excretion by 96%. This may contribute to nephrotoxicity.

Although amounts of contrast present and the kinetics of distribution in various tissues differ widely, there seem to be few if any differences among the agents themselves (1). However, this is generally of no consequence

to standard cardiac imaging, as the images are made in real time and immediately after injection. Even with signal-averaging imaging techniques, the imaging times are soon enough after injection for distribution kinetics not to significantly influence results.

Materials that are added to preserve or stabilize the radiocontrast agents also vary among preparations and contribute to their differences (e.g., ethylenediamine tetraacetic acid (EDTA) to prevent metal-catalyzed deiodination). The major additives bind calcium. Different contrast agents contain different additives that bind calcium differently and, thus, have a different effect on the coronary venous calcium levels after intracoronary injection. Binding of calcium contributes to adverse hemodynamic effects noted with intracoronary injection. Data suggest that the negative inotropic effects caused by calcium-binding actions of these agents can be reduced by adding calcium to the media (2). Data from animal studies with Urografin-76™, iopamidol, ioxaglate, and iohexol show that the agents with the lesser calcium-binding effect (i.e., iohexol, iopamidol, and ioxaglate) cause less of a decrease in coronary sinus calcium (3, 4). How calcium binding interacts with lower osmolarity to produce fewer hemodynamic effects is not clear, but several studies have noted fewer hemodynamic alterations using noncalcium-binding nonionic agents (5, 6). In addition to adverse hemodynamic alterations, ventricular fibrillation that can occur with intracoronary injection is also increased with contrast agents that bind calcium (7-10). Repolarization is altered by calcium binding that contributes to the occurrence of ventricular fibrillation. Addition of calcium to the agents will decrease the incidence of ventricular fibrillation. Serum calcium will decrease transiently (11) when agents with these additives are administered, but this is unlikely to have important clinical implications.

Sodium content is likewise important. It was once assumed that the lower the sodium, the safer the intracoronary injection, based on the fact that higher content sodium agents were very toxic. Other data, however, suggest that no sodium in the medium is also toxic, and it appears that sodium content is optimal when it is near the physiologic level (12). Nonionic agents may change coronary venous sodium concentration less than conventional agents. How this contributes to the lower toxicity of these agents is not known.

ADVERSE EFFECTS

Adverse effects of contrast agents generally fall into two categories, anaphylactoid and toxic. Anaphylactoid reactions include urticaria, cardiovascular collapse, angioedema, and bronchospasm. Toxic reactions include hot flushing sensation, nausea, metallic taste, arrhythmias, vascular congestion, and renal failure. Anaphylactoid reactions generally are idiosyncratic, whereas toxic effects occur in most patients to some degree. These will be discussed separately.

Anaphylactoid

Anaphylactoid reactions are of two types, major and minor, depending on the severity and what needs to be done therapeutically. Often allergic in nature, these include bronchospasm, urticaria, angioedema, and shock. These reactions are neither dose- nor injection rate-related. There are a number of hypotheses as to why these reactions occur but some, if not all, are immune (IgE)-mediated. There is some evidence that complementary, alternate pathways and kinin activation occur in these patients, but this does not occur consistently and may occur in the absence of an adverse reaction (13). Regardless of the mechanism involved, there appears to be at least some increased risk of a repeat adverse reaction when one has occurred previously. Skin testing for these reactions is generally not felt to be useful (14) and may be misleading. A repeat reaction may be of a lesser nature and may be obviated by various pretreatment regimens. However, an essential indicator of the angiographic procedure should be clearly documented, and emergency equipment should be available in the event the repeat anaphylactoid reaction is severe.

Toxic

As opposed to anaphylactoid reactions, toxic reactions are due to the inherent physical or chemical properties and toxicity of contrast agents and the substances added to them. The majority of toxic effects probably occur as a result of hyperosmolality. Major physiologic effects occur as a result of the hyperosmolality of contrast agents when they are injected into the blood stream. Locally, erythrocytes lose cellular water very rapidly and increase internal viscosity. The cells are then unable to deform appropriately to cross the capillary beds, and acute capillary plugging can occur. This can particularly be a problem in patients with pulmonary hypertension or sickle cell anemia when a high osmolar agent is used. Endothelial damage can also occur as a result of the high osmolality of contrast injected near the endothelium, with resultant thrombophlebitis and thrombosis in the veins utilized. Hyperosmolality can result in a major increase in intravascular volume by drawing in extravascular water. The vasodilation that occurs also seems to be directly related to the osmolality. Neurotoxicity may also be related to the capillary damage that can occur from the hyperosmolar contrast injection.

Hypotension

Cardiovascular collapse can occur without anaphylactoid characteristics. Hypotension and cardiovascular collapse that can occur in relation to contrast media administration may be anaphylactoid-type reactions, may be due to the direct toxic effects of the agent, or may be vasovagal in nature. It is obvious that recognition of the cause is essential if appropriate therapy is to be administered. Anaphylactoid reactions usually get worse quickly despite efforts to raise blood pressure. When this occurs, it is best to insert multiple, large-bore, intravenous lines and administer fluids, colloids, and vasopressors as rapidly as possible. The blood pressure decline is often very resistant to these measures, and it may take many liters of fluid and up to an hour or two of vasopressor support to raise and maintain the blood pressure. In the cardiac patient this can be hazardous because these patients are frequently those in whom a fall in blood pressure is poorly tolerated. Direct toxic effects of the agent refer primarily to the hyperosmolality-induced drop in blood pressure. This is usually transient and generally does not require any treatment. In circumstances where treatment is necessary, oxygen administration and leg elevation will usually rapidly reverse the hypotension. If the hypotension persists or worsens despite these measures, other mechanisms should be considered. Vagal reactions should be considered, especially if there is also a decline in heart rate, although this is not universal, and a pure vasodepressor reaction can occur. These reactions are usually reversed promptly by atropine and fluids.

Nephrotoxicity

Contrast nephrotoxicity is one of the most commonly discussed adverse effects of radiographic contrast media. The acute incidence of acute renal insufficiency after intravascular contrast administration is unknown. Various studies have reported different incidences, depending on how renal toxicity is defined, which population is studied, and how the contrast is administered. Rates vary between 0 and 92%, but realistically, a significant rise in serum creatinine probably occurs in <5% of patients with normal renal function, when standard contrast agents and volumes are used. It seems that intraarterial administration has a higher rate of nephrotoxicity (15-20). Whether this is related to patient selection, disease state, contrast volume, direct renal injection, or other factors is not clear.

Risk factors for contrast nephrotoxicity appear to include advanced age, underlying renal insufficiency, dehydration, hyperuricemia, diabetes mellitus, congestive heart failure, and multiple contrast exposures over a brief period of time. Whether these are independent risk factors depends on the study, but many patients who develop nephrotoxicity have multiple risk factors, with a recent study finding 3.67 (mean) risk factors per patient (21). In a study limited to cardiac angiography and conventional contrast agents in patients with abnormal renal function, the incidence of worsening renal function was 23% (18). Class IV heart failure, multiple contrast studies within 72 hours, insulin-dependent diabetes mellitus, and contrast dose were significant risk factors. In the absence of other risk factors, the incidence was 2% in patients who received <125 ml of contrast agent, whereas in those who received >125 ml the incidence was 19%.

Possible mechanisms for contrast-induced renal toxicity include direct contrast toxicity, renal hemodynamic changes, tubular obstruction by protein or uric acid crystals, immune reactions, or red cell sludging. While data exist to support all of these potential mechanisms, most agree that the injury is related to a combination of direct toxicity and changes in renal blood flow.

Patients who experience nephrotoxicity usually, but not always, present with oliguria within the first 24 hours after contrast administration. This lasts for only 2 to 4 days, with the serum creatinine peaking at approximately 7 days with a gradual return to baseline levels in the large majority of cases. Occasionally, hemodialysis is necessary, but this is unusual. Occasionally, recovery may be delayed for several weeks. Several guidelines should be followed in patients at risk for this complication. These include adequate hydration before and after exposure, limiting contrast load to 0.88 mg of iodine/kg, and limiting the number of contrast studies within any 24- to 48-hr period in patients at high risk. All high-risk patients should be observed for urine output and serum creatinine after study for at least 24 hrs. While it may be helpful, use of either mannitol or diuretics to maintain urine flow is controversial (22).

Whether there are any differences between conventional and newer agents in the degree of renal dysfunction produced has not been completely resolved. Some data suggest less renal toxicity occurs with the nonionic agent iopamidol (23). Iopamidol may also produce less protein aggregation in the tubules than diatrizoate, thus limiting any potential for nephrotoxicity from this mechanism (23). The reader is referred to a recent review (22) for further discussion of this topic as it relates to cardiac angiographic procedures.

Thromboembolism

Data regarding the thromboembolic complications of contrast agents must be interpreted in conjunction with the techniques utilized to perform the catheterization procedure and the type of patient studied. Use of systemic anticoagulation, the use of heparin-bonded catheters, the time the catheters are in the vascular system, and the amount of flushing of catheters all will affect the incidence of thromboembolic problems. It appears that low osmolar contrast agents do not have the same inhibitory effects on blood clotting and platelet aggregation that the conventional agents do. At least one report involving three patients (24) suggests that use of a nonionic agent may have contributed to major thromboembolic complications during coronary angiography. It is our opinion that these problems result from breakdown in meticulous technique rather than the contrast agent. When using low osmolar contrast agents, the operator should strongly consider systemic anticoagulation during cardiac angiographic procedures, avoid leaving blood and contrast mixtures in syringes for prolonged periods, and maintain a meticulous routine of flushing catheters and cleaning guidewires. Others have suggested adding heparin to the contrast agent (24).

Incidence of Adverse Effects

While not limited to only cardiac applications, the most comprehensive data regarding adverse reactions to intravascular administration of contrast agents have been collected by the Committee on Safety of Contrast Media of the International Society of Radiology (14, 25). These data were collected when only conventional agents were used, and it is difficult to prove that serious adverse reactions will be reduced by newer agents because of the low incidence and recurrence of reactions. The overall incidence of adverse reactions is approximately 5%, but with arterial injection it is only about one-half of that. In patients with a history of allergy, the incidence is 10 to 12%, with the risk being highest in those with a shellfish or saltwater fish allergy, followed by various other food allergies, asthma, hay fever, and penicillin, in descending frequency. In those with a prior history of contrast reaction the frequency of adverse reaction is only 15 to 16%, with serious reactions rarely recurring. Mild adverse reactions for which no treatment is required and moderate ones for which treatment but not hospitalization is required comprise the overwhelming majority of adverse reactions. Occasionally, severe reactions occur for which hospitalization is necessary (0.007%). The incidence of death following conventional contrast agent administration is estimated to be between 1/10,000 and 1/40,000.

Handling the "Contrast Allergic" Patient

Exactly how patients with a history of contrast reaction should be managed with repeat administration is not clear. Management of this problem has ranged over the years from complete avoidance of contrast to skin testing and test dosing to various premedication regimens and finally to doing nothing at all

because of the relatively low incidence of severe repeat reactions. None of these approaches is totally satisfactory, but pharmacotherapy regimens for premedication appear to be the safest.

Greenberger et al. (26) reported on a series of 857 contrast media administrations to patients who had a prior history of anaphylactoid reactions to contrast media undergoing repeat studies after various pretreatment regimens. In 695 cases, prednisone and diphenhydramine were administered, and there was a 10.8% reaction rate with 0.7% developing transient hypotension. Subsequently, 180 procedures were performed with ephedrine added to the regimen, and only a 5% rate was noted. Further addition of cimetidine did not change the rate significantly.

In another study reported by Ring et al. (27), various combinations of steroids and histamine H-1 and H-2 receptor antagonists or normal saline were given prospectively to 800 patients undergoing intravenous contrast administration for renal study. In the normal saline group, the incidence of adverse effects, excluding heat sensation, was 12.9%, whereas, in the combined H-1 and H-2 blocker group the incidence was 6.1% ($p < 0.05$). Nausea, urticaria, and angioedema were significantly less with this treatment. There were no other significant differences noted. Only one type of contrast agent was used, so comparison among agents is not possible.

Lasser et al. (28) reported on a series of 6763 patients who never had experienced a reaction to contrast agents. These patients were given either two doses of methylprednisolone (or placebo) 12 and 2 hr prior or one dose of methylprednisolone (or placebo) 2 hr prior to contrast administration. They found that the incidence of contrast reactions was significantly less using the two-dose regimen, as compared with the one-dose regimen (6.4 vs. 9.4%). Moreover, the adverse reaction rate in the placebo group was no different, as compared with the one-dose regimen (9.9 vs. 9.4%). Comparing their data with uncontrolled data using nonionic contrast agents, they found no difference in the rate of reactions between the 2-dose methylprednisolone regimen group and the nonionic contrast group. They suggested that nonionic agents did not provide any benefit in routine use for preventing adverse effects to contrast agents.

From a practical standpoint, how should these data be applied to the patient undergoing cardiac angiography? There are a number of factors that make available data somewhat less relevant to the average patient undergoing cardiac catheterization. First, most of the available studies are in a broad group of patients receiving contrast for a variety of procedures, not just those receiving arterial injection for angiography. Reaction rates with arterial, as opposed to venous, injection may be different. Patients undergoing cardiac catheterization tend to be older than the population at large receiving contrast agents, making them somewhat less likely to have a reaction. However, the type of patient undergoing cardiac catheterization and angiography is less likely to tolerate a severe "allergic-type" reaction. For the population at large, it is the authors' practice not to premedicate with steroids but only with diphenhydramine orally 30 min before the procedure. As more patients are done as outpatients, the administration of steroids 12 hr before contrast administration, as the data reviewed above suggest is necessary, presents some practical problems.

In the patient who has a history of severe reaction to contrast agents, we believe that premedication with steroids (60 mg of prednisone or the equivalent) the night before and immediately prior to the procedure is appropriate. In addition, diphenhydramine (50 mg) and cimetidine (300 mg) should also be given because these agents are very well tolerated and may provide some additional protection. Routine use of β-adrenergic agonist drugs, such as ephedrine, is potentially dangerous in the cardiac patient and should not be used routinely. While the data are not clear that this regimen is necessary or effective, it is imperative that reasonable measures be taken to avoid contrast reactions in such a patient.

CARDIAC EFFECTS
Electrocardiographic Changes and Arrhythmias

The major change that occurs in the ECG as a result of intracoronary administration of contrast agents is sinus node slowing. This effect occurs 5 to 10 sec after injection and persists for approximately 60 sec. It occurs somewhat more frequently with right coronary than left coronary injection. This is probably due to direct effects on the sinus node, as well as to reflex vagal suppression. In addition, there is shifting of the QRS axis, increasing QRS duration, ST segment depression, T wave inversion or peaking, and increased AV conduction as manifested by P-R prolongation and occasionally development of higher degrees of heart block. Some degree of ECG change is almost universal, especially with high osmolar ionic agents, and follows the same time course as the sinus slowing but may persist for a slightly longer period. These ECG changes appear to be related to the osmolality and probably the electrolyte balance. These changes are markedly attenuated with the newer nonionic agents.

Ventricular arrhythmias also may occur, and these appear related to sodium and calcium content as mentioned previously. These effects occur irrespective of the coronary anatomy and do not seem any more frequent in patients with severe coronary artery disease than in normal patients, although they may not be as well tolerated in the more severely ill patients. The incidence and severity of both the ECG effects and the rhythm disturbances depend to a great extent on the contrast agent used. Among the agents in general use today, diatrizoate seems to cause much more severe effects on these parameters than do the lower osmolality agents, but with all of these agents the safety is markedly improved over the older agents used for coronary angiography that had ventricular fibrillation rates as high as 11%.

Effects on Systemic Hemodynamic Parameters

Administration of contrast media generally causes some transient decrease in both systemic vascular resistance and blood pressure. This may be mild or marked, but the degree to which it occurs probably is related to the osmolarity of the agent utilized, with the conventional higher osmolar agents having a greater effect. It occurs with systemic injection, suggesting peripheral vasodilation. But intracoronary administration also causes a decrease in systemic blood pressure. This latter effect is probably related to effects of the contrast agent on left ventricular function and various reflexes.

The effect of angiographic contrast media on ventricular function seems to be related to the method of administration. When conventional agents are given directly into a coronary artery, there is a consistent rise in left ventricular end-diastolic pressure, but ejection fraction and ventricular volume are not affected to any major degree. Following left ventricular angiography, the left ventricular end-diastolic pressure generally rises, especially with the use of conventional ionic, high osmolar contrast agents. Data comparing contrast agents and their effect on left ventricular hemodynamics conflict, but there appears to be less of an effect when lower-osmolarity agents are used (29-32). Ejection fractions and ventricular volumes seem to exhibit only minor changes, at least in the early period after angiography (33). This may be more pronounced in patients with abnormal ventricular function. It may be related to a direct toxic effect (e.g., effect of calcium-binding), an abnormality of the calcium/sodium relationship, enhanced myocardial ischemia causing compliance changes, an increase in intravascular volume secondary to the osmotic load, or some combination of these factors. Time after angiography is an important determinant in the responsible mechanism. There is evidence to support all of these ideas, and in any given patient the mechanism probably differs.

Effects on Coronary Flow and Dilation

Injection of conventional contrast agents into a coronary artery causes a transient increase in coronary flow and decrease in coronary resistance within seconds of injection (34). This appears similar in magnitude to the reactive hyperemia response secondary to release of acute coronary occlusion and thus is probably related to coronary vascular reserve. This flow increase is primarily due to the hyperosmolality as the changes appear less with lower osmolar agents and can be reproduced by higher osmolar saline. This transient increase in coronary blood flow does seem to cause only a small change in large coronary artery size. Using standard doses of diatrizoate sodium meglumine and high magnification 105-mm photospot coronary angiograms, we (35) have found only minimal changes in epicardial coronary artery size, using a magnify-

ing optical measuring device. This technique has magnification and precision capabilities far in excess of standard magnification and measuring techniques. It is unlikely that the minimal coronary dilating effects of contrast agents will alter interpretation of angiograms for diagnostic purposes.

GUIDELINES FOR USE

A general principle of cardiac catheterization is that the procedure should be performed as safely as possible while obtaining the necessary diagnostic information. There is no value to performing multiple procedures when it can be determined that one provides all the necessary information. Use of contrast agents should be viewed in the same way. It is preferable to do one diagnostic angiogram rather than to have to repeat an angiogram because of inadequate visualization. Angiography should also be performed in order of decreasing clinical importance. The angiogram (site and projection) that will yield the most diagnostic information should be the first one obtained, especially if the patient has the potential to tolerate only a small volume of contrast. This way, if the procedure needs to be aborted, useful information has been obtained.

The amount of contrast administered for any angiogram depends on a variety of factors, including the type of catheter used, the vessel or chamber to be visualized, rate of blood flow in the vessel, size of the patient, tissue density, total amount necessary for all of the angiograms to be performed, and type of contrast agent used. Likewise, rate of injection is related to many factors, the most important of which are the vessel or chamber to be visualized, the flow rate in the vessel, and the type of catheter. Guidelines are provided in Table 10.2. It must be remembered, however, that these guidelines should be individualized to the patient undergoing study and that it is always better to have one diagnostic angiogram than two of less than optimal quality.

Choosing a Contrast Agent

It is apparent that there are a number of different contrast agents that are suitable for cardiac angiography. Choosing among the different agents is, to a certain extent, a matter of personal preference. The major differences

Table 10.2
Guidelines for Administration of Contrast Agents

Type of Angiography	Dose (ml)	Rate of Injection (ml/sec)
Coronary artery		
Right	3–6	2–3
Left	4–7	2–3
Bypass grafts	4–7	2–3
Left ventricular	30–45	10–15
Aortic	30–60	15–30
Right ventricular	30–45	10–15
Pulmonary artery	30–60	15–30

have been discussed, and this information can be used to guide choice. There has been some debate regarding the appropriate utilization of the newer nonionic, low-osmolar contrast agents. This discussion stems from the fact that these agents are considerably more expensive than conventional agents, and so a significant anticipated benefit should be demonstrated before these agents are routinely administered. There are considerable data available that suggest that these newer agents are safe and provide diagnostic quality angiography similar to that of conventional agents. They are unquestionably better tolerated by patients, particularly those that are "high risk," according to both subjective and objective measures (36) (Fig. 10.1).

Feldman et al. (37) randomized 82 patients with unstable ischemic syndromes or heart failure to receive either ioxaglate or diatrizoate sodium meglumine during cardiac catheterization. This group of patients was chosen because it was an unstable group in which contrast-related complications would be least tolerated. Clinical diagnosis, hemodynamics before contrast administration, left ventricular ejection fraction, case duration, contrast volume, and cinefilm quality were not significantly different. A total of 10 contrast-related adverse reactions occurred, 3 of which were minor. Of the seven severe adverse reactions, such as acute pulmonary edema and prolonged systemic hypotension (<100 mm Hg systolic pressure), six were in the diatrizoate group, and only one was in the ioxaglate group, a significant difference.

Roubin et al. recently (38) randomized 925 patients undergoing percutaneous transluminal coronary angioplasty (PTCA) who received either iopamidol ($n = 445$) or diatrizoate ($n = 480$). Sixty-seven percent of the patients were either New York Heart Association (NYHA) class 3 or 4, and 45% had multivessel coronary artery disease (CAD). They found a significantly lower incidence of ventricular tachycardia or fibrillation with iopamidol, as compared with diatrizoate (2.3% vs. 0.7%). There was significant difference in the incidence of either hypotension or ischemic complications. Gertz et al. (30) reported data from a group of patients undergoing catheterization, showing more severe hypotension and ECG changes in the group receiving diatrizoate, as compared with those receiving iopamidol. In a crossover trial,

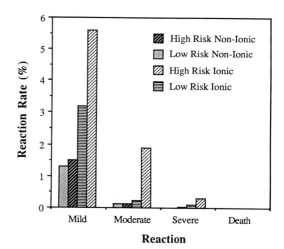

Figure 10.1. Reaction rates observed in 61,000 patients from the R.A.C.R. survey of ionic and nonionic intravenous contrast use. Patients who were high risk and received a nonionic agent had a lower reaction rate than those who were low risk and received an ionic agent. (Modified from Palmer FJ. The R.A.C.R. survey of intravenous contrast media reactions: a preliminary report. Australas Radiol 1988;32:8-11.)

Ciuffo et al.(39) reported similar findings. Iohexol was likewise found to cause less severe changes, as compared with diatrizoate (32). Lambert et al. have recently demonstrated a more stable course during catheterization in 15 patients with severe aortic stenosis, using iopamidol, as compared with a similar group using diatrizoate (40).

In a recent clinical evaluation of iopamidol, 76%, 9239 patients undergoing contrast administration were evaluated (Squibb Diagnostics, unpublished data). The overall incidence of contrast-related side effects was 614:9239 (0.066%). Of these 9239 patients, 8874 (96%) underwent cardiac angiographic procedures. There was an 0.065% incidence of side effects in this group. Of the patients studied, 61.1% had unstable angina, 20.2% had impaired left ventricular function, 10.6% had recurrent ventricular arrhythmias, and 23.2% were felt to be at risk for renal complications. Of the side effects experienced during the procedure, bradyarrhythmias accounted for 26.9%, angina for 27.4%, ventricular fibrillation for 4.1%, nausea and vomiting for 18.1%, systemic hypotension for 20.4%, hives for 5.4%, death for 1.5%, and assorted other complications for the rest. The overall incidence of death was 9/9239 (0.00097%). This incidence of death is comparable to available statistics for administration of conventional contrast agents in the population at large.

The guidelines listed in Table 10.3 provide a profile of indications for the routine use of nonionic, low-osmolar contrast agents. However, many laboratories, including ours, have begun to utilize nonionic or low-osmolar contrast agents routinely in all patients undergoing cardiac angiography. Cost appears to be the major limiting factor to their more widespread use. How the operator chooses to utilize these agents should be based on the clinical situation and assessment of patient status. Gertz and colleagues compared ionic and nonionic contrast media in cardiac angiography and found that nonionic agents were essentially devoid of important changes in the ECG and systemic blood pressure. (41)

CONCLUSIONS

Contrast agents for intravascular administration have been refined so that they can provide diagnostic quality angiography with minimal risk. Low osmolar agents, many of which are nonionic, are available which offer an excellent alternative to conventional high osmolar agents, especially in unstable high-risk patients. Currently, the need is not for agents that will lower risk further while providing needed contrast but for a safer way to administer them.

Table 10.3
Generally Accepted Indications for Use of Low Osmolar Contrast Agents

Unstable ischemic syndromes
Congestive heart failure
Diabetes mellitus
Renal insufficiency
Hypotension
Severe bradycardia
History of contrast allergy
Severe valvular heart disease
Need for internal mammary artery injection
History of transient ischemic attack or recent cerebrovascular accident
Percutaneous transluminal coronary angioplasty

References

1. Morris TW, Fischer HW. The pharmacology of intravascular radiocontrast media. Annu Rev Pharmacol Toxicol 1986;26:143-160.
2. Hanley PC, Holmes DR, Julsrud PR, Smith HC. Use of conventional and newer radiographic contrast agents in cardiac angiography. Prog Cardiovasc Dis 1986;28:435-448.
3. Thomson KR, Evill CA, Firzsche J, Benness G. Comparison of iopamidol, ioxaglate and diatrizoate during coronary arteriography in dogs. Invest Radiol 1980;115:234-241.
4. Bourdillon PD, Bettmann MD, McCracken S, Poole-Wilson PA, Grossmann W. Effects of a new nonionic and a conventional ionic contrast agent on coronary sinus ionized calcium and left ventricular hemodynamics in dogs. J Am Coll Cardiol 1985;6:845-853.
5. Murdock DK, Walsh J, Euler DE, Kozeny G, Scanlon P. Inotropic effects of ionic contrast media: the role of calcium binding additives. Cathet Cardiovasc Diagn 1984; 10:455-463.
6. Higgins CB, Gerber KH, Mattrey RF, Slutsky RA. Evaluation of the hemodynamic effects of intravenous administration of ionic and nonionic contrast materials. Radiology 1982;142:681-686.
7. Zukerman LS, Friehling TD, Wolf NM, Meister SG, Nahass G, Kowey PR. Effect of calcium binding additives on ventricular fibrillation and repolarization changes during coronary angiography. J Am Coll Cardiol 1987;10:1249-1253.
8. Murdock DK, Johnson SA, Loeb HS, Scanlon PJ. Ventricular fibrillation during coronary angiography: reduced incidence in man with contrast media

lacking calcium binding additives. Cathet Cardiovasc Diagn 1985;59:153-159.

9. Murdock DK, Euler DE, Kozeny G, Murdock JD, Loeb HS, Scanlon PJ. Ventricular fibrillation during coronary angiography in dogs: the role of calcium binding additives. Am J Cardiol 1984;54:897-901.

10. Violante MR, Thomson KR, Fischer HW, Kenyon T. Ventricular fibrillation from diatrizoate with and without chelating agents. Radiology 1978;128:497-498.

11. Berger RE, Gomez LS, Mallette LE. Acute hypocalcemic effects of clinical contrast media injections. Am J Roentgenol 1982;138:282-288.

12. Paulin S, Adams DF. Increased ventricular fibrillation during coronary arteriography with a new contrast medium preparation. Radiology 1971;101:45-50.

13. Goldberg M. Systemic reactions to intravascular contrast media. Anesthesiology 1984;60:46-56.

14. Shehadi WH. Adverse reactions to intravascularly administered contrast media. Am J Roentgenol 1975;124:145-152.

15. Berkseth RO, Kjellstrand CM. Radiologic contrast induced nephropathy. Med Clin North Am 1984;68:351-370.

16. Mason RA, Arbeit LA, Giron F. Renal dysfunction after arteriography. JAMA 1985;253:1001-1004.

17. D'Elia JA, Gleason RE, Alday M, et al. Nephrotoxicity from angiographic contrast material. Am J Med 1982;72:719-725.

18. Taliercio CP, Vlietstra RE, Fisher LD, Burnett JC. Risks for renal dysfunction with cardiac angiography. Ann Intern Med 1986;104:501-504.

19. Swartz RD, Rubin JE, Leeming BW, Silva P. Renal failure following major angiography. Am J Med 1978;65:31-37.

20. Martin-Paredero V, Dixon SM, Baker JD, et al. Risk of renal failure after major angiography. Arch Surg 1983;118:1417-1420.

21. Byrd L, Sherman RL. Radiocontrast induced acute renal failure: a clinical and pathophysiologic review. Medicine 1979;58:270-278.

22. Taliercio CP, Burnett JC. Contrast nephropathy, cardiology and the newer radiocontrast agents. Int J Cardiol 1988;19:145-151.

23. Humes HD, Cielinski DA, Messana JM. Effects of radiocontrast agents on renal tubule cell function: implications regarding the pathogenesis of contrast induced nephrotoxicity effects of contrast agents on renal function. Cardio 1988;5:14-18.

24. Grollman JH, Liu CK, Astone RA, Lurie MD. Thromboembolic complications in coronary angiography associated with the use of nonionic contrast medium. Cathet Cardiovasc Diagn 1988;14:159-164.

25. Shehadi WH. Contrast media adverse reactions: occurrence, recurrence and distribution patterns. Diagn Radiol 1982;143:11-17.

26. Greenberger WA, Patterson R, Tapio CM. Prophylaxis against repeated radiocontrast media reactions in 857 cases. Arch Intern Med 1985;145:2197-2200.

27. Ring J, Rothenberger K-H, Clauss W. Prevention of anaphylactoid reactions after radiographic contrast media infusion by combined histamine H1 and H2 receptor antagonists: results of a prospective controlled trial. Int Arch Allergy Appl Immun 1985;78:9-14.

28. Lasser EC, Berry CC, Talner LB, et al. Pretreatment with corticosteroids to alleviate reactions to intravenous contrast material. N Engl J Med 1987;317:845-849.

29. Salem DN, Konstam MA, Isner JM, Bonin JD. Comparison of the electrocardiographic and hemodynamic responses to ionic and nonionic radiocontrast media during left ventriculography: a randomized double blind study. Am Heart J 1986;111:533-536.

30. Gertz EW, Wisneski JA, Chiu D, Akin JR, Hu C. Clinical superiority of a new nonionic contrast agent (iopamidol) for cardiac angiography. J Am Coll Cardiol 1985;5:250-258.

31. Bettmann MA, Higgins CB. Comparison of an ionic with a nonionic contrast agent for cardiac angiography. Cardiac Angiography 1985;29:S70-S74.

32. Mancini GBJ, Bloomquist JN, Bhargava V, et al. Hemodynamic and electrocardiographic effects in man of a new nonionic contrast agent (iohexol): advantages over standard ionic agents. Am J Cardiol 1983;51:1218-1222.

33. Stern L, Firth BG, Dehmer GJ, et al. Effect of selective coronary arteriography on left ventricular volumes and ejection fraction in man. Am J Cardiol 1980;46:827-831.

34. Kloster FE, Griesen WG, Green GS, Judkins MP. Effects of coronary arteriography on myocardial blood flow. Circulation 1972;46:438-444.

35. Hill JA, Feldman RL, Conti CR, Pepine CJ. Effects of selective injection of contrast media on coronary artery diameter. Cathet Cardiovasc Diagn 1982;8:547-552.

36. Palmer FJ. The R.A.C.R. survey of intravenous contrast media reactions: a preliminary report. Australas Radiol 1988;32:8-11.

37. Feldman RL, Jalowiec DA, Hill JA, Lambert CR. Contrast media related complications during cardiac catheterization using HexabrixTM or RenografinTM in high risk patients. Am J Cardiol 1988;61:1334-1337.

38. Lembo NJ, Roubin GS, Chin HK, Black AJ, Douglas JS, King SB. Does nonionic contrast media decrease the incidence of PTCA related complications? (Abstr) Circulation 1988;78:II-378.

39. Ciuffo AA, Fuchs RM, Guzman PA, et al. Benefits of nonionic contrast in coronary arteriography: preliminary results of a randomized double-blind trial comparing iopamidol and renografin-76. Invest Radiol 1984;19:S197-S202.

40. Lambert CR, Pepine CJ. Hemodynamic effects of high versus low-osmolar contrast media for ventriculography in severe aortic stenosis. Cardiovasc Intervent Radiol 1988;11:10-13.

41. Wisneski JA, Gertz EW, Dahlgren M, Muslin A. Comparison of low osmolality ionic (ioxaglate) versus nonionic (iopamidol) contrast media in cardiac angiography. Am J Cardiol 1989, in press.

11

Cinefilm and Processing

Arnold Auger, M.D.

INTRODUCTION

Assuming that procedures outlined in Chapter 8 have been employed to optimize the x-ray system so that the best image that the equipment is capable of producing at the surface of the film is created, it is appropriate to direct attention to cinefilm and its processing. The correct combination of film, chemistry, and processor to give the final image desired must be chosen and constantly maintained in order to achieve excellent diagnostic film quality. The physician practicing in the cardiac catheterization laboratory should have an understanding of these areas to optimize the results of his studies.

CINEFILM

Cinefilm is produced by many companies for many purposes, none of which is coronary cineangiography. Therefore, a film that will satisfy the requirements for coronary angiography without making major compromises must be chosen from among these commercially available. What exactly are these requirements?

In cineangiography the image is produced by light on an image intensifier tube, which uses ionizing radiation as its exciting source. This means that the patient is being exposed to both primary and secondary (scattered) radiation, while others in the laboratory are exposed to scattered radiation. The amount of radiation is directly proportional to the amount of energy used to excite the tube to produce the diagnostic image. Safety dictates that the diagnostic image be produced with

the least amount of radiation exposure for both the patient and those in the laboratory who absorb scattered radiation on a daily basis. Hence, choosing a "fast" film (i.e., one that requires a minimum amount of light to produce a properly exposed image), should reduce the amount of light needed, and therefore the amount of radiation. Although on first observation this seems to be a reasonable assumption, since the cinefilm camera records the image from the image intensifier with an input screen made of crystals that are activated by the x-ray photons, it is mandatory that enough photons strike the screen to reduce the quantum mottle to a level low enough to render the finished product diagnostic. Because cinefilm speed is increased by increasing the grain size of the silver in the emulsion, fast film tends to exaggerate the quantum mottle (large grain size) to the point that the film may be unacceptably "noisy." Detail is reduced to such an extent that the picture produced may not be of diagnostic quality. This problem can be negated by decreasing the aperture size of the lens on the cinecamera. However, this move will require an increase in x-ray exposure to the patient and personnel in order to reduce the quantum mottle to an acceptable level. A "slower" film would not exaggerate the mottle but would require a higher radiation exposure to obtain enough light. Hence, a compromise between the level of quantum mottle and an acceptable radiation level must always be made by those involved in cineangiography. Diagnostic quality angiography should be achieved at the lowest possible risk to patient and personnel.

Characteristics of Currently Available Cinefilm

What are the characteristics of the products that are currently available? In answering this question the individual manufacturers of the films will not be considered, but rather film in its generic sense will be discussed. As noted above, the faster the film, the larger the size of the silver particle in the emulsion and the grainier the film appears. Grainy film records less detail. Thus, as grain size decreases, the speed of the film slows, but its ability to record detail increases. Under most circumstances, the larger the grain size, the higher the contrast of the film or the steeper its exposure-density curve or characteristic curve. The exposure-density curve indicates in graphic form the effect of exposure levels and developing time on the density produced in the emulsion of a given film. These curves are available from the film producers and act as a handy guide to the capabilities of a given film product. The smaller the grain size, the flatter the exposure-density curve, with a corresponding decrease in contrast. Characteristics of fast and slow film are summarized and compared in Table 11.1.

Taking the compromises discussed earlier into consideration, it would seem that choosing a film that is somewhere between slow and fast film would be optimal. The type of film preferred will also depend on some other considerations since cinefilm has certain other characteristics. These are listed below.

1. D_{max} is the maximum density that a fully exposed and optimally processed film can produce.
2. **Amount of light that is available to project the film**. This factor will depend upon the cinefilm projection and circumstances used for film review (individual reviewing film in darkened room, panel reviewing film projected in light room, carbon arc projection, etc). This factor governs the total extent of the film's capabilities.
3. **Inherent fog level**. Fog is inherent in all film and increases with age and storage conditions as well as processing conditions. The higher the fog level, the less the contrast will be for any given D_{max} for any film type.
4. **Contrast characteristics**. This factor controls the ability of the film to allow differentiation between shades of gray that are relatively similar. High contrast film would allow visualization of a vessel with very little contrast material in it. However, due to the grain size the image quality still might not be diagnostic.
5. **Film speed**. Speed of the film governs the amount of light needed to properly expose the film to the density requirements of the laboratory.

Density-Exposure Relationship

The density log-exposure relationship (i.e., D log E curve) (Fig. 11.1) is another name for the exposure-density curve. Density is a logarithmic measure of the light-absorbing characteristics of an image. Figure 11.2 illustrates the effect of varying development time on the density-log-exposure relationship of black-and-white film. Such data graphically show how developing time, exposure, and different developers influence the quality (density) of the finished cinefilm. There is a wide latitude for densities available over the range of exposures. Increasing development time makes this relationship shift so that even wider densities are available at lower exposures.

Influence of Developer Chemistry

The latitude in film density may be markedly reduced by using inappropriate developers (Fig. 11.2). Film characteristics may be so compromised that the end result is not likely to be optimal and, indeed, is nondiagnostic.

Influence of Film Speed and Developer

Figure 11.3 illustrates density-exposure data for a relatively fast film. Under these processing conditions this faster film requires less exposure to achieve the same density as the slower film shown in Figure 11.1. This faster film, however, will have a larger grain size, as noted above. Therefore, the final result might

Table 11.1
Characteristics of Fast and Slow Films

Fast Film	Slow Film
Large grain	Fine grain
High contrast	Low contrast
Quantum mottle: high-low resolution	Quantum mottle: low-high resolution

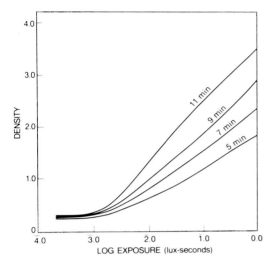

Figure 11.1. Effect of varying development time (in minutes) on density log-exposure relationship for a typical black-and-white negative film.

not fit the laboratory's needs, even though the x-ray exposure to all concerned would be considerably less. Under other circumstances (Fig. 11.4) the same fast film used in Figure 11.3 was developed in a different developer (used for Fig. 11.2). An examination of the curves shows that this film now develops like a much slower film. So now the advantages of the fast film (i.e., lower radiation dose) may be lost.

Influence of Developing Time

The effect of developing time on density and base plus fog level of a given film are illustrated in Figure 11.5. An increase in development time to increase density will increase fog density. The relationship between density increase and log exposure increase is termed gamma (γ). As this relationship increases, fog increases (*inset*).

Characteristic Density-Exposure Relation for a Given Film

Figure 11.6 indicates the area of densities of a given film that most closely approaches a straight line (*B–C*). Use of a film on this straight line portion of the curve provides the maximum contrast between adjacent shades of gray. The toe and shoulder areas of this relationship are those that fall outside of the straight line portion and do not provide as high a level of contrast between adjacent shades of gray for a given change in exposure.

However, exposures on these areas do have the capacity to store some useful information. Thus, it is imperative that the choice of film, chemistry, temperature, and time be considered carefully when selecting films that are going to be used in the catheterization laboratory. These figures also illustrate how

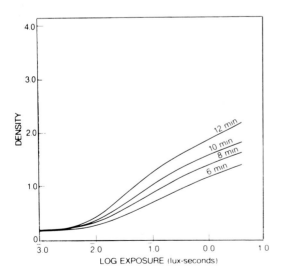

Figure 11.2. Effect of using inappropriate developer for the film shown in 11.1.

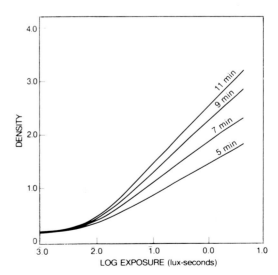

Figure 11.3. Density-exposure curves for various development times for a relatively fast film.

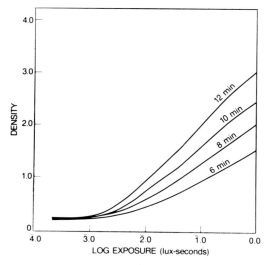

Figure 11.4. Data for a fast film processed using inappropriate developer.

vulnerable the cinefilm is to a variety of factors and the need for rigid day-to-day control over these factors.

FILM PROJECTOR

Figures 11.1 through 11.4 are graphs obtained from a film that has the ability to develop densities of 3, which most catheterization laboratories will not be able to use since their projectors will not have light sufficient to penetrate the denser portions of the film. The logical question at this point would be: Why are these projectors used if they are not representative of usable densities? Older projector light sources could only penetrate 1.4 or less. Newer projectors can penetrate densities of 1.9 to 2 routinely. With continuing development, densities of 3 or more should be routinely penetrated in the future.

Figures 11.5 and 11.6 were generated from films that are more in keeping with the types of film that can be used on equipment in operation in today's catheterization laboratory. Notice that these curves start at the bottom at the base-plus-fog level and curve upward in a manner quite similar to that of the other film. However, when a D_{max} of about 1.25 (see Fig. 11.6) is approached, the curve tends to flatten out, and further exposure has less and less effect on the total density produced by this type of film. Curves such as those seen in

Figure 11.6 are representative of those we are going to be using. Therefore, it is important to understand how best to use these films to get the desired results. Since the maximum amount of contrast between the different cardiovascular structures to be filmed is desirable, structures of maximum interest should fall on the D log E curve where the greatest change is achieved with the least change in exposure (e.g., highest γ). This is what is meant by putting the tissue density of interest in the flat region of the D log E curve. On most film used today this flat region falls somewhere between 0.6 and 2.0 on the density scale. Thus, projection equipment should operate with film densities between 0.0 and 2.2. However earlier equipment and faulty or poorly maintained newer equipment fall short of these limits and lead to problems discussed later in the chapter.

CINECAMERA

The first device that the cinefilm comes into contact with as it travels from can to projector is the cinecamera. The cinecamera is considered in its generic sense, as almost all

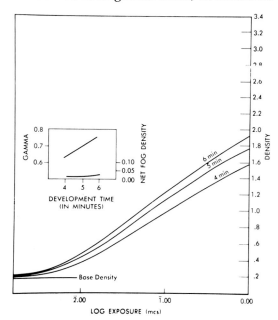

Figure 11.5. Effect of development time on fog density as described in the text. Curves for a development-time series on a typical black-and-white negative film.

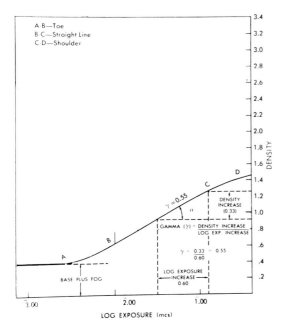

Figure 11.6. Characteristic curve for a typical black-and-white negative film. Description of various areas on a typical density-exposure curve as described in the text.

manufacturers of cardiac catheterization laboratory equipment use the same camera purchased from the same manufacturer. The film format used universally is 35-mm that is supplied with either 200- or 400-ft magazines.

The cinecamera, as used in most catheterization laboratories today, consists of a high-speed drive mechanism that is synchronized to the line frequency of the power supply line. This drive mechanism, through a system of gear reductions, pulls the film through the camera at speeds of 7.5, 15, 30, 60, and 90 frames/sec. Need for the wide range of frame speeds is dictated by the speed at which the part under examination moves and the blood flow. For example, if the gastrointestinal system were being imaged, 7.5 or 15 frames/sec would be satisfactory. Whereas in cardiovascular imaging, 30, 60, and even 90 frames/sec are sometimes needed. A magazine is used to hold and protect the film so that it can be transported to and from the place of use in ordinary light without fogging the film.

Last but not least, a lens which focuses the image on the film in the camera is required. Prior to purchase of equipment a decision

must be made relative to the desired framing of the cine image. This refers to the filling of the frame on the cinefilm. Since the frame on the standard 35-mm cinecamera is wider than it is tall, a 3:4 aspect ratio, the decision must be made as to whether to fill the frame vertically, leaving an area on each side unexposed, or whether to try to fill the frame from side to side, thereby "overframing" top to bottom. It is standard in most cardiac catheterization laboratories today to overframe top and bottom about 25% to fill the cineframe side to side. This is done by a lens with a focal length that is different from the one that would be used if one only fills the frame vertically. One word of caution is needed with respect to vertical overframing. Unless the automatic shutters on the collimator are set so that they collimate to the vertical size covered by the cineframe, a portion of anatomy that can be seen on the TV monitor may not be recorded on film because the TV displays a larger area.

There is no set focal length that can be recommended because the total lens component within the system must be taken into consideration. However, the manufacturers can make recommendations in the selection of the lens that will frame the image to the size desired.

Routine Maintenance Procedures

The film magazines should be inspected daily to remove film chips and dust and dirt that inevitably collect in them. The film plane in the camera (the shiny surface that the film is held against by the spring-loaded pressure plate), must also be cleaned and inspected regularly to remove the buildup of emulsion that gradually will deposit on the frame plate. This deposit causes scratches on the film. These scratches, unlike those produced by the processor, will always be in exactly the same place on each cineframe for every film recorded by a given magazine. Scratches caused by the processor will move within the frame.

Another caution point is the size of the loop that is left outside the magazine when it is loaded. If this loop is either too large or too small, the film may be damaged. The wrong size loop usually produces a nonlinear scratch on each frame that is always in the same spot. Most available camera magazines are supplied with loop formers to guarantee the correct loop size. There are still some, however, that do not, and these are the ones that require that great care be taken to assure the correct loop size.

PROCESSING

The processing of black-and-white film is usually a very simple procedure. Processing involves developing, stopping, fixing, washing and drying the film. However, many properly exposed films are ruined in processing. The essentials for the **developer** to process a silver halide film include:

1. Correct developer for the film being used, or one that fits other specific needs even though it may not be the specific one recommended.
2. Correct developer temperature.
3. Correct amount of agitation of the developer. This assures that fresh developer reaches the emulsion to develop it sufficiently during the time that it dwells in developer solution.
4. Correct developing dwell time. Manufacturers of film design emulsion to be processed in a specific manner, and any variation from their specifications will usually result in degraded image quality in some manner. For example, if a film that is designed to dwell in developing solution for 7 min at a temperature of 75° F does so for only 5 min at the same temperature, the film will be slightly underdeveloped and the desired density will not have been reached. Also the gray scale will have been shortened. The exposure-density curve will have flattened out, thereby providing lower contrast between the limited shades of gray that do exist on the film. Since the contrast between adjacent structures is what allows the eye to differentiate one from the other, anything that decreases contrast is not acceptable. Conversely, a situation where-in the dwell time is correct but the developer temperature has increased to 78° F will have the same effect as developing the film for a longer period of time. The density will increase and the number of shades of gray will also increase. While this sounds like a good situation, something else will also have happened that is not as acceptable. All the shades of gray in the image will have shifted toward the black end of the gray scale. If the light source for viewing the finished film is not bright enough to penetrate the darker shades of gray, then some of the diagnostic information will be lost. A situation

like this can easily happen when the temperature of the developer solution is either not properly set or not precisely controlled. The proper dwell time at the proper temperature combined with the correct amount of agitation of the solution at the surface of the emulsion is absolutely essential to bring out the optimum image on any film.

After the developer, the next chemical in the processing sequence is the **fixer** bath. Its purpose is to: (*a*) remove the undeveloped silver from the emulsion of the film; (*b*) fix the residual metallic silver in the emulsion, thus preserving the captured image; (*c*) harden the emulsion, making it less likely to be damaged in subsequent handling; and (*d*) clear the antihalation back, if present. This opaque backing material eliminates back scatter of light that has penetrated the emulsion and would otherwise bounce back, in a random pattern from the rear surface of the film or the mirror-like pressure plate that holds the film flat in the focal plane. This reflected light would degrade the image made by the incident light on the first pass through the emulsion. This opaque backing material must be removed to prepare the film for viewing. Again, as with developer, the fixer solution is made to work best at a given temperature and immersion time. The prime prerequisite is that the film remain in the fixer long enough to be adequately fixed to preserve its archival value. In most films this time period will equate to twice its clearing time. That is the time it takes an unexposed film to become transparent when held in fixing solution. Although the temperature of the fixer is not as critical as with the developer, it must be warm enough to adequately fix the film and not cause reticulation, with crinkling of the emulsion due to too drastic a temperature change.

The final bath through which the film must pass is the **wash** bath. This wet process is critical to the archival value of the finished film. If not properly washed, the film will look fine when first viewed; however, if 2 or 3 years later it were to again be viewed, underwashed film will have turned brown, losing its diagnostic value. Therefore, it is mandatory that enough fresh water be supplied at all times to the wash bath in order to dilute the residual chemistry in the wash tank to a concentration well below that which will have an adverse

Table 11.2
Some Commonly Used Cinefilm Processors: Comparison of Their Characteristics

Feature	Allen[a]	Jamison[a]	Cinerex[b]	Odelca[c]	Fisher[d]
Variable speed	Y[e]	Y	Y	Y	Y
Leader	F	F	F	P	F
Developer time variable	Y	Y	N	Y	Y
Film speed	N/A	0/70	Fixed	0/15	0/24
Automatic replenishment	Y	Y	N/A	Add on	N
Power supply	220/30a	220/30a	N/A	220/16a	220/30a
phase	1	1		1	1
Daylight load	Y	Y	Y	Y	Y
Reel capacity (ft)	2000	2000	400	400	400
Water flow (gal/min)	2	2	N/A	5.51/m	N/A
Darkroom needed	Y	Y	Y	Y	Y
Single or multistrand	S	S	S	S	M
Attendant needed	Y	Y	N	N	N

[a] High-capacity, single-strand, needs attendant to splice leader at end of film run.
[b] Low-capacity, with no need for attendant but must be rethreaded at each use.
[c] Low-capacity, needs no attendant, self-threading with short leader that is supplied.
[d] (Medium-capacity because of its ability to run parallel strands of film simultaneously. Unit must be rethreaded after all strands have been run.
[e] F, full; M, multistrand; N/A, not applicable; N, no; P, partial; Y, yes.

effect on the archival value of the finished film. The tank which holds the wash water must also be free of algae and dirt present in most public water supplies. An adequate filtering system should be installed if the local water supply has a tendency to be dirty. Again, the manufacturers' instructions for both the film and the processor should be closely followed.

Once the film exits the wash, the residual water globules must be removed to prevent spots produced by dirt that is in the water. Manufacturers of processors have tried many ways to remove the residual water from the film surface. Squeegees, air knives, buffer wheels, and sponges, all work to a more or less satisfactory degree, but important problems exist with each.

1. Squeegees are usually made of rubber or soft plastic and are designed to drag on the surface of the film to strip residual water from the surface. This works well as long as the squeegee is properly cleaned and adjusted; however, if the squeegee is allowed to become encrusted with dirt or crystalline debris from the processing chemistry, it may produce linear scratches on the film.
2. Air knives consist of a blower which sends a thin stream of high velocity air at an angle against the film. This stream of air blows the residual water from the film surface. Two major problems with this device are (a) it is so noisy that it may be detrimental to the hearing of those subjected to it for long periods of time, and (b) it will leave occasional water on the film that was probably blown off but then bounced back.
3. Buffer wheels consist of two wheels that look like cut off paint rollers that are mounted on spindles in such a manner as to allow the bristles to come lightly into contact with the film surface. The buffer wheels are turned at high speed so that they buff the film surface counter to the direction of film travel. The buffing action strips residual water from the film, and as long as the bristles remain in contact with the film surface, they do a very good job. With this device attention to the light contact with the film surface must be stressed, as the ability to strip the water from the buffing on the film surface. The buffer wheels must be checked often to assure that the bristles are still standing erect and touching the film surface since they tend to bend backwards and lose contact over time. New buffers should be on hand to replace them. It might be mentioned here that in the past it has been difficult to obtain these special wheels from the distributor of the processor, and therefore a stock should always be maintained.

Table 11.3
Essential Processor Maintenance Tasks and Frequency of Their Performance

Task	Frequency
Sensitometric strip	Daily before schedule begins
Clean squeegees	When daily schedule is over
Clean top rollers	When daily schedule is over
Check solution level	Every morning prior to startup
Check replenisher levels	Daily before schedule begins
Check transport speed	Daily with surface distance meter/map meter
Check water flow	Weekly, this is a visual check to be sure that flow filters are still allowing enough flow
Drain & clean tanks	Monthly; check wash for algae
Change water filters	When visible flow decreases and weekly
Check temperature accuracy	Monthly or if films are light or variable
Check buffer contact	Daily, adjust for light contact, replace if matted
Check air filter	Weekly; replace when matted with dust
Check replenisher	Weekly; good quality films depend on correct replenishment rate

4. Sponges used for removing water from film are flat and of high quality. The sponges are rinsed in a solution consisting of water and a wetting agent, such as "Kodak photoflo," then placed in a holder which keeps the sponges in contact with the film surface. The sponge tends to absorb excess water, and the wetting agent reduces the surface tension of any water that remains on the surface so that it forms a film instead of a globule, thereby eliminating water marks. Most manufacturers do not advocate the use of sponges. However, they are quite useful for removing water, and some companies have even designed special holders so that they remain in contact with the film. These holders can be obtained from at least two manufacturers (Chem Arts & Associates and Perkins Diagnostic Imaging, Inc.).

One of the most important elements in total quality control within the catheterization laboratory environment is a good system for maintaining the film-processing quality. A good densitometer and sensitometer are some of the best investments that can be made when starting up a laboratory. Daily checking of the processing system must be instituted. Prior to use a sensitometric strip should be run through the processor and compared with the standard. Such routine will assure you that at least this portion of the total catheterization laboratory system is operating properly.

PROCESSORS

Processors that are employed in most catheterization laboratory settings are manufactured specifically for catheterization laboratory use (Table 11.2). They may be divided into two general types: those that do not require someone to be in attendance to couple the leader to the film once the end of the film has been reached and those that do require attendance. The type that do not require the attendance of someone to stand by listening for the warning bell are lower volume units that should fit the needs of a smaller laboratory without someone assigned to continuous processing duty. The other units resemble larger commercial systems in that they require an attendant at all times when processing and are designed for higher throughput. Some very large laboratories have even installed commercial units. But in general, the needs of the average-sized laboratory will be well-served with the purchase of one, two, or three of the units designed for cinefilm processing. A partial list of these units is provided in Table 11.2.

Processor Setup

The following is a relatively simple series of steps to follow when first setting up the processor in any laboratory.

1. Choose the film and chemistry that are going to be used to begin.
2. Refer to the exposure-density curve for this film, and choose the correct dwell time and the correct temperature for this dwell time.
3. Set processor speed to assure that the film rests in the developer the length of time indicated.
4. Set the temperature so that the developer is maintained at the temperature indicated on the exposure-density curve. This temperature must be checked with a good quality laboratory thermometer as the built-in thermostats might be calibrated incorrectly.
5. Expose a sensitometric strip on a piece of the same film that is going to be used.
6. Process the strip by running it through the processor in the same manner as will be done with the cinefilm.
7. Read the processed strip, and if the middle density of all the densities is between 0.9 and 1.1, then the processor is ready to begin processing the actual **phantom** films made in the catheterization laboratory.

This film strip should also be projected through the same projector that is going to be used for the cinefilm. The grain, as seen on this strip, represents the actual inherent grain of the film itself, whereas, the film done on the laboratory unit will show film grain plus the quantum mottle of the system. The myocardium area of the phantom should be between 0.9 and 1.1 when measured. The catheterization laboratory system should be adjusted to bring the myocardium area of the phantom to within these parameters with an acceptable amount of mottle. Suggested routine processor maintenance is outlined in Table 11.3.

VIEWERS AND PROJECTORS

There are many types of projectors that have been used for the viewing of the finished film. These range from conventional movie projectors in the early days to the specialized units of today, which are made to project the film with little or no flicker between frames, regardless of the speed at which the film is viewed.

Any one of the newer projectors will allow flicker-free viewing; however, depending upon the wattage of the lamp in the projector that is chosen, it is possible to find it limited relative to the D_{max} that can be used. This is because the darker the film, the more light needed to be able to see all of the information that has been captured within the emulsion on the film. If the light source is too weak, it will quite drastically limit the number of shades of gray that are visible. Another consideration is the distance that will have to be used if the image is to be projected. What might be totally adequate for the laboratory, such as an underexposed film, which will look quite acceptable on low-light-powered projectors, will look washed out when viewed on a high-light-powered projector. This same low-light-powered projector will not allow projection of an acceptable image more than a few feet without its becoming so dim that it is totally useless. Therefore, the location where the projector is to be used must be considered when choosing one. The minimum that should be acceptable is a unit that will penetrate a film exposed and processed to a D_{max} of 2.2 with enough lamp brightness to project a diagnostic image that will cover a 6-inch × 8-inch screen with enough brilliance so that it can be seen without having to completely darken the room. Several manufacturers make projectors that will meet these requirements and will be readily serviced by the sales organization that sells them.

SUMMARY AND CONCLUSIONS

In order to produce optimum results in any catheterization laboratory, it is mandatory to have x-ray equipment that has adequate power to penetrate the large patient; an x-ray tube unit that has enough capacity to supply the needed photons without overheating so quickly that time is wasted waiting for it to cool; and an imaging system that has the proper characteristics to give the degree of contrast and spatial resolution desired. It should be so adjusted that all lenses within the system are operating at, or as close to, infinity as they can be set in order to minimize vignetting. This is the "falloff" in intensity of transmitted light due to absorption of light that is passing through the lenses as it strikes the inside of the lens barrel. The closer a lens setting gets to infinity, the less of its transmitted light will strike the inside of the lens barrel, since an infinity setting means that the lens is looking at a parallel light bundle that does not depend so drastically upon the lens to correct it; a processing system that will properly process the exposed film; and a projector that will meet the needs of the particular method of operation.

For those who are anticipating opening a catheterization laboratory but do not have either the background knowledge or inclination to acquire the necessary knowledge about film and film processing, there two alternatives.

1. Go to a laboratory that is producing results that are considered acceptable and start with the combination of film, chemistry, developing time, and temperature that is being used there. Insist that the catheterization laboratory equipment be made to produce acceptable films at these processing and exposure factors.

2. Choose a film that is producing the type of results desired and is being used on equipment of the same type. Insist that the film manufacturer's representative and equipment manufacturer's representative combine their resources to produce the results that are desired. These two representatives are usually more than willing to help achieve the best results that can be produced. It will benefit all parties to produce top quality cinefilms. Most x-ray equipment and cinefilm producers have specialists that do nothing but assist customers in this endeavor.

12

Ventriculography

J. Ward Kennedy, M.D.
Florence H. Sheehan, M.D.

HISTORICAL BACKGROUND

As the emphasis in adult cardiology drifted away from congenital heart disease and considerable experience was gained in the catheterization of patients with valvular heart disease, interest increased in more detailed assessment of ventricular function through the use of angiography. In the late 1950s Dodge and colleagues in this country and Ardvisson, working in Sweden, began to develop methods for measurement of cardiac chamber volumes using rapid 6 and later 12 frames/sec, biplane cut, or roll film contrast angiograms (1, 2). Dodge and colleagues established methods for determination of left ventricular stroke volume, left ventricular muscle mass, and left atrial volume (3-5). By determining end-diastolic and end-systolic volume, it was possible to calculate stroke volume and minute output of the left ventricle. By comparing left ventricular output with forward cardiac output, as measured by standard dye dilution or Fick techniques, left ventricular regurgitant stroke volume and minute output could be calculated. It also became possible to integrate pressure and volume information during the cardiac cycle to better understand pressure-volume relationships. With knowledge of the ventricular pressure, chamber dimensions, and left ventricular wall thickness, it was then possible to measure left ventricular wall stress (6). While initially impressive, with development of catheter-tip pressure manometers and rapid biplane cine-filming techniques, precise simultaneous pressure and volume information became available, and the mechanics of left ventricular performance could be determined in various types of heart disease in humans.

This type of information gradually became available in relatively large numbers of patients, as well as in a number of individuals found to have no anatomic or physiologic evidence of heart disease following careful study. The data from these normal persons were accumulated and eventually provided reference standards for normal chamber size and function, in addition to the mass of the left ventricular myocardium for both men and women (7).

With further experience in evaluating left ventricular size and performance in patients with heart disease, various investigators began to appreciate the importance of the relationship between left ventricular stroke volume and end-diastolic volume. It became clear that the ratio of stroke volume to end-diastolic volume, i.e., left ventricular ejection fraction, was of great value for assessment of left ventricular pump function (8, 9). Now, nearly 2 decades later, the ejection fraction is still the most frequently used method for assessing global left ventricular function. This measurement is most useful in evaluation of left ventricular function in patients with valvular heart disease and cardiomyopathy, but it is also useful in assessing patients with ischemic heart disease (10).

In the mid- and late 1960s, with widespread use of selective coronary arteriography and development of coronary artery bypass surgery, evaluation of left ventricular function became essential. This was because it became apparent that ventricular performance was a major independent predictor of surgical risk and long-term survival in patients with ischemic heart disease. With simple visual assessment of ventricular size and distribution of regional contraction abnormalities it was possible to divide patients into low-, medium-, and high-risk categories (11). Angiographers also noted that there were several different types of abnormalities in regional wall motion both in the sequence of regional contraction and in the extent of wall movement. Herman et al. defined abnormalities of extent of contraction as **hypokinesis** for reduced movement, **akinesis** for loss of contraction, and **dyskinesis** for paradoxical outward motion during systole (12). These terms have become the reference standards for describing abnormalities of contraction.

TECHNIQUE OF LEFT VENTRICULAR ANGIOGRAPHY

The left ventricle can be evaluated angiographically by injection of contrast material into the right side of the heart, and filming the contrast material as it enters the left ventricle, and by injection of contrast material into the left atrium, the left ventricular chamber, or even the ascending aorta in patients with aortic valvular regurgitation. In most instances, optimal examination is obtained when contrast material is injected directly into the left ventricular chamber. The techniques for catheterization of the left ventricle are detailed in Chapter 6. Briefly, a pigtail catheter is usually placed in the left ventricle retrograde through the aortic valve. Other multiple-hole catheters may be used (multipurpose, Sones, NIH, etc.).

CONTRAST INJECTION TECHNIQUES

To obtain high-quality angiograms for analysis of wall motion and mitral insufficiency, ventricular ectopic rhythms must be avoided by placing the catheter in the area of the ventricular cavity that is least likely to cause ectopy during power injection. This is often midway between the apex of the ventricle and the aortic valve, with the loop directed backward toward the mitral valve. In some patients

it may be necessary to move the catheter tip to another location until a region free of ectopy is found during test injection. This is done by a forceful test injection using 5 to 10 ml of contrast material to see if ectopy occurs and to assess the contrast material distribution. This information is also used to determine how much contrast material should be injected.

When an appropriate injection site is selected, a power injection of 30 to 50 ml of contrast material is made into the ventricular chamber at a rate of 10 to 20 ml/sec. The volume and rate of injection of contrast material will vary, depending on the size of the patient, size of the chamber, function of the ventricle, hemodynamic state of the patient, and other factors. Larger volume and more rapid injection are required in large, hyperdynamic ventricles, seen in patients with aortic or mitral regurgitation. Smaller volume and slower injections are appropriate in small or hypokinetic ventricles. In patients with very poor left ventricular function and dilated ventricles, contrast material mixes slowly in the chamber so that a relatively small amount of contrast material injected rapidly and allowed to mix over three to five cardiac cycles often provides excellent ventriculograms. In patients with recent anterior or apical myocardial infarction and those with ventricular aneurysms, the possibility that a mural thrombus in the ventricle may be dislodged during manipulation of the catheter must be considered. In these patients the experienced angiographer will place the catheter so as to avoid the area of possible mural thrombus, which is likely to be attached to the area of the wall that is most akinetic or dyskinetic.

FILMING TECHNIQUES

During the early years of cardiac angiography, direct x-ray exposure of large cut or roll filming at 6 or 12 frames/sec was utilized. Since the development of high-quality image intensifiers and cinerecording and television monitoring systems adapted for angiocardiography, these cumbersome devices have been replaced by cinefilming in either single or biplane projections at 30, 50, 60, or 90 frames/sec. For visual and most quantitative analysis of left ventricular angiograms, 30 frames/sec is adequate, but many laboratories prefer to film at 60 frames/sec to provide for a more pleasing image of ventricular filling and ejection and more frames for analysis. For patients with tachycardia 60 frames/sec is a more desirable filming rate.

FILMING PROJECTION

The left ventricle has been traditionally viewed by single-plane angiography in the 30° right anterior oblique (RAO) projection. With biplane filming, anteroposterior and lateral or RAO and left anterior oblique (LAO) projections have been used. Although biplane filming is ideal, the greater expense of biplane cineradiographic equipment and increased radiation exposure for the patient and operators militates against routine use of biplane cineradiography for most examinations in adults. In patients with valvular and congenital heart disease and in most with nonischemic cardiomyopathies, ventricular contraction is relatively symmetrical and reasonably represented in the RAO view. In patients with ischemic heart disease who have a prior myocardial infarction or ongoing ischemia at the time of study, segmental wall motion defects may not be adequately represented in a single view.

The location of coronary obstructions can help guide the angiographer in selecting the best single view for left ventriculography. In patients with major obstruction in the left anterior descending and/or right coronary arteries, the RAO view is preferable. In patients in whom the circumflex artery is the major site of obstruction, the LAO view is best. In patients with diffuse three-vessel disease the RAO view usually provides adequate information for assessment of surgical risk, as well as acting as a guide for the surgeon for the placement of revascularization conduits. In a minority of patients, it is necessary to perform either biplane or two serial contrast injections with filming in both RAO and LAO views. In these circumstances the most important view should be done first, and the second injection should be deleted in patients who respond unfavorably to the first. Fortunately, there are now many ways to evaluate regional ventricular contraction can now be evaluated noninvasively with echocardiography or radionuclide angiography so that unstable patients almost never need to be subjected to more than one

left ventriculogram. Some may not need ventriculography at all if they are at extremely high risk and have been adequately evaluated by another technique.

Recently, investigators have proposed using sagittal plane angulated views of the left ventricle in order to improve examination of certain portions of the wall (13–15). The most common is the cranial LAO view, which provides better definition of the lateral wall, septum, and outflow tract than standard 60° LAO or 90° lateral projections. Although there are times when this view is desirable, **we do not use it routinely** for biplane cineangiography.

QUALITATIVE ASSESSMENT OF LEFT VENTRICULAR ANGIOGRAMS

Although we advocate quantitative assessment of left ventricular contraction and valvular regurgitation, a great deal of information can be derived from subjective visual evaluation of left ventricular contraction patterns in patients with all types of heart disease. The angiographer must appreciate the way the ventricle responds to acute and chronic changes in both pressure and volume. These differences are most notable in patients with acute vs. chronic volume overload. In chronic volume overload of the left ventricle, such as occurs in aortic or mitral regurgitation, ventricular septal defect, and patent ductus arteriosus, the ventricle responds by progressive increase in end-diastolic volume and stroke volume and maintains a normal cardiac output at rest. So the **ratio of stroke volume to end-diastolic volume (ejection fraction)** remains normal or only modestly decreased in the patient with normal left ventricular function. When symptoms of congestive heart failure develop, however, angiography usually demonstrates an increase in end-diastolic volume and a fall in ejection fraction. Thus, in well-compensated patients, the enlarged end-diastolic volume is an index of the severity of volume overload and is not an indication of diminished left ventricular performance.

Because of these relationships, the ejection fraction is of great value in assessing the patient with volume overload of the left ventricle. There is, however, a special situation in which care must be taken in the interpretation of the ejection fraction. In patients with chronic severe mitral regurgitation, the left ventricle ejects a large portion of its stroke volume into the low-pressure left atrium. Since this results in a reduction in ventricular afterload, the ejection fraction is often higher for a given degree of left ventricular dysfunction than it would be under other circumstance without mitral regurgitation. This finding may mislead the physician into believing that left ventricular function or functional reserve is better than it actually is. In one small series of patients in whom the ejection fraction was measured before and several months following mitral valve surgery for severe mitral insufficiency, the ejection fraction deteriorated in half of the patients in whom it was abnormal preoperatively and in all of those in whom it was below 50% prior to surgery (16). This experience suggests that only a normal or high ejection fraction (>65 to 75%) reliably indicates relatively normal left ventricular function in patients with severe mitral insufficiency. This topic is discussed in more detail in Chapter 27.

In patients with acute volume overload, as seen in mitral or aortic valve endocarditis or ruptured mitral valve chordae tendineae, the patient has often had normal left ventricular function prior to the acute illness. In this situation, the ventricle is unprepared for the acute volume overload and responds by minimal dilation, increase in ejection fraction, and marked increase in filling pressure. The majority of these patients in whom regurgitation is severe will present with acute pulmonary edema. Under most circumstances the appropriate therapy is early surgical correction of the valvular lesion. In patients who survive without surgery, the ventricle gradually dilates, the myocardium hypertrophies, and the filling pressure decreases so that after several months the patient acquires characteristics of those with chronic volume overload.

The response of the patient with chronic pressure overload of either the right or left ventricle, as occurs in either pulmonic or aortic stenosis, is one of progressive myocardial hypertrophy without chamber dilation. These patients who present prior to the development of congestive heart failure have normal-sized heavily trabeculated chambers with relatively normal contractile function and thick walls. However, since the presence of significant hypertrophy usually results in decreased compliance, the left ventricular end-diastolic pressure is usually elevated despite normal end-diastolic volume. When these patients develop congestive heart failure, the end-diastolic and end-systolic volumes increase, and the stroke volume and ejection fraction fall. Fortunately, in patients with aortic stenosis the ejection fraction usually improves following successful valve replacement (8, 17).

Today, idiopathic hypertrophic subaortic stenosis and other forms of hypertrophic cardiomyopathy are most often evaluated by echocardiography, but in the past left ventriculography was the standard method of evaluation. In these patients the end-diastolic volume is normal or small, and the ventricle often has a thick free wall and an increased ejection fraction. This may result in obliteration of the apical portions of the chamber. In a 60° LAO or lateral view during systole, the anterior leaflet of the mitral valve can often be seen moving forward and even touching the septum. While simultaneous injections of contrast material in the right and left ventricles are not necessary for clinical purposes, these biventricular angiographic studies can identify the markedly thickened basal portion of the interventricular septum that is characteristic of patients with outflow obstruction. If only a single-plane RAO view is available, idiopathic hypertrophic subaortic stenosis can be suspected by the presence of a high ejection fraction, apical cavity obliteration, and a reduction in the density of the contrast material as a band separating the upper third of the chamber from the apex. This angiographic appearance is caused by the anterior leaflet of the mitral valve abutting the septum during systole.

Another condition which is usually evaluated with echocardiography is mitral valve prolapse. This condition is well demonstrated angiographically in the RAO projection. The mitral valve plane is easily appreciated in this view as nonopacified blood enters the contrast-filled ventricle during diastole. With the onset of systole, the mitral valve moves posterior and closes along the plane of the annulus. In patients with mitral valve prolapse, the valve leaflets outlined by contrast behind them prolapse backward beyond the annulus into the left atrium. In its most severe form this appears as a large ring of contrast material

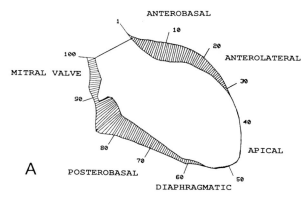

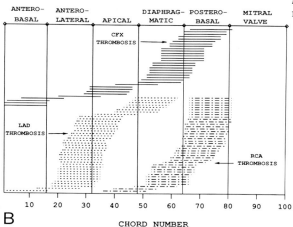

Figure 12.1. *A,* Left ventricular segments 1 to 5 analyzed from the right anterior oblique ventriculogram as defined in the CASS report (18). *B,* Quantitative analysis was performed using the centerline method to locate the most hypokinetic one-fifth of the ventricle in patients with single-vessel coronary artery disease studied during acute myocardial infarction. The location of hypokinesis is highly variable; as a result, attempts to measure wall motion in predefined segments will underestimate abnormality (35). *CFX,* circumflex; *LAD,* left anterior descending; *RCA,* right coronary artery.

extending around the annulus. Severe prolapse is nearly always associated with significant mitral regurgitation, while minor degrees of prolapse are usually not.

LEFT VENTRICULAR CONTRACTION PATTERNS IN ISCHEMIC HEART DISEASE

The most characteristic angiographic feature of the left ventricle in ischemic heart disease is the segmental localization of contraction and even relaxation abnormalities. Although many patients with severe coronary artery stenosis have normal left ventricular contraction patterns when observed in a resting state, most patients with totally obstructed vessels or a history of or ECG evidence of myocardial infarction have clear and distinct segmental contraction abnormalities. A very useful method of locating these segments and

quantifying the severity of contraction abnormality was developed for the Coronary Artery Surgery Study (CASS), as shown in Figure 12.1 (18). This method requires that 10 different segments of the left ventricle, five in the RAO and five in the LAO projection, be scored 1 through 6 as: (1) normal, (2) mild hypokinesia, (3) severe hypokinesia, (4) akinesia, (5) dyskinesia, and (6) aneurysm. The segment scores are then added so that when the method is applied to a single-plane RAO ventriculogram, a normal score is 5, and the most abnormal score is 30. This semiquantitative method of evaluating left ventricular function is superior to use of ejection fraction in defining surgical risk in patients with coronary artery disease (19).

Location of wall motion abnormalities relative to location of artery stenosis as viewed from the RAO projection, occlusion of the left anterior descending coronary artery, and development of Q wave infarction result in

A. LAD

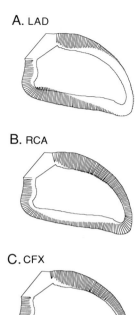

B. RCA

C. CFX

Figure 12.2. The location of hypokinesis due to isolated thrombosis of the left anterior descending (*LAD, N* = 185), right (*RCA, N* = 132), and left circumflex (*CFX, N* = 57) coronary arteries. In each panel, the mean motion of the infarct patients is indicated by the lengths of the chords. For comparison the normal mean motion is presented by the solid end-diastolic/contour.

abnormalities of the anterolateral and apical segments (Fig. 12.2). In very proximal left anterior descending obstruction, the apical portion of the anterobasal segment may be involved. If the anterior descending artery extends around the apex, the wall motion abnormality may also extend to involve the inferior portion of the apex as well. The severity of wall motion abnormality may vary from hypokinesis to dyskinesis, which is indicative of ventricular aneurysm. In nearly all patients, motion of the basal portion of the anterobasal segment is preserved.

In inferior myocardial infarction due to occlusion of either the right coronary artery or anatomically dominant left circumflex artery, the inferior basal and inferior apical segments show contraction abnormalities. The extent of the abnormality will depend upon the

distribution of the posterior descending. In some patients it extends to or around the apex, and in others it is short and does not reach the apex. Although akinesis is frequently present after inferior infarction, dyskinesis is distinctly uncommon, and development of a large ventricular aneurysm is rare. This difference in severity of wall motion abnormalities between the inferior and anterior wall may also relate to "splinting" of the inferior wall by the diaphragm.

Wall motion abnormalities associated with myocardial infarctions resulting from circumflex coronary artery occlusion are often more subtle in their appearance when observed in the RAO view than those associated with either left anterior descending or posterior descending occlusion. These wall motion abnormalities appear as a hypokinetic region at the junction between the anterolateral and anterior apical segments and are often associated with a similar abnormality in the inferoapical segment of the wall. In high-quality angiocardiograms, a double density may be appreciated due to normal contraction of the anterior lateral segment with a hypokinetic or akinetic segment behind.

The LAO projection best allows observation of septal wall motion abnormalities resulting from anterior infarctions. This projection also provides an end-on view of inferior wall contraction abnormalities resulting from infarcts due to right coronary artery occlusions. The LAO projection best demonstrates the posterior wall motion abnormalities often seen in segments 9 and 10 in patients with posterior infarctions associated with left circumflex artery occlusion.

A **left ventricular aneurysm** may be defined as a region of the left ventricular wall that extends beyond the expected location of the wall during diastole and is akinetic or dyskinetic during systole. In other words, this abnormality distorts the diastolic contour of the chamber, as well as having no contractile function. They most often occur following Q wave infarctions of the anterior free wall and apex, especially when the anterior descending coronary artery is occluded proximal to the first diagonal branch of that vessel. Ventricular aneurysms frequently have mural thrombus attached, which may be seen as a mass projecting into the chamber and, occasionally, moving separately from the wall with each cardiac contraction. Mural thrombus is often seen more easily by echocardiography than by cardiac angiography. Older aneurysms may contain calcified layers of thrombus which are visible by fluoroscopy. This distortion of the left ventricular cavity by a large aneurysm often makes application of mode-dependent equations for calculation of ejection fraction difficult, if not impossible.

LEFT ATRIAL ANGIOGRAPHY

The left atrium is often visualized during left ventricular angiography because of the presence of mitral regurgitation. It may be selectively opacified by transseptal catheterization or may be seen during right atrial angiography in patients with congenital heart disease and right-to-left shunts. The left atrium may also be visualized by filming the levophase of a pulmonary artery injection. The left atrium is normally a relatively small structure containing about one-half the volume of the left ventricle in diastole. In the absence of mitral regurgitation, left atrial angiography may be useful for the identification of atrial mural thrombi and for the detection of left atrial myxomas, but both of these entities are usually best identified by echocardiography and transseptal catheterization should not be done when these entities are suspected.

QUANTITATIVE VENTRICULAR ANGIOGRAPHY AND WALL MOTION ANALYSIS

Regional and global left ventricular function is commonly estimated by visual inspection of the contrast ventriculogram. However, quantitative analysis provides precise measurement of the severity of ventricular dysfunction, the ventricle's compensatory response, the effect of treatment in enhancing functional recovery, and a prognostic index. Furthermore, quantitative analysis permits objective comparisons between patients and also between observers. The most commonly measured parameters are **left ventricular chamber volume** and **ejection fraction**. However, since coronary artery stenosis causes local dysfunction, when coronary artery disease is present, measurement of regional wall motion is more sensitive in reflecting the function of ischemic and nonis-

chemic myocardium. Although fewer studies have been performed on the right ventricle, its volume, ejection fraction, and wall motion can be measured using methods similar to those for the left ventricle.

DETERMINATION OF LEFT VENTRICULAR VOLUME

Because of its high degree of accuracy, measurement of left ventricular volume from contrast angiograms is the reference standard by which other imaging modalities are judged. This accuracy has been repeatedly verified by comparing the end-diastolic volumes calculated from angiograms of cadaver hearts with their directly measured volumes. In vivo validation has also been performed by comparing angiographic stroke volumes with volumes calculated using Fick or indicator-dilution techniques (1, 2, 20). Volumes calculated from ventriculograms using the area-length method agree closely with the known volumes ($r = 0.995$, standard error of the estimate = 8.2 ml) (1).

With the area-length method, the projected image is likened to an ellipse, and the ventricular chamber to an ellipsoid of revolution. The short-axis diameter of each ventricular image is calculated from the measured area and long axis length as $D = 4A/\pi L$, in which D is the diameter, A is the area of the projected image, and L is the length of the chamber. Volume (V) is then computed as $V = (\pi/6)(L)(D_a)(D_b)$, in which L is the longer measured length of two orthogonal projections, and D_a and D_b are the calculated transverse diameters. Although volume can also be calculated with comparable accuracy using Simpson's rule, the area-length method has found greater acceptance due to its computational simplicity.

Calculated volumes are consistently larger than true volumes, due to the volume of the papillary muscles, trabeculae carneae, and chordae tendineae. Therefore regression equations are used to correct for this systematic error. Equations have been developed for each of the standard biplane projections (Table 12.1). Volume can also be determined accurately from single-plane images in the anteroposterior or 30° RAO projections because the transverse or short-axis diameter, calculated

Table 12.1
Regression Equations For Left Ventricular Volume Determination

Projection	Regression	Number of Observations	Standard Error of Estimate (ml)	Reference Standard	Reference
AP/lateral[a]	$V' = 0.928 V - 3.8$	54 (9)[b]	8.2	Casts	Dodge et al. (1)
AP	$V' = 0.951 V - 3.0$	1204 (55)	15.0	Biplane	Sandler & Dodge (3)
AP	$V' = 1.00 \ V + 9.6$	15[c]	24.0	Biplane	Kennedy et al. (21)
AP	$V' = 0.788 V + 8.4$	16[c]	28.8	Biplane	Kasser & Kennedy (22)
RAO 30°	$V' = 0.81 \ V + 1.9$	15	24.0	Biplane	Kennedy et al. (21)
RAO 30°	$V' = 0.938 V - 5.7$	11	5.5	Casts	Wynne et al. (13)
RAO 30°/LAO 60°	$V' = 0.989 V - 8.1$	11	8.0	Casts	Wynne et al. (13)

[a] *AP*, anteroposterior; *V*, volume computed from the cineimage using the area-length method;
  V', volume after correction by regression equation.
[b] Parentheses indicate the number of subjects if multiple images/subject were studied.
[c] These studies had 10 patients in common.

using the area-length method, is similar in orthogonal views (3, 13, 21, 22). The ventricle is usually foreshortened in the 60° LAO projection, which some investigators correct by adding 15 to 30° cranial angulation (14, 15).

Correction must also be made for **magnification** and **pincushion distortion** in the imaging system. This is usually accomplished by filming a grid of known dimension, such as a 10 cm × 10 cm Plexiglas plate with fine wires embedded at 1-cm intervals at the midchest level with the same imaging mode (intensifier magnification) and table-to-tube positions used during ventriculography. When the ventriculogram is projected for tracing, the grid film is also examined. A correction factor is derived from the ratio of the number of grid squares spanning the ventricle to their measured width (22). The correction factor can also be determined by measuring the distance between metallic bands on "banded" pigtail catheters (23); however, biplane imaging is required. Since the correction factor is applied to the diameters and long-axis length in the volume equation, errors as well as corrections are cubed.

In practice, the quality of the image, and the care and confidence with which the ventricular endocardial contours are traced, are very important factors influencing the accuracy of volume determination. Reproducibility studies have shown that interobserver variability ranges from 6.6 to 20 ml for end-diastolic volume, from 5.7 to 10 ml for end-systolic volume, and from 0.04 to 0.05% for ejection

fraction (24-27). For patients who are in a regular rhythm beat-to-beat variability is also low (24). The effect of contrast medium on volume and function is insignificant until seven beats after injection (28). Variability is greatest between serial studies, even in clinically stable patients (24). This is probably due to changes in the patient's hemodynamic condition between studies.

Calculation of left ventricular volume is the basis for the derivation of many other clinical parameters. Besides the end-diastolic volume, end-systolic volume, stroke volume, ejection fraction, cardiac output, and their indices (Fig. 12.3), the mass of the myocardium can also be computed by adding a measurement of wall thickness (4). The area-length method has also been applied to calculation of right ventricular and left and right atrial volumes (5, 29, 30), but these measurements are not often made for clinical purposes.

METHODS OF WALL MOTION ANALYSIS

The endocardial contours that were delineated for calculation of chamber volume can also be used to quantify regional wall motion. In patients with coronary artery disease (CAD) there may be dysfunction in nonischemic as well as ischemic regions (30, 31). Regional hypokinesis has also been observed in patients with valvular heart disease and in those with nonischemic cardiomyopathy (32,

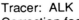

ID #	LAST, FIRST	CATH DATE

Hospital: University
Lab #:   2
Attending: Doe, M.D.
Height: _____cm   Weight: _____kg

Tracer: ALK
Correction factor: RAO = 0.542, LAO = 0.561
Frame: ED =   , ES =

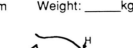

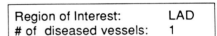

Measure	Value	Value / BSA
EDV (cc)		
ESV (cc)		
SV (cc)		
C.O. (L/min)		
Mass (gm)		
RRI (sec)		
HR (bpm)		
EF		
BSA (m^2)		

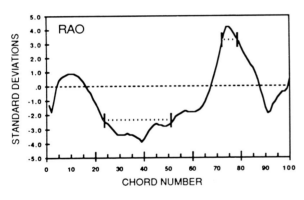

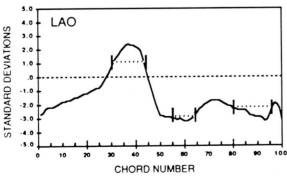

Region of Interest:	LAD
# of diseased vessels:	1

Hypokinesis, SD/chord: -3.097
Hyperkinesis, SD/chord: +3.765

% Akinetic: 24
% Hypokinetic (<-1SD):   46
% Hyperkinetic (>+1SD): 16

Location of significant WMA (<-2SD):
   Anterior ▣
   Inferior ☐
   Diffuse ☐

Hypokinesis, SD/chord: -2.889
Hyperkinesis, SD/chord: +1.746

% Akinetic: 16
% Hypokinetic (<-1SD):   54
% Hyperkinetic (>+1SD): 13

Location of significant WMA (<-2SD):
   Septal   ▣
   Posterior ☐
   Diffuse ☐

Figure 12.3.   Cardiac catheterization report listing the results of quantitative angiographic analysis. The volumes are presented in the *upper box* on the *right: EDV,* end-diastolic volume; *ESV,* end-systolic volume; *SV,* stroke volume; *CO,* cardiac output; *RRI,* R to R interval or cycle length; *HR,* heart rate; *EF,* ejection fraction; *BSA,* body surface area. Wall motion analysis by the centerline method is presented below. *WMA,* wall motion abnormality.

33). In addition to measuring the severity of such abnormalities in ventricular function for evaluation of disease progression or effect of therapy, regional wall motion analysis is useful for assessing prognosis (19, 33).

The methodology used for analyzing regional wall motion is less universally accepted than those techniques used to determine ventricular volume and ejection fraction. This is due in part to the lack of a standard for testing the accuracy of wall motion measurements. As a result, a large number of methods have been developed and validated empirically, using criteria such as accuracy in distinguishing the function of diseased patients from that of normal subjects or homogeneity of function in normal subjects. Although these methods vary in the assumptions made concerning the directionality of regional motion, they fall into two categories, depending on whether or not the motion vectors derive from a coordinate system. The earliest methods were based on a rectangular coordinate system in which motion was measured along a hemiaxis constructed perpendicular to the long axis (12). Another frequently used approach is motion measurement along radii from a central point in the ventricular chamber, such as the center of mass or a point on the long axis. In these methods, motion is usually expressed as a shortening fraction. Some investigators use the coordinate system to subdivide the ventricle into a number of regions and express wall motion in terms of an area or regional ejection fraction. This approach reduces variability in the measurement (34), but the severity of a regional abnormality may be underestimated if it spans more than one region (35).

Two coordinate system methods are based on observations in selected patient populations. Slager and co-workers analyzed the ventriculograms of normal subjects and used automated border recognition to track motion of endocardial irregularities frame-by-frame throughout the cardiac cycle (36). After analyzing the trajectories of these "landmarks," they defined 20 pathways in a rectangular coordinate system (36), along which they measured wall motion. Ingels and co-workers selected the origin of their radial coordinate system after analyzing the motion of metallic markers implanted in the midwall in patients undergoing coronary artery bypass graft surgery (37).

There are several problems associated with coordinate system methods. First, they constrain all motion to proceed toward a single origin or long axis, which is probably invalid (36, 38, 39). Second, they use the apex as a landmark on which the coordinate system is constructed, which is unwise because the apical contour is often less well opacified and more difficult to identify reproducibly (40, 41). Also, since the ventricle is usually foreshortened in the LAO projection, methods that require identification of the apex cannot be accurately applied to this view. Because of the irregular shapes of projections of the right ventricle, which may be triangular or indented, neither radial nor rectangular coordinate system methods are applicable.

In view of these problems, more recently developed methods have focused on alternate approaches to defining motion vectors. One approach is to divide the end-diastolic and end-systolic contours evenly into an equal number of points and measure motion as distance between corresponding points on the two contours. However, the implicit assumption that the ventricular contour shortens homogeneously is invalid since ischemia causes regional dysfunction.

The Centerline Method of Wall Motion Analysis

The centerline method was developed to address many of these issues (Fig. 12.4) (35). Motion is measured along 100 chords constructed perpendicular to and evenly distributed along a "centerline" drawn midway between the end-diastolic and end-systolic contours. Thus, the method makes no reference to any geometric figure, coordinate system, long axis, or apical landmark. Normalization for patient-to-patient differences in heart size is accomplished by dividing each chord's motion by the length of the end-diastolic perimeter to yield 100 **shortening fractions**.

The shortening fractions are converted into units of standard deviation from the mean motion of a normal reference population. This expresses the abnormality in terms of significance and allows comparison of function in different regions (42). Since the normal

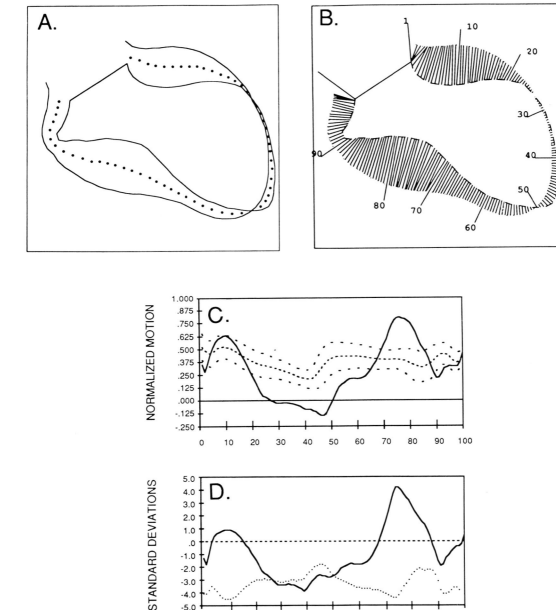

Figure 12.4. Centerline method of wall motion analysis. *A,* A centerline is constructed midway between the end-diastolic and end-systolic endocardial contours. *B,* Motion is measured along 100 chords constructed perpendicular to the centerline. *C,* Motion at each chord is normalized by the end-diastolic perimeter length to yield a shortening fraction. The patient's motion + SD measured in a normal population (*dashed line*). D, the patients wall motion is plotted in units of standard deviations (SD) from the normal mean (dashed line). Wall motion abnormality in the central infarct region, peripheral infarct region, and noninfarct region is calculated by averaging the motion of chords lying within these regions.

range for wall motion varies considerably from region to region around the ventricular contour (42-45), any attempt to define a threshold for hypokinesis (e.g., shortening fraction ≤0.25) would erroneously include normally functioning myocardium at the apex and select only very severely dysfunctional myocardium at the anterobasal wall. This is not a problem when the threshold is defined in standard deviations from normal, since all chords have comparable units for motion.

This "standardization" not only provides a uniform measure of motion around the contour but also allows calculation of an average motion value for chords lying within a region of interest (Fig. 12.3). The ability to measure function over a region is important, because it is more sensitive in detecting motion abnormalities than measuring the function of discrete points on the ventricular contour (42). The greater sensitivity of area methods can be explained by their lesser variability, since averaging the motion of a sequence of chords significantly reduces point-to-point variability (41). For these reasons, the centerline method calculates the severity of hypokinesis due to stenosis of a coronary artery by averaging the motion of chords lying in the most hypokinetic part of that artery's territory. This approach not only yields an "area" measurement but also focuses on the portion of the ventricle having the most abnormal function. Although coordinate system-based methods subdivide the ventricle into discrete regions, these predefined regions usually do not coincide with the part of the ventricle where motion is most depressed and often include either part of the "border zone" of intermediate dysfunction or a portion of normal ventricular wall (41).

Another advantage of the centerline method is its ability to calculate the circumferential extent of hypokinesis or hyperkinesis. That is, the number of chords having hypokinesis more severe than a given threshold can be easily determined and expressed as a percentage of the contour. Commonly used thresholds of hypokinesis are 1 SD below normal and 2 SD below normal, with ≥3 SD below normal being classified as akinesis.

Validation studies have demonstrated the sensitivity and specificity of the centerline method for identifying both hypokinesis and hyperkinesis (35, 46, 47) and its reproducibility (41). It should be noted that none of the methods of wall motion analysis, including the centerline method, can distinguish the motion of the ventricular walls from the motion of the heart within the chest. Methods of realigning the end-diastolic and end-systolic endocardial contours have been developed using empirical criteria but have no theoretical validity and may introduce systematic error and exacerbate variability (41).

Application of the Centerline Method in Ischemic Heart Disease

Because ischemic heart disease is inherently a regional disorder, analysis of wall motion is a very useful adjunct to calculating the global ejection fraction. The severity of hypokinesis measured by the centerline method has been correlated significantly with the minimum cross-sectional area of the respective stenosed coronary artery, and with infarct size measured from creatine phosphokinase release (35), intracoronary thallium scintigraphy (48), antimyosin antibody uptake (49), and magnetic resonance imaging (MRI) (50) in patients studied after acute myocardial infarction (AMI). Several studies have demonstrated the importance of measuring wall motion in both the ischemic region, as well as the other regions. In patients with AMI, the noninfarct region may be hypokinetic due to previous infarction or multivessel disease and thus contribute to lowering the ejection fraction. In other patients hyperkinesis in the noninfarct region may be an acute compensatory mechanism to maintain the ejection fraction at a normal level (51, 52). Later on, chronic hyperkinesis may develop, particularly in those with single-vessel disease (53, 54). Since the ejection fraction integrates the effect of wall motion abnormalities in the ischemic and noninfarct regions, this parameter of global function may not sensitively reflect the severity of hypokinesis in either the ischemic or infarcted region. Likewise, the ejection fraction may not reflect the effects of therapeutic interventions in salvaging myocardium (55-57). For these reasons, the measurement of regional as well as global left ventricular function is particularly useful in evaluating response to treatment in patients with AMI and other ischemic syndromes.

NEWER APPROACHES TO IMAGING THE LEFT VENTRICLE

Digital subtraction techniques are being used increasingly to facilitate the tedious task of delineating the endocardial contour of the left ventricle (see Chapter 29). The use of this and other image-processing techniques offers distinct advantages over the use of routine contrast cineventriculography. If injected into the left ventricle, the volume of contrast required is much smaller, as little as 7 to 10 ml (58-60). This reduces arrhythmias during injection and depression of myocardial function caused by the contrast material. Because of the lower contrast volume load, it is possible and safe to perform repeated injections and serial studies to evaluate the effect of acute interventions on left ventricular performance. The addition of digital processing to a full-volume contrast injection yields excellent images suitable for frame-by-frame analysis of function throughout the cardiac cycle. It is also possible to image the left ventricle after an intravenous injection of contrast material, but some patients are unable to suspend respiration until the end of the levophase, which is required to prevent motion artifact (58, 61).

Regardless of the quality of the image obtainable from contrast angiography, the accuracy of the volume, or the resolution of the wall motion analysis, the inescapable restriction is the invasiveness of the procedure. Two-dimensional echocardiography, radionuclide angiography, MRI, and cine-CT all can be used to obtain images of the cardiac chambers and evaluate ventricular function. All have their limitations and advantages. As nonangiographic methods are developed for the evaluation of cardiac performance, the standard by which these new techniques are evaluated will be cardiac angiography for some years to come.

The many investigators who helped develop quantitative methods to assess cardiac functions have laid the groundwork from which less invasive methods have been developed. As the invasive angiographic methods reviewed in this chapter are gradually replaced, it will be a credit to those investigators who developed our basic knowledge of cardiac function using invasive and, at times, difficult and complex procedures.

References

1. Dodge HT, Sandler H, Ballew DW, Lord JD. The use of biplane angiocardiography for the measurement of left ventricular volume in man. Am Heart J 1960;60:762–776.
2. Arvidsson H. Angiocardiographic determination of left ventricular volume. Acta Radiol 1961;56:321–339.
3. Sandler H, Dodge HT. The use of single plane angiocardiograms for the calculation of left ventricular volume in man. Am Heart J 1968;75:325–334.
4. Rackley CE, Dodge HT, Coble YD Jr, Hay RE. A method for determining left ventricular mass in man. Circulation 1964;29:666–679.
5. Sauter HJ, Dodge HT, Johnston RR, Graham TP. The relationship of left atrial pressure and volume in patients with heart disease. Am Heart J 1964;67:635–642.
6. Gault JH, Ross J, Braunwald E. Contractile state of the left ventricle in man: instantaneous tension–velocity–length relations in patients with and without disease of the left ventricular myocardium. Circ Res 1968;22:451–463.
7. Kennedy JW, Baxley WA, Figley MM, Dodge HT, Blackmon JR. Quantitative angiocardiography. I. The normal left ventricle in man. Circulation 1966;34:272–278.
8. Kennedy JW, Twiss RD, Blackmon JR, Dodge HT. Quantitative angiocardiography. III. Relationships of left ventricular pressure, volume and mass in aortic valve disease. Circulation 1968;38:838–845.
9. Kennedy JW, Yarnall SR, Murray JA, Figley MM. Quantitative angiocardiography. IV. Relationships of left atrial and ventricular pressure and volume in mitral valve disease. Circulation 1970;41:817–824.
10. Hamilton GW, Murray JA, Kennedy JW. Quantitative angiocardiography in ischemic heart disease. The spectrum of abnormal left ventricular function and the role of abnormally contracting segments. Circulation 1972;45:1065–1080.
11. Kennedy JW, Kaiser GC, Fisher LD, et al. Clinical and angiographic predictors of operative mortality from the Collaborative Study in Coronary Artery Surgery (CASS). Circulation 1981;63:793–802.
12. Herman MV, Heinle RA, Klein MD, Gorlin R. Localized disorders in myocardial contraction: asynergy and its role in congestive heart failure. N Engl J Med 1967;277:222–232.
13. Wynne J, Green LH, Mann T, Levin D, Grossman W. Estimation of left ventricular volumes in man from biplane cineangiograms filmed in oblique projections. Am J Cardiol 1978;41:726–732.
14. Als AV, Paulin S, Aroesty JM. Biplane angiographic volumetry using the right anterior oblique and half–axial left anterior oblique technique. Radiology 1978;126:511–514.
15. Rogers WJ, Smith LR, Bream PR, Elliott LP, Rackley CE, Russell RO. Quantitative axial oblique contrast left ventriculography: validation of the method by demonstrating improved visualization of regional wall motion and mitral valve function with accurate volume determinations. Am Heart J 1982;103:185–193.

16. Kennedy JW, Doces JG, Stewart DK. Left ventricular function before and following surgical treatment of mitral valve disease. Am Heart J 1979;97:592–598.

17. Kennedy JW, Doces JG, Stewart DK. Left ventricular function before and following aortic valve replacement. Circulation 1977;56:944–950.

18. Principal Investigators of CASS and Their Associates. The National Heart, Lung, and Blood Institute Coronary Artery Surgery Study. A multi–center comparison of the effects of randomized medical and surgical treatment of mildly symptomatic patients with coronary artery disease, and a registry of consecutive patients undergoing coronary angiography. Circulation 1981;63:I–1–81.

19. Kennedy JW, Kaiser GC, Fisher LD, et al. Multivariate discriminant analysis of the clinical and angiographic predictors of operative mortality from the collaborative study in coronary artery surgery (CASS). J Thorac Cardiovasc Surg 1980;80:876–887.

20. Hugenholtz PG, Wagner HR, Sandler H. The in vivo determination of left ventricular volume: comparison of the fiberoptic–indicator dilution and the angiocardiographic methods. Circulation 1968;37:489–508.

21. Kennedy JW, Trenholme SE, Kasser IS. Left ventricular volume and mass from single–plane cineangiocardiogram: a comparison of anteroposterior and right anterior oblique methods. Am Heart J 1970;80:343–352.

22. Kasser IS, Kennedy JW. Measurement of left ventricular volumes in man by single–plane cineangiocardiography. Invest Radiol 1969;4:83–90.

23. Cha SD, Incarvito J, Maranhao V. Calculation of magnification factor from an intracardiac marker. Cathet Cardiovasc Diagn 1983;9:79–87.

24. Cohn PF, Levine JA, Bergeron GA, Gorlin R. Reproducibility of the angiographic left ventricular ejection fraction in patients with coronary artery disease. Am Heart J 1974;88:713–720.

25. Rogers WJ, Smith LR, Hood WP Jr, Mantle JA, Rackley CE, Russell RO Jr. Effect of filming projection and interobserver variability on angiographic biplane left ventricular volume determination. Circulation 1979;59:96–104.

26. Dodge HT, Sheehan FH, Stewart DK. Estimation of ventricular volume, fractional ejected volumes, stroke volume, and quantitation of regurgitant flow. In: Just H, Heintzen PH, eds. Angiocardiography: Current status and future developments. Berlin: Springer–Verlag, 1986;99–108.

27. Chaitman BR, DeMots H, Bristow JD, Rosch J, Rahimtoola SH. Objective and subjective analysis of left ventricular angiograms. Circulation 1975;52:420–425.

28. Vine DL, Hegg TD, Dodge HT, Stewart DK, Frimer M. Immediate effect of contrast medium injection on left ventricular volumes and ejection fraction: a study using metallic epicardial markers. Circulation 1977;56:379–384.

29. Lange PE, Onnasch D, Farr FL, Heintzen PH. Angiocardiographic right ventricular volume determination. Accuracy, as determined from human casts, and clinical application. Eur J Cardiol 1978;8:477–501.

30. Graham TP Jr, Atwood GF, Faulkner SL, Nelson JH. Right atrial volume measurements from biplane cineangiocardiography. Circulation 1974;49:709–716.

31. Lang T–W, Corday E, Gold H, et al. Consequences of reperfusion after coronary occlusion: effects on hemodynamic and regional myocardial metabolic function. Am J Cardiol 1974;33:69–81.

32. Thompson R, Ahmed M, Seabra–Gomes R, et al. Influence of preoperative left–ventricular function on results of homograft replacement of the aortic valve for aortic regurgitation. J Thorac Cardiovasc Surg 1979;77:411–421.

33. Wallis DE, O'Connell JB, Henkin RE, Costanzp–Nordin MR, Scanlon PJ. Segmental wall motion abnormalities in dilated cardiomyopathy: a common finding and good prognostic sign. J Am Coll Cardiol 1984;4:674–679.

34. Gelberg HJ, Brundage BH, Glantz S, Parmley WW. Quantitative left ventricular wall motion analysis: A comparison of area, chord and radial methods. Circulation 1979;59:991–1000.

35. Sheehan FH, Bolson EL, Dodge HT, Mathey DG, Schofer J, Woo HW. Advantages and applications of the centerline method for characterizing regional ventricular function. Circulation 1986;74:293–305.

36. Slager CJ, Hooghoudt TEH, Serruys PW, et al. Quantitative assessment of regional left ventricular motion using endocardial landmarks. J Am Coll Cardiol 1986;7:317–327.

37. Ingels NB Jr, Daughters GT II, Stinson EB, Alderman EL. Evaluation of methods for quantitating left ventricular segmental wall motion in man using myocardial markers as a standard. Circulation 1980;61:966–972.

38. Goodyer AVN, Langou RA. The multicentric character of normal left ventricular wall motion. Implications for the evaluation of regional wall motion abnormalities by contrast angiography. Cathet Cardiovasc Diagn 1982;8:225–232.

39. McDonald IG. The shape and movements of the human left ventricle during systole. Am J Cardiol 1970;26:221–230.

40. Sandor T, Paulin S, Hanlon WB. Left ventricular wall motion analysis using operator–independent contour positioning. Comput Biomed Res 1984;17:129–142.

41. Sheehan FH, Stewart DK, Dodge HT, et al. Variability in the measurement of regional ventricular wall motion from contrast angiograms. Circulation 1983;68:550–559.

42. Gelberg HJ, Brundage BH, Glantz S, Parmley WW. Quantitative left ventricular wall motion analysis: a comparison of area, chord and radial methods. Circulation 1979;59:991–1000.

43. Harris LD, Clayton PD, Marshall HW, Warner HR. A technique for the detection of asynergic motion in the left ventricle. Comput Biomed Res 1974;7:380–394.

44. Stewart DK, Dodge HT, Frimer M. Quantitative analysis of regional myocardial performance in

coronary artery disease. Cardiovasc Imaging Image Processing 1975;72:217–224.

45. Ingles NB Jr, Daughters GT II, Stinson EB, Alderman EL. Measurement of midwall myocardial dynamics in intact man by radiography of surgically implanted markers. Circulation 1975;52:859–867.

46. Sheehan FH, Bolson EL, Dodge HT, Mitten S. Centerline method — Comparison with other methods for measuring regional left ventricular motion. In: Sigwart U, Heintzen PH, eds. Ventricular wall motion. Stuttgart: Georg Thieme Verlag, 1984:139–149.

47. Ginzton LE, Berntzen R, Lobodzinski S, Thigpen T, Laks MM. Computerized quantitative segmental wall motion analysis during exercise: radial vs. centerline left ventricular segmentation. In: Computers in Cardiology. Long Beach, CA: IEEE Computer Soc, 1985:157–160.

48. Schofer J, Sheehan FH, Spielmann R, Wygant J, Bleifeld W, Mathey DG. Early intracoronary thallium/technetium–pyrophosphate scintigraphy is a reliable method to predict myocardial salvage (abstr). Circulation 1986;74:II–273.

49. Khaw BA, Gold HK, Yasuda T, et al. Scintigraphic quantification of myocardial necrosis in patients after intravenous injection of myosin–specific antibody. Circulation 1986;74:501–508.

50. Johns JA, Yasuda T, Gold HK, et al. Estimation of site and localization of myocardial infarction by magnetic resonance imaging (abstr). J Am Coll Cardiol 1986;7:196A.

51. Stamm RB, Gibson RS, Bishop HL, Carabello BA, Beller GA, Martin RP. Echocardiographic detection of infarct–localized asynergy and remote asynergy during acute myocardial infarction: correlation with the extent of angiographic coronary disease. Circulation 1983;67:233–244.

52. Sheehan FH, Szente A, Mathey DG, Dodge HT. Assessment of left ventricular function in acute myocardial infarction: the relationship between global ejection fraction and regional wall motion. Eur Heart J 1985;6:E117–125.

53. Martin GV, Sheehan FH, Ritchie JL, et al. Beneficial effects of streptokinase on function of non–infarct regions (abstr). Circulation 1987;76:IV–180.

54. Serruys PW, Simoons ML, Suryapranata H, et al. Preservation of global and regional left ventricular function after early thrombolysis in acute myocardial infarction. J Am Coll Cardiol 1986;7:729–742.

55. Stack RS, Phillips HR III, Grierson DS, et al. Functional improvement of jeopardized myocardium following intracoronary streptokinase infusion in acute myocardial infarction. J Clin Invest 1983;72:84–95.

56. Sheehan FH, Mathey DG, Schofer J, Krebber HJ, Dodge HT. Effect of interventions in salvaging left ventricular function in acute myocardial infarction: a study of intracoronary streptokinase. Am J Cardiol 1983;52:431–438.

57. Sheehan FH, Mathey DG, Schofer J, Dodge HT, Bolson EL. Factors determining recovery of left ventricular function following thrombolysis in acute myocardial infarction. Circulation 1985;71:1121–1128.

58. Tobis JM, Nalcioglu O, Johnston WD, et al. Correlation of 10–milliliter digital subtraction ventriculograms compared with standard cineangiograms. Am Heart J 1983;105:946–951.

59. Nichols AB, Martin EC, Fles TP, et al. Validation of the angiographic accuracy of digital left ventriculography. Am J Cardiol 1983;51:224–230.

60. Mancini GBJ, Hodgson JM, Legrand V, et al. Quantitative assessment of global and regional left ventricular function with low–contrast dose digital subtraction ventriculography. Chest 1985;87:598–602.

61. Nissen SE, Booth D, Waters J, Fassas T, DeMaria AN. Evaluation of left ventricular contractile pattern by intravenous digital subtraction ventriculography: comparison with cineangiography and assessment of interobserver variability. Am J Cardiol 1983;52:1293–1298.

13

Coronary Angiography

Carl J. Pepine, M.D.
Charles R. Lambert, M.D., Ph.D.
James A. Hill, M.D.

INTRODUCTION

Coronary angiography is the only method generally available to study intraluminal anatomy of the coronary arteries in living persons. The introduction of a widely applicable and safe selective coronary angiographic technique approximately 30 years ago, the development of high-quality magnification cineradiography, and the advent of practical catheter-based intervention have led to incredible growth of coronary angiography, both as a clinical and research tool. This procedure represents a benchmark in medicine for diagnosis, treatment, and research and has probably made more important contributions in these areas than any other laboratory-based procedure. Before addressing the conduct of this procedure, it seems appropriate to review its indications.

GOALS OF CORONARY ANGIOGRAPHY

As stated by Gensini, "The primary goal of coronary angiography is identification, localization and assessment of obstructive lesions within the arteries of the heart" (1). Congenital anomalies (e.g., anomalous coronary artery origin, myocardial bridges, atresia, fistulae) as well as other acquired disorders (e.g., spasm, thromboembolus, traumatic injury) can also be detected.

Specifically, coronary angiography is performed to determine the presence or absence of atherosclerotic coronary artery disease

(CAD) and to define its severity (i.e., degree of stenosis) and extent (i.e., number of artery segments involved).

INDICATIONS FOR CORONARY ANGIOGRAPHY

General

Indications for this study are discussed in Chapter 2 of this text. Indications currently used in the authors' laboratories are best summarized in the ACC/AHA Task Force guidelines for coronary angiography. Most cardiovascular specialists agree that knowledge of the presence or absence of CAD and its severity and extent are extremely helpful in directing patient management and formulating **prognosis** for patients with symptoms or other findings suggesting the presence of myocardial ischemia. The technique may be useful for patients with either typical or atypical clinical syndromes. More recently, use of coronary angiography to identify spasm and/or thrombus has added to its diagnostic usefulness in these patients.

The "Need to Know"

The general indication for coronary angiography is the "**need to know**" (2), which obviously covers a wide range of circumstances. This largely depends on the physician-patient relationship and is dictated, to some extent, by the availability of the technique and its risks and costs in a given locality or practice setting (see Chapter 2). The most common need for coronary angiography relates to evaluation of patients with known or suspected symptomatic ischemic heart disease for therapeutic procedures. These procedures have rapidly expanded to include coronary artery bypass grafting (CABG), percutaneous transluminal coronary angioplasty (PTCA), thrombolysis, valvuloplasty, and numerous other cardiac procedures, as well as noncardiac procedures (e.g., vascular surgery) in which the risk of the procedure is substantially increased in patients with severe CAD.

For example, coronary angiography is indicated to define the basis for signs and symptoms of ischemia in certain patients with **either stable or unstable angina**, as well as in selected patients with **complicated or uncomplicated myocardial infarction** (see Chapters 25 and 26). Coronary angiography may identify anatomic patterns associated with a high risk of death or infarction (e.g., left main coronary stenosis, severe three-vessel CAD with abnormal left ventricular function) that can be modified by an appropriate revascularization procedure. Knowledge of the presence or absence of CAD can be of considerable help to surgeons operating on patients with valvular or congenital heart disease, as well as aortic root or pericardial disease. It is the authors' practice to perform coronary angiography in all adult male patients over the age of 35 and female patients older than 40 years of age in whom any type of cardiac surgery is contemplated.

Coronary angiography is often useful in patients who are **incapacitated by chest pain syndromes** that are **not typical** of ischemia-related symptoms. Demonstration of no important coronary artery obstruction or spasm excludes, with certainty, the possibility that CAD is the basis for these patients' chest pain syndrome. In addition, specialized measurements of coronary flow and vasodilator reserve can be performed during catheterization to evaluate abnormalities that may affect the coronary microcirculation. These are important initial steps to take before pursuit of an alternate diagnosis that may identify an esophageal, respiratory, or musculoskeletal origin for chest pain. In such patients this information may eliminate the need for recurrent and costly admissions to coronary care units and expedites the patient's return to an active and normal life.

The High Risk Patient and the Asymptomatic Patient

More recently, patients with indicators of **"high risk"** for events (death, myocardial infarction, etc.), based upon noninvasive study, have comprised an increasing number of those patients referred for coronary angiography. Some of these patients may be only mildly symptomatic or even asymptomatic. Recommendations for coronary angiography in asymptomatic patients require additional comment. Recent widespread use of treadmill exercise and other forms of noninvasive testing has identified a subset of patients with ischemic electrocardiographic responses but without symptoms attributable to ischemia (i.e., possible silent myocardial ischemia). At present, it is apparent that the outcome of these patients depends upon the presence of CAD and characteristics of the ischemic response and not absence of pain. When these abnormalities occur in patients who are at high risk for the presence of CAD (e.g., hypercholesteremia, hypertension, cigarette smoking, male) or in the presence of another independent noninvasive test that is also abnormal (e.g., abnormal treadmill ECG plus redistribution abnormalities on stress thallium-201 scanning), these abnormalities are most likely related to coronary artery disease. The severity of the CAD determines the prognosis of these asymptomatic patients, but coronary disease and its severity can be readily identified with certainty only by selective coronary angiography. This area is discussed in detail in Chapter 25.

Other patients who warrant mention are those individuals with abnormal resting electrocardiograms or chest pain of uncertain etiology who have jobs that involve the safety of others. This group includes airline pilots, bus drivers, policemen, and firemen. Here, the physician might utilize knowledge of the presence or absence of coronary artery disease to help counsel the patient. Based on this information, the patient and employer can be encouraged to modify the patient's occupation and work-related stress.

To summarize, in 1962 Sones stated that "coronary arteriography is indicated when a problem is encountered which may be resolved by objective demonstration of the coronary artery tree, providing competent personnel and medical facilities are available and the potential risks are acceptable to the patient and his physician" (2). Indications for coronary angiography have not changed significantly since this statement was published.

PREPARATION OF THE PATIENT FOR CORONARY ANGIOGRAPHY

The patient's primary or hospital attending physician should not refer a patient for coronary angiography without first explaining the procedure in broad terms. Several preliminary studies, in addition to the usual clinical examination, are required. These include a recent chest x-ray and several other clinical laboratory tests. The latter tests are a complete blood count, blood urea nitrogen, and creatinine. An evaluation of clotting function is **not** routinely needed unless there is a history suggesting that there is a bleeding disorder or that the patient is taking **oral** anticoagulants. Likewise, blood typing and cross matching are not routinely needed unless the patient is going to surgery or is bleeding.

A member of the catheterization team, in addition to the cardiologist performing the procedure, should visit the patient prior to catheterization to familiarize the patient with the procedure and acquaint him with some of the personnel performing the test. This visit is best done on the afternoon or evening prior to scheduled catheterization if the patient is hospitalized. If the patient is an outpatient, we schedule this visit several days to weeks before the planned procedure. The patient's fear of the unknown, the awesome equipment in the catheterization laboratory, and other uncertainties can be very frightening. It is helpful that he or she be comforted by familiar faces in addition to the physician performing the procedure (who may be masked during the procedure). Videotape or slide programs are also very helpful to describe and preview the procedure for the patient. These are available free of charge upon request from the American College of Cardiology. In certain selected instances it may also be helpful to have the patient visit the laboratory to allay his or her anxieties.

In most instances, the procedure should be performed in a **fasting postabsorptive state**, since either contrast material or vagal reactions may induce nausea or vomiting.

Also, there may be a small possibility that the patient will be a candidate for emergency surgery. If the patient's procedure is performed at noon or after noon, it is the authors' practice to feed the patient a light liquid breakfast before 8 AM. Of course, if the procedure is urgently indicated (e.g., aortic root dissection, postmyocardial infarction angina, cardiogenic shock), the study can be done without these precautions.

Written informed consent should be obtained by the physician who will perform the study. It is important that the physician obtaining consent indicate in the patient's chart by a written note what was explained to the patient and the patient's level of understanding.

Many patients scheduled to undergo coronary angiography are receiving potent **pharmacologic agents**. Guidelines relating to discontinuation of these agents must be **individualized** based upon assessment of each patient. For example, oral anticoagulants need not be discontinued if cutdown technique is used. For a percutaneous procedure oral anticoagulants should be stopped approximately 2 days prior to catheterization. It is often not necessary to discontinue heparin in patients prior to coronary angiography by either cutdown or percutaneous technique. Problems with bleeding in the heparinized patient can be handled by administration of intravenous protamine or stopping heparin for several hours. Digitalis and diuretics need not be discontinued prior to the procedure, particularly if the patient has heart failure or atrial fibrillation. Digitalis toxicity, however, must be avoided, as these patients may have increased ventricular irritability and cardioversion is not without risk in the digitalis toxic patient. Aspirin and antiischemic agents (e.g., calcium antagonists, nitrates, and β-adrenergic blockers) need not be discontinued, particularly if a patient has unstable rest angina. However, if there is a need to document coronary artery spasm, it is important to discontinue calcium antagonists and long-acting nitrates four to five half-lives before the procedure. If ischemic episodes occur during this interval, they are best managed by sublingual or intravenous nitroglycerin.

Sedation and analgesia may be helpful, particularly in patients who are apprehensive about the procedure. While it has been the authors' practice over the years to eliminate or reduce premedication to a minimum, particularly when the possibility of coronary spasm is suspected or when coronary angiography is done on an outpatient basis, premedication is still in use by many operators. When premedication includes more than antihistamines, the authors prefer to use a short-acting benzodiazepine. Prophylactic antibiotics are not routinely used.

Some patients present with a **history of allergic reaction** to contrast agents or related iodine-containing materials. Reactions which are probably allergic include rash, hives, transient hypotension, or bronchospasm. Most commonly, when the history is carefully reviewed, the reactions do not actually resemble allergic reactions and seem to consist of flushing or vagal-mediated nausea or vomiting. This poses a dilemma for the physician performing coronary angiography. Indications for the procedure must be reviewed and weighed against the possible risks of precipitating an anaphylactic reaction. The frequency of flushing, nausea, vomiting, hypotension, and arrhythmias can be markedly reduced with use of a nonionic contrast agent (see Chapter 10). Fortunately, in most instances these reactions in patients with a previous history of allergy to contrast material can be prevented or minimized by pretreatment with antihistamines (H_1 blockers) and glucocorticosteroids. We use 60 mg of prednisone orally the night before the procedure and repeat this dose 1 hr before the procedure along with 50 mg of diphenhydramine. An H_2 histaminergic receptor blocker may also be useful on occasion. These premedications may not prevent true anaphylactic reactions.

NORMAL RADIOGRAPHIC CORONARY ARTERY ANATOMY (FIGS. 13.1–13.5)

Knowledge of the anatomic distribution of the coronary arteries is important for the physician participating in the care of patients undergoing cardiac catheterization. For the physician planning to perform coronary angiography, the **radiographic anatomy must be committed to memory** before the first patient is approached. The brief summary to follow is intended as an introduction for

physicians participating in the practice of coronary angiography. Each operator must be very familiar with normal, as well as abnormal, radiographic anatomy of the coronary arteries. He should develop his own protocol for radiographic projections that is modified for more optimal visualization of specific areas in a given patient's coronary system as the need arises (Fig. 13.1).

Left Coronary Artery

The ostium of the left coronary artery usually arises from the superior portion of the left coronary sinus, somewhat anterior to the coronal plane from a position between the pulmonary artery and left atrial appendage (Figs. 13.2 and 13.3). The proximal portion of the left main coronary artery continues for a variable distance before it divides into its anterior descending and circumflex branches. The left main coronary artery may terminate in a trifurcation, with an intermediate branch bisecting the angle between the left anterior descending and left circumflex coronary arteries. The left main artery regularly does not supply secondary branches. The ostium and proximal portions of the main left coronary artery are often best visualized in the shallow (20 to 30°) left anterior oblique projection (LAO) (Fig. 13.1). Minimal (10 to 15%) cranial angulation in the sagittal plane may be helpful. The distal portion of the left main artery and bifurcation are best viewed in the shallow (20°) right anterior oblique projection (RAO) with minimal (0 to 15°) caudal or moderate (20 to 30°) cranial angulation. A secondary view for the distal left main and bifurcation is the 30 to 45° LAO with about 25° of caudal angulation.

Left Anterior Descending Artery

The left anterior descending artery originates at an obtuse angle from the left main artery and courses anteriorly, inferiorly, and toward the patient's right to emerge from behind the pulmonary artery and descend in the anterior intraventricular groove (Figs. 13.2 and 13.3). In most patients this vessel continues to the apex and in some it also supplies the inferior apical region. Occasionally, the left anterior descending courses in an intramyocardial position. Sometimes, systolic compression from **muscular bridges** over the artery can be

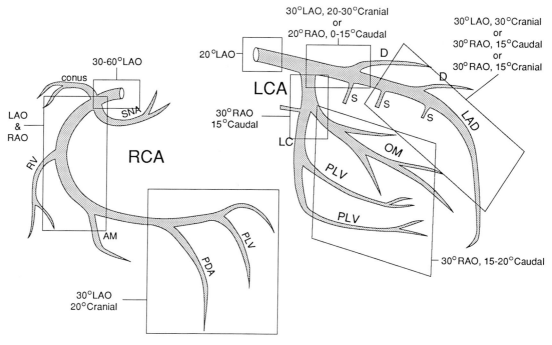

Figure 13.1. Schematic representation of the right (*RCA*) and left (*LCA*) coronary arteries depicted in the left anterior oblique (*LAO*) and right anterior oblique (*RAO*) projections, respectively. Approximate frontal and sagittal plane projections and angulations for visualization of various portions of the coronary arteries are indicated. The LCA branches are noted as: *SNA*, sinus node artery; *RV*, right ventricular; *AM*, acute marginal; *PDA*, posterior descending artery; *PLV*, posterior left ventricular; *LC*, left circumflex; *OM*, obtuse marginal; *S*, septal; *D*, diagonal; *LAD*, left anterior descending.

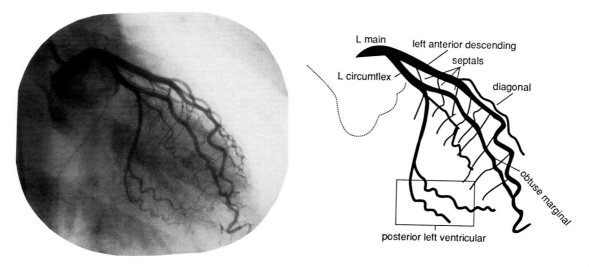

Figure 13.2. Normal radiographic anatomy of the left coronary artery and its branches, as seen in the right anterior oblique projection with slight (15°) caudal angulation.

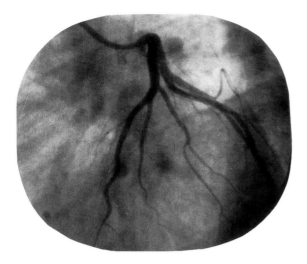 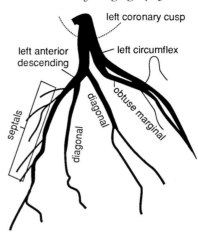

Figure 13.3. Normal radiographic anatomy of the left coronary artery and its branches, as seen in the left anterior oblique projection with cranial (20°) angulation.

observed obstructing flow of contrast in systole. In a few such cases obstruction during diastole is also present over several centimeters. Systolic compression caused by muscular bridges is usually accentuated after nitroglycerin. Recognition of these features helps to distinguish the bridge from other forms of obstruction, such as that caused by a pericardial band or CAD.

The proximal left anterior descending is best visualized in LAO projections (30 to 60°) with cranial angulation (20 to 30°) (Figs. 13.1 and 13.3). The mid and distal portions are better seen in LAO projections without cranial angulation and RAO projections (Fig. 13.2). In the RAO projections some caudal or cranial angulation (15 to 30°) may be used to minimize overlap of the mid left anterior descending with diagonal branches.

Septal Perforating and Diagonal Branches

Septal branches arise at right angles from the left anterior descending and course deep into the intraventricular septum. Septal branches vary in number, and the first branch is sometimes large enough for angioplasty or bypass considerations. Sometimes a large septal perforating trunk arises from the first or second septal branch position and supplies multiple secondary branches. Septal left anterior descending branches supply the anterior two-thirds of the septum and form potential for anastomosis with septal perforating branches

derived from the posterior descending branch of the right or left circumflex arteries. The proximal septal perforators are often large (1 to 1.5 mm in diameter), and their proximal portions are best visualized in the shallow (30°) LAO projection with cranial angulation (30°) and shallow (30°) RAO projection with caudal angulation (Fig. 13.2).

Diagonal Branches

The diagonal branches arise at oblique angles to the left anterior descending continuing on the epicardial surface to descend diagonally towards the obtuse margin of the heart. Diagonal branches vary in number and size, but usually the first two or three are large enough for angioplasty or bypass consideration. On rare occasions a diagonal branch can be quite large and even supply septal perforating branches. The proximal parts of the diagonal branches are usually best viewed in the 30 to 45° LAO projection with 30° cranial angulation (Fig. 13.3). The 30° RAO projections with caudal (15°) or cranial (30°) angulation will minimize overlap of the diagonal branches.

Left Circumflex Artery

The left circumflex artery continues often in the same general direction as the left main coronary artery, under the left atrial appendage to enter the left atrial-ventricular groove. The left circumflex then continues toward to the patient's left and posteriorly at an oblique angle. After providing several posterior lateral ventricular branches, which parallel the left anterior descending diagonal branches in their direction toward the obtuse margin, the left circumflex supplies an obtuse marginal branch, which continues along the obtuse margin of the heart. The continuation of the left circumflex coronary in the atrialventricular groove is highly variable. In some patients with anatomically dominant left circumflex artery circulations, the left circumflex continues to supply a large posterior descending branch. In the more common variety the left circumflex continues as a small terminal posterior left ventricular branch(es) and does not reach the posterior intraventricular groove.

The proximal portion of the left circumflex is best visualized in the RAO projection (30°) with about 15° caudal angulation (Fig. 13.2). A secondary view is the steep LAO projection (30 to 45°) with cranial angulation (15 to 20°). The obtuse marginal branch is best viewed in the RAO projections (30°) with 15 to 20° of caudal angulation.

Right Coronary Artery

The ostium of the right coronary artery (RCA) usually arises from an anterior position at approximately the middle portion of the right coronary sinus (Figs. 13.4 and 13.5). It is usually somewhat lower in position than the left coronary ostium. The RCA ostium is always more anterior than the left coronary ostium. From this position the RCA descends to the patient's right in the anterior right atrioventricular (AV) groove. The conus branch to the proximal pulmonary conus and right ventricular outflow region is its first branch. Alternatively, the conus artery may originate from a separate ostium and will not be visualized when the RCA ostium is selectively engaged as in Figures 13.4 and 13.5. Regularly, there are also two or three large right ventricular branches that arise in an anterior direction and course diagonally over the right ventricle. A sinus node branch usually originates posteriorly and courses in a cranial direction to encircle the superior vena cava. A major branch is provided at the acute margin, which usually supplies only right ventricular

myocardium. On occasion this branch may continue to supply the apex. In the majority of individuals the RCA artery continues along the diaphragmatic surface of the heart in the AV groove to reach the crux. The RCA continues to supply, in the majority of instances (90%), a branch to the AV node and then descends in the intraventricular groove to provide the posterior descending artery (PDA) branch. This PDA branch is variable in size but in the majority of individuals remains quite large. It courses in an anterior direction in the inferior intraventricular groove to supply septal perforating branches. These ascend at right angles to supply the inferior third of the septum. These branches can provide a rich collateral pathway via septal perforating arteries to the left anterior descending.

The right ostium and most proximal RCA is best viewed in the relatively steep (45 to 60°) LAO projections (Fig. 13.4). The midportion of the RCA is well seen in most LAO and RAO projections. The part of the RCA continuing along the diaphragmatic surface is best seen in the LAO projections. The RCA at the crux and PDA are best seen in the 30° LAO projection with cranial (20 to 30°) angulation (Fig. 13.4). A secondary view would be the 20° RAO projection with cranial angulation.

TECHNIQUES FOR SELECTIVE CORONARY ARTERY OPACIFICATION

Current visualization techniques provide excellent resolution of large- and medium-sized coronary vessels and even vessels as small as 100 μm in diameter. Repeated injections in multiple projections are needed for most diagnostic studies. Because of the potential for thromboembolism or thrombus formation at or distal to the site of catheter insertion, anticoagulation is used routinely in the authors' laboratories in patients undergoing coronary angiography. Heparin is administered intraarterially or intravenously shortly after the first catheter enters a peripheral artery. The dose varies but usually ranges from 3000 to 5000 units. The authors operate on the axiom that bleeding can readily be controlled during or following catheterization but that thromboembolism can not and results in

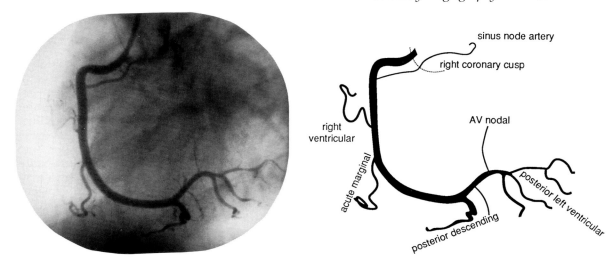

Figure 13.4. Normal radiographic anatomy of the right coronary artery and its branches, as seen in the left anterior oblique projection.

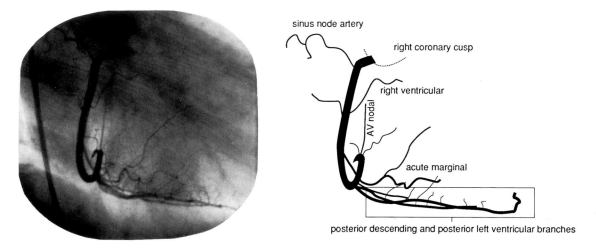

Figure 13.5. Normal radiographic anatomy of the right coronary artery and its branches, as seen in the right anterior oblique projection.

devastating consequences. In the authors' experience, heparin use appears to reduce the incidence of rare but major thromboembolic complications of coronary angiography. The nonionic contrast agents do not have either the anticoagulant or antiplatelet aggregation properties that the ionic agents exert. Nor do the nonionic agents potentiate the anticoagulant effects of heparin, as is seen with the ionic agents. Thus, in our opinion when nonionic contrast agents are used for

coronary angiography, heparin should always be used. Furthermore, use of these newer contrast agents demands even more meticulous attention to the safety details of the coronary angiographic procedure. Blood in connecting tubes, manifolds, or syringes must not be left in contact with these agents. Manifolds with a port for heparinized flush solution are essential. Contrast agents and their use are discussed in more detail in Chapter 10.

There are two general approaches used for selective coronary angiography. These are the **femoral artery approach** and the **brachial artery approach**. Each approach may be used with several techniques, and each has its proponents. Many angiographers routinely use several techniques in a very capable fashion. It is our belief, however, that an angiographer should attempt to achieve expertise with one technique and use it routinely while reserving alternate techniques for instances in which certain problems preclude use of his/her primary technique. If the frequency of need for an alternate technique is not sufficient to maintain skills for its use in a safe and time-effective manner, cases requiring an alternate technique should be referred to colleagues who are using the alternate technique on a regular basis.

Femoral Artery Approach

The femoral artery approach is the most widely used. It requires complete familiarity with the anatomy of the peripheral circulation and expertise in a technique for percutaneous vascular catheterization (3). The percutaneous technique is used to introduce the femoral artery catheter in almost all cases except for that of small children and other very special cases in which femoral artery cutdown may be needed.

The technique for percutaneous catheter insertion and the needles and wires used are described in detail in Chapter 6 and Chapter 7. Because it is essential that this technique be mastered in order to do coronary angiography in a rapid, safe, and efficient manner, it will be reviewed in brief here. A special needle with a **blunt bevel** and appropriate obturator is introduced through the femoral artery. When adequate arterial blood flow is observed, it is advanced, and the obturator or stylet is removed. Alternately, a **sharp 18-gauge needle** without obturator or stylet is introduced through only the outer wall of the femoral artery. The authors prefer the latter alternative for introduction of catheters for coronary angiography. We feel that the sharp needle, without obturator, has the potential to cause less damage to diseased, calcified, femoral arteries. Furthermore, the sharp needle permits single puncture through only the anterior part of the artery wall and minimizes

bleeding during the procedure when patients are anticoagulated. This is especially important in the setting of thrombolytic therapy. The sharp needle technique is also more rapid.

When good pulsatile flow is observed, a guidewire (usually 0.035 inches in diameter) is introduced through the needle and advanced into the arterial system. After a fluoroscopic check to ensure that the guidewire has advanced in retrograde fashion (i.e., into the iliac artery and aorta), pressure is maintained on the artery proximal to the insertion site with the left middle and fourth fingers, and the needle is removed with the right hand as the guidewire is wiped with a heparinized saline sponge held by the right thumb and forefinger. The guidewire is coiled as it is wiped, and the coil is secured by the left forefinger and thumb. Alternately, an assistant may control the guidewire. A preselected coronary angiographic catheter is threaded over the guidewire and advanced to the appropriate artery. The authors prefer to modify the procedure by introduction of an appropriate arterial dilator and **valved catheter sheath**. The latter facilitates catheter exchanges and minimizes damage to the artery. Selective coronary angiography is then done using special catheters (4, 5) and techniques described below.

Judkins Catheters and Technique

These preformed right and left coronary catheters are usually made of polyurethane or polyethylene with stainless steel wire mesh or bands (see Figs. 7.20 and 7.21). The coronary artery catheters are usually 100 cm in length, 5 to 8 Fr in diameter, and taper approximately to 5 Fr diameter at their tips. They have only an end hole and are made in multiple different preformed variations. The preformed curves are designed on the principle that the proximal and transverse portions of the aortic arch, ascending aorta, and left coronary ostium lie in approximately the same plane. The body of a catheter advanced to the aortic root from below tends to lie against the lateral wall of the aorta opposite the direction of its tip (Fig. 13.6). Thus, the operator should select the appropriately sized catheter prior to attempted engagement. This is done by evaluating the patient's body habitus, associated clinical findings (i.e., aortic stenosis), and aortic root size and shape from either chest film or fluoroscopic examination. Information about root size is also obtained from the behavior of the pigtail catheter, which may have been advanced to the left ventricle prior to coronary angiography.

An assessment is made as to whether the ascending aorta is normal in size, uncoiled, dilated, or markedly dilated. **Left coronary Judkins catheters** have primary (90°), secondary (180°), and tertiary curves (5) (Fig. 13.6). The radius of curvature for the tertiary curve is about 10 cm. The distance between primary and secondary curves varies from approximately 3.5 to 6 cm (Fig. 7.27). The size of the left coronary catheter is determined by the distance between primary and secondary curves (e.g., 4, 5, or 6), and this also determines the angle that the distal segment forms with the coronary artery. For example, the longer the distance (e.g., 5 vs. 4), the greater the angle that the distal segment forms with the left coronary ostium. A No. 4 left Judkins has a distance of approximately 4 cm between the secondary and primary curves. This catheter size is applicable for most normal

aortas and can be used in the large majority of patients. The distance between primary and secondary curves is approximately 5 cm, for the No. 5 Judkins. This size is useful for the uncoiled or slightly enlarged aortas of hypertensive male patients. The No. 6 size has a primary-secondary curve distance of approximately 6 cm and is useful for the large post-stenotic dilated aorta of the patient with aortic valve stenosis or aortic root disease (e.g., patients with Marfan's syndrome or syphilis). Occasionally, catheters as large as No. 7 are needed and may be made by heat gun. A No. 3 or 3.5 catheter is used in children and/or smaller adults, particularly young women. The **right coronary Judkins catheter** has a secondary curve of 135° with a radius of 5 to 6 cm for the small and medium sizes and about 11 for the large size (Fig. 13.7). The reader is referred to Chapter 7 of this text for a more detailed discussion about these catheters, their construction, and selection.

The left Judkins catheter is usually used first (following ventriculography). As the catheter is advanced in the aortic arch, pressure is monitored. With the patient in a

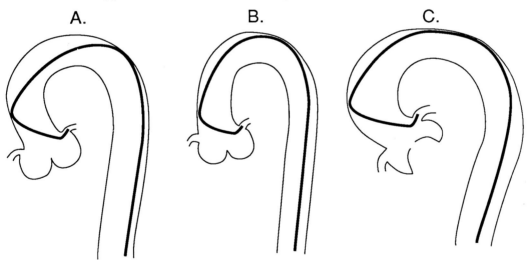

Figure 13.6. Approach to the left coronary artery using Judkins catheters. Examples of catheter position in various types of aortic roots are shown in the LAO projection. When the catheter is advanced into the ascending aorta, the catheter tip will move along the left wall of the aorta to "drop into" the left coronary ostium. The secondary bend of the catheter will touch the right lateral aortic wall. In the normal sized aortic root (*A*), this is accomplished using a No. 4 left series catheter. In the small aortic root (*B*) a No. 3.5 catheter may be used. In the dilated aortic root (*C*) a No. 5 or 6 catheter is used as shown. Particular attention must be paid to the position of the catheter within the left coronary ostium. The catheter size should be appropriate so that withdrawal of the catheter allows the angle between the distal segment of the catheter and the main left coronary artery to be minimal, so that the tip does not touch the coronary artery wall.

shallow LAO projection the catheter is advanced, and the tip moves down the left wall of the ascending aorta until it "drops into" the sinus of Valsalva and left coronary ostia (Fig 13.6). The pressure wave is inspected for alterations or "damping." When these are absent, a test injection (1 to 2 cc) is observed on fluoroscopy. During this test, the operator must pay particular attention to the position of catheter in left coronary artery. The angle that the Judkins catheter tip makes with the direction of the proximal coronary artery must be minimal to ensure that the tip does not touch the artery wall. This is very important in order to avoid dissection of the coronary artery, should the catheter move unexpectedly to a deeper position within the artery, for example, when the patient exhales. If there is any suspicion of left main coronary artery obstruction (e.g., calcification, unstable angina, marked ECG changes during ischemia, or damping of systolic pressure on engagement), a cusp flush is essential before selective opacification.

After multiple injections are made with filming in different views, the left catheter is exchanged for the right coronary catheter (Fig. 13.7). This catheter is usually advanced so that its tip lies in the upper portion of the left sinus. Clockwise rotation is then used to move the tip anteriorly until it enters the right ostia. This maneuver is best done in the 20° LAO projection.

If the operator has difficulty engaging either coronary artery ostia with the preselected catheter, it is important that time not be wasted attempting to manipulate an improperly sized catheter into a coronary orifice. A test injection should be done near the coronary ostia to help assess its position and size as well as the desired catheter size and shape. The catheter should then be replaced with one of a different size or shape. Selective engagement of the coronary arteries is generally easy and can be performed rapidly (within 1 min) even by less experienced operators using the Judkins catheter.

The major advantage of the Judkins technique is its simplicity. It requires less dexterity and training than other techniques. Since the catheters have only an end hole, obstruction at the tip produces alteration of the pressure waveform. Recognition of pressure wave change may prevent the operator from injecting or embolizing a clot or damaging the intima of the coronary artery.

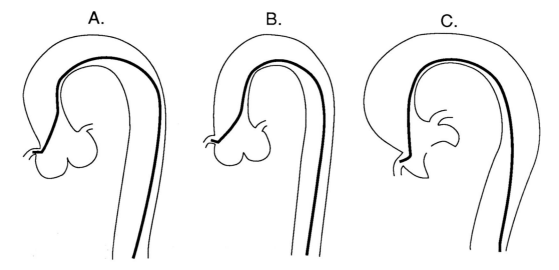

A.   **B.**   **C.**

Figure 13.7. Approach to the right coronary artery using Judkins catheters. The catheter is advanced to a point approximately 2 cm above the left coronary ostium and pointed toward the left ostium. From this position it is rotated in a clockwise fashion until it enters the right coronary orifice. The figures illustrate the importance of catheter size relative to the aortic root in the LAO projection. In the normal-sized aortic root (*A*) a medium right catheter is used; in smaller aortas a smaller catheter may be needed (*B*); and in the larger poststenotic dilated aortas (*C*), a larger or longer configuration is required.

A disadvantage is that the technique is, for practical purposes, applicable only from the femoral arteries; although on rare occasions, we have used it from the left brachial artery. Thus, obstructive disease of the descending aorta, iliac, or femoral vessels can make catheterization impossible or difficult and/or high-risk for arterial damage, thrombosis, and cholesterol (athero) embolization. Multiple catheters must be used, thus increasing the chance of arterial damage and/or embolization. If one needs to reexamine both coronary arteries, for example, after nitroglycerin and ergonovine, or during chest pain, catheters must be exchanged. This limitation is minimized in our laboratories by use of a valved sheath. In some cases when it is important to rapidly repeat either right or left coronary angiography several times during the procedure, we will use the contralateral groin to introduce the other coronary artery catheter. One catheter is then kept in the ascending aorta while the other is being used. Deliberate left ventricular catheterization, between coronary injections, to examine left ventricular end-diastolic pressure or perform a ventriculogram, cannot be done easily using the left coronary catheter. Usually a guidewire is needed. The right coronary catheter can usually be guided into the left ventricle on clockwise rotation from the left cusp, but a guidewire may also be needed on occasion. In either case the Judkins coronary catheter must then be exchanged for another catheter for ventriculography. Finally, if one suspects an aberrant coronary artery origin, either congenital or secondary to disease of the aortic root, Judkins catheters may have to be abandoned.

Amplatz Catheters and Technique

This preformed catheter series is available in four left coronary tip sizes and the right catheters in three sizes (Figs. 7.29 and 7.30). These catheters have "hook" shapes, which are very pronounced for the left coronary artery and less pronounced for the right coronary artery (5). The right coronary catheter also has an additional curve to conform to the aortic arch. Again, as with Judkins catheters, selection of proper catheter size is essential and depends upon the size and shape of the ascending aorta and aortic sinuses. Size 1 is for the smallest aortic root, 2 for normal, and 3

for large roots. Attempts at trying to forcibly engage a preformed catheter that does not conform to a particular aorta, aortic root, or aortic sinus only results in wasted time and increases risk of complication.

The left Amplatz catheter is advanced to the noncoronary cusp. The bottom of the "hook" is "braced" in this cusp in the LAO projection (Fig. 13.8*A*). The tip is rotated until it enters the left ostium and displacement is prevented by slight withdrawal of the catheter body. If the tip does not reach the ostium (i.e., lies below), the catheter size is too small and should be replaced with the next larger size. If the tip lies above the ostium, the catheter is too large. After filming the left coronary artery, the catheter is exchanged for the right coronary catheter. In the LAO projection the

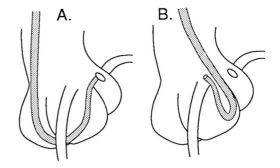

Figure 13.8. *A*, Approach to the left coronary artery using Amplatz catheters. The left coronary artery is approached by pointing the tip of the large hook-shaped left coronary catheter toward the patient's left and advancing until the catheter lies on the posterior or noncoronary cusp. From this position if the catheter is appropriately sized for the aortic root, the tip will be easily engaged in the left coronary ostium with only slight withdrawal. If the tip lies below the left coronary ostium, the catheter size is too small. If the hook cannot be opened, the catheter size is too large. *B*, A similar approach can be used for the right coronary artery if the right ostium is high, and the root is moderately large, as shown. As the left catheter is advanced to touch the noncoronary cusp the catheter is rotated until it is engaged into a high right coronary artery. For arteries that lie in the midportion of the right sinus or lower, a right coronary catheter with a much smaller hook (not shown) must be used. The tip of the small hook is pointed leftward. This catheter generally is braced against the left aortic cusp and therefore lies directly opposite to the right coronary artery orifice.

right catheter is "braced" in the left coronary cusp as it is rotated slightly to secure the tip in the right coronary ostium (Fig. 13.8*B*). When the right coronary ostium is very high, the left Amplatz catheter may be used to engage the right ostium.

Some advantages of Amplatz catheters are as follows: (*a*) The catheters can be used percutaneously from either the leg or the brachial artery. The brachial 2 and 3 catheters are variations of the left Amplatz design. (*b*) Attempts to seek a coronary ostium require less operator training and for some operators less time than with nonpreformed catheters. (*c*) They have only an end hole; thus, immediate dampening of the pressure waveform is produced when the tip is obstructed.

A disadvantage of the Amplatz technique is that multiple catheters must be used. Also, the left coronary artery may be difficult to engage with the left catheter, particularly in smaller aortic roots and patients with short left main stem or low ostium. Subselective catheterization of either the left anterior descending or left circumflex may be unavoidable in some cases. If the coronaries need reexamination after pharmacologic interventions, physiologic maneuvers, or pain, the operator may find that multiple catheter exchanges become an important inconvenience.

Multipurpose Catheter and Technique

This single catheter technique usually utilizes a 7 or 8 Fr, 100-cm polyurethane or woven Dacron catheter with stainless steel wire incorporated that (Fig. 7.31) resembles Gensini and some Sones catheters (6). The tip is a more flexible tip than that of the Gensini or even some Sones catheters. The different manufacturers have developed tips with different characteristics.

Torque control is very good, and the catheter tip usually can be manipulated into either coronary ostia or the left ventricle by maneuvers that are somewhat similar to those employed with the Sones (see below) technique (Figs. 13.9 and 13.10). Most operators advocate starting from the posterior sinus or noncoronary cusp in the 30° RAO position (Fig. 13.9*A*). The catheter is advanced with the tip pointed toward the spine. When a loop has been formed, with slight clockwise rotation the tip will "flip" to the left cusp and point toward the ostium (Fig. 13.9*B*). The tip is then maneuvered into the left ostium by slight withdrawal or advancement of the catheter. Breathing maneuvers may also be helpful. The catheter is then withdrawn slightly to secure the tip, and injections are

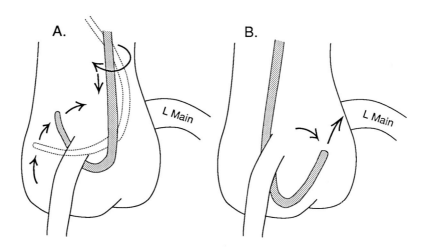

Figure 13.9. Approach to the left coronary artery using the multipurpose catheter. This is best done in the 30° *RAO* (right anterior oblique) projection with the tip pointed posteriorly. Advancement of the catheter allows a loop to be formed in the noncoronary or posterior sinus. From this position the catheter is rotated clockwise until the tip points toward the left coronary ostium. The catheter is advanced, the ostium is engaged; and then as the patient inspires, the catheter is withdrawn slightly to secure the tip in the ostium of the left coronary artery.

made. The right coronary artery is approached in the 45° LAO position. From the left cusp the catheter is rotated clockwise (Fig. 13.10). The tip is directed anterior and to the patient's right. The catheter is then slightly withdrawn to engage the right coronary ostium.

The multipurpose catheter technique requires more operator training than the other percutaneous techniques that use preformed catheters. The multipurpose catheter technique has the major advantage of using the same catheter for both right and left coronary arteries and left ventricular angiography. In routine practice, however, our experience has been that only about 80% of cases can be completed optimally with the single catheter and that ectopy during left ventriculography is common. The left coronary artery may require a preformed catheter for good selective visualization in the remainder of cases.

Brachial Approach
Sones Catheter and Technique

Through a small antecubital cutdown, the brachial artery is isolated by blunt dissection (2). The right brachial artery is preferred, but on occasion (e.g., prior scarring, brachial, or axillary-subclavian artery obstruction) the left arm can be used. One of several varieties of

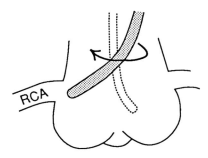

Figure 13.10. Approach to the right coronary artery using the multipurpose technique. This is best done in the LAO projection and begins, in a manner similar to the approach to left coronary artery; however, once the catheter tip points toward the left coronary artery, continued rotation in a clockwise direction is used until the tip is oriented anteriorly toward the right coronary orifice. From this position the catheter is then advanced and withdrawn until the tip is secured in the ostium.

catheters, which range in diameter from about 6 to 8 Fr and in length from 80 to 125 cm, is employed (see Fig. 7.19) (see Chapter 7 for details about the construction of these catheters). The advantage of these catheters is that their shafts are relatively rigid at body temperature. This provides excellent torque control for maneuvering the tip through the subclavian artery and maintaining tip control in the high velocity blood flow stream immediately above the aortic valve to cannulate the coronary ostia.

The tip of each Sones catheter tapers to about 5.5 Fr diameter over the distal 1 to 2 cm, depending upon the type used with type 1 longer than type 2. The two types have tapered sections of different lengths. This tapering makes the distal portion much more flexible and favors directing the catheter tip toward the coronary ostium by enabling this portion to be formed in a "J shape." Each Sones catheter has an end hole, and either two or four side holes that help stabilize the tip during injections. The tapered section of the catheter is generally maintained in an angled bend by a rigid wire before the catheter is used so that the distal section maintains an obtuse angle with the main catheter body. The tapered tip is relatively more flexible than the main body of the catheter, allowing manipulation of the catheter from the subclavian artery into the ascending aorta and formation of a loop in the left aortic sinus. It is usually helpful to flex the catheter about 3 inches from its tip several times prior to insertion to facilitate building a loop on the left cusp.

To accomplish time-efficient use of the catheter, it must be advanced to the ascending aorta without introducing major distortions in the tip or the plane of the angle that the tip makes with the body of the catheter. When difficulty is encountered at the subclavian brachiocephalic trunk, we recommend that a guidewire be used. In addition, the technique of building a loop in the left coronary cusp is important to master. This is accomplished by directing the tip of the catheter to the patient's left toward the left sinus as it enters the ascending aorta. When the tip touches the left cusp, the catheter is advanced to from a loop with its tip in the left sinus (Fig. 13.11). The catheter is advanced and withdrawn with short movements that are sometimes rapid. Advancement and counterclockwise rotation

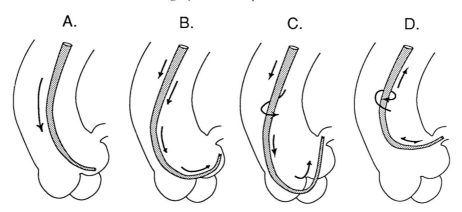

Figure 13.11. Approach to the left coronary artery using Sones technique. This is best done in the LAO projection. The key to success with this technique is to advance the Sones catheter to the ascending aorta and position the tip in the left coronary cusp without major distortions of the primary angle. (*A*) From this position gentle advancement (*B*) allows formation of a loop utilizing the floor of the left cusp. When the loop begins to climb the left sinus and point upward, gradual additional advance and withdrawal manipulation and counterclockwise torque will produce posterior movement of the tip. From this position (*C*) advance and withdrawal movement to transmit the torque will help transmit movement of the tip to the left coronary ostium. When the catheter reaches this point and further advancement simply enlarges the loop, the tip can be firmly engaged in the left ostium by withdrawing the catheter while the patient inspires, and adding clockwise torque. This secures the catheter tip in the ostium of the left coronary artery (*D*).

of the catheter will usually permit the tip to move in a superior and somewhat posterior direction to point toward and then enter the left ostium. Slight withdrawal and clockwise rotation of the catheter will usually secure the tip in the left main coronary artery. This movement of the catheter tip is often enhanced if it is done as the patient is directed to inspire deeply.

After filming the left coronary artery, the tip is withdrawn. The most reliable approach to the right coronary artery is to again build a loop in the left cusp (Fig. 13.12). While the tip is still relatively horizontal and anterior to the left ostium, the catheter is rotated clockwise. Again, using short advance-withdrawal motions to help transmit this torque to the tip, the tip will rotate anteriorly to cross the commissure between the left and right aortic cusps and enter the right ostium.

When the procedure is completed, the catheter is removed, and the arteriotomy repaired when good antegrade and retrograde backflow are observed. Usually a "purse-string" or some form of "everting mattress" suture technique is employed using vascular suture (6-0 or 7-0 Tevdeck or Proline).

Modified Brachial Technique

The brachial artery approach may be modified so that **percutaneous technique** is used with or without a sheath. We prefer a short 7 Fr valved sheath with modified catheters (7). This entry technique is particularly useful for patients with large muscular arms or previous scarring, or for outpatient procedures. The sheath is secured to the arm, and maneuvers similar to those noted above with the Sones technique are followed. However, because the percutaneous modification restricts catheter movement and the "feel" obtained with the cutdown technique, modified catheters are sometimes helpful. A brachial 2 catheter may be used for the left coronary artery.

The brachial approach with Sones-type catheters has some advantages. A single catheter can be used in most cases for catheterization of both coronary arteries, left ventriculography, and selective coronary artery bypass graft angiography. Obstructive disease of the abdominal aorta or iliofemoral arteries poses no problem. If brachial artery occlusion should occur, there is usually sufficient collateral circulation around the

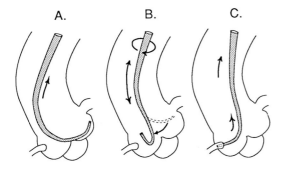

Figure 13.12. Approach to the right coronary artery using the Sones catheter. Again the right coronary artery is most readily approached from the initial configuration used for the left coronary artery (i.e., the catheter tip is positioned in the left cusp (*A*) with the patient in the LAO projection). From the left cusp a small loop is formed, and when the tip begins to climb the left sinus, but is relatively horizontal, the catheter is rotated clockwise. Slow advance and withdrawal movements will again transmit this torque to the tip and also allow the tip to traverse the commisure between the left and right aortic cusps. When this occurs, it is often necessary to provide reverse torque (counterclockwise) to check the movement of the tip (*B*). From this position slightly withdrawing the catheter usually engages the tip in the ostium of the right coronary artery (*C*). Again, inspiration is helpful to secure the tip.

elbow to prevent tissue loss. If ischemic symptoms develop, they rarely persist after a few months. If they do persist, the artery can be repaired using simple local surgical techniques often as an outpatient. If bleeding occurs, for example, after thrombolytic therapy or during anticoagulation, the arm is easier to tamponade than the groin. The latter makes the technique attractive for outpatient catheterization.

There are also disadvantages to the technique. Because of the multiple side holes, a clot can form at the tip of Sones-type catheters or in one of the side holes without producing an altered pressure waveform. With subsequent injection, the clot can dislodge and embolize. An aberrant or tortuous subclavian artery or distortion of the aortic root can make the technique difficult or impossible. But most importantly, the cutdown, arteriotomy, manipulation of a nonpreformed catheter, and subsequent arterial repair require considerable operator dexterity if the technique is to be employed in a time-efficient manner at a minimum risk to the patient.

OTHER ANGIOGRAPHIC PROCEDURES FOR THE CORONARY CIRCULATION

Saphenous Vein Bypass Graft Angiography

The increasing numbers of patients returning for evaluation following revascularization has made saphenous vein bypass graft angiography an essential procedure for the coronary angiographer. The techniques used are essentially the same as those used for selective coronary angiography, except that different catheters may be required.

Saphenous vein grafts are usually attached to the anterior portion of the aorta well above the coronary sinuses. Generally, we use the right Judkins catheter to selectively enter these grafts. If the aortic anastomosis can be localized from a radiopaque marker used at surgery or an aortic root angiogram, the catheter is positioned at this level or slightly above it. By rotating the catheter clockwise the tip can usually be engaged in the bypass orifice. The left anterior oblique view is most helpful for catheterization of these grafts. If the right Judkins is unsuccessful (usually because the graft is very high, the root is dilated, or the graft exits the aorta at a very obtuse angle), a right or left saphenous vein bypass graft catheter may be used.

If the Sones or multipurpose catheter technique is used, these grafts are usually accessible, with the same catheter used for selective coronary angiography. A larger, longer loop is formed. Again the tip is positioned at or slightly above and to the left of the aortic anastomosis. By rotating the catheter clockwise, the tip can be engaged.

Internal Mammary Artery Graft Angiography

Internal mammary artery grafts (IMA) are used with increased frequency, and this has made techniques to visualize the IMAs a necessity for coronary angiographers. In our experience, the IMA is best approached with a special preformed catheter made for this purpose. From either groin either mammary artery is approached with a guidewire advanced ahead of the catheter tip. The wire is first directed to the innominate and then to the subclavian artery. The internal mammary catheter is advanced over the wire, and when the tip reaches the subclavian artery, the wire is removed. The catheter tip then returns to its preshaped right angle configuration, and the tip is directed inferiorly as the catheter is slowly withdrawn to engage the orifice of the internal mammary artery. For test injection and selective angiography a nonionic contrast agent should be used to minimize the intense burning chest pain perceived by patients with intact chest wall branches. Nitroglycerin should also be given into this arterial graft if its full potential size is to be evaluated.

In patients with severe iliofemoral atherosclerosis and for those using the brachial artery approach alternate techniques are required. Either the right or left IMA can be rapidly canulated from their respective brachial arteries using the same preshaped IMA catheter described above for the femoral approach. The catheter is introduced, either percutaneously or via cutdown, into the respective brachial artery. If cutdown or sheath technique is used for the brachial approach, the IMA catheter must be "preloaded" with an 0.035-inch J wire to protect the brachial, axillary, and subclavian arteries because of the sharply angled tip. When the proximal subclavian is entered, the wire is removed, and the catheter is withdrawn and rotated to engage the IMA. This is a very simple and rapid procedure for the ipsilateral IMA. The contralateral IMA can be approached by reintroduction of the catheter on that side. Alternatively, techniques to maneuver a guidewire and catheter into the aortic arch and to the contralateral IMA may be used. One technique is to advance a Simmons (sidewinder) catheter to the aortic root over a preloaded guidewire (8). When the wire is removed, the catheter assumes its preformed large "hook-like" shape. Selection of the size of the Simmons catheter depends upon the size and configuration of the aortic root. Usually the medium or large size is used. The tip is rotated toward the contralateral shoulder and advanced into the subclavian artery. When it is introduced from the right brachial artery, it will now lie in the left

subclavian artery, and this position should be confirmed by a small volume contrast injection. An exchange guidewire (0.035-inch diameter, 260-cm length) is advanced through the catheter into the left subclavian artery. The Simmons catheter is then exchanged for a preshaped IMA bypass catheter. When the tip of this catheter is inserted into the contralateral subclavian artery beyond the IMA origin, the guidewire is removed. The catheter is slowly withdrawn and rotated until the IMA is engaged. After left IMA angiography the catheter is withdrawn to the ipsilateral subclavian artery, and the ipsilateral IMA (in this case right) is visualized.

Ventricular Angiography

Ventriculography (discussed in detail in Chapter 22) provides information that complements the coronary angiogram and assists in patient evaluation. Wall motion, aneurysm, septal perforation, and mitral insufficiency can be documented and quantified. Also, consider a patient in whom transient, ischemic-type, ST segment depression (spontaneously or during stress) develops in electrocardiographic leads I, AVL, and V_{5-6}. These changes may result from ischemic myocardium perfused by a diseased anterior descending, diagonal, or circumflex marginal branch of the left coronary artery branch. In many instances, an RAO ventriculogram may reveal a localized area of hypokinesis in the anterior lateral region. Thus, the relationship of the ischemia, regional wall motion abnormality, and coronary occlusive disease, viewed by coronary angiography, is helpful in deciding which coronary narrowing is responsible for production of ischemia.

Motion of hypokinetic myocardial regions can be improved by nitroglycerin (9) or during postextrasystolic beats. It is possible to detect functionally jeopardized reversible ischemic or hibernating myocardium. Many laboratories, including ours, perform ventricular angiography before and after sublingual nitroglycerin in patients with motion abnormalities. Since radiographic contrast material injected into the coronary circulation may alter left ventricular performance, many perform the left ventriculogram prior to coronary angiography. However, if one wishes to evoke areas of potential motion abnormality, induced perhaps by marginal areas of perfusion, it may be wise to consider performing coronary angiography before left ventriculography as a form of "stress." Abnormalities in wall motion that are potentially reversible can then be assessed on postextrasystolic beats or after nitroglycerin administration. Very sick patients tolerate coronary angiography much better than left ventriculography. Therefore, it is sometimes clinically useful to perform coronary angiography early in the course of the procedure, attempting to obtain maximal information before performing the higher-risk ventriculographic procedure.

GENERAL PRINCIPLES APPLICABLE TO ALL TECHNIQUES

The operator must know the radiographic anatomy of the heart and coronary circulation in order to choose the appropriate view required. In general, views should be chosen to minimize overlap of major vessels while avoiding the vertebra and lungs. Appropriate shutter/collimator position should frame the area of interest. This minimizes radiation exposure and will reduce scatter to improve the quality of the images. All filming should be done during inspiration with the diaphragm in its most inferior position. This may require a slow inspiration with initiation of injection just before maximum inspiration is reached, as some patients will perform a Valsalva maneuver when told to inspire maximally. The Valsalva maneuver defeats the purpose by causing the diaphragm to move superiorly while reducing coronary perfusion pressure. The pressure from the catheter tip must be evaluated immediately before each injection of contrast. If damping of pressure is observed, before any contrast material is injected the catheter should be withdrawn slowly until a normal pressure waveform is observed. A small volume (1 to 2 cc) test injection should be made to determine the position of the tip and the status of the coronary artery. If attenuation of the pressure waveform is due to ostial obstruction or catheter-related dissection, an injection made when pressure is damped may enlarge the tear and create an occlusive dissection. In an extremely small coronary artery in which repeated damping is observed on entry, injection of 200 μg of

nitroglycerin near the ostium often will produce sufficient dilation to permit entry without pressure damping. If damping is still observed, a different shaped catheter should be used.

Before any injections are made into the coronary arteries, the system (syringe, manifold, and catheter) must be free of air and blood. We recommend a **closed manifold system** filled with heparinized saline flush. This step helps prevent air or blood from entering the system. This setup helps provide adequate transmission of pressure to permit recognition of waveform attenuations that may arise due to catheter-tip impaction in the artery wall or obstruction of the coronary orifice. Once these steps are mastered, they require only a few seconds and will help avoid serious morbidity.

After the above measures are completed, contrast injection is made of sufficient volume and flow rate to opacify the artery under study. Inadequately opacified vessels generally result in overestimation of stenosis severity due to contrast "streaming" as it forms a layer with unopacified blood. When the heart rate is high and the coronary arteries are large, a higher contrast flow rate is needed, as compared with that required for slow heart rate and small coronary arteries. Generally, we use 3 to 4 cc injected over approximately 2 cardiac cycles for the right coronary artery and 4 to 6 cc for the left. Occasionally, larger volumes may be needed. Cinefilming should be started before contrast leaves the catheter tip and continued until most of the arterial phase of opacification is completed. In patients with obstruction at least one filming run for each artery should be continued well after the arterial phase to look for collateral filling. Repeat filming after intracoronary nitroglycerin is always helpful in the evaluation of stenosis, coronary spasm, and collaterals (10).

With the use of an image intensifier field of 4.5 to 6 inches to provide optimal magnification of the coronary arteries and a collimator to minimize spine, lung, and diaphragm, the "field of view" will be considerably smaller than the myocardial distribution covered by the branches of either coronary artery. Accordingly, the tabletop or image intensifier tube must be moved to follow the distribution of a coronary artery and its branches filled with contrast media. This movement, called

"panning," is a learned procedure that follows a specific pattern for each coronary artery in each projection. The initial field of view should permit optimal visualization of the ostium and proximal part of the coronary artery understudy. From this position the field should follow the distribution of the artery and its major branches. Since most of the coronary artery obstructions of interest (e.g., for revascularization) will be located in the proximal and midportions of the artery understudy, the time spent with these proximal portions in the field of view should occupy most of the duration of a cinefilm run. The remaining portion of the film run should be reserved to include the distal segments of the artery and possible collateral channels which might fill to supply segments of other arteries or branches. But the field of view should return to include the catheter tip at the end of each filming run. This permits identification of "contrast staining" at sites of intimal flaps, thrombus, or even catheter-related dissection.

PERSONNEL

Coronary angiography must be performed by experienced, skilled operators in order to minimize possible major complications and ensure adequate study of the coronary arteries and deal with the relatively infrequent complications when they do occur. This includes physicians who are highly trained and experienced in all aspects of cardiac anatomy, physiology, radiography, and resuscitation techniques. We strongly support the training guidelines outlined in the Bethesda Conference on Cardiovascular training (11, 12). Well-trained nurses, technicians, and other paramedical aides are an essential part of the catheterization team. The ability to work together and in harmony is a necessary requirement to perform this highly complex procedure efficiently.

EQUIPMENT

Radiographic technique and equipment are addressed in detail in Chapter 8, and only some important points will be reviewed here. In order to obtain adequate visualization of the coronary arteries in a safe manner, several important technical factors must be considered. A high-resolution image intensifier system with magnification (5- or 6-inch) and a high-quality television viewing system are absolutely mandatory. This fluoroscopic system forms the mainstay of a catheterization laboratory planning to perform coronary angiography. When equipment is not operating properly, scheduled procedures should not be performed until maintenance has been completed. **Suboptical diagnostic studies blamed on equipment inadequacies can not be justified.** Regardless of the technique employed for opacifying the coronary arteries and recording the angiograms for future viewing, the image intensifier x-ray system must be of high resolution (≥ 2.8 line pairs/mm) for proper catheter guidance and positioning within a reasonable period of time. Operators using old, poorly maintained equipment or equipment with low-quality films must resort to making many more selective injections and to taking many more cinefilms to be certain that they have not missed something. This practice contributes to increasing the risk of the procedure.

Image intensifiers of different sizes are particularly useful for various types of patients and heart sizes. Some image fields are dual; some are triple. The smaller image field systems (4.5- to 6-inch) provide optimal magnification and detail for coronary angiography. Automatic kV and mA control systems provide optimal brightness over a wide range of patient and exposure fields. Because multiple projections in several planes must be used, either the x-ray tube-image tube or the table must facilitate these views. Multiple-plane angulation systems are essential. The radiographic view must be changed quickly, so that the various degrees of obliquity desired can be obtained and maintained in either the frontal or sagittal planes. A 35-mm cinecamera, capable of at least 60 frames/sec filming, usually with an optimal overframing lens, is considered by the authors to be the minimum necessary for adequate recording of the fluoroscopic image of the coronary arteries. "Zoom lenses" are also becoming popular to improve image magnification and reduce radiation exposure for coronary angiography. The cameras use large-capacity film magazines (200 to 400 ft) that can be preloaded. To minimize delays while catheters are in place additional preloaded magazines must always be at hand for quick changing. If larger-format serial radiographic filming techniques are used, they should complement cineangiography and not be used instead of cinetechnique.

Choice of film type depends upon the individual characteristics of the system and operator preference. This area is reviewed in detail in Chapter 11 of this text. Briefly, optimal speed, contrast, and detail are important prerequisites and are much more important for high-quality coronary angiography than any other radiographic procedure due to cardiac motion and the small size of the coronary artery. A highly efficient, cinefilm processor is also required to optimally process large quantities of film rapidly. Fresh film, optimally processed and viewed, and routine dosimetry and sensitometry studies provide for the best quality control.

A high-quality videotape recorder is an important aid during coronary angiography, providing the operator with an immediate review of selected injections in slow motion. Videodisk recorders also provide excellent quality images with single-frame "instant replay" capabilities. These playback units help the operator to limit the number of coronary injections in a given patient. Study of these tape- or disk-recorded images also helps to optimize patient positioning and other technical aspects during the procedure so that appropriate corrections or repeat injections can be made to clarify the findings. These recordings provide backup in the event of cinefilm "loss." Some laboratories have recently employed an "all-digital" image storage mode. While this is, no doubt, the future of all angiographic laboratories, limitations in data storage, resolution, and signal-to-noise ratios of digital systems currently prevent such systems from displacing film-based cineangiography as the standard for coronary angiography.

Although most coronary injections are done with a hand-controlled syringe, a pressure injection syringe or a "gun-controlled" syringe may be useful in special situations (e.g., aortic stenosis, aortic insufficiency, or hyperkinetic circulatory states (tachycardia, etc.)) in which the blood flow rate in the coronary arteries is extremely high. Angioplasty guide catheters that have a larger lumen may also be helpful in such circumstances.

Additional equipment (e.g., surgical instruments, drapes, syringes) must be on hand and already prepared for use. The laboratory must be equipped with appropriate safety devices that include a defibrillator charged and ready for use. The defibrillator must be tested daily, prior to entrance of patients into the catheterization laboratory, and must be kept in close range for prompt use. Appropriate electrocardiographic and pressure-monitoring systems are essential. The monitor screen must be in clear view of the operator at all times. Well-positioned electrocardiographic leads on skin areas that have been appropriately prepared are required for an artifact-free signal. This is essential to assess possible ST segment shifts that may occur during the procedure and to evaluate arrhythmias. At least three electrocardiographic leads should be monitored continuously during coronary angiography, and other leads must be available for use when needed to help document the presence of transient myocardial ischemia. Radiolucent electrode systems should be used for the precordial leads, and the modified limb leads must be positioned out of the fluoroscopic field of the heart. Nothing is more annoying than to have an important area of a coronary artery obscured by an ECG lead or electrode. We prefer to monitor standard leads I, II, and V_5 or V_2. These ECG signals must be calibrated and free of distortion introduced by inappropriate filtering or improperly applied leads. Additionally, appropriate drugs to control possible ischemia (intravenous and sublingual nitroglycerin, intravenous verapamil), hypertension (nitroprusside nifedipine, phentolamine), hypotension (dopamine, phenylephrine), pain (morphine), tachyarrhythmias (lidocaine, procainamide, propranolol, bretylium), and bradyarrhythmias (atropine, isoproterenol); oxygen, airway, and suction apparatus; and other emergency items must be kept immediately available and in good working order. Other medications (e.g., antihistamines and aspirin) are essential.

SPECIAL TESTS DURING CORONARY ANGIOGRAPHY

Coronary Artery Spasm

Although noninvasive tests are used to document transient myocardial ischemia and to formulate a working diagnosis, visualization of coronary spasm during **coronary angiography is the reference standard** for this diagnosis. Angiographic evidence for coronary spasm must be associated with objective evidence for myocardial ischemia in order to be separated from catheter-related spasm. Catheter-related spasm occurs at or within 1 centimeter of the catheter tip and does not cause transient ischemia. If one believes that catheter-related spasm is causing ischemia, the most likely situation is that coronary artery dissection has been overlooked. In the ideal situation, when spontaneous ischemia (i.e., pain, ST segment changes) occurs in the catheterization laboratory, the angiographer should attempt to visualize each coronary artery. If he documents coronary obstruction and its resolution with intracoronary nitroglycerin, the diagnosis of spasm as the basis for ischemia is established (10). In other cases, without a spontaneous ischemic episode in the laboratory provocative testing may be required. A number of provocative tests have been used, but only **ergonovine** is now in widespread use (13). Ergonovine is a nonspecific vasoconstrictor with structural similarities to several neurotransmitters.

Intravenous Ergonovine

The response to intravenous ergonovine in patients without coronary spasm is minimal generalized vasoconstriction. This is manifest by coronary diameter reduction (approximately 15%), associated with a small increase in both systemic and left ventricular end-diastolic pressures. Coronary diameter reduction after a low dose of ergonovine (≤0.2 mg), accompanied by objective evidence for ischemia with or without chest pain, but without important increases in heart rate or blood pressure that can be reversed by intracoronary nitroglycerin, fulfills criteria for coronary spasm.

We use a low total cumulative dose protocol. Calcium antagonists and long-acting nitrates are withheld for 48 hours before angiography. **No premedications, atropine, or nitrates are given.** Nitroglycerin is on hand for parenteral use. A nonionic angiographic contrast agent is used to minimize effects on coronary size, ECG, and ventricular pressure. Baseline coronary angiographic, hemodynamic, and multiple-lead ECG recordings are

obtained in a pain-free period. If preformed catheters are used, the catheter for the coronary artery most likely to be involved in spasm (based on location of previous ECG changes or the baseline angiogram) is advanced to the left ventricle to monitor pressure. If the patient does not have a spontaneous ischemic episode (i.e., ST shifts and/or angina) and the operator has a strong index of suspicion that spasm may contribute to the clinical findings, ergonovine 0.025 or 0.05 mg is injected intravenously as a bolus. Initial dose size is based on clinical findings and presence of severe CAD (e.g., 0.025 mg in unstable patients). Heart rate, blood pressure, ECG, and possible onset of symptoms are observed for approximately 2 min. This waiting period is important because there is often a delay after the injection before spasm occurs in patients who have positive responses. If no changes occur, an additional 0.05 mg of ergonovine is administered. This procedure is repeated until a total dose of 0.2 mg is reached. Should symptoms occur or hemodynamic or ischemic ECG changes result, recordings are repeated, and both left and right coronary angiograms are performed. Intracoronary nitroglycerin (100 μg) is given promptly, and angiography is repeated. Intracoronary nitroglycerin is very specific for coronary artery spasm at these low doses and will have little influence on esophageal spasm. If hypotension occurs or spasm does not reverse promptly, nitroglycerin is given in larger doses (200 to 300 μg) into the artery(s) involved. This immediately reverses the ischemia-related findings without producing further hypotension (10). When a very proximal newly observed stenosis does not respond to intracoronary nitroglycerin, coronary dissection should be suspected. An example of coronary spasm provoked in a patient with rest angina appears in Figure 13.13.

Others employ larger doses, but the majority of patients with coronary spasm who respond to ergonovine do so at a dose ≤0.2 mg. We limit the total dose because of concern for safety and to avoid possible provocation of an angiographic response not due to spasm (i.e., "false-positive" response) in patients with severe coronary stenosis. In a patient with subtotal obstructive coronary atherosclerosis, larger doses of a

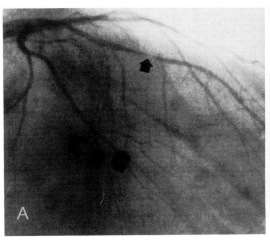 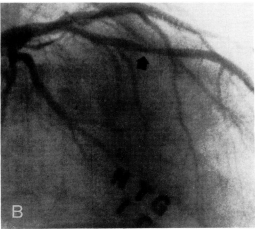

Figure 13.13. An example of ergonovine-provoked spasm of the left anterior descending coronary artery (A) promptly relieved by intracoronary nitroglycerin (B).

vasoconstrictor, like ergonovine, could produce total occlusion.

Major risks of provocative testing include the usual complications of myocardial ischemia, such as ventricular arrhythmias, heart block, myocardial infarction, and death. Patients who develop a positive response are those at risk for complications, but the incidence of either death or myocardial infarction is very, very low. Ventricular arrhythmias are not uncommon.

Ergonovine produces chest pain with ST segment elevation in the vast majority of variant angina patients who are in an active phase of their disease and in 2 to 5% of patients with more classical effort angina syndromes (13). In these cases localized reversible severe coronary narrowing occurs usually at doses between 0.05 and 0.20 mg. In our experience with this test over 12 years in a large number of patients, we know of no patient who failed to respond to a total cumulative dose of 0.2 mg of ergonovine (provided there were no confounding medications) and was found to have coronary spasm at a later date.

Intracoronary Ergonovine

Recently, ergonovine has been given directly into each coronary artery (5 to 10 μg, total cumulative dose of 50 μg) as a test for spasm (14). This has the advantage of eliminating systemic vasoconstriction and esophageal smooth muscle stimulation, while allowing specific separation of the right and left coronary responses. We use 25 μg doses repeated over 2 to 3 min when we use intracoronary administration.

Other Tests

More recently, low doses (10 to 100 μg) of **acetylcholine,** have been given directly into each coronary artery as a test for spasm (15). This causes coronary constriction at sites of endothelial disruption where endothelium-dependent relaxant factor production may be deficient. The response seen with this agent is very transient and reverses spontaneously within 20 to 30 sec. **Methacholine,** another cholinergic agonist, has also been used as a test for coronary spasm. The **cold pressor test** (i.e., hand immersion in ice water), **hyperventilation, histamine**, and **exercise** may be useful in selected cases to provoke coronary spasm. Experience with these tests is limited, and we believe that they should be used only when a patient's history suggests that these conditions are likely to evoke signs and/or symptoms of ischemia.

ASSESSING THE PRESENCE OR ABSENCE OF CORONARY OCCLUSIVE DISEASE AND ITS SEVERITY

The authors cannot adequately emphasize the importance of high-quality films to reduce the possibility of misleading or hazardous errors in interpretation. It is not the purpose of this chapter to describe, in detail, the radiographic anatomy and pathology of the coronary tree. (The reader is referred to texts by Gensini, Soto, etc.)

This description is what a coronary angiographer looks for during an appropriate angiographic study. The angiographer must systematically evaluate each individual major coronary artery. First, the anatomic position, size, and course of each of the coronary vessels and their major branches are examined beginning at the ostium. Next, the degree of any observed coronary lumen diameter reduction is assessed. The extent of any CAD (i.e., single, double, triple, or number of segments involved) is noted. The exact diameter narrowing used to define a hemodynamically significant coronary narrowing varies from 50 to 70%, depending on the operator, but these data must be quantified. The subject of quantification of CAD continues to undergo study and controversy and is discussed in Chapter 23. More accurate characterization of each coronary artery obstruction is desirable to help minimize observations and to evaluate possible interventions and/or the course of the disease process.

The **location** of the coronary artery narrowings are noted, i.e., proximal, mid, or distal. Narrowings are considered proximal if they are located in the right coronary artery before the acute marginal branch, the left main coronary, the anterior descending branch before the first septal perforator, or the circumflex branch before the obtuse marginal branch. In addition to estimating the location and magnitude of any coronary narrowing, it is important to indicate its length. Other findings (e.g., areas of spasm, major diameter changes reversed by nitroglycerin, myocardial bands or bridges, anomalous coronary origins) must be noted and distinguished from atherosclerotic or other types (emboli, thrombosis, etc.) of organic obstructions.

The angiographic anatomy of **coronary spasm** is characterized by dynamic lumen obstruction that often changes from minute to minute. The process is almost always localized to the larger artery segments, and the right coronary artery is most frequently involved. The left anterior descending is next most frequently involved. Rarely, saphenous vein and internal mammary bypass grafts may be involved. In some cases spasm appears focal or localized to only a small segment of one artery. In others spasm appears multifocal with several localized sites in either the same or different arteries. In still others a much more diffuse process occurs, manifested by generalized narrowing of one or multiple coronary arteries. A few patients may have focal or multifocal spasm in one artery branch with diffuse spasm in another branch. Finally, some show a migratory process when repeated angiograms are done. Determinants of this variable anatomic pattern are unknown. As a general rule, however, spasm involves segments with lumen irregularities, rather than the very smooth segments, supporting the post-mortem descriptions of atherosclerosis. However, spasm does not necessarily localize at sites of most severe atherosclerotic obstruction. When spasm is relieved, either spontaneously or by nitroglycerin, the lumen-endothelial border often appears hazy, suggesting that this layer of the vessel wall may be thickened, edematous, or contain mural thrombus. Occasionally, nonocclusive intraluminal thrombus is present at or just distal to a site of coronary spasm. Collaterals may appear during spasm and disappear when spasm is relieved.

It is also helpful for the coronary angiogram reader to illustrate and report the location and extent of individual coronary narrowings in diagrammatic fashion. Diagrams that we have found to be useful are pictured in Figure 13.14. Here the diagram of the coronary arterial tree can be used to indicate the location of various coronary narrowings. The degree of narrowing can be recorded, and vessel diameter at the narrowing and the length of narrowing can be noted. While determining the exact location, degree, and length of narrowing is important, it is only part of the evaluation of the coronary circulation. Distal vessel anatomy must be considered in addition to the condition of the ventricle perfused by that vessel. The latter is assessed by the left ventricular angiogram, an integral part of every evaluation for suspected CAD (see Chapter 22).

PHYSIOLOGIC MEASUREMENTS

Physiologic measurements are discussed in detail in Chapter 18. Essential elements of the

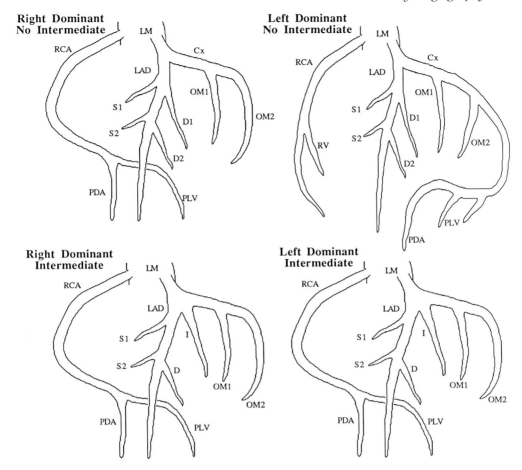

Figure 13.14. Coronary arterial diagrams useful for preliminary reporting of angiographic results.

coronary angiography procedure include measurements of pressure before coronary angiographic study. These data complement the anatomic information obtained from the angiographic procedures. Left ventricular and aortic pressures should be measured to determine the presence or absence of valvular or subvalvular pressure gradients. Left ventricular end-diastolic pressure at rest should always be measured. Right heart catheterization is also useful in selected patients to evaluate the presence of coexisting cardiac abnormalities. Combined with measurements of cardiac output, oximetry, and other measurements (i.e., pulmonary artery pressure), right-sided catheterization studies provide a useful complement to the total patient evaluation, when other cardiac problems are suspected. In addition, right heart catheterization provides an easy method of stressing the heart during the

catheterization procedure in the form of an atrial pacing stress test. The electrocardiogram recorded during and immediately after pacing-induced tachycardia can provide additional quantitative data (heart rate, ST segment depression, angina) relative to the functional significance of any coronary artery narrowings. The authors find this test useful for patients who perform inadequately on the treadmill, or who are limited in achieving maximum heart rates (i.e., physical handicaps or deconditioning).

COMPLICATIONS OF CORONARY ANGIOGRAPHY

Risks of coronary angiography are discussed in detail elsewhere (Chapter 3). Briefly, major complications of coronary angiography include death, myocardial infarction, stroke, and peripheral vascular problems. In general, the incidence of these complications is related to the operator's experience, number of studies done by a laboratory, and severity of the disease process. Physicians referring patients for cardiac catheterization must be aware of a particular laboratory's complication rate. Published figures suggest that reputable laboratories can achieve a death rate of 0.1% or less and a myocardial infarction rate of approximately the same order. Peripheral arterial problems occur at a higher frequency (approximately 0.1 to 1%). It is important also to consider incomplete studies as a complication.

MANAGEMENT OF COMPLICATIONS OF CORONARY ANGIOGRAPHY

Some complications occurring in the catheterization laboratory produce permanent damage to an organ system and thus, only supportive measures can be used. In the central nervous system, complications such as stroke due to thromboembolism may result in dense functional loss. Occasionally, occipital blindness, which is probably due to hyperosmolarity of contrast material, occurs but is usually transient. This problem disappears within a few hours after appropriate hydration and maintenance of blood pressure. Air emboli into the central nervous system can also produce an agitated, confused, or comatose state, but in general, it does not result in permanent damage. Hyperbaric oxygen chambers may be used to treat air embolism patients.

Myocardial infarction occurring during coronary angiography may be the result of embolism (e.g., air, thrombus) or arterial damage by the catheter (e.g., dissection), in addition to possible toxic effects of the contrast material. In any patient developing signs and symptoms of severe ischemic injury during a coronary angiographic procedure, both coronary arteries should be rapidly visualized to identify the location and severity of the obstruction. In most instances, the ischemic injury is treatable. When possible, reperfusion should be attempted if new complete obstruction is identified. First, **intracoronary nitroglycerin** should be given to determine if

spasm is present. **Thrombolytic agents** may be given into the artery involved. In cases associated with extensive occlusive dissection of an artery supplying a large amount of functional myocardium, prompt revascularization (PTCA or CABG) should be attempted. Support with the intraaortic balloon pump or autoperfusion or "bailout catheter" may be advisable in some cases.

Ventricular fibrillation must be treated immediately by electrical defibrillation. Heart block or asystole occurring without myocardial infarction is relatively infrequent. If it occurs, a temporary pacing wire can be inserted, and pacing can be commenced from either a right or left ventricular site if a vein is not handy. External cardiac pacing can also be used. If asystole is persistent, intravenous epinephrine might be helpful. In all of these situations cardiopulmonary resuscitation must be carried out until a stable rhythm and circulation are established.

Vasovagal attacks can produce bradycardia as slow as 20 beats/min and profound hypotension. Heart rate and blood pressure can be restored by rapid administration of a bolus of atropine. Pyrogen reactions (e.g., shaking chills followed by hyperpyrexia) can result from injection of foreign particles into the circulation. Prompt use of antihistamines and antipyretics will help modify this uncomfortable but usually benign complication. Hypotension secondary to nitroglycerin administration or contrast-induced vasodilation usually responds to elevation of the legs. Prolonged hypotension may require administration of fluid and/or a vasoconstrictor (e.g., phenylephrine, dopamine). Allergic reactions to contrast material are discussed in Chapter 10.

Arterial complications must be treated promptly. Loss of a distal pulse due to thrombosis, arterial damage, or hematoma usually can be restored by appropriate surgical procedures. In all patients in whom limb symptoms (i.e., pain, anesthesia, weakness) are present, surgical repair should be attempted.

In established, well-functioning busy laboratories, the incidence of these complications is usually exceedingly low. However, it cannot be overemphasized that the operator must pay meticulous attention to all aspects of the procedure, as well as to patient needs, in order to perform coronary angiography successfully.

FUTURE DIRECTIONS

Although the basic practice of coronary angiography is most likely to continue to be founded upon the methodologies outlined previously in this chapter, new technology will no doubt change certain aspects of the procedure in coming years. As noted elsewhere in this volume, new catheter design and construction are allowing use of smaller and smaller systems for both the femoral and brachial approaches. The use of smaller catheter systems and less toxic contrast media will facilitate outpatient studies and make studies in more critically ill patients safer. In the next 5 to 10 years, advances in both analog and digital components of imaging chains will enable the filmless cardiac catheterization laboratory to become reality. Indeed, the entirety of data processing in the catheterization laboratory from the technician's flow sheet to image acquisition and report generation will probably become computer based. These innovations will obviate the need for many ancillary paper-based procedures and support personnel currently used in day-to-day operations. Coronary angiography will continue to be closely allied with therapeutic catheter techniques, as outlined elsewhere in this volume. These will include coronary angioplasty, catheter-based atherectomy devices, and laser angioplasty. Mastery of the basic principles of coronary angiography will continue to be a must for operators involved in any aspect of interventional work and especially these newer methodologies. In this regard, more rigorous credentialing will be required to maintain an acceptable standard of care in diagnostic and interventional practice as this field continues to rapidly evolve.

References

1. Gensini GG. Coronary Arteriography. Mount Kisco, NY, Futura, 1975.
2. Sones FM, Shirey FK. Cine coronary arteriography. Mod Concepts Cardiovasc Dis 1962;31:735–738.
3. Seldinger ST. Catheter replacement of the needle in percutaneous arteriography: a new technique. Acta Radiol 1953;39:368–376.
4. Judkins MP. Selective coronary arteriography. 1. A percutaneous transfemoral technique. Radiology 1967;89:815–824.
5. Amplatz K, Formanek G, Stanger P, Wilson W. Mechanics of selective coronary artery catheterization via femoral approach. Radiology 1967;89:1040–1047.
6. Schoonmaker FW, King SB. Coronary arteriography by the single catheter percutaneous femoral technique. Experience in 6800 cases. Circulation 1974;50:735–740.
7. Pepine CJ, von Gunten C, Hill JA, et al. Percutaneous brachial catheterization using a modified sheath and new catheter system. Cathet Cardiovasc Diagn 1984;10:637–642.
8. Dorros G, Lewin R. Angiography of the internal mammary artery via the contralateral brachial artery. Cathet Cardiovasc Diagn 1987;13:138–140.
9. Pepine CJ, Feldman RL, Ludbrook P, et al. Left ventricular dysdinesia reversed by intravenous nitroglycerin: a manifestation of silent myocardial ischemia. Am J Cardiol 1986;58:38B–42B.
10. Pepine CJ, Feldman RL, Conti CR. Action of intracoronary nitroglycerin in refractory coronary artery spasm. Circulation 1982;65:411–414.
11. Schlant R. 17th Bethesda Conference: adult cardiology training. Introduction. J Am Coll Cardiol 1986;7:1195.
12. Conti CR, Faxon D, Gruentzig A, et al. Task Force III: training in cardiac catheterization. J Am Coll Cardiol 1986;7:1205–1206.
13. Pepine CJ, Feldman RL, Conti CR. Recommendations for use of ergonovine to provoke coronary artery spasm (letter). Cathet Cardiovasc Diagn 1980;6:423–426.
14. Hackett D, Larkin S, Chierchia S, et al. Induction of coronary artery spasm by a direct local action of ergonovine. Circulation 1987;75:577–582.
15. Yasue H, Horio Y, Nakamura N, et al. Induction of coronary artery spasm by acetylcholine in patients with variant angina: possible role of the parasympathetic nervous system in the pathogenesis of coronary artery spasm. Circulation 1987;74:955–963.

14

Noncardiac Angiography

Jeffrey Brinker, M.D.
Stephen Kaufman, M.D.

INTRODUCTION

While the cardiologist is most concerned with imaging the heart and coronary arteries, he frequently has the need to visualize other vascular structures. Whether the result of necessity or opportunity, traditional procedural boundaries that have existed between cardiologist and vascular radiologist have become less distinct. A growing number of the former are becoming angiographic-interventional specialists whose full-time activities revolve around a sophisticated angiographic suite with the physical capabilities of performing many types of radiographic studies. Rather than attempting to review every aspect of vascular radiology, this chapter will be primarily concerned with those situations most commonly encountered in the practice of adult invasive cardiology. It may be worth emphasizing that no text is an adequate substitute for experience. If need arises for extension of a procedure to an area not within the angiographer's expertise, appropriate radiologic consultation must be obtained. This is especially true when combined procedures (e.g., coronary angiography and digital carotid angiography) are considered. While one may be sympathetic with attempts to avoid a second procedure for the patient, a poorly performed study may be worse than no study at all. Furthermore, interpretation of the angiograms is often more demanding than its performance, and it is unjustifiable for this to rest with a physician who is unable to name the vessels he has opacified.

Extracardiac structures most often requiring angiographic definition by the cardiologist are the pulmonary vessels and the aorta. There are a number of clinical scenarios in which the need for contrast injection at these sites may arise:

1. Evaluation of cardiac disease: ascending aortography or pulmonary angiography may be necessary or desirable for visualization of the heart itself. Pulmonary arterial injection, for example, may be used to provide a levophase study of the left atrium or ventricle while aortography allows for evaluation of the stenotic aortic valve and, in the presence of aortic regurgitation, the left ventricle and mitral valve.
2. Evaluation of noncardiac pathology in a patient presenting with cardiac symptoms: Extension of the catheterization procedure may be necessary to document unsuspected disease such as aortic dissection in a patient with chest pain.
3. Evaluation because of difficulty or anomaly encountered during an otherwise routine cardiac investigation: Peripheral angiography is often helpful when there is trouble negotiating tortuous and stenotic vessels. Aortography may also be indicated for evaluation of the distal aorta, iliac, and femoral arteries prior to a contemplated procedure, such as intraaortic balloon placement or passing a balloon catheter for aortic valvuloplasty.
4. Anatomic assessment of a possible complication encountered on this or a previous catheterization: Peripheral arterial injection may reveal a dissection, pseudoaneurysm, or A-V fistula.

5. Screening of noncardiac anatomy: During intravascular catheterization, a central injection of contrast may be used to obtain a relatively low risk study, such as digital carotid angiography in a patient with a neck bruit.
6. Combining procedures to avoid an additional angiographic study: Descending aortography to evaluate an abdominal aneurysm may be added to a cardiac study, obviating the need for a second invasive procedure.
7. Evaluation of postoperative anatomy: One may need to visualize the site of previous vascular surgery as an addendum to a cardiac procedure, such as the aortography to view a coarctation repair in a patient now presenting with aortic stenosis.
8. Angiography primarily directed at noncardiac disease: Cardiologists may have or share responsibility for angiographic evaluation of pulmonary embolic disease or dissecting aneurysm.

GENERAL GUIDELINES

Since no angiographic procedure is entirely without risk, careful consideration must be given to each. No matter how routine the study appears, each patient presents with unique circumstances that may require a specialized procedure. It may be helpful to adopt a systematic approach similar to that outlined in Table 14.1 for every study. While the best views, injection rates, and imaging modalities vary with each area of interest and, indeed, with each case, there are some common principles applicable to most angiographic procedures (Table 14.2).

PULMONARY ANGIOGRAPHY

Contrast material injection in the pulmonary artery provides important information concerning the pulmonary arterial and venous system. It may also allow for visualization of the left atrium, left ventricle, and ascending aorta when more direct injection is difficult or risky. Pulmonary angiography is indicated in the evaluation of a variety of congenital and acquired diseases, including pulmonary arterial branch stenosis, pulmonary arteriovenous malformations, anomalous pulmonary venous connections, and obstructive venous disease. It is, however, most frequently performed in the setting of suspected pulmonary embolic disease. The general approach to this procedure will be discussed within the con-

TABLE 14.1.
General Guidelines for Preparation for Angiographic Study

1. What is (are) the problem(s)?
2. What is (are) the angiographic goal(s)?
3. Is there need for hemodynamic evaluation?
4. Is the study necessary?
   a. Will treatment strategy be made or changed based on its results?
   b. Are there other diagnostic procedures that can supply the needed information at lower risk?
   c. Are there special risks (allergy, renal disease, peripheral vascular disease) that must be considered?
5. What is the optimal radiographic procedure (cine, serial cut film, 105-spot film, digital, biplane)?
6. What vascular access is necessary or available?
7. What is the specific sequence of contrast injections (sites, projections, filming modalities)?
8. Do I need help in performance or interpretation?

text of embolic disease, although it is also applicable to the other disorders.

Pulmonary Angiography for Suspected Embolic Disease

Physiologic Monitoring

Performance of pulmonary angiography requires a catheter to be manipulated through the chambers of the right heart and positioned in the pulmonary artery. Adherence to proper cardiac catheterization technique, including attention to hemodynamic data, is essential. Determination of the overall hemodynamic profile of the patient may add information important to his care (1, 2), including the suggestion of alternative diagnoses, such as left ventricular failure, pulmonary venous disease, and pericardial disease. In those without preexistent cardiopulmonary disease the mean pulmonary artery pressure correlates well with the degree of embolic obstruction (3,4), and the presence of right ventricular failure (especially if the end-diastolic pressure is above 20 mm Hg) indicates a poor prognosis (5). The risk of pulmonary angiography is increased in patients with

TABLE 14.2.
Suggestions for Performance of Angiographic Procedures

1. The most important information should, in most cases, be obtained first.
2. Record hemodynamics prior to, as well as after, contrast material administration, when possible.
3. Test inject under fluoroscopy with low pressure prior to power injection.
4. Ensure that all areas of interest are within the radiographic field.
5. Optimal opacification is achieved by injection upstream as close to the area of interest as possible.
6. When using serial cut film, check technique with scout films.
7. Limit contrast material and radiation exposure to that level compatible with a diagnostic study.
8. Coordinate injection rate and filming technique so that optimal opacification is achieved.
   a. High flow through a vascular bed requires injection of larger volumes of contrast material over shorter intervals and rapid filming.
   b. Delayed imaging may be necessary for collateral or venous phase visualization.
9. Contrast material injection may produce motion artifact if painful or cough provoking. Consider low-osmolar agents, anesthesia, or the addition of lidocaine.
10. Catheters should be frequently flushed especially when nonionic contrast is utilized, or if systemic anticoagulation is omitted.
11. Catheters selected must be adequate for desired injection rate.
12. Anticipate effects of catheter recoil.
13. Position catheter to limit potential for migration into a smaller branch.

pulmonary hypertension, especially if the right heart is failing (6). These findings will alert the physician to take special precautions (reduced amounts of contrast material, low osmolar contrast material, subselective injections) when angiography is necessary.

Pressure monitoring is helpful to verify the location of the catheter during manipulation. Fluoroscopy in the anterior-posterior view is not always adequate to define catheter position; for example, the coronary sinus, which is not uncommonly entered when the brachial or subclavian technique is utilized, may be indistinguishable from the right ventricular outflow tract. Recognition of a right atrial pressure waveform from a catheter so placed will make this differentiation. Observation of the pressure tracing provides a measure of safety as one advances the catheter through the heart. This is most pertinent when using stiff catheters that are capable of perforating the heart. Loss of pressure should caution the operator against advancing the catheter, especially when resistance is felt or the catheter appears to be "hung up." Continuous ECG monitoring is essential and should start as soon as the patient arrives in the laboratory. Sinus bradycardia or heart block may occur as a vagal response while gaining vascular access. Supraventricular as well as ventricular arrhythmias may be provoked during the procedure, either of which may be poorly tolerated. Attention to the rhythm during catheter manipulation may allow for the early detection of irritability and prevent production of sustained tachycardias.

Vascular Access

In many institutions the percutaneous femoral venous approach to pulmonary angiography has supplanted the antecubital technique. In addition to speed and simplicity, another advantage of this approach is the relative ease with which one may enter pulmonary artery branches, since selective or subselective injections are often preferred for evaluation of pulmonary emboli. Entry into the left pulmonary artery is difficult when approached from the arm, and catheter placement in specific segments may be impossible. The right femoral vein offers a more direct path to the heart and is preferred over the left, which may enter the inferior vena cava at an abrupt angle.

The principal drawback of femoral venous catheterization for performance of pulmonary angiography is the potential for dislodging thrombi from the iliac veins or the vena cava (7). This is more a theoretic than a real disadvantage (8), and we have yet to encounter a clinically evident complication of this type. However, when performing pulmonary angiography for suspected embolic disease, we routinely hand inject 10 cc of contrast material into the femoral vein and follow it fluoroscopically through the iliac vein and into the vena cava. If there is a suggestion of abnormality, an inferior vena cavogram, using a mechanical injector and serial cut films, is performed. If no thrombi are seen within the iliac vein or vena cava, the guidewire and catheter are advanced through the system and into the right atrium.

There are a number of catheter types available for pulmonary angiography. The Grollman pulmonary artery seeking catheter (Cook Inc., Bloomington, IN) is used in most of our cases (Fig. 14.1) (9). This polyethylene pig-tailed catheter has a gentle reverse secondary curve proximal to the distal 3 cm that is angled 90° from the shaft. Its configuration facilitates passage through the heart and limits the likelihood of the tip becoming caught in the trabeculated right ventricle. The characteristics of this soft material, combined with the catheter's other attributes, essentially eliminate the possibility of cardiac perforation.

The catheter may be introduced percutaneously over a guidewire. The ability to accept a guidewire also facilitates the catheter's manipulation into essentially any pulmonary arterial segment. The catheter is stable and does not recoil during injection of contrast material. The standard catheter is available in 6.7 and 8.3 Fr diameters. The former is used most frequently and allows for a high enough flow rate (20 ml/sec) for selective angiography. While injection in the main pulmonary artery is rarely performed for assessment of embolic disease, if required for other studies, the larger catheter having a higher flow rate (up to 45 ml/sec) may be used. A 7 Fr Grollman polyurethane catheter (Cook, Inc., Bloomington, IN) has recently been introduced and has a single 90° curve 6 cm from its pigtail ring. This catheter has 12 side holes, good torque control, and has been used with success (10).

The technique of pulmonary artery catheterization with the Grollman catheter is shown in Figure 14.2. The anteromedial portion of the right atrium is probed with the tip of the catheter until entry into the right ventricle is achieved. This is marked by a change in pressure and perhaps elicitation of ventricular ectopy. Counterclockwise rotation should then direct the distal curve upwards toward the ventricular outflow tract. From this point gently advancing the catheter will allow it to enter the pulmonary artery. On occasion, the catheter may get "hung up" in the outflow tract and buckle at the tricuspid valve when

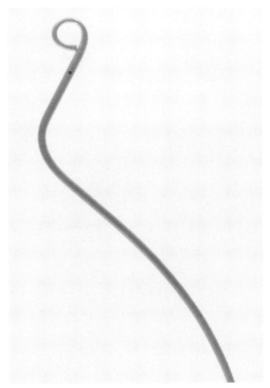

Figure 14.1. Standard Grollman pulmonary artery seeking catheter.

force is applied. Having the patient take a deep breath orients the heart more vertically and may allow the catheter to advance into the pulmonary artery. If this is not successful, a guidewire may be used to help prevent buckling by stiffening the catheter.

In patients with right atrial enlargement, the distal tip of the catheter may be too short to enter the right ventricle directly. One may then bend the "stiff" end of a guidewire into a curve approximately 4 cm in diameter (11) and advance it into the catheter to a point just proximal to the pigtail. Care must be taken to ensure that this stiff end of the guidewire is never advanced beyond the tip of the catheter. The guidewire generally adds enough additional curvature to allow the catheter to be directed through the tricuspid valve and into the right ventricle. The catheter may then be advanced into the pulmonary artery, as described above (Fig. 14.3). A tip-deflecting guidewire system (Cook Inc., Bloomington, IN) may also be successful in these situations

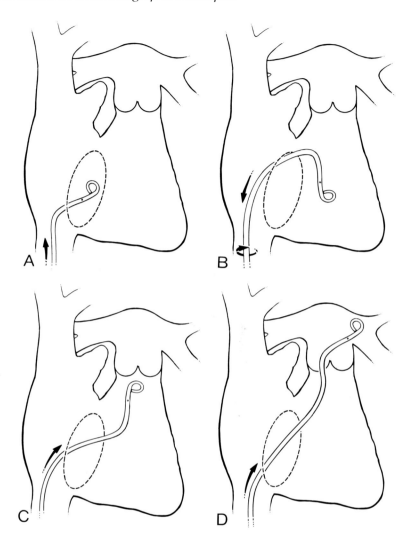

Figure 14.2. Procedure for catheterization of the pulmonary artery using the femoral approach with the Grollman catheter. When in the right atrium the catheter is directd towards the tricuspid valve *(A)*. With further advancement the right ventricle is entered *(B)*. The catheter is then withdrawn slightly and rotated so that the distal segment is directed toward the right ventricular outflow tract *(C)*, from which it can be easily positioned in the pulmonary artery *(D)*.

and offers an alternative to using the stiff end of the guidewire.

Catheters inserted from the femoral vein usually enter the left pulmonary artery preferentially. If subselective injection of the left lower lobe branches is necessary, further advancement of the catheter is usually all that is required. For selective right pulmonary angiography, withdrawal of the catheter into the main pulmonary artery, rotation of the

tip toward the right side, and advancement will usually be successful. If not, a J-tipped guidewire may be directed into the right pulmonary artery and the catheter threaded over it.

Balloon-tipped angiographic catheters may also be used from the femoral approach. The Berman (Critikon Inc., Tampa, FL) catheter allows for some flow direction while maintaining torque control. This device may

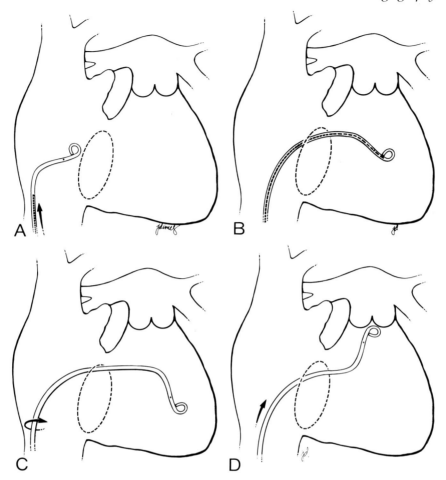

Figure 14.3. Pulmonary artery catheterization in patient with cardiomegaly. The curved back end of a guidewire is inserted to the catheter's pigtail *(A)*, allowing the catheter to be advanced through the tricuspid valve and into the right ventricle *(B)*. The guidewire is then removed, and right ventricular pressure is measured *(C)*. Rotation of the catheter directs it to the outflow tract and into the pulmonary artery *(D)*.

facilitate catheterization of the pulmonary artery in some cases, although the balloon may be a hindrance in the presence of significant tricuspid regurgitation. Since it has no end hole, it must be introduced through a sheath. A 7 Fr catheter will deliver flows of 20 ml/sec and will fit through a 7 Fr sheath. This catheter may be manipulated into the pulmonary artery in either of two ways. Once through the sheath, the balloon is inflated with air or carbon dioxide and advanced into the right atrium. The latter should be used if an abnormal communication between the venous and arterial systems is suspected. The

catheter may then be directed through the tricuspid valve and rotated to point up towards the outflow tract. A deep breath at this time will augment pulmonary flow, which is especially helpful with balloon catheters. Advancement will then cause the catheter to enter the pulmonary artery. Usually the catheter is directed towards the left pulmonary artery. If right pulmonary artery injection is required, one may enter the right ventricle by looping the catheter around the lateral wall of the right atrium in a counterclockwise direction so that it crosses the tricuspid valve pointing up. Advancement of this loop will cause the catheter tip to preferentially enter the right pulmonary artery in much the same way it does coming from the brachial approach (Fig. 14.4). This method may also be helpful in the presence of tricuspid regurgitation by adding support and, in effect, stiffening the catheter. One should position the Berman angiographic catheter somewhat more distally to compensate for recoil which occurs during contrast injection.

The pulmonary artery angiography may also be done using venous access in either upper extremity or the neck (see Chapter 6). These sites may be considered in cases of clinically recognized thrombosis of the iliofemoral veins or inferior vena cava (IVC), previous IVC ligation or umbrella placement, or groin infection. Percutaneous technique is utilized when using the neck and may be employed in the arm if an antecubital vein of sufficient size is recognizable from the surface. The brachial approach requires accessing a medially directed vein in order to enter the axillary and subclavian system directly. Laterally directed antecubital veins usually lead to the cephalic system, which enters the axillary vein at an unfavorable angle for the manipulation required for pulmonary artery catheterization. In most cases an antecubital cutdown readily reveals an adequately sized median cubital vein.

There are a variety of catheters available for pulmonary artery catheterization from the brachial approach. The traditional woven Dacron catheters have given way to the balloon-tipped angiographic catheters at our institution because of the latter's lessened likelihood of myocardial perforation and ease of use. Pigtail catheters may be introduced for use via the brachial approach. These include a modified Grollman catheter without the reverse curve (12) and a 5 Fr multiple-bend pigtail catheter (Cordis Corp, Miami, FL), available in three configurations. The latter are said to have a maximum injection rate of 22 ml/sec and have good torque control, especially when used with a guidewire (13).

In planning pulmonary angiography one should consider that entry into the left pulmonary artery is difficult when the brachial approach is used. If selective left pulmonary angiography is required and catheterization must be from the arm, one may form the proximal stiff end of a guidewire into an

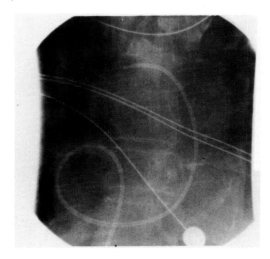

Figure 14.4. Pulmonary artery catheterization in the setting of tricuspid regurgitation. Balloon catheter was looped around the lateral wall of the right atrium allowing support for crossing the tricuspid valve. When introduced in this fashion the catheter commonly enters the right pulmonary artery.

S-shaped curve and advance it into the Berman catheter placed in the main pulmonary artery. This may allow the catheter to be directed into the left pulmonary artery. Alternatively, torqueable guidewires may be used with end-hole angiographic catheters.

Angiographic Technique

The diagnosis of pulmonary embolic disease requires selective or subselective angiography. Injection of contrast material into the main pulmonary artery is often less sensitive (14, 15), requires larger volumes of contrast material, and is rarely indicated for evaluation of either pulmonary emboli or arteriovenous malformations. Selective angiography is performed on the side of maximum abnormality revealed on the ventilation-perfusion lung scan (14, 16, 17). Subselective injections using oblique projections and/or magnification techniques (14, 17) are used when the scan defects are small, or if the initial selective angiogram is equivocal.

Seventy-six percent iodinated contrast material is injected with a flow rate determined by the site of injection and the pulmonary artery pressure. If the latter is less than 40 mm Hg systolic, 20 ml/sec for 2 sec is used in the right or left pulmonary artery and 15 ml/sec for 2 sec if the catheter is placed more selectively. If the pulmonary arterial systolic pressure is between 40 and 70 mm Hg, injection rates are reduced to 15 ml/sec and 10 ml/sec over 2 sec for the two sites, respectively. Pulmonary angiography should be performed with more caution when the systolic pressure is greater than 70 mm Hg because contrast material may acutely elevate the pressure and/or produce right heart failure (6, 18). Subselective catheter positioning and small volumes of low osmolar contrast material should be employed in this situation. The presence of right heart failure, as evidenced by a right ventricular end-diastolic pressure of 20 mm Hg or greater, is associated with an increased risk of death for pulmonary angiography (6), and this finding should cause the operator to reconsider the absolute necessity of angiography. If deemed essential, subselective techniques using very small doses of low-osmolar contrast material (5 to 10 ml total) should be employed. Digital pulmonary angiography, with the use of dilute contrast material (19), or wedged pulmonary angiography, with the use of balloon-tipped end-hole catheters should also be considered (20).

Although large field (9- or 12-inch image intensifier) cineradiographic technique has been advocated in selected situations (21), we still prefer cut films (14 inch x 14 inch) because they have greater spatial resolution and cover a larger area of the lung. Cinetechnique, on the other hand, allows examination of contrast flow and is a technique that all adult catheterization laboratories have. Filming, using cutfilm, is carried out at a rate of 3 films/sec for 3 sec and then 1 film/sec for an additional 3 sec for a total of 12 exposures. An exposure time of no greater than 20 msec should be used to minimize motion. For nonmagnification angiography, a kVP of 70 to 75 at 1000 mA is used for maximum contrast resolution. A 1.2-mm x-ray tube focal spot is usually employed; however, magnification angiography requires a 0.3 mm-focal spot. In the latter situation a kVP of 90 to 95 is used to compensate for the lower milliamperage (approximately 150 mA) necessitated by the small focal spot. Depending upon the x-ray tube heat capacity and the size of the patient, magnification angiography may require a filming rate slower than 3/sec.

Digital Pulmonary Angiography

Digital subtraction angiography (DSA) has recently been advocated for pulmonary angiography (19, 22-24), especially in those patients who are hemodynamically unstable, have pulmonary hypertension, or who are suspected of having large emboli. This technique does not require placement of a catheter in the pulmonary artery and thus avoids potential complications of right heart catheterization (see Chapter 9). Adequate studies may be obtained by the injection of 20 ml of contrast material per second for a total of 30 ml into the superior vena cava or right atrium. Digital angiograms may also be obtained by injecting contrast material (5 ml/sec for 2 sec) through the end hole of an indwelling balloon-tipped pulmonary arterial pressure monitoring catheter (19). Location of the catheter tip determines the lung imaged. The opposite lung may be visualized by injecting contrast material (10 ml/sec for 2 sec) through the proximal port of the thermodilution catheter.

The major disadvantage of DSA is the requirement for the patient to remain motionless; patients suspected of having pulmonary emboli are rarely able to suspend respiration long enough to complete a digital study. Cardiac motion itself makes evaluation of the vessels adjacent to the heart difficult, although gating techniques have been introduced to minimize this problem. As compared with standard pulmonary angiography, digital angiography has less resolution, and emboli may be detected only in the main right or left pulmonary arteries and their primary or secondary branches (19, 22, 24). Emboli in smaller peripheral branches cannot be completely excluded. Digital imaging of selective pulmonary arterial injections of dilute contrast is advantageous, however, in the evaluation and treatment of patients with pulmonary arteriovenous malformations with embolization techniques (25). These patients are able to suspend respiration for a sufficient period of time for such procedures, and DSA has adequate resolution, can be performed quickly, and requires less contrast material than conventional filming techniques.

Wedged Pulmonary Angiography With Balloon Flotation Catheters

Balloon occlusion pulmonary angiography, utilizing an indwelling flow directed catheter, has been suggested for the diagnosis of pulmonary emboli in patients thought too ill to undergo conventional angiography (20, 24, 26, 27). The procedure may be performed at the bedside in unstable patients, using portable chest films, or in the catheterization laboratory in patients with severe pulmonary hypertension in an effort to limit contrast material exposure.

The technique requires an end-hole balloon flotation catheter, such as a Swan-Ganz or Berman type. The balloon is inflated, and the catheter is advanced to a wedge position. This is followed by a hand injection of 10 cc of a mixture composed of 8.5 cc of contrast material and 1.5 cc of 2% lidocaine. The latter is used to suppress the cough response initiated by the contrast material. Low-osmolar agents may also be beneficial in this regard. A single radiograph is taken at the conclusion of the injection, after which the balloon is deflated. This procedure is easily accomplished with minimal risk but has a low sensitivity (28). Although a positive study may be taken as indicative of pulmonary emboli, a negative examination has little meaning since only a small area of the pulmonary circulation is seen with each injection, and emboli in other areas can not be excluded. In as much as the balloon catheter cannot be easily directed to selected parts of the pulmonary circulation, its position proximal to an embolus would indeed be fortuitous. While pulmonary emboli most often occur in the lower lobes, and flow-directed catheters commonly are carried there (27), pulmonary blood flow is reduced in embolized beds, thereby lessening the likelihood of the catheter entering those segments. This method of establishing the diagnosis of embolic disease is therefore of limited value.

Complications of Pulmonary Angiography

Although pulmonary angiography is relatively safe when performed by an experienced team, it is an invasive technique often utilized in compromised patients, and complications may occur. The overall incidence of significant morbidity ranges between 1 and 4% with a mortality rate of 0.2 to 0.4% (1, 6, 29, 30). Complications may be classified as being due to the right heart catheterization or those secondary to contrast material injection. The former include atrial and ventricular extrasystoles, sustained tachycardia (supraventricular and ventricular), ventricular fibrillation, right bundle branch block (which may result in complete heart block if there is preexisting left bundle branch block), and myocardial perforation with or without pericardial tamponade. Digitalis intoxication, recent myocardial infarction (1), and blood gas and electrolyte abnormality may all predispose to malignant arrhythmia. Intense anticoagulation or thrombolytic therapy increase the risk of pericardial bleeding, should perforation occur.

Contrast material injection may be accompanied by allergic reaction, cardiac depression, or an acute increase in pulmonary vascular resistance. The latter may be particularly risky in patients with marked pulmonary hypertension and/or right ventricular failure.

Role of Pulmonary Angiography in Suspected Embolic Disease

Pulmonary embolism is a common disorder with a mortality as high as 30% in untreated patients (29, 31, 32). If diagnosed and properly treated, risk of death is reduced to about 8% (29, 32). There are hazards associated with overdiagnosis of this entity since heparin therapy is one of the leading causes of drug-related complications, with significant hemorrhagic complications occurring in as many as 15% of those so treated (33).

Clinical recognition of pulmonary embolism may be difficult. Symptoms and common laboratory tests (arterial oxygen saturation and electrocardiography) may be suggestive but are not specific. Ventilation-perfusion lung scanning and pulmonary angiography are the two imaging modalities used for the detection of embolism. Lung scanning is non-invasive, easily performed, and highly sensitive for embolism. A normal perfusion scan excludes the diagnosis (33, 30, 34, 35). Other disease states, however, may result in diminished regional pulmonary arterial flow and limit the specificity of the perfusion scan. Combined ventilation-perfusion scanning is generally (36-40), although not universally (33), considered to improve specificity and should be performed whenever possible. A high quality chest x-ray is important in the interpretation of scans and should always be available (41).

The characteristic findings of pulmonary embolism are perfusion defects in segmental areas of the lung that are normally ventilated and appear normal on the chest radiograph (39, 40). If such defects are present in two or more lung segments, there is a "high probability" (86 to 100%) of pulmonary embolism (37, 38, 40-42). Subsegmental defects on perfusion scanning associated with normal ventilation scans and chest film are considered to have a "moderate probability" (27 to 50%) of pulmonary embolism (37, 38, 41, 42). Scans showing small perfusion defects and normal ventilation, or those having matched perfusion-ventilation defects of any size and a normal chest radiograph, have been termed "low probability" (0 to 5%) (37, 38, 41). A recent prospective study, however, has shown a 23% incidence of pulmonary embolism in patients with large matched perfusion-ventilation defects (42).

It is especially difficult to exclude pulmonary embolism in patients with severe chronic obstructive pulmonary disease having extensive ventilation defects (43). Lung scanning is usually indeterminate in such cases as it is when perfusion-ventilation defects occur in areas of abnormality on the chest x-ray (37, 38, 42, 44). Unfortunately, abnormal chest films are not infrequent in patients with embolic disease (29, 41). The findings (consolidation, pleural effusion, and atelectasis) are nonspecific while similar findings, when not due to embolic disease, may result in defects on lung scans. Therefore, lung scans with corresponding ventilation-perfusion abnormalities and chest radio-graphic abnormalities cannot exclude the possibility of pulmonary embolism.

In the patient clinically suspected of having pulmonary embolism a ventilation-perfusion lung scan and a chest radiograph should be the initial screening procedures. A normal perfusion scan eliminates the possibility embolism (30, 33-35). Patients with a high probability scan generally do not require pulmonary angiography unless there is a strong contraindication to heparin, or unless thrombolytic therapy or invasive intervention is contemplated (2, 34, 40). Patients with low probability scans may require angiography if the clinical impression of embolism is highly suggestive and if there is risk of heparinization. A moderate probability or "indeterminate" scan most often result in angiography.

Pulmonary angiography when required should be performed within the first few days after the clinical episode suggesting embolization. Resolution of emboli may begin within a day of their occurrence and may be complete by 1 to 2 weeks (29, 31, 45, 46). Although the patient may be anticoagulated prior to angiography, heparin should be suspended for at least 2 hr before the procedure if the procedure is done percutaneously.

Angiography should be directed by results of the lung scan. With large lobar defects selective right or left pulmonary angiography should be performed first. For smaller segmental or subsegmental defects, subselective angiography in the lobar or segmental arterial branch corresponding to the abnormality may be performed to enable the diagnosis of small peripheral emboli (14, 17). Selective injections reduce dilution of contrast material and provide for minimal overlapping of pulmonary vessels from adjacent portions of the lung. Use of oblique projections when the initial angiogram is equivocal further reduces superimposition of vessels (15, 47). Magnification angiography may also be performed to further improve resolution of small emboli (14, 17). Once emboli are detected, the procedure is terminated. If angiography is negative in one area of scan defect, selective angiography must be performed in other areas of scan abnormality, if present. There is no need to image areas shown to be normal by perfusion scan.

Venography of the lower extremities is not an adequate substitute for pulmonary angiography in the diagnosis of pulmonary embolus. It may be negative in up to 30% of the patients with documented emboli (42), and venous thrombosis may occur in patients with abnormal lung scans not due to emboli. Bilateral leg venography has been recommended, however, to improve the detection of "thromboembolic disease" in patients with lung scan defects and negative angiography (42).

Interpretation of the Pulmonary Angiogram

Demonstration of an intraluminal filling defect within the pulmonary arteries establishes pulmonary embolism angiographically (Fig. 14.5) (47-49). If complete obstruction to blood flow is present, the proximal end of the clot must be demonstrated to protrude into the lumen of the artery (Fig. 14.6). Vascular

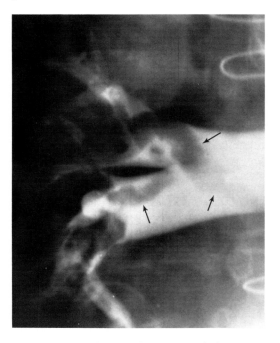

Figure 14.6. A large pulmonary embolus is seen obstructing the right upper and lower lobe pulmonary arteries. Proximal to the occlusion thrombus is seen within the arterial lumen *(arrows).*

occlusion without evidence of a filling defect is nonspecific. Abrupt cutoff of pulmonary vessels has been seen with pulmonary abscess, neoplasm, and tuberculosis (21). Slow or diminished flow in a localized area is also nonspecific and may be seen in a multitude of other conditions. Selective angiography has diminished the incidence of equivocal angiography, which was not uncommon when injections were made only in the main pulmonary artery (Fig. 14.7) (1).

The syndrome of chronic pulmonary embolism (50) occurs when pulmonary emboli organize and become fibrotic. This may come about as a result of repeated bouts of emboli over a period of years, or because large emboli fragment but do not completely lyse. These patients may have chronic dyspnea and suffer from recurrent thrombophlebitis. In most cases pulmonary hypertension is present. The angiographic manifestations include occluded vessels, as well as those with stenoses and webs (Fig. 14.8). Although these angiographic findings

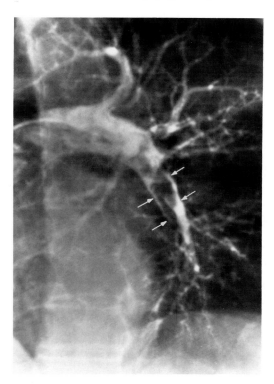

Figure 14.5. Pulmonary embolus. An intraluminal filling defect *(arrows)* is demonstrated within the left lobe pulmonary artery.

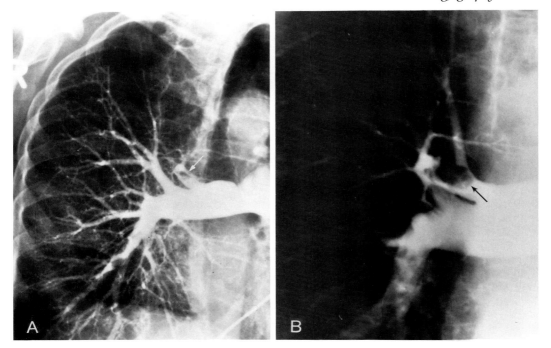

Figure 14.7. Embolus confirmed by subselective injection. The right pulmonary angiogram shows a possible defect in an upper lobe branch *(arrow)* *(A)*. Subselective angiography *(B)* demonstrates an intraluminal filling defect *(arrows)* diagnostic of embolus.

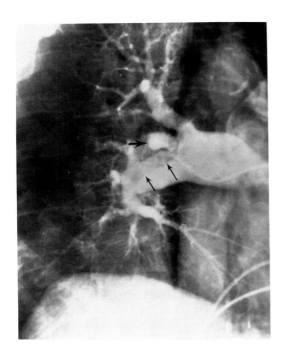

Figure 14.8. Chronic pulmonary embolus. A 74-year-old woman with previous pulmonary emboli and severe exercise intolerance. There is an old adherent thrombus *(small arrows)* within the right lower lobe pulmonary artery. An occluded branch is seen *(large arrow)*. Peripheral right lower lobe vessels are abruptly tapered. The pulmonary arterial pressure was 110/40 mm Hg, and the angiogram was performed with an injection of 20 ml of contrast over 2 sec.

are not entirely specific, this syndrome should be considered in patients with the appropriate clinical setting.

Pulmonary Angiography for Nonembolic Disorders

Pulmonary Arteriovenous Malformation

Pulmonary arteriovenous malformations (PAVMs) are congenital abnormalities that may occur as an isolated entity but are commonly associated with the Osler-Weber-Rendu syndrome (51, 52). Clinical manifestations include dyspnea and cyanosis due to shunting of nonoxygenated blood through the lung. The disorder may be complicated by brain abscess, paradoxical embolization, stroke, or hemoptysis with a substantial risk of mortality. About 80% of PAVMs consist of a single pulmonary arterial branch communicating directly with a drain-

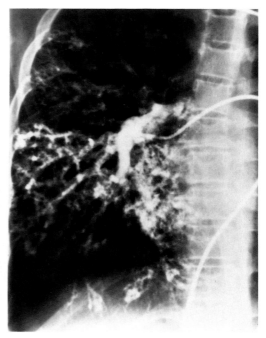

Figure 14.10. Complex pulmonary arteriovenous malformations. Multiple diffuse arteriovenous communications exist throughout the right lower lobe.

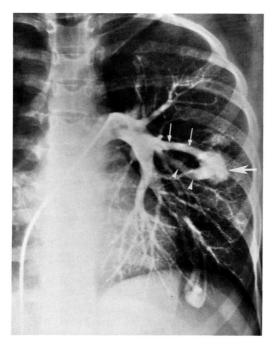

Figure 14.9. Pulmonary arteriovenous malformations. Simple type PAVMs demonstrated in lower lobe and lingula. Each malformation consists of a single feeding artery *(small arrows)*, aneurysmal segment *(large arrow)*, and a draining vein *(arrowheads)*.

ing vein through an aneurysmal vascular segment (Fig. 14.9)(25). The remaining cases are more complex, consisting of several arterial branches communicating with a septated aneurysmal segment and two or more draining veins (Fig. 14.10). Pulmonary angiography is diagnostic and is a necessary prerequisite for **transcatheter embolization**, which has become the treatment of choice for PAVM (25, 53–57). The latter procedure eliminates the need for thoracotomy and preserves maximal lung function. It is indicated in all patients with symptoms and in those with lower lobe PAVMS greater than 3 mm in diameter, regardless of symptoms because of the risk of paradoxical embolization, brain abscess, and stroke.

Therapeutic embolization of PAVMs has been performed using steel coils (Cook Inc., Bloomington, IN) (55, 56) and detachable silicone balloons (Becton-Dickinson, Inc., Rutherford, NJ) (Fig. 14.11) (25, 53, 54). The latter are particularly advantageous since they can be positioned precisely within the feeding

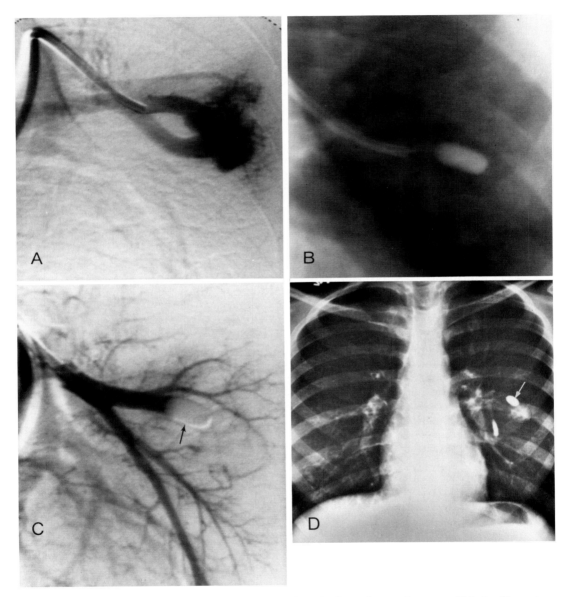

Figure 14.11. Balloon occlusion of PAVM. Selective digital subtraction angiogram within feeding artery of malformation *(A)*. The balloon is inflated within feeding artery *(B)* and is seen occluding the malformation *(arrow)* *(C)*. Follow-up chest film *(D)* shows balloon in place *(arrow)*, as well as a second balloon occluding the feeding artery to a lower lobe PAVM.

artery and repositioned if necessary prior to final detachment.

Diagnostic pulmonary angiography of both lungs is required before embolotherapy. Selective right and left pulmonary angiograms in several projections are necessary to localize the feeding vessels. This is usually performed at a separate session in order to limit the dose of contrast material. In the largest series reported to date (25) therapeutic embolization, using detachable balloon technique, was successful in 14 of 17 patients with an increase in arterial PO_2 from a mean of 44 mm Hg to 65 mm Hg. Recurrence due to collateral development has not been a problem, and complications have been few.

Pulmonary Branch Stenosis

Stenosis of the pulmonary artery may occur either in a diffuse or focal pattern. The latter exists as discrete obstructions with relatively normal-sized vessels before and beyond while the former is manifest by abrupt tapering of vessels that remain small in their peripheral distribution.

Angiography plays an important role in the diagnosis of pulmonary branch stenosis and is necessary for performance and evaluation of **catheter balloon dilatation**, should it be considered. Pressure recordings are necessary to establish the hemodynamic importance of the stenoses. Complete cardiac catheterization should be considered to exclude associated congenital defects. We have encountered a case with unilateral peripheral pulmonic stenosis associated with scimitar syndrome on the contralateral side (Fig. 14.12)(57). Magnetic resonance imaging may also contribute to the diagnosis of this disorder (Fig. 14.13).

Partial Anomalous Pulmonary Venous Return

Partial anomalous pulmonary venous return most frequently occurs in association with atrial septal defect. On occasion, however, it may exist as an isolated entity. This often presents as an abnormal finding on chest x-ray or with the clinical picture of an atrial septal defect (ASD). A solitary left anomalous pulmonary venous connection is particularly unusual and may pose a diagnostic puzzle

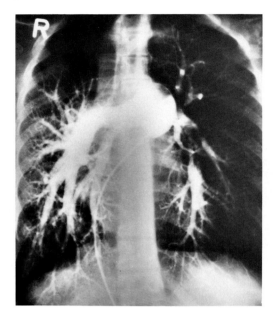

Figure 14.12. Pulmonary artery branch stenosis. Multiple discrete stenoses involving the left pulmonary artery. (From Platia EV, Brinker JA. Scimitar syndrome with peripheral left pulmonary artery branch stenoses. Am Heart J 1984; 107:594–596).

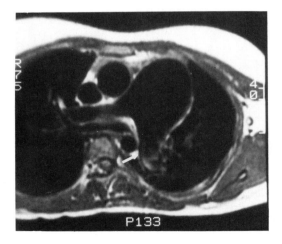

Figure 14.13. Pulmonary artery stenosis. Diffuse pulmonary arterial stenoses demonstrated by MRI. Transition from dilated proximal pulmonary artery to hypoplastic branch vessel (*arrow*).

being missed at catheterization unless the oxygen saturation run includes samples from the high superior vena cava and left innominate vein (58). Analysis of dye dilution curves obtained by selective injection in both the right and left pulmonary arteries is also helpful. Pulmonary angiography with delayed filming to include the venous phase is diagnostic (Fig. 14.14). Digital subtraction angiography (DSA) and computed tomography (CT) with contrast provide less invasive alternatives (59) but may offer little benefit if pulmonary arterial access is necessary for hemodynamic characterization and oximetry.

When occurring in association with atrial septal defect, anomalous veins most often enter in or near the right atrium, and the condition is easily identified at surgery when both defects are corrected. Thus, demonstration of an atrial septal defect at catheterization usu-

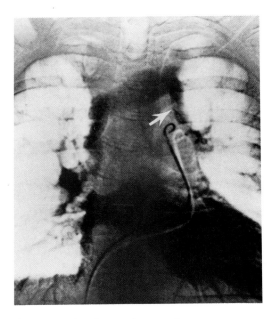

Figure 14.14. Anomalous pulmonary venous return. Venous phase of pulmonary angiogram demonstrating anomalous vein from left lung *(arrow)*. This was an isolated finding in a patient thought to have atrial septal defect. (From McGaughey MD, Traill TA, Brinker JA. Partial left anomalous pulmonary venous return: a diagnostic dilemma. Cathet Cardiovasc Diagn 1986;12: 110–115.)

ally precludes the need to angiographically define all of the pulmonary veins. Rarely, an anomalous vein enters the systemic venous circulation remote from the atria and is not identified at the time of atrial septal defect repair. While this does not justify routine pulmonary angiography or selective dye curves for every patient with atrial septal defect, abnormalities on chest x-ray or oximetry suggesting such a problem should be pursued at catheterization.

Other Indications for Pulmonary Angiography

There are a number of other congenital and acquired abnormalities of the pulmonary vascular system that may be revealed angiographically. While the need for angiography has been reduced in some instances by availability of other diagnostic techniques, such as magnetic resonance imaging (MRI) and CT scanning, the angiogram is still the "reference standard" and is usually required if surgical intervention is being considered. Demonstration of unilateral absence of a pulmonary artery (60, 61), pulmonary artery to atrial shunt (62), pulmonary artery sling (63), and pulmonary arterial aneurysm (64-66) can be achieved by routine pulmonary angiography. Sarcoma of the pulmonary artery may be visualized by contrast material injection in the right ventricle or pulmonary artery (67). Pulmonary venous obstruction may be documented by wedge and subselective pulmonary angiography (68, 69).

On occasion, it is necessary to visualize the pulmonary arterial system by other than routine techniques. In patients with a variety of congenital heart defects pulmonary blood flow is maintained by surgical shunts or systemic to pulmonary collateralization. In some, the opportunity for surgical intervention depends upon assessment of a confluence between the right and left pulmonary arteries, size of the pulmonary vessels, pressure in the pulmonary circulation, and the presence and extent of collateralization. Enlargement of small pulmonary arteries by a palliative procedure may be documented by angiography (70). Patency of a surgical shunt, as well as collateralization, may be assessed (Fig. 14.15). Cranial angulation (about 40°) provides optimal visualization of the pulmonary artery bifurcation.

Access to the pulmonary arterial system may require catheterization of the shunt or a bronchial collateral. We have been successful in negotiating Blalock-Taussig shunts and bronchial collaterals with standard Judkins right coronary angiography catheters. Pressure measurements and contrast material injections can be performed through this catheter, or if necessary, an exchange guidewire will enable other catheters to be positioned properly.

A portion of the lung may receive its blood supply from a systemic artery. Frequently, this is in association with bronchopulmonary sequestration, although it rarely may occur without sequestration. The anomalous systemic artery may be documented angiographically or by less invasive imaging techniques (71).

Pulmonary Angiography to Visualize the Left Heart

Injection of contrast material into the pulmonary artery allows visualization of the left atrium, ventricle, and ascending aorta. We have used this technique to evaluate left ventricular function in situations in which direct injection was thought to be associated with

increased risk, such as that in the presence of left ventricular thrombus, in aortic valvular endocarditis, and in patients with aortic valve prosthesis. This technique has been suggested as a means of demonstrating cardiac thrombi in patients with cerebral infarction (72). Aortic dissection may also be visualized by cineangiography following pulmonary arterial injection, and this may be useful in selected cases.

The disadvantages of this approach include dilution of contrast material as it passes through the pulmonary circulation, additional radiation dosage given as one "follows" the contrast material through the lungs, or chance of missing information by delaying imaging by means of an arbitrary time period (usually 3 to 5 sec), direct exposure of contrast material to the lungs, and inability to assess valvular regurgitation. In addition, there are alternative imaging techniques such as echocardiography, gated blood pool scanning, MRI, CT, and DSA, which can be applied with less risk.

AORTOGRAPHY

The aortogram has been an important tool in the diagnosis and follow-up evaluation of a number of disorders (Table 14.3). While the

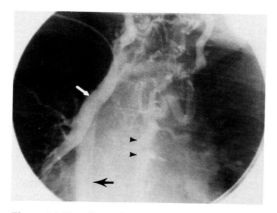

Figure 14.15. Superior vena cavogram in patient with Glenn shunt. The right pulmonary artery is opacified, as is a network of collaterals to the azygos *(arrow)* and hemiazygos *(arrowheads)* veins. The superior vena cava is delineated by the *white arrow.*

TABLE 14.3.
Indications for Aortography

1. Aortic valve integrity
2. Nonselective views of coronary arteries or grafts
3. Supravalvular aortic stenosis
4. Disease of the brachiocephalic and other branch vessels
5. Aortic aneurysm
6. Aortic dissection
7. Coarctation
8. Detection of systemic-to-pulmonary communications
9. Definition of pulmonary circulation by shunts or collaterals
10. Postvascular surgery
11. Posttrauma
12. Aortic or para-aortic neoplasia
13. Arterial thromboembolic disease
14. Atherosclerotic narrowing
15. Inflammatory arterial disease

remarkable advances attained in noninvasive imaging have lessened the need for this procedure, aortography still plays an important role in the delineation of anatomy and is especially useful if surgery is contemplated.

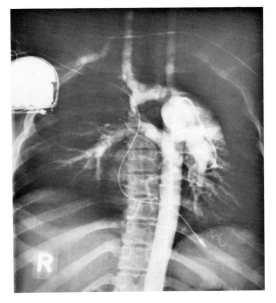

Figure 14.16. Aortography to delineate pulmonary circulation. Aortogram demonstrates pulmonary arterial system via functioning Blalock-Taussig shunt. Patient has single ventricle with atretic pulmonary valve.

Contrast radiograms of the aorta and its branches may be recorded in a variety of ways, including cinefilms, serial cut films, 105-mm photofluorography, and digital acquisition. Each has advantages and disadvantages. Cineangiography is logistically simple, views structures in motion, and allows one to pan areas of interest without introduction of motion artifact. This technique is ideal for evaluation of aortic regurgitation and may be helpful in dissection by revealing the motion of an intimal flap. We have found it useful for visualizing the distal aorta and iliofemoral system, when necessary, as part of a cardiac catheterization, although it lacks the field size and resolution of serial cut filming. The latter is the technique of choice when fine anatomic detail is required and when there is a large field of interest. It is routinely used in the study of aortic aneurysm and dissection, and when the pulmonary arterial system is filled by systemic flow (Fig. 14.16).

Digital subtraction angiography is usually reserved for the evaluation of discrete sites, especially when there is a need to limit contrast exposure. It is of value in interventional procedures and has proved helpful in locating a radiolucent intravascular foreign body (Fig. 14.17) (73). We also use DSA in screening for carotid disease at catheterization, achieving satisfactory opacification of these vessels with ascending aortic injections of diluted contrast.

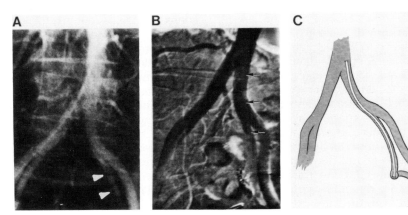

Figure 14.17. Detection of a nonradiopaque foreign body. A radiolucent angioplasty catheter sheath accidentally dislodged in the ascending aorta was searched for angiographically. Cineangiography performed in the descending aorta revealed a straightening of the left internal iliac vessel *(A, arrowheads).* Digital angiography revealed the sheath to extend proximally into the descending aorta *(B).* The foreign body was removed using a snare introduced from the right femoral artery. (From McIvor ME, Kaufman SL, Satre S, Porterfield JK, Brinker JA. Search and retrieval of an unidentifiable foreign object. Cathet Cardiovasc Diagn, in press, 1988.)

Digital angiography has largely replaced use of 105-mm photofluorography in our laboratory; however, this latter technique can yield excellent studies, especially when there is a need to perform selective injections of smaller vessels. It provides better resolution with less total radiation than cineangiography and may be available in laboratories that lack the ability to perform serial cut filming or DSA.

Ascending Aortography

Contrast material injection of the ascending aorta is performed to assess the anatomy of the aortic root, arch, and branch vessels, to locate coronary bypass grafts, and to quantitate aortic insufficiency. Since optimal opacification requires a relatively large amount of contrast material to be delivered over a short time, pigtail catheters capable of handling high flow rates are most often used. These have the advantage of accepting a guidewire, allowing for safe and easy placement, especially in cases where the aortic wall is fragile (e.g., Marfan's syndrome or aortic dissection). In addition, the pigtail dissipates the pressure of the injection without a "jet" of contrast material exiting the end hole. This prevents recoil and the possibility of damage, should the catheter migrate towards a small branch or a weakened area of aorta. Since the aortogram is commonly performed as part of a more complete diagnostic catheterization, one can use a pigtail catheter of the same outer diameter as the other arterial catheters used during the procedure (usually 7 or 8 Fr). Catheters designed to handle high flow while maintaining a small outside diameter (O.D.) may be considered when aortography alone is performed. It should be remembered that the newer low osmolar contrast agents have relatively high viscosity, especially at room temperature, and adequate flow rates may require high pressure. It is important that the catheter handle this pressure and flow. The pigtail is placed a few centimeters above the aortic valve in order to opacify the entire aortic root and yet not interfere with the valve itself, possibly inducing artifactual regurgitation. While angiography can safely be performed in most patients, there are rare instances in which even obtaining arterial access may pose a risk. In these patients intravenous digital subtraction angiography may be particularly helpful (Fig. 14.18) (74).

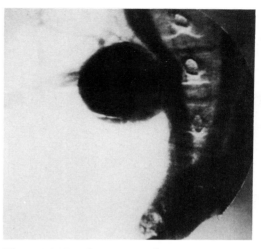

Figure 14.18. Aneurysm of innominate artery. Digital angiogram following intravenous contrast injection in a patient with Ehlers-Danlos syndrome IV in whom arterial access was thought too risky. (From Pyeritz RE, Stolle CA, Parfrey NA, Myers JC. Ehlers-Danlos syndrome IV due to a novel defect in type III procollagen. Am J Med Genet 1984;19:607–622.)

Optimal positioning of the patient for aortography depends upon the clinical objectives. In general the ascending aorta is best visualized in the steep left anterior oblique (LAO) projection. This allows assessment of aortic insufficiency and spreads out the ascending aorta and arch. Supravalvular aortic stenosis, coarctation, and aortic-pulmonary communications are well seen. Aortocoronary grafts may also be detected in this view. On occasion, when there is significant aortic regurgitation, better functional assessment of the left ventricle may be obtained from an right anterior oblique (RAO) projection. This view is also helpful in locating grafts to the left anterior descending system that may be foreshortened and overlapped in the LAO. In these special instances biplane cineangiography is often utilized.

Serial cut films are utilized for aortic aneurysms and dissections as well as for the evaluation of aorta to pulmonary artery shunts, be they iatrogenic or congenital. Most often biplane aortograms in the anterior-posterior and lateral projections are obtained. This, however, limits the total number and rate of images that can be recorded because of the need to alternately expose the films in order to avoid image degradation by x-ray scatter. If faster filming or a greater number of images are required, a single-plane steep LAO projection may be substituted. The programming of serial films depends upon the information desired. The ascending aorta is best visualized during the first 2 sec of injection, and the filming rate should be 2 to 3 films/sec over this time. The total number of images recorded and programming of the remaining films varies. Late filming is necessary to visualize the collaterals in coarctation, a false lumen in cases of dissection, and pulmonary anatomy in the presence of systemic-to-pulmonary communications. We usually obtain a total of 12 to 15 films in each view with an exposure rate of 1 film/sec after the first 2 to 4 sec.

The rate and amount of contrast material needed for aortography depends upon the size of the patient, the cardiac output, and the specific anatomy. Usually, 50 to 70 cc of contrast material delivered over 2 to 3 sec suffices. Larger amounts of contrast material are needed in patients with large aortic aneurysms (such as are occasionally encountered in the Marfan's syndrome) and those with high blood flow rates. Use of nonionic contrast material is recommended for those patients who are hemodynamically precarious, are otherwise at increased risk, or who will require a great deal of contrast material to complete the study.

In general, less contrast material is needed and better pictures are obtained if the injection is made as close as possible to the area of interest. While the ascending aortogram gives information about the origins of the brachiocephalic vessels, digital subtraction techniques or selective injections provide better definition. Similarly, there may be little reason to inject contrast material in the ascending aorta if the object of the study is to evaluate a descending aortic aneurysm or to assess the pulmonary arterial system via bronchial collateralization. Proximal or distal injections may be necessary, however, to fully define the extent of the disease process, other pathology, or collateralization.

Aortic Dissection

While the patient with aortic dissection may often present with a characteristic clinical picture, this is not always the case (75). Similarly,

a variety of other disorders can present with signs and symptoms compatible with acute dissection (76). The definitive diagnosis of dissecting aneurysm of the aorta has traditionally rested with aortography, and this is still the "reference standard" required by many surgeons before operation is considered (see Chapter 32). Goals of aortography in patients with the clinical suspicion of dissection are to establish the diagnosis and to identify whether the dissection involves the ascending aorta or arch (proximal, Fig. 14.19) or exists solely distal to the left subclavian artery (distal, Fig. 14.20). Secondary objectives would be to evaluate the integrity of the aortic valve and determine patency of major branch vessels (Fig. 14.21). In older patients or those with a history of coronary artery disease there may be a need to assess coronary anatomy for atherosclerotic obstruction so that a combined surgical procedure may be performed. Rarely,

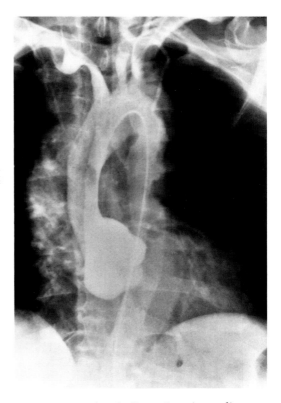

Figure 14.19. Aortic dissection. Ascending aortography reveals dissection involving proximal aorta and extending into brachiocephalic vessels.

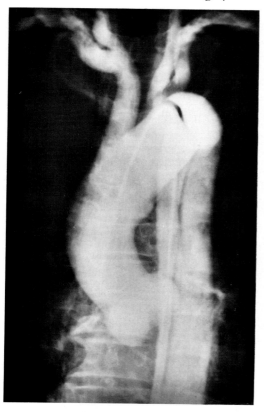

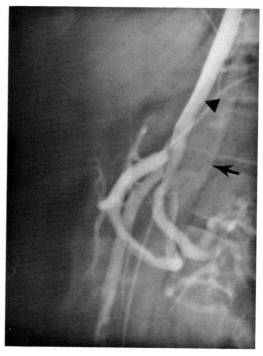

Figure 14.21. Aortic dissection. Lateral view of descending aortogram demonstrating true lumen compressed *(arrowhead)* and then occluded by false lumen *(arrow).*

Figure 14.20. Aortic dissection. Angiography demonstrates dissection limited to distal aorta.

rupture into a contiguous structure may need documentation (Fig. 14.22).

Angiographic diagnosis of dissection rests with demonstration of a false lumen and/or an intimal flap. Occlusion of branch vessels and compression of the contrast-filled aorta by intramural clot are highly suggestive. Noninvasive imaging techniques vary in their sensitivity and specificity when compared with aortography, and each have some limitations. Echocardiography can be quickly obtained at the patient's bedside if necessary, but adequate studies can not be recorded in many patients. Dissections limited to the descending thoracic aorta are rarely diagnosed by transthoracic sonography (77). While traditional M-mode echocardiography appears to lack the sensitivity and specificity of CT or MRI (78), two-dimensional, transesophageal, and Doppler echocardiography offer significant

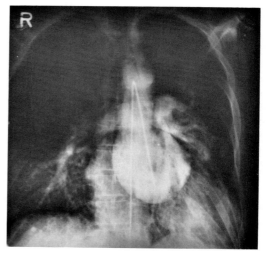

Figure 14.22. Aortic dissection. Ascending aortography revealing a rupture of dissecting aneurysm into pulmonary artery in a patient with Marfan's syndrome.

improvement and may reveal dissection missed by other techniques, including aortography (79-81).

Contrast-enhanced CT has been proven of value in diagnosis of thoracic aortic disease and in expert hands appears to be as efficacious as aortography in diagnosing dissection (82). The finding of a dual lumen with an intervening intimal flap is diagnostic (Fig. 14.23) while intimal calcification displaced by the false lumen (Fig. 14.24), a thickened aortic wall, disparity between the ascending and descending aorta, and compression of the true lumen are suggestive (83). Dynamic CT and reformatted images add to the study (Fig. 14.25) (84). Pitfalls may exist in the CT diagnosis of dissection (85, 86), including differentiation of an intramural hematoma from mural thrombus in an aneurysm (87).

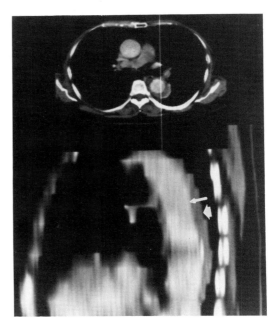

Figure 14.25. Aortic dissection. Reformatted CT demonstrating true *(arrow)* and false *(arrowhead)* lumens.

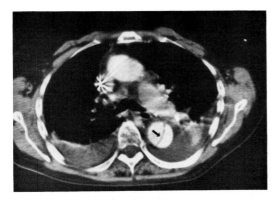

Figure 14.23. Aortic dissection. Contrast enhanced CT demonstrates intimal flap *(arrow)*.

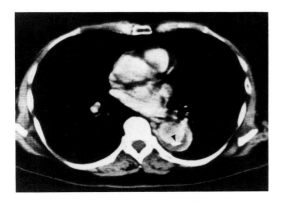

Figure 14.24. Aortic dissection. CT scan reveals medial displacement of intimal calcification *(arrowhead)*.

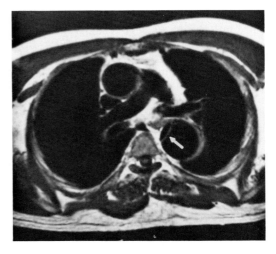

Figure 14.26. Aortic dissection. MRI revealing intimal flap *(arrow)* in descending aorta.

Magnetic resonance imaging is capable of providing a diagnosis of dissection by demonstrating an intimal flap and double lumen (88) (Fig. 14.26). It does not require contrast injection and may be superior to CT in assessment of aortic branches (89, 90). Since MRI does not image calcium, it cannot detect its displacement, however. Other limitations are present with MRI, including difficulty imaging acutely ill patients and patients having pacemakers or requiring artificial ventilation.

There is growing enthusiasm to screen patients for dissection with one of the less invasive modalities. Angiography may then be reserved for those cases having negative screens but in whom there remains a high clinical suspicion and those cases in which there are specific surgical considerations. While one would agree that noninvasive techniques are desirable, especially in the acutely ill patient, the catheterization laboratory is often better prepared to care for such an individual. In addition, use of nonionic contrast material and small pigtail catheters has probably reduced the risks associated with angiography.

Aortic Aneurysm

Aneurysmal dilatation of the aorta may be "true" (containing all three layers of the vessel wall) or "false" (encapsulated only by elements of the adventitia and reactive fibrosis). Causes of the former include atherosclerosis, inflammation, infection, or congenital defects. False aneurysms usually result from trauma but may occur as a result of infection, especially with the tubercle bacillus. While aneurysms of the ascending and descending aorta may remain clinically silent for long periods of time, those involving the arch become evident earlier by compression of a structure in the thoracic outlet. The objective of angiography in the evaluation of aortic aneurysms is to demonstrate the extent of the process, involvement of major branches, and presence of additional pathology (e.g., other aneurysms, stenoses, shunts). Thus, thoracic aortic aneurysms are usually approached with an initial ascending aortic injection in the LAO projection. A second injection may be required for adequate visualization of the descending aorta.

Atherosclerotic aneurysms are most common; they are usually fusiform but occasionally are saccular and are most often located in the arch or descending portions of the aorta (Fig. 14.27). The atherosclerotic processes produce elongation as well as dilatation of the aorta and may effect multiple locations of this

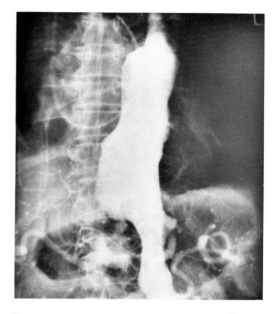

Figure 14.27. Aortic aneurysm. Atherosclerotic aneurysm of thoracic aorta.

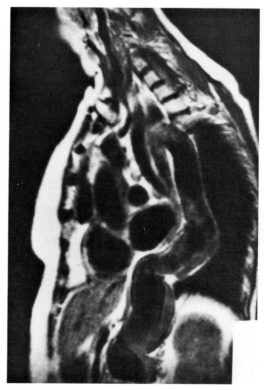

Figure 14.28. Aortic aneurysm. Atherosclerotic aneurysmal dilation of the thoracic and abdominal aorta demonstrated by MRI.

vessel along its entire course (Fig. 14.28). The presence of calcification in an ascending aortic aneurysm had in the past suggested syphilitic involvement. At present, however, such a finding is most frequently the result of atherosclerosis. While not common, luetic aortitis may be suggested by a thin deposition of calcium limited to the ascending aorta, aortic regurgitation, and serologic evidence of the disease. The coronary ostia may be narrowed by the process as well.

Aneurysms caused by infection (Fig. 14.29) (mycotic aneurysms) may be classified as primary (not associated with an identifiable intravascular source) or secondary (due to an intravascular or contiguous extravascular source of infection)(91). Mycotic aneurysms now are most commonly associated with arterial trauma or endocarditis, involve the abdominal aorta or femoral artery, and, if an etiologic agent is identified, are most likely due to *Staphylococcus aureus* or *Salmonella species* (92).

Sinus of Valsalva aneurysms may be congenital or acquired (due to endocarditis). They usually involve the right or noncoronary aortic

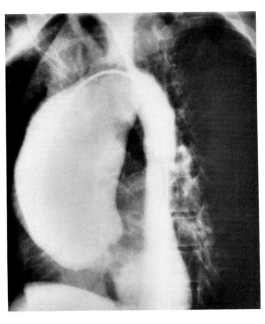

Figure 14.30. Marfan's syndrome. Massive dilation of the ascending aorta associated with moderate aortic regurgitation.

sinus and produce signs and symptoms when they rupture into a cardiac chamber, although rarely they may produce symptoms by obstructing the right ventricular outflow tract. Echocardiography has proven valuable in diagnosis of these aneurysms (93-95), with angiography usually reserved for those in whom a complication has occurred and surgery has been considered.

Dilation of all three aortic sinuses and the ascending aorta may occur in **Marfan's syndrome** (Fig. 14.30). When such aortic dilation occurs without involvement of other organs, the term idiopathic annuloaortic ectasia may be used (96). Aortic dilation may be accompanied by regurgitation, dissection, or rupture, and these conditions account for the vast majority of deaths in patients with Marfan's syndrome (97). This poor prognosis has prompted an aggressive approach to the management of the disorder that includes, in selected patients, insertion of a composite graft consisting of a prosthetic valve, to which one end of a woven vascular graft is sutured (98). This replaces as a unit the aortic valve and sinuses of Valsalva. Coronary flow is established by anastomosing side holes in the graft to the intraaortic origins of the coronary

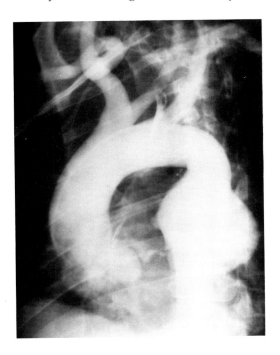

Figure 14.29. Aortic aneurysm. Mycotic aneurysm of descending aorta in a young drug addict. Culture revealed *Staphylococcus.*

arteries, or if this is not feasible, by constructing bypass grafts from the prosthesis to the coronaries. Patients with proximal aortic dissections, severe aortic regurgitation, and

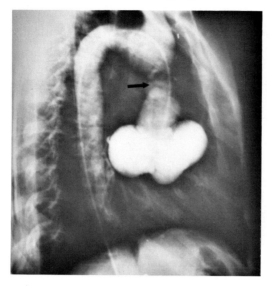

Figure 14.31. Marfan's syndrome. Previous surgery to replace portion of the ascending aorta above aortic sinuses with subsequently dramatic enlargement of the latter. Distal anastomosis of graft with aorta *(arrow)* appears restrictive; however, no gradient was detected.

those having marked dilation of the aortic root (in excess of 5.5 to 6 cm) may be considered for this procedure. Echocardiography, MRI or CT scanning can be used to follow the dilation of the ascending aorta and to document the occurrence of dissection. Aortography is reserved for those patients thought to require surgery on the basis of the noninvasive workup. Usually, angiography is part of a complete catheterization including coronary angiography. The degree of dilation of the sinuses and the location of the origins of the coronary arteries with respect to this dilation is of surgical importance. Angiography also plays a role in the evaluation of postoperative patients who are thought to have a complication (99) (Figs. 14.31 and 14.32).

There are a variety of other disorders that may be associated with aneurysms of the aorta or its major branches. These include Takayasu's arteritis, rheumatoid arthritis and ankylosing spondylitis, giant cell arteritis, relapsing polychondritis, Reiter's syndrome, and Kawasaki's disease. Each of these entities has other features that afford distinction.

Traumatic aneurysms may be due to blunt or penetrating injuries. The locations most frequently afflicted by traumatic aneurysm are those in which the aorta undergoes transition from being relatively free to being fixed. These

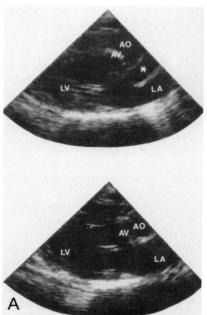

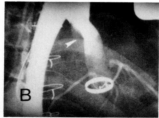
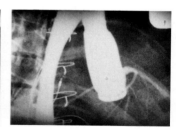

Figure 14.32. Dehiscence of valve prosthesis. Asymptomatic patient with Marfan's syndrome. Status postcomposite valve-graft insertion. Routine two-dimensional echocardiography revealed space between the aorta and the left atrium during ventricular systole *(asterisk)* that disappears in diastole *(A, top* and *bottom,* respectively). Ascending aortography demonstrates systolic collapse of graft *(B),* the cause of which was partial dehiscence of the valve prosthesis from annular insertion site. (From Josephson RA, Singer I, Levine JH, et. al. Systolic expansion of the aortic root: An echocardiographic and angiographic sign of aortic composite graft dehiscence. Cathet Cardiovasc Diagn 1988:14:105–107.)

include the aortic isthmus (the area just beyond the origin of the left subclavian artery) and the site of attachment of the aorta to the-heart. Angiography plays a major role in the evaluation of the patient thought to have a traumatic injury to the aorta and may be accomplished by the techniques described above. There may be an advantage to the utilization of intraarterial digital subtraction angiography, which may be performed faster, with less contrast material, and at a lower cost than conventional aortography (100). While aortography is considered the method of choice in evaluation of aortic laceration and is relatively safe, fatal complications may occur. It has been suggested that attempts to pursue aortography by the retrograde approach be abandoned if difficulty is encountered in passage of the guidewire or catheter in cases with suspected aortic trauma (101) (see Chapter 32).

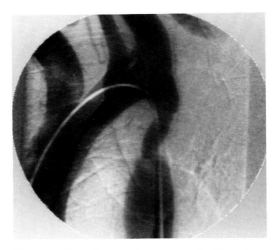

Figure 14.33. Coarctation restenosis. Digital angiogram revealing restenosis of a coarctation. Gradient across stenosis was 60 mm Hg.

Coarctation of the Aorta

Diagnosis of coarctation of the aorta in the adolescent and adult can usually be made clinically, although it may on occasion be missed when the patient presents with an associated disorder. We have "discovered" at catheterization significant coarctations in two such patients presenting with severe aortic insufficiency. Angiography is used to assess the precise location and length of the coarcted segment, the extent of collateral vessels, and the presence and significance of other cardiovascular abnormalities. Angiography is obviously necessary if percutaneous angioplasty is being considered and may be helpful in assessment of postsurgical or postangioplasty restenosis or aneurysm formation (102) (Fig. 14.33).

The coarcted segment of the aorta can often be negotiated from the retrograde approach using a soft steerable guidewire. In lieu of this, brachial arterial catheterization may be accomplished with relative ease. The aortic narrowing is well visualized by ascending aortography in the steep LAO projection. Evaluation by DSA may be helpful as might assessment of a transcoarctation pressure gradient that is a function of the severity of the narrowing and adequacy of collateralization. Magnetic resonance imaging has been shown to be useful in the diagnosis of coarctation and appears superior to the echocardiogram in children with this defect (103).

Systemic to Pulmonary Shunts

Communications from the systemic to pulmonary circulation may be congenital or acquired. Patent ductus arteriosus is the most common example of the former and is usually easily diagnosed on the basis of clinical and noninvasive study. Most adults with this disorder should probably undergo catheterization for hemodynamic and angiographic characterization. In many cases it is easy to pass through the ductus from either the pulmonary or aortic side. Ascending aortography filmed in the steep LAO projection demonstrates the defect well and affords evaluation of the length and width of the connection, which is of some importance to the surgeon.

Abdominal Aortography

Angiography of the abdominal aorta may be considered in the evaluation of abdominal aortic aneurysms (Fig. 14.34), dissections, stenosis (Fig. 14.35), clot, or branch integrity (Fig. 14.36). We most frequently perform this procedure to evaluate the distal circulation either because of a planned procedure (e.g., intraaortic balloon placement, aortic valvuloplasty, angioplasty) in a patient having clinical suspicion of disease or because of difficulty

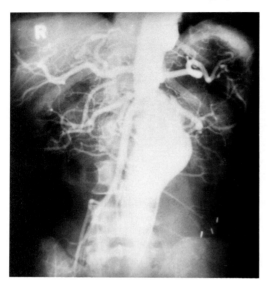

Figure 14.34. Abdominal aortic aneurysm. Aneurysm of the abdominal aorta with involvement of the renal arteries.

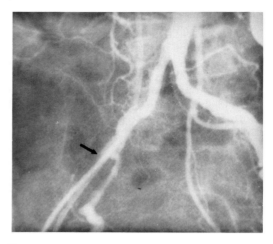

Figure 14.36. Cineangiographic frame revealing occlusion of the right external iliac artery by indwelling arterial sheath in a patient with right lower extremity pain following aortic valvuloplasty.

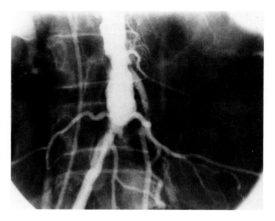

Figure 14.37. Occlusion of left iliac artery. Cineangiographic frame from distal aortogram obtained because of difficulty encountered during arterial entry in a patient undergoing coronary angiography. Total occlusion of the left iliac artery and atherosclerotic disease of the distal aorta and right iliac artery are noted.

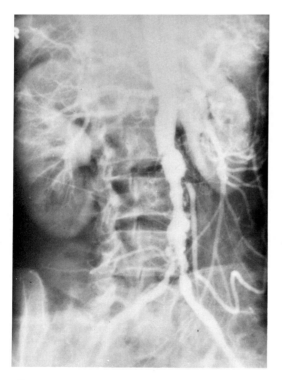

Figure 14.35. Atherosclerosis of aorta. Diffuse atherosclerotic narrowings in a patient with abdominal angina.

negotiating the lower aorta during routine catheterization (Fig. 14.37).

The role of routine abdominal aortography in evaluation of aneurysm is controversial (104-107). The diagnosis of this disorder and estimation of its size certainly does not rest with angiography, since physical examination, plain films of the abdomen, and ultrasonography are often adequate and have less risk.

More recently CT (108), MRI (109), and DSA (110) have been shown to be helpful and perhaps more advantageous than angiography in sizing the aneurysm. The angiogram does give information concerning extent of the aneurysm and the associated atherosclerotic process, including involvement of major branch vessels, such as the renal arteries, superior mesenteric, and iliofemoral system. The risk of the procedure is relatively small and may be successfully performed via the femoral retrograde approach. A pigtail catheter advanced over a wire may be used and is positioned at the level of the 12th thoracic vertebra. Alternatively, one of a number of catheters capable of providing aortic as well as more selective injections may be selected (111, 112).

Injection of 40 to 50 ml of contrast material over 2 sec is usually adequate with filming performed in the anterior-posterior and lateral views. On occasion, a repeat injection filmed in the right posterior oblique is necessary to evaluate the renal arteries properly (113). Serial cut filming may be superior to cineangiography, and the exposure sequence should stress early acquisition, with a total of 12 films recorded in each plane.

We have found cineangiography adequate and logistically simpler for the evaluation of the distal aorta and iliofemoral system, however. An injection of 8 to 15 cc/sec for a total of 20 to 40 cc is performed, depending on the size of the vessel and its run off. The anterior-posterior projection is utilized and filming at 30 to 60 frames/sec. The catheter is placed distal to the renal arteries, and the contrast material is followed down the iliofemoral system. Since these studies are painful, the use of low-osmolar contrast material is suggested. It is anticipated that there will be a growing interest in performance of peripheral vascular angioplasty to include the distal aorta (114, 115) by radiologists and cardiologists alike. Use of cineangiography and DSA will be applicable to these interventions. Although noninvasive techniques have been used to screen for aortoiliac disease, they are not as helpful as angiography (116).

ANGIOGRAPHY OF THE BRACHIOCEPHALIC SYSTEM

Suspected disorders of the brachiocephalic and extracranial cerebrovascular system may be evaluated angiographically as part of a cardiac catheterization procedure. We have used DSA to delineate the carotid arteries in patients with symptomatic cerebrovascular disease as well as those with asymptomatic neck bruits. While this technique does not achieve the resolution of selective carotid angiography, it may suffice to reveal or exclude hemodynamically significant stenoses (Fig. 14.38). Upon completion of the cardiac procedure, a pigtail catheter is placed in the ascending aorta, and the digital study is performed by injection of dilute contrast material that limits the total dye exposure to an acceptable dose. A 50% dilution of 60% sodium meglumine diatrizoate with 5% dextrose in water is most commonly used, although a similar dilution of a low-osmolar agent may by substituted. A total of 40 cc injected over 2 sec is used for each injection. The aortic arch and origin of the great vessels are imaged first in the 45° LAO view. To adequately evaluate the carotid arteries it is necessary to visualize these vessels in two projections in which the vertebral arteries have been rotated so that there is no overlap of the carotid bifurcations. This is accomplished by obtaining both RAO and LAO views (45 to 60°) of the neck. The success of this technique depends upon the ability of the patient to cooperate. Images may be severely degraded if the patient is unable to suspend respiration or refrain from swallowing during the examination.

The increased utilization of the internal mammary artery as a conduit for coronary bypass makes it essential that the cardiologist be able to perform selective angiography of this vessel in postoperative studies, as well as preoperatively if its integrity is suspect (see Chapter 13). Flow through the mammary may be compromised by disease proximal to its origin, and assessment of the subclavian artery may be indicated during catheterization, especially if there is a significant blood pressure differential (117)(Fig. 14.39).

MISCELLANEOUS ANGIOGRAPHY

The cardiologist may have need to visualize vessels for reasons other than those delineated above. This can usually be safely and easily performed utilizing the same general principles. Angiography may be used to

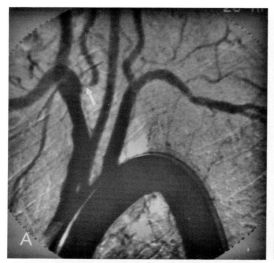

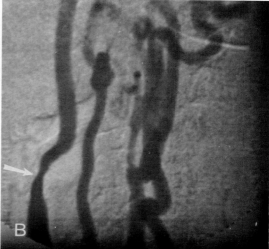

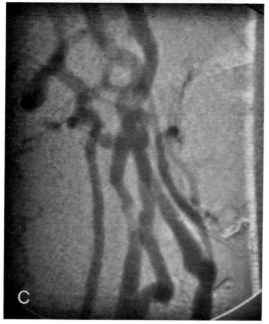

Figure 14.38. Sequence of intraarterial digital carotid angiography. Aortic arch, imaged first, reveals stenosis of right vertebral artery (*A, arrow*). LAO view of carotids (second injection, *B*) reveals stenosis of right internal carotid (*arrow*) and flush occlusion of external carotid. Third injection filmed in the RAO view "unwraps" left carotid system (*C*).

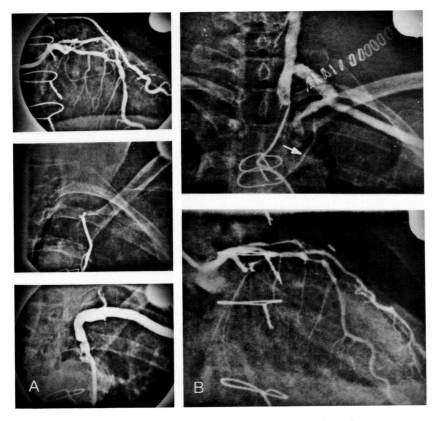

Figure 14.39. Subclavian artery stenosis. Patient with angina postinternal mammary artery bypass to left anterior descending artery (LAD). Injection of the left coronary artery demonstrated retrograde filling of the graft to the subclavian artery. Selective injection of the subclavian artery revealed stenosis with no antegrade flow through the left internal mammary artery (LIMA) (*A, top, middle,* and *bottom,* respectively). After carotid-to-subclavian shunting, there is antegrade flow through the mammary (*B, arrowhead*) while it fails to opacify via native coronary injection. (From McIvor ME, Williams GM, Brinker JA. Subclavian-coronary steal thorugh a LIMA-to-LAD bypass graft. Cathet Cardiovasc Diagn 1988;14:100–104.)

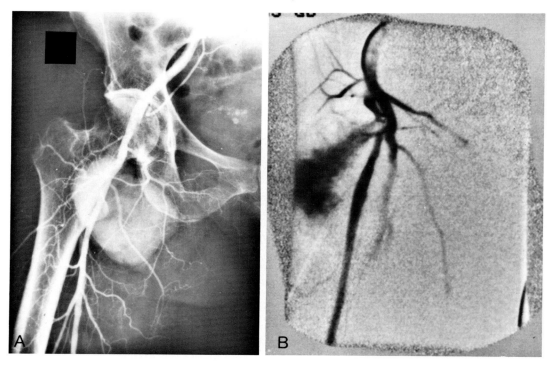

Figure 14.40. False aneurysm of the superficial femoral artery. Patient developed expanding hematoma after withdrawal of intraaortic balloon. Contrast is seen entering hematoma on femoral angiography *(A)* and DSA *(B).*

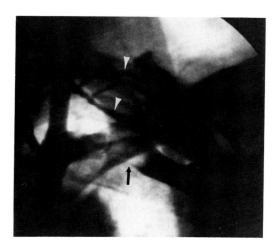

Figure 14.41. Thrombotic occlusion of right subclavian vein. Venography was obtained by injection of contrast through indwelling antecubital IV after unsuccessful percutaneous attempts to enter subclavian vein for pacemaker insertion. Subclavian occlusion *(arrow)* and collaterals *(arrowheads)* are well seen in this digital fluoroscopic image.

evaluate a complication of a previous interventional procedure (Fig. 14.40), and it may be of assistance in performance of other procedures. We have, for instance, found it helpful during permanent pacemaker implantation to inject contrast material through a peripheral vein in order to visualize the subclavian system when the latter could not be entered by "blind" puncture. Digital acquisition of the image may allow roadmapping and facilitate the procedure, or may document occlusion, thereby preventing potentially dangerous persistent attempts at entry (Fig. 14.41).

References

1. Dalen JE, Brooks HL, Johnson LW, Meister SG, Szucs Jr MM, Dexter L. Pulmonary angiography in acute pulmonary embolism: indications, techniques, and results in 367 patients. Am Heart J 1971; 81: 175–185.
2. Moser KM. Pulmonary embolism. Am Rev Respir Dis 1977; 115: 829-852.
3. McIntyre KM, Sasahara AA. Hemodynamic alterations related to extent of lung scan perfusion defect in pulmonary embolism. J Nucl Med 1971; 12: 166-170.

4. McIntyre KM, Sasahara AA. The hemodynamic response to pulmonary embolism in patients without prior cardiopulmonary disease. Am J Cardiol 1971; 28: 288-294.
5. Alpert JS, Smith R, Carlson J, Ockene IS, Dexter L, Dalen JE. Mortality in patients treated for pulmonary embolism. JAMA 1976; 236: 1477-1480.
6. Mills SR, Jackson DC, Older RA, Heaston DK, Moore AV. The incidence, etiology, and avoidance of complications of pulmonary angiography in a large series. Radiology 1980; 136: 295-299.
7. Ferris EJ, Athanasoulis CA, Clapp PR. Inferior vena cavography correlated with pulmonary angiography. Chest 1971; 59: 651-653.
8. Stein MA, Winter J, Grollman JH Jr. The value of the pulmonary artery-seeking catheter in percutaneous selective pulmonary arteriography. Radiology 1975; 114: 299-304.
9. Grollman JH Jr, Gyepes MT, Helmer E. Transfemoral selective bilateral pulmonary arteriography with a pulmonary artery-seeking catheter. Radiology 1970; 96: 202–204.
10. Mills CS, Van Aman ME. Modified technique for percutaneous transfemoral pulmonary angiography. Cardiovasc Intervent Radiol 1986; 9: 52-53.
11. Courey WR, de Villasante JM, Waltman AC. A quick, simple method of percutaneous transfemoral pulmonary arteriography. Radiology 1974; 113: 475-477.
12. Grollman JH, Renner JW. Transfemoral pulmonary angiography: update on technique. AJR 1981; 136: 624-626.
13. Tempkin DL, Ladika JE. New catheter design and placement technique for pulmonary arterography. Radiology 1987; 163: 275-276.
14. Bookstein JJ. Segmental arteriography in pulmonary embolism. Radiology 1969; 93: 1007-1013.
15. Johnson BA, James AE, White RI Jr. Oblique and selective pulmonary angiography in diagnosis of pulmonary embolism. AJR 1973; 118: 801-808.
16. Bookstein JJ, Feigin DS, Seo KW, Alazraki NP. Diagnosis of pulmonary embolism: experimental evaluation of the accuracy of scintigraphically guided pulmonary arteriography. Radiology 1980; 136: 15-23.
17. Novelline RA, Baltarowich QH, Athanasoulis CA, Waltman AC, Greenfield AJ, McKusick KA. The clinical course of patients with suspected pulmonary embolism and a negative pulmonary arteriogram. Radiology 1978; 126: 561-567.
18. Watson J. Severe pulmonary hypertensive episodes following angiocardiography with sodium metrizoate. Lancet 1964; 2: 732-733.
19. Goodman PC, Brant-Zawadzki M. Digital subtraction pulmonary angiography. AJR 1982; 139: 305-309.
20. Bynum LJ, Wilson JE, Christensen EE, Sorensen C. Radiographic techniques for balloon-occlusion pulmonary angiography. Radiology 1979; 133: 518-520.
21. Meister SG, Brooks HL, Szucs MM, Banas JS Jr, Dexter L, Dalen JE. Pulmonary cineangiography in acute pulmonary embolism. Am Heart J 1972; 84: 33-37.
22. Pond GD, Ovitt TW, Capp MP. Comparison of conventional pulmonary angiography with intravenous digital subtraction angiography for pulmonary embolic disease. Radiology 1983; 147: 345-350.
23. Ludwig JW, Verhoeuen LA, Kersbergen JJ, Overtoom TT. Digital subtraction angiography of the pulmonary arteries for the diagnosis of pulmonary embolism. Radiology 1983; 147: 639-645.
24. Ferris EJ, Holder JC, Lim WM, et al. Angiography of pulmonary emboli: digital studies and balloon-occlusion cineangiography. AJR 1984; 142: 369–373.
25. White RI Jr, Mitchell SE, Barth KH, et al. Angioarchitecture of pulmonary arteriovenous malformations: an important consideration before embolotherapy. AJR 1983; 140: 681-686.
26. Greene R, Zapol WM, Snider MT, et al. Early bedside detection of pulmonary vascular occlusion during acute respiratory failure. Am Rev Respir Dis 1981; 124: 593-601.
27. Dougherty JE, LaSala AF, Fieldman A. Bedside pulmonary angiography utilizing an existing Swan-Ganz catheter. Chest 1980; 77: 43-46.
28. LePage JR, Garcia RM. The value of bedside wedge pulmonary angiography in the detection of pulmonary emboli: a predictive and prospective evaluation. Radiology 1982; 144: 67-73.
29. The urokinase pulmonary embolism trial. Circulation 1973; 47: II1-108.
30. Bell WR, Simon TL. A comparative analysis of pulmonary perfusion scans with pulmonary angiograms. Am Heart J 1976; 92: 700-706.
31. Dalen JE, Alpert JS. Natural history of pulmonary embolism. Prog Cardiovasc Dis 1975; 17: 259-270.
32. Alpert JS, Smith R, Carlson J, Ockene IS, Dexter L, Dalen JE. Mortality in patients treated for pulmonary embolism. JAMA 1976; 236: 1477-1480.
33. Robin ED. Overdiagnosis and overtreatment of pulmonary embolism: the emperor may have no clothes. Ann Intern Med 1977; 87: 775-781.
34. Stein PD, Willis PW, Dalen JE. Importance of clinical assessment in selecting patients for pulmonary arteriography. Am J Cardiol 1979; 43: 669-671.
35. Kipper MS, Moser KM, Kortman KE, Ashburn WL. Longterm follow-up of patients with suspected pulmonary embolism and a normal lung scan. Perfusion scans in embolic suspects. Chest 1982; 82: 411-415.
36. Alderson PO, Doppman JL, Diamond SS, Mendenhall KG, Barron EL, Girton M. Ventilation-perfusion lung imaging and selective pulmonary angiography in dogs with experimental pulmonary embolism. J Nucl Med 1978; 19: 164-171.
37. McNeil BJ. A diagnostic strategy using ventilation-perfusion studies in patients suspected for pulmonary embolism. J Nucl Med 1976; 17: 613-616.
38. Biello DR, Mattar AG, McKnight RC, Siegel BA. Ventilation-perfusion studies in suspected pulmonary embolism. AJR 1979; 133: 1033-1037.
39. Alderson PO, Rujanavech N, Sicker-Walker RH, McKnight RC, et al. The role of 133 Xe ventilation studies in the scintigraphic detection of pulmonary embolism. Radiology 1976; 120: 633-640.
40. Neumann RD, Sostman HD, Gottschalk A. Current status of ventilation-perfusion imaging. Semin Nucl Med 1980; 10: 198-217.

41. Moses DC, Silver TM, Bookstein JJ. The complimentary role of chest radiography, lung scanning and selective pulmonary angiography in the diagnosis of pulmonary embolism. Circulation 1974; 49: 179-188.

42. Hull RD, Hirsh J, Carter CJ, et al. Pulmonary angiography, ventilation lung scanning, and venography for clinically suspected pulmonary embolism with abnormal perfusion lung scan. Ann Intern Med 1983; 98: 891-899.

43. Alderson PO, Biello DR, Khan AR, Barth KH, McKnight RC, Siegel BA. Scintigraphic detection of pulmonary embolism in patients with obstructive lung disease. Radiology 1981; 138: 661-666.

44. Cavaluzzi JA, Alderson PO, White RI. Pulmonary embolism with unilateral lung scan defects and matching infiltrates. J Can Assoc Radiol 1979; 30: 162-164.

45. Fred HL, Axelrad MA, Lewis JM, Alexander JK, et al. Rapid resolution of pulmonary thromboemboli in man. An angiographic study. JAMA 1966; 196: 1137-1139.

46. Murphy ML, Bullock H. Factors influencing the restoration of blood flow following pulmonary embolization as determined by angiography and scanning. Circulation 1968; 38: 1116-1126.

47. Weidner W, Swanson L, Wilson G. Roentgen techniques in the diagnosis of pulmonary thromboembolism. AJR 1967; 100: 397-407.

48. Sagel SS, Greenspan RH. Non-uniform pulmonary artery perfusion. Radiology 1971; 99: 541-548.

49. Bookstein JJ, Silver TM. The angiographic differential diagnosis of pulmonary embolism. Radiology 1974; 110: 25-33.

50. Mills SR, Jackson DC, Sullivan DC, et al. Angiographic evaluation of chronic pulmonary embolism. Radiology 1980; 136: 301-308.

51. Dines DE, Arms RA, Bernatz PE, Gomes MR. Pulmonary arteriovenous fistulas. Mayo Clin Proc 1974; 49: 460-465.

52. Fox LS, Buntain WL, Brasfield D, Tiller R, Lynn HB, Longino LA. Pulmonary arteriovenous malformations in children. J Pediatr Surg 1979; 14: 53-57.

53. Terry PB, Barth KH, Kaufman SL, White RI. Balloon embolization for treatment of pulmonary arteriovenous fistulas. N Engl J Med 1980; 302: 1189-1190.

54. Barth KH, White RI Jr, Kaufman SL, Terry PB, Roland JM. Embolotherapy of pulmonary arteriovenous malformations with detachable balloons. Radiology 1982; 142: 599-606.

55. Taylor BG, Cockerill EM, Manfredi F, Klatte EC. Therapeutic embolization of the pulmonary artery in pulmonary arteriovenous fistula. Am J Med 1978; 54: 360-365.

56. Jonsson K, Hellekant C, Olsson O, Holen O. Percutaneous transcatheter occlusion of pulmonary arteriovenous malformation. Ann Radiol 1988; 23: 335-337.

57. Platia EV, Brinker JA. Scimitar syndrome with peripheral left pulmonary artery branch stenoses. Am Heart J 1984; 107: 594-596.

58. McGaughey MD, Traill TA, Brinker JA. Partial left anomalous pulmonary venous return: a diagnostic dilemma. Cathet Cardiovasc Diagn 1986; 12: 110-115.

59. Arlart IP, Bargon G, Sigel H. Anomalous intrapulmonal vein drainage and pulmonary vein connection in DSA. Eur J Radiol 1986; 6: 12-14.

60. Kucera V, Fiser B, Tuma S, Hucin B. Unilateral absence of pulmonary artery: a report on 19 selected clinical cases. Thorac Cardiovasc Surg 1982; 30: 152-158.

61. Kleinman PK. Pleural telangiectasia and absence of a pulmonary artery. Radiology 1979; 132: 281-284.

62. Lekuona I, Cabrera A, Inguanzo R, Cid C, Agosti J. Direct communication between the right pulmonary artery and left atrium. Thorax 1986; 41: 78-79.

63. Stone DN, Bein ME, Garris JB. Anomalous left pulmonary artery: two new adult cases. AJR 1980; 135: 1259-1263.

64. Davis SD, Neithamer CD, Schreiber TS, Sos TA. False pulmonary artery aneurysm induced by Swan-Ganz catheter: diagnosis and embolotherapy. Radiology 1987; 164: 741-742.

65. Dillon WP, Taylor AT, Mineau DE, Datz FL. Traumatic pulmonary artery pseudoaneurysm simulating pulmonary embolism. AJR 1982; 139: 818-819, 1982.

66. Arom KV, Richardson JD, Grover FL, Ferris G, Trinkle JK. Pulmonary artery aneurysm. Am Surg 1978; 44: 688-692.

67. Hynes J, Smith HC, Holmes DR, Edwards WD, Evans TC Jr, Orszulak TA. Preoperative angiographic diagnosis of primary sarcoma of the pulmonary artery. Circulation 1982; 66: 672-674.

68. Bowen JS, Bookstein JJ, Johnson AD, Peterson KL, Moser KM. Wedge and subselective pulmonary angiography in pulmonary hypertension secondary to venous obstruction. Radiology 1985; 155: 599-603.

69. Tadavarthy SM, Klugman J, Castaneda-Zuniga WR, Nath PH, Amplatz K. Systemic-to-pulmonary collaterals in pathological states. A review. Radiology 1982; 144: 55-59.

70. Kirklin JW, Bargeron LM, Pacifico AD. The enlargement of small pulmonary arteries by preliminary palliative operations. Circulation 1977; 56: 612-617.

71. Flisak ME, Chandrasekar AJ, Marsan RE, Ali MM. Systemic arterialization of lung without sequestration. AJR 1982; 138: 751-753.

72. Eriksson S, Osterman G, Asplund K, et al. Pulmonary-artery cineangiocardiography to demonstrate cardiac thrombi in patients with cerebral infarction. Acta Neurol Scand 1984; 69: 27-33.

73. McIvor ME, Kaufman SL, Satre S, Porterfield JK, Brinker JA. Search and retrieval of an unidentifiable foreign object. Cathet Cardiovasc Diagn, in press, 1988

74. Pyeritz RE, Stolle CA, Parfrey NA, Myers JC. Ehlers-Danlos syndrome IV due to a novel defect in type III procollagen. Am J Med Gen 1984; 19: 607-622.

75. White TJ, Pinstein ML, Scott RL, Gold RE. Aortic dissection manifested as leg ischemia. AJR 1980; 135: 353-356.

76. Eagle KA, Quertermous T, Kritzer, et al. Spectrum

of conditions initially suggesting acute aortic dissection but with negative aortograms. Am J Cardiol 1986; 57: 322-326.

77. Bondestam S, Hekali P, Landtman M. Sonographic diagnosis of dissection of the descending thoracic aorta. Ann Chir Gynaecol 1981; 70: 210-212.

78. Matsumoto M, Matsuo H, Ohara T, Yoshioka S, Abe H. A two-dimensional echoaortocardiographic approach to dissecting aneurysms of the aorta to prevent false-positive diagnoses. Radiology 1978; 127: 491-499.

79. Erbel R, Borner N, Steller D, et al. Detection of aortic dissection by transoesophageal echocardiography. Br Heart J 1987; 58: 45-51.

80. Goldman AP, Kotler MN, Scanlon MH, Ostrum B, Parameswaran R, Parry WR. The complementary role of magnetic resonance imaging, Doppler echocardiography, and computed tomography in the diagnosis of dissecting thoracic aneurysms. Am Heart J 1986; 5: 970-981.

81. Hitter H, Ranquin R, Mortelmans L, Parizel G. Diagnosis of aortic dissection. Comparison of investigatory methods—case report. Angiology 1987; 38: 859-863.

82. White RD, Lipton MJ, Higgins CB, et al. Noninvasive evaluation of suspected thoracic aortic disease by contrast-enhanced computed tomography. Am J Cardiol 1986; 57: 282-290.

83. Heiberg E, Wolverson M, Sundaram M, Connors J, Susman N. CT findings in thoracic aortic dissection. AJR 1981; 136: 13-17.

84. Godwin JD, Herfkens RL, Skioldebrand CG, Federle MP, Lipton MJ. Evaluation of dissections and aneurysms of the thoracic aorta by conventional and dynamic CT scanning. Radiology 1980; 136: 125-133.

85. Hekali P, Velt P, Gutierrez O, Tottemann S, Mare K. Radiology of aortic dissection: pitfalls in diagnosis. Eur J Radiol 1986; 6: 314-318.

86. Goodwin JD, Breiman RS, Speckman JM. Problems and pitfalls in the evaluation of thoracic aortic dissection by computed tomography. J Comput Assist Tomogr 1982; 6: 750-756.

87. Egan TJ, Neiman HL, Herman RJ, Malave SR, Sanders JH. Computed tomography in the diagnosis of aortic aneurysm dissection or traumatic injury. Radiology 1980; 136: 141-146.

88. Pernes JM, Grenier P, Desbleds MT, de Brux JL. MR evaluation of chronic aortic dissection. J Comput Assist Tomogr 1987; 11: 975–981.

89. Dinsmore RE, Wedeen VJ, Miller SW, et al. MRI of dissection of the aorta: recognition of the intimal tear and differential flow velocities. AJR 1986; 146: 1286–1288.

90. Amparo EG, Higgins CB, Hricak H, Sollitto R. Aortic dissection: magnetic resonance imaging. Radiology 1985; 155: 399-406.

91. Crane AR. Primary multiocular mycotic aneurysms of the aorta. Arch Pathol 1937; 24: 634-641.

92. Brown SL, Busuttil RW, Baker JD, Machleder HI, Moore WS, Barker WF. Bacteriologic and surgical determinants of survival in patients with mycotic aneurysms. J Vasc Surg 1985; 1: 541-548.

93. Desai AG, Sharma S, Kumar A, et al. Echocardiographic diagnosis of unruptured aneurysm of

right sinus of Valsalva: an unusual cause of right ventricular outflow obstruction. Am Heart J 1985; 109: 363-364.

94. Terdjman M, Bourdarias J-P, Farcot H-C, et al. Aneurysms of sinus of Valsalva: two-dimensional echocardiographic diagnosis and recognition of rupture into the right heart cavities. J Am Coll Cardiol 1984; 3: 1227-1235.

95. Sakakibara S, Donno S. Congenital aneurysm of sinus of Valsalva. A clinical study. Am Heart J 1962; 63: 708-719.

96. Lemon DK, White C. Annuloaortic ectasia: angiographic, hemodynamic and clinical comparison with aortic valve insufficiency. Am J Cardiol 1978; 41: 482-486.

97. Murdoch JL, Walker BA, Halpern BL, Kuzma JW, McKusick VA. Life expectancy and causes of death in the Marfan's syndrome. N Engl J Med 1972; 286: 804-808.

98. Bentall H, Debono A. A technique for complete replacement of the ascending aorta. Thorax 1968; 23: 338-339.

99. Nath PH, Zollikofer C, Castaneda-Zuniga WR, et al. Radiological evaluation of composite aortic grafts. Radiology 1979; 131: 43-51.

100. Josephson RA, Singer I, Levine JH, et al. Systolic expansion of the aortic root: An echocardiographic and angiographic sign of aortic composite graft dehiscence. Cathet Cardiovasc Diagn 1988; 14: 105-107.

101. Mirvis SE, Pais SO, Gens DR. Thoracic aortic rupture: advantages of intraarterial digital subtraction angiography. AJR 1986; 146: 987-991.

102. LaBerge JM, Jeffrey RB. Aortic lacerations: fatal complications of thoracic aortography. Radiology 1987; 165: 367-369.

103. Clark RA, Colley DP, Siedlecki E. Late complications at repair site of operated coarctation of aorta. AJR 1979; 133: 1071-1075.

104. Fletcher BD, Jacobstein MD. MRI of congenital abnormalities of the great arteries. AJR 1986; 146: 941-948.

105. Baur GM, Porter JM, Eidemiller LR, Rosch J, Keller F. The role of arteriography in abdominal aortic aneurysm. Am J Surg 1978; 136: 184-189.

106. Bell DD , Gaspar MR. Routine aortography before abdominal aortic aneurysmectomy. A prospective study. Am J Surg 1982; 144: 191-193.

107. Nuno IN, Collins GM, Bardin JA, Bernstein EF. Should aortography be used routinely in the elective management of abdominal aortic aneurysm? Am J Surg 1982; 144: 53-57.

108. Eriksson I, Forsberg JO, Hemmingsson A, Lindgren PG. Preoperative evaluation of abdominal aortic aneurysms: Is there a need for aortography? Acta Chir Scand 1981; 147: 533-537.

109. Johnson WC, Paley RH, Castronuovo JJ, et al. Computed tomographic angiography. Am J Surg 1981; 141: 434-440.

110. Flak B, Li DKB, Ho BYB, et al. Magnetic resonance imaging of aneurysms of the abdominal aorta. AJR 1985; 144: 991-996.

111. Passariello R, Simonetti G, Rossi P, et al. Angiographic characterization of aortic aneurysms by digital intravenous angiography. Ann Radiol 1983; 26: 599-600.

112. Hawkins IF, Haseman MK, Gelfand FN. Single mini-catheter technique for abdominal aortography and selective injection. Radiology 1979; 132: 755-757.

113. Kogutt MS, Jander H. Use of a curved multi-hole catheter for abdominal and femoral arteriography. Radiology 1978; 128: 817-818.

114. Gerlock AJ, Goncharenko V, Sloan OM. Right posterior oblique: the projection of choice in aortography of hypertensive patients. Radiology 1978; 127: 45-48.

115. Grollman JH, Del Vicario M, Mittal AK. Percutaneous transluminal abdominal aortic angioplasty. AJR 1980; 134: 1053-1054.

116. Khalilullah M, Tyagi S, Lochan R, et al. Percutaneous transluminal balloon angioplasty of the aorta in patients with aortitis. Circulation 1987; 76: 597-600.

117. Limpert JD, Vogelzang RL, Yao JST. Computed tomography of aortoiliac atherosclerosis. J Vasc Surg 1987; 5: 814-819.

118. McIvor ME, Williams GM, Brinker J. Subclavian-coronary steal through a LIMA-to-LAD bypass graft. Cathet Cardiovasc Diagn 1988; 14: 100-104.

15

Coronary Angioplasty

George N. Vetrovec, M.D.

INTRODUCTION

Coronary angioplasty has made a major impact on the management of coronary artery disease. Beginning as a procedure for patients with very specific, ideal lesions, the technique has evolved dramatically. With evolution of more sophisticated equipment and increased operator experience, there has been greater applicability of angioplasty in the management of coronary artery disease. Thus selected patients with multiple vessel disease, total occlusions, tandem lesions, and complex branch disease are now potential candidates for angioplasty. Operator experience and skill in catheter and guidewire manipulation clearly contribute to the high success rates in complex anatomy. However, an equally important component is appropriate case selection principally based on careful angiographic review of lesion morphology, as well as extent of coronary artery disease and left ventricular function. Furthermore, during and after angioplasty, high quality coronary angiography is important to define lesion morphology, branch anatomy, and adjacent vessels. Thus, the outcome of coronary angioplasty is the product of multiple factors, including operator technical skill, appropriate case selection, familiarity and use of equipment to expedite and facilitate the procedure, as well as the use of high quality angiographic techniques to identify vessel anatomy and lesion morphology.

This chapter will present a rational approach to case selection, equipment utilization, and patient management for coronary angioplasty.

PATIENT SELECTION

Patient selection is the most important aspect of coronary angioplasty. Recognizing high risk patients, equipment limitations, and extent of operator experience are all important. Although applications of angioplasty have expanded dramatically, these advances have principally been accomplished in centers with significant experience and expertise. Operator training, experience, and procedure volume must be considered as parts of case selection. Early angioplasty experience documented the impact of a "learning curve" on angioplasty outcome in routine, principally single-vessel disease patients (1, 2). The concept continues to apply particularly to more complex procedures today. Thus, the following patient selection description must be viewed as representing an "ideal" for experienced operators, emphasizing the wide range of potential applications in appropriate circumstances.

Routine Angioplasty

Ideal indications for coronary angioplasty remain as described by Andreas Gruentzig (3): discrete, noncalcified, isolated, proximal, single-vessel lesions in symptom-limited patients who are good candidates for bypass surgery. Today, such lesions have success rates of 90 to 95% while serious complications, such as need for emergency coronary bypass surgery, are infrequent ($\pm 4\%$) (4, 5). These very favorable results have lead to the practice of recommending that patients with single-vessel disease be managed with angioplasty while coronary bypass surgery is recommended for patients with more extensive disease. The number of "ideal" candidates for routine coronary angioplasty represents a small portion of the overall coronary artery disease population.

Complex Coronary Angioplasty

The marked increase in use of angioplasty in the management of coronary artery disease has resulted from inclusion of patients with more complex disease. For example at the Medical College of Virginia, the overwhelming majority of angioplasty procedures are performed on patients with complex anatomic disease. Complex disease is defined as tandem lesions, branch obstructions, nonacute total occlusions, long or diffuse lesions, and multivessel obstructions. Expanded applications for "complex" coronary angioplasty are summarized in Table 15.1.

Table 15.1.
Expanded Applications for Elective Coronary Angioplasty: "Complex" Coronary Angioplasty

Multivessel disease
Tandem lesions
Long lesion or diffuse-vessel disease
Complex branch lesions
Nonacute total occlusions
High-risk "salvage" angioplasty
   Nonsurgical candidates
   Severe left ventricular depression
Postbypass surgery
   Grafts
   Native arteries

Important principles regarding patient selection for complex angioplasty are summarized in Table 15.2. The goal of angioplasty is to revascularize all major areas of the myocardium. Thus, all lesions should be technically feasible. Likewise, to maximize safety, the risk of cardiogenic shock associated with acute vessel occlusion should be minimized by avoiding dilatation of single lesions supplying most of the myocardium through collaterals to other occluded vessel segments. Such lesions can become a "left main" equivalent in terms of relative risk. However, risk can often be reduced by a logical lesion dilatation sequence. Likewise, to avoid multiple-vessel acute closure, staged procedures frequently increase safety. An example is a patient with

recent left anterior descending occlusion, but with residual anterior myocardium in jeopardy, whose distal anterior descending is collateralized from the right coronary artery, which has a proximal 80% stenosis. Here, left anterior descending dilatation should be attempted first. If successful, the patient should be observed for approximately 24 hours and then only after angiographic documentation of a persistently adequate anterior descending dilatation should the right coronary artery lesion be attempted. Use of these principles significantly enhances the safety and adequacy of angioplasty, particularly in patients with complex or multiple-vessel disease.

Tandem or Long Lesions

With currently available steerable guidewires and low profile balloon catheters, most patent lesions can be traversed despite their length, tortuosity, or calcification. One exception is a patent but long recanalized lesion. This may be very difficult or impossible to cross. Such lesions are frequently seen late in patent but previous infarction-related arteries and are characterized angiographically by very narrow, irregular, tortuous channels. However, for most tandem or long lesions, success is only slightly lower and acute complications slightly higher, as compared with that of routine lesions.

Although dilatation of long or diffusely diseased lesions is frequently feasible, important aspects of patient selection also include the patient's response to medical treatment, the extent of myocardium in jeopardy, and the feasibility of bypass surgery for revascularization of the same vessel. Many times the diffuse disease, which makes angioplasty less ideal, may likewise reduce the feasibility of bypass surgery. So the risk/benefit ratio of angioplasty vs. other treatments like bypass

Table 15.2.
Complex Angioplasty Selection Factors

Technical feasibility of each lesion
Limited or protected myocardium in distribution
   of each lesion attempted
Feasibility of bypass surgery as an alternative
   treatment
General factors: age, activity, and response to
   medical treatment

surgery is an important concept in case selection of patients with complex disease. Such choices frequently involve multiple factors, only one of which is the potential success of lesion dilatation.

Branch Lesions

Risk of damage to lesion-associated branches during major vessel dilatation may be 25 to 30% if the ostium of the branch is involved in the disease process (6, 7). In contrast, branches without ostial disease or branches in the area of balloon inflation but not in the lesion itself are at relatively low risk (4%, <1%, respectively) (6, 7) for damage during angioplasty. Protection of major branch vessels, using techniques for simultaneous primary vessel and branch access with dual wires and/or balloons, is necessary in many circumstances (see Figs. 15.1–15.3). Dual access techniques provide a safe and effective means to maximally revascularize complex Y lesions (8, 9), although the expected success rate may be slightly lower than for routine angioplasty.

Nonacute Total Occlusions

Successful dilatation of nonacute total occlusions is frequently possible, but the success rate is lower than for stenotic lesions (10, 11). Success rates for total occlusions differ, based on the duration of occlusion. More recent total occlusions, usually measured in days, have a much higher success rate, often approaching the success rate for patent lesions. More chronic total occlusions have a substantially lower success rate of 50 to 60%. Success is primarily determined by the ability to freely cross the lesion with a guidewire. Ischemia-related complication rates are low, as the vessel is already occluded, although potential risks include adjacent vessel occlusion secondary to dissection or embolization of clot dislodged from the occluded artery (12). The latter is more common in recent total occlusions. Finally, restenosis rates appear somewhat higher in nonacute total occlusions (10). Despite these limitations, many patients, particularly those with recent total occlusions and significant amounts of myocardium in

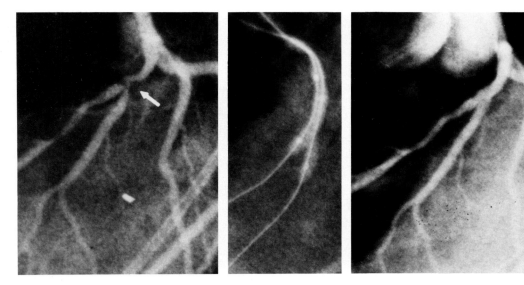

Figure 15.1. Complex angioplasty. Management of branch lesions using two balloons and two guiding catheters. *Left panel* reveals a severe stenosis involving both the left anterior descending and diagonal branches with a secondary or tandem lesion in the midanterior descending. *Middle panel* reveals a simultaneous "kissing" balloon inflation, utilizing a dual-wire technique. *Right panel* illustrates the final result.

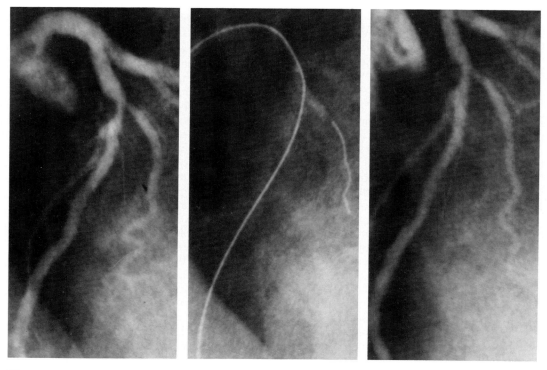

Figure 15.2. Complex angioplasty. Management of branch disease, utilizing a single guiding catheter, with an alternate balloon inflation, combining an "over-the-wire" balloon system for the anterior descending (*middle panel*) with a "nonover-the-wire," steerable balloon for the diagonal branch. The *right* and *left panels* illustrate the pre- and postdilatation findings, respectively.

Figure 15.3. An unusually complex dilatation involving bifurcation disease of the distal right, posterior descending, and posterolateral bifurcation stenosis. A dual guiding catheter approach permitted simultaneous balloon inflation. Newer large, lumen guide catheter and/or small steerable balloon systems allow dual inflation procedures without need for dual arterial access.

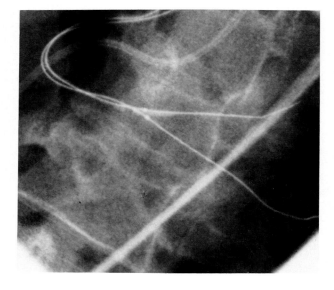

jeopardy can benefit from angioplasty. However, performing the procedure as early as possible following suspected total occlusion is important. Hopefully, newer modalities, such as laser angioplasty and/or atherectomy will enhance success rates, particularly in patients with the more chronic total occlusions.

High-Risk Angioplasty

A major component in patient selection for "high-risk" or "salvage" angioplasty is the risk/benefit ratio of alternative treatment. The historical and angiographic findings of high-risk patients should be reviewed by a cardiac surgeon and the interventionalist. There should be agreement on the plan, particularly with regard to any circumstance in which the patient would be considered for emergency surgery. Furthermore, the patient and family must understand and agree to the potential risks. However, in patients with disabling ischemia-related symptoms, unresponsive to medical management, who have other major life-threatening diseases that increase the risk or preclude long-term benefits from surgical revascularization, coronary angioplasty provides a useful alternative.

A subcategory of high-risk angioplasty includes patients for whom the risk of surgical revascularization appears inordinately high because of severe depression of ventricular function, with ejection fractions frequently <25%. For example, 15 patients with a <30% ejection fraction who were considered poor candidates for bypass surgery underwent high-risk angioplasty at the Medical College of Virginia in the last year. Successful dilatation was achieved in all 24 lesions attempted in 20 vessels. This was a highly selected population of patients with refractory unstable angina despite aggressive medical management and ideal anatomy for angioplasty. During hospitalization after angioplasty, all patients experienced less or no angina with only one in-hospital death secondary to pulmonary edema without myocardial infarction. Thus, in highly selected patients with depressed left ventricular function, angioplasty can provide revascularization with clinical stabilization. As success rates for angioplasty continue to improve, the potential application of angioplasty in patients with poor left ventricular function may increase. As the risk of bypass surgery is also higher in patients with abnormal ventricular function (13), angioplasty may become a more frequently recommended treatment in carefully selected patients with severe depression of left ventricular function.

Angioplasty following Bypass Surgery

Dilatation of postbypass surgery patients is quite useful to extend the effectiveness of the operation (14, 15). Angioplasty is potentially effective to dilate graft body lesions, graft insertion site lesions, and particularly, native vessel coronary stenoses, either distal to the graft insertion or in previously ungrafted

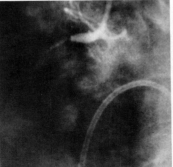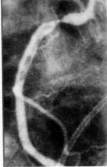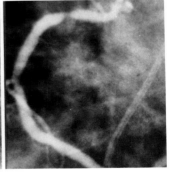

Figure 15.4. Intracoronary thrombolysis during acute myocardial infarction. *Left panel* illustrates total right coronary artery occlusion shortly after the onset of acute myocardial infarction. After 125,000 units of intracoronary streptokinase, there is reperfusion with significant residual thrombus remaining (*middle panel*). Finally, *right panel* illustrates resolution of the large thrombus. A severe residual stenosis that is a cause of early reclosure in many instances following thrombolytic therapy remains. (From Vetrovec GW: Thrombolysis in early transmural myocardial infarction. Postgrad Med 1985;77:60.)

arteries (16). The latter lesions are associated with success and restenosis rates that are comparable to routine angioplasty. However, graft ostial and body stenoses have a high early recurrence rate approaching 50%. Furthermore, dilatation of diffusely diseased or long, irregular graft lesions should be avoided because of the high risk that local-lipid laden and thrombotic material may embolize distally. This material is less amenable to thrombolytic therapy than is the more usual arterial thrombus seen in a native vessel. Avoiding patients at risk for graft debris embolization significantly reduces the risk of graft body angioplasty. Finally, angioplasty is most effective at distal insertion site lesions, which frequently develop soon after the bypass procedure. Success rates in this area are comparable to success rates for native arterial dilatation.

Thus, angioplasty has changed the approach to recurrent angina in the postbypass patient. In the past, there has been reluctance to be as aggressive with these patients because documentation of disease progression frequently led to reoperation. Consequently, these bypass patients often were treated medically for some time until they developed intractable symptoms before they were referred for repeated coronary angiography. However, with the availability of angioplasty, a much more aggressive diagnostic approach is warranted. Prompt referral for coronary angiography is indicated when signs or symptoms of ischemia reappear. Documentation of an insertion site lesion, or a graft lesion before the graft occludes, provides an opportunity for revascularization of that vein graft while it is still patent. Dilatation of the native vessel might not be possible because of a long segmental occlusion. Thus, a much more aggressive diagnostic approach to recurrent angina in postbypass surgery patients may extend the benefits of surgery by preserving the life of the graft.

Acute Myocardial Infarction

Potential applications for coronary angioplasty in patients with acute transmural myocardial infarction are summarized in Table 15.3. These are discussed in detail in Chapters 5 and 26. Primary or immediate indications for angioplasty include patients with significant contraindications to thrombolytic therapy, failure to reperfuse to thrombolytic therapy, and/or patients in cardiogenic shock (17, 18).

The more common potential use for angioplasty in patients with acute myocardial infarction is in the 25 to 35% of **patients who fail to reperfuse with systemic thrombolytic therapy**. Angioplasty is feasible and has a high probability of success in such patients, although the risk of complications appears somewhat higher than for routine angioplasty. Time is extremely important, with the benefits of revascularization being quite limited beyond 4 to 6 hours after the onset of symptoms (see Chapter 5). Another indication for acute angioplasty is in patients with cardiogenic shock. Primary treatment of patients who have acute myocardial infarction with angioplasty seems restricted. Only 20% of hospitals have catheterization laboratories, and not all of these perform coronary angioplasty (19). Immediate thrombolytic therapy in community hospitals is associated with earlier potential reperfusion than when patients are transported to angioplasty facilities (20). Thus, angioplasty for acute myocardial infarction, except in special centers, will continue to be utilized only for selected patient problems (e.g., the acute infarction patient with a contraindication to thrombolytic therapy). The limited ability to determine successful reperfusion in the early hours following myocardial infarction using only clinical criteria, however, is a problem. Some advocate bringing all

Table 15.3.
Applications of Coronary Angioplasty in Acute Myocardial Infarction[a]

Primary (immediate)
   Contraindications to thrombolytic therapy
   Failure to reperfuse with thrombolytic therapy
   Cardiogenic shock
Secondary (during hospitalization)
   Anatomy
      Severe stenosis postthrombolytic therapy in infarction-related artery
   Ischemia
      Infarction-related artery and/or additional lesions in coronary circulation

[a] See Chapter 5 for a more detailed discussion of percutaneous transluminal coronary angioplasty in acute myocardial infarction.

patients who appear to be evolving large infarcts, particularly anterior ones, to the catheterization laboratory to perform acute angiography to determine vessel patency (21).

Secondary angioplasty is the more important application of angioplasty in patients with acute myocardial infarction. Indications include patients with severe residual stenoses and/or continued ischemia, either because of the infarction-related artery or because of other potentially dilatable vessels. (Fig. 15.4).

TECHNIQUE

Another major component of successful angioplasty is technique. Important parts of the technique include excellent angiography pre- and postdilatation, adequate in-laboratory fluoroscopy, availability of and knowledge of the dilatation equipment, and operator experience.

Angiographic Assessment

Information derived from coronary angiography that impacts on the angioplasty outcome is summarized in Tables 15.4 and 15.5. Before angioplasty, the severity and length of coronary stenoses must be assessed. Equally important, however, in predicting outcome and facilitating the procedure is lesion morphology, including eccentricity, thrombus, and calcification. Recognizing eccentricity is important to delineate the channel through a lesion that facilitates guidewire or balloon pas-

Table 15.4.
Angiographic Assessment before Angioplasty

Lesion severity
  Degree of stenosis length
Lesion morphology
  Eccentricity, thrombus, calcium complex
    lesions
Branches
  Lesion-associated branches with or without
    disease
  Vessel-associated branches potentially
    affecting guidewire passage
Collateral supply
  Presence and extent of collaterals
  Presence and extent of disease in collaterals
    supplying the artery
Proximal artery characteristics
  Origin and course of artery containing lesion
    potentially influencing guide catheter
    selection

Table 15.5.
Angiographic Assessment after Angioplasty

Resultant stenosis
  Percent residual lesion with or without
    flow compromise
Lesion morphology
  Split dissection
  Thrombus
Distal/adjacent vessels
  Associated branch damage
  Emboli

sage. Likewise, presence of thrombus, frequently seen in patients with recent onset of unstable ischemic syndromes, suggests possible higher risks for embolization and/or acute closure following successful dilatation.

Excellent visualization of branches in arteries to be dilated is essential. Lesion-associated branches of significant size need to be identified and assessed for associated disease. It is important to identify branches proximal and distal to the dilatation lesion to enhance the ease and success of guidewire passage through the vessel.

Specialized views are sometimes necessary to provide appropriate lesion or branch delineation (see Chapter 13). The left lateral projection is extremely helpful pre- and postcoronary angioplasty for proximal and mid right coronary artery lesions (22). This particular view clearly identifies the orientation of right ventricular marginal branches, which frequently expedites guide-wire passage across the lesion. The midsegment of the right coronary artery is also well visualized in the lateral projection to assess lesion morphology and dissection pre- and postangioplasty. Complementary left and right coronary injections in the left lateral projection are particularly helpful in determining the potential channel and length of the "skip area" for a mid right coronary artery total occlusion being considered for angioplasty. Supplemental views useful to augment more standard views when either lesion morphology or branch orientation is not satisfactory for assessment before or after angioplasty are listed in Table 15.6. The presence, extent, and origin of collateral arteries, as well as any significant disease in the originating arteries is also important. The origin and proximal part of the vessel to be dilated should be assessed for selection of the guide catheter. Thus, careful angiographic definition and review prior to angioplasty is most important to facilitate the procedure and enhance safety.

Likewise, follow-up angiography after completion of the dilatation procedure is important. A radiographic view should be selected that least foreshortens the dilated segment and provides minimal overlap for accurate assessment of the residual percent stenosis, as well as lesion morphology with regard to localized dissection and/or thrombus. Any contrast flow compromise should be noted. While minor lesion dissection is common and is seen in at least 50% of our patients, major dissection, particularly when either the lumen or contrast flow is compromised, suggests possible high risk for acute reocclusion (23). Likewise, filling defects consistent with thrombus seen immediately following successful dilatation are significantly associated with acute reclosure. In the first 1000 patients dilated at the Medical College of Virginia, acute closure occurred in 25, or approximately 4% of the population (23). Intracoronary, lesion-associated filling defects suggestive of thrombus were seen in nearly two-thirds of these patients, and 80% of reclosures occurred within 15 min while the patient was still in the laboratory. Thus, in patients with a history of recent unstable angina or infarction, particularly with angiographic evidence suggestive of thrombus, predilatation and postdilatation in-lab observation with sequential angiography at 5 and 10 min is warranted in order to docu-

ment impending acute closure manifested as progressive lesion deterioration. Early recognition of impending acute closure allows for reaccess of the vessel for either repeat dilatation and/or to provide access for a perfusion catheter prior to urgent coronary artery bypass surgery.

Following angioplasty, angiography should include careful review of distal and/or adjacent vessels for evidence of lesion-associated branch damage or distal emboli. Recognition of major vessel occlusions is generally easy and is associated with definitive clinical findings. However, smaller branch emboli or dilatation-associated occlusion may be the source of acute or subacute ischemic chest discomfort. Recognition of branch vessel occlusion may explain periprocedure symptoms without major ECG changes and, thus, be useful in management of postangioplasty patients.

Dilatation Equipment

Angioplasty equipment continues to evolve at a rapid rate. One of the reasons for the dramatic expansion of angioplasty into more complex diseases has been the availability of improved devices, which have enhanced the safety and facility of dilatation procedures. Rapid changes continue. Catheter manufacturers believe that the average useful life of a new catheter design is less than 2 years. An outline of some of the types and

Table 15.6.
Supplemental Views Helpful in Angiographic Assessment of Lesions before and after Coronary Angioplasty[a]

Coronary Zone	Views
Proximal-mid LAD[b] and Diagonals	90–110° LAO
	RAO/cranial
	AP/cranial
Proximal intermediate marginal	LAO/caudal
	LAO 110°/caudal
Proximal and midmarginals	RAO/caudal
	AP/caudal
Ostial and proximal RCA	LAO/caudal
Proximal mid RCA	Lateral
Distal RCA and PDA-PLB bifurcation	AP/cranial
	Lateral/cranial

[a] See Chapter 13 on coronary angiography.
[b] LAD, left anterior descending; AP, anteroposterior; LAO, left anterior oblique; PDA-PLB, posterior descending artery, posterior left ventricular branch; RAO, right anterior oblique; RCA, right coronary artery.

characteristics of guiding catheters, balloon dilation catheters, and guidewires currently in use appears in Tables 15.7–15.9.

Guiding Catheters

Guiding catheters are important for coronary access and back-up support. Most of the standard shapes parallel diagnostic coronary angiographic catheter shapes (Table 15.7). However, some differences exist, as many left Judkins type guides tend to be more "open" and, thus, require smaller sizes to access the coronary ostia than are required for a diagnostic catheter. For instance if a standard left Judkins diagnostic catheter is difficult to engage because of a relatively small aortic root, it may be wise to choose the smaller 3.5 left guiding catheter to provide more ready access to the left ostium. The 4.0 size left guide catheter may not access the coronary at all. For dilations in the circumflex coronary artery, the left Amplatz-type catheters frequently provide the greatest support for guidewire steering and vessel crossing, particularly in patients with short left main coronary arteries.

Access of the right coronary artery with a standard Judkins catheter frequently requires more patience and skill in rotating the catheter into the right coronary ostium. This can be facilitated by very gently moving the guiding catheter backwards and forwards in the sheath while rotating the catheter. This maneuver helps transmit torque to the catheter tip, thus reducing the possibility of kinking the guiding catheter at the sheath. Likewise, wetting the catheter with saline at the sheath will decrease rotational friction. Special consideration must be given to the tortuous or "shepherd's crook" right coronary artery. To enhance support and "straighten" the vessel for guidewire and balloon passage, utilization of the left I or II Amplatz, Arani, or multipurpose catheters may be helpful. Side holes in the guide catheter are particularly useful in the right coronary artery. The right coronary ostium is frequently smaller than the left, and the deeper access required in many instances for the right is associated with antegrade flow occlusion. Not only does acute ischemia result but also marked bradycardia and even ventricular fibrillation can occur as the result of ischemia and/or contrast material injections. Although side holes slightly reduce coronary visualization, reducing ischemia and bradycardia by utilizing guide catheters with side holes is, overall, helpful.

Inexperienced operators frequently begin with the more standard Judkins catheter and only go to specialized catheters after failure. More experienced operators tend to choose the catheter most likely to provide the most efficient dilatation success. However, this is no replacement for experience in coronary

Table 15.7.
Representative Types of Angioplasty Guiding Catheters[a]

Catheter	Type	Available Curve Size
Standard coronary (comparable to diagnostic catheters in shape)	Left Judkins	3.5–5 cm
	Right Judkins	
	Left Amplatz	I, II
	Right Amplatz	I, II
Brachial	Stertzer brachial	Multipurpose
		Bent tip
Special use	Left bypass	
	Right bypass	
	Internal mammary	
	El Gamal coronary bypass	
	King multipurpose	
	Arani double loop	90°, 75°angle
		Short and long tip

[a] Standard curves are generally available from Advanced Cardiovascular Systems (ACS™), Cordis, Interventional Medical (IM), and CR Bard, Inc. (USCI™), and brachial and special use are from CR Bard, Inc. (USCI™). All catheters are available in 8 Fr (current predominant size). IM has recently introduced very large lumen 9 Fr guides, while all other companies are introducing larger internal lumen 8 Fr guides.

Table 15.8.
Representative Types of Coronary Angioplasty Guidewires

Type	Diameter (inches)	Tip
USCI[a]		
Standard steerable	0.014	Straight, J
	0.016	
Flexible (flex)	0.014	Straight, J
	0.016	
Very flexible (veriflex)	0.014	Straight, J
ACS[b]		
High torque floppy	0.014	Straight
	0.018	
High torque intermediate	0.014	Straight
	0.018	
High torque standard	0.014	Straight
	0.018	

[a] USCI™, registered trademark of CR Bard, Inc. All USCI™ wires are 180 cm in length but are "extendible" with a 0.016, 122 cm attachable wire.
[b] ACS, registered trademark of Advanced Cardiovascular Systems Inc., a subsidiary of Eli Lilly and Company. All ACS™ wires are extendible using the DOC system.

Table 15.9.
Representative Types of Balloon Angioplasty Catheters

Type	Material	Inflated Size (mm)	Average Deflated Profile (inches)	Distal Dye/Pressure	Guidewire Maximum Size (inches)	Maximum Inflation Pressure (atm)
USCI[a]						
LPS II	PVC	2 – 4	0.050	+/+	0.016	9.5
Simplus Profile	PET	2 – 4	0.036	–/–	0.016	9.5
Plus	PET	2 – 4	0.039	+/+	0.016	12.0
Probe[b]	PET	2 – 3	0.030	–/–	–	12.0
ACS						
Simpson	PE	2 – 4	0.055	+/+	0.018	9.0
Simpson Ultra-low	PE	2 – 4	0.049	–/–	0.014	9.0
Hartzler LPS[b]	PE	2 – 4	0.046	–/–	–	9.0
Hartzler Micro[b]	PE	2 – 4	0.048	–/–	–	9.0
Delta	PE	2 – 4	0.054	–/–	0.018	9.0
Mansfield						
ProAct	PE	2 – 4	0.042	–/–	0.014	13.0
Max Trak	PE	2 – 4	0.051	+/+	0.018	13.0
Heart Trak	PE	2 – 4	0.051	+/+	0.018	13.0
Sci Med						
Skinny	PC	2 – 3	0.037	–/–	0.014	10.0
Trac Plus	PC	2 – 4	0.049	+/+	0.018[c]	12.0
DGW[b]	PC	1.5	0.018	–/–	–	8.0

[a] USCI, registered trademark of CR Bard, Inc. ACS, registered trademark of Advanced Cardiovascular Systems Inc., a subsidiary of Eli Lilly and Company.; DGW, dilating guidewire; PET, polyethylene terephthalate; PC, polyolifin copolymer; PE, polyethylene; PVC, polyvinyl chloride; Sci Med, registered trademark of SciMed Life Systems, Inc.; –, not applicable.
[b] Steerable balloon devices, nonover-the-wire.
[c] Accepts dilating guidewire.

angioplasty. Amplatz catheters may be associated with a slightly higher risk of coronary vessel dissection. However, the tradeoff in shortening overall procedure time, by assuring the highest probability of success in crossing lesion in the first attempt, far outweighs the minimal additional risk of dissection. Amplatz-type guiding catheters should be removed from the coronary artery only under fluoroscopy because withdrawing the Amplatz left guiding catheter may paradoxically advance its tip further down the coronary artery. When this appears to occur, the guide catheter should be advanced first, which will cause the catheter to "fall" out of the coronary, frequently into the left ventricle. Then it can be safely withdrawn.

Guiding catheters continue to evolve. Current changes include the adding of a soft tip end to potentially decrease ostial damage. Thinner materials with adequate stiffness or support provide for either slightly tapered tips or larger internal diameters. Increased internal diameters are important for providing improved contrast opacification with balloon catheters still in the coronary artery. Larger internal diameters also allow easier dual access of complex branch stenoses and even "kissing-balloon" techniques through a single-guide catheter.

Guidewires

Guidewires have a variety of tips that range from minimally flexible and very steerable to more flexible and less steerable and even very "floppy" tips, which have little steering capability (Table 15.8). The more rigid, steerable wires are particularly useful for steerability (torquability) and for crossing total occlusions and/or recanalized channels that often require some ability to push the guidewire to cross the lesion. Conversely, the more flexible and floppy wires are less steerable but also less traumatic for crossing complex unstable lesions, graft stenoses, or for recrossing lesions immediately after dilatation. Another advantage of the extremely flexible wire is that the soft tip frequently will avoid some of the difficulty associated with traversing multiple branches by simply forming a tip loop which then passes freely down the vessel.

The tip of a guidewire may become lodged in a small branch inadvertently, and continu-

ing to force the wire forward may cause it to become embedded in the vessel wall. On attempting to retract the wire the tip may remain lodged, and the tip ribbon may fracture. Then the wire will begin to uncoil and, if pulled briskly, may fracture, leaving behind a wire segment. **Tip ribbon fracture** is easily recognized by failure to visualize movement of the wire tip on manipulation of the guidewire in the operator's hand. Once this is recognized, the balloon catheter should be advanced as far as possible to the tip end of the wire, and then the balloon and wire should be retracted together with slow but firm force. This technique can prevent wire fracture (24). Should the wire fracture, surgical or percutaneous removal of the wire may be necessary. Obviously, large fragments need to be removed because of the risk of systemic and/or coronary emboli. However, very small distal fragments have been left in place without major difficulties (25).

Another useful technical modification of guidewire technology is the long or extendible guidewire (26). These wires allow exchange of balloon catheters for either larger or smaller sizes without having to recross coronary lesions with the wire. An extendible or long wire allows retraction of the balloon catheter after dilatation removing the major mechanical obstruction to contrast material injection through the guide catheter. This technique has become routine for many operators to provide high-quality angiographic definition after dilatation before guidewire removal.

Balloon Catheters

Balloon catheters are predominantly of two types (Table 15.9). **"Over the wire" systems** utilize freely movable, steerable guidewires and have the advantage of being able to be exchanged while maintaining translesion guidewire access. Generally, the profile of such balloons is slightly larger than "nonover-the-wire," steerable balloon systems. **Nonover-the-wire** steerable balloon systems tend to be of lower profile but do not allow translesion pressure gradient assessment. Just as steerable systems en-hanced the success rate of coronary angioplasty, the continued development of lower profile balloon systems has progressively enhanced the ability to more predictably cross severely stenotic lesions, as well as to successfully dilate more distal coronary lesions.

The occasional unreliability of pressure gradients, as compared with angiographic lesion assessment and reduced procedure time associated with steerable balloons, have contributed significantly to the popularity of nonover-the-wire steerable balloon catheters. The lower profile construction of these catheters also enhances the ability to test inject through the guiding catheter while the balloon is still across the stenosis. However, these systems do require recrossing lesions to up or downsize balloons as necessary to either initially traverse or adequately dilate very severe stenosis. Although there are long-standing theoretical concerns regarding inability to recross a dilated lesion, in reality most lesions can be repeatedly crossed without producing dissection or causing acute vessel closure. Thus, there seems to be a growing trend towards the use of nonover-the-wire steerable systems, as opposed to over-the-wire steerable systems.

FACILITATING THE PROCEDURE

Patient Preparation

While single-vessel dilatation of isolated proximal stenoses may require minimal time, complex angioplasty can be very time-consuming and, thus, requires careful planning with regard to patient management, contrast utilization, and overall efficiency of operation. Because complex procedures take a longer time than diagnostic catheterizations and frequently patients are more anxious, effective patient sedation is important to allow the operator to comfortably perform the procedure. Multiple sedatives are available, but one effective regimen is to pretreat patients with 1 to 2 mg of lorazepam and 4 mg of parenteral morphine. This combination is similar to the regimen used for preinduction sedation for patients undergoing cardiac surgery and will not interfere with emergency bypass if required. Once in the laboratory, the sedation may be extended and/or enhanced by incremental 2- to 3-mg dosages of intravenous morphine. Other premedications should include aspirin, along with a calcium channel antagonist. Systemic heparinization is important during the actual procedure. Sublingual nifedipine may be given to assure antispasm protection prior to balloon inflations. Likewise intracoronary or intravenous nitroglycerin may be utilized prophylactically or in response to acute spasm (see Fig. 15.5).

Most patients undergoing angioplasty have had recent diagnostic angiography and, thus, unless clinical events suggest a major change, angiography at the time of the

Figure 15.5. Acute coronary artery spasm (*left panel*) identified after balloon inflation but with guidewire access. Following intracoronary nitroglycerin, there is resolution of the spasm (*right panel*).

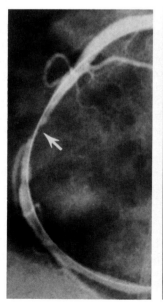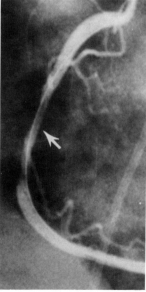

angioplasty procedure can be limited to identifying important angiographic details as outlined above. Projections utilized can be limited to those particularly useful for the lesions in question, based on the preliminary angiogram.

In contrast, there is so-called "ad hoc" angioplasty or dilatation performed at the time of the diagnostic catheterization. Although this technique may be efficient from a physician, patient, and laboratory standpoint, one must be certain that additional lesions or other important angiographic findings are not overlooked by elimination of careful angiographic review before dilatation. However, in urgent or emergency circumstances patients requiring immediate angioplasty should have discussed the possibility of angioplasty before arriving in the catheterization laboratory. Finally, in patients with suspected restenosis, it is still important to be certain that new or progressive disease that might affect the outcome has not developed in other areas of the coronary system.

Dilatation

Once the guiding catheter is seated, the balloon catheter with guidewire is advanced. The guidewire should always be advanced beyond the balloon catheter by several centimeters in over-the-wire systems to provide maximum flexibility of the wire. However, because "tractability" of the balloon over the guidewire may at times create difficulties in traversing severely tortuous coronary vessels, an over the wire balloon system can be utilized as a "fixed" wire system by advancing the balloon and the extended guidewire as a single unit while steering the guidewire. Once the guidewire or steerable balloon reaches the lesion, it is important to move slowly with gentle advancement of the wire or balloon while gently rotating the guidewire so that the appropriate channel is found. With markedly eccentric stenoses, it is useful to work in a projection which identifies the direction of the channel and to steer the wire in that direction.

Advancing the balloon itself across the lesion may require considerable guidewire support in severely stenotic lesions. In many instances, to achieve adequate support, the guiding catheter must be advanced into the coronary ostium. In so doing, it is important

to advance the guiding catheter slowly and to be certain that it is advancing over the balloon-catheter system to provide stability. Care should be taken to observe arterial pressure to be sure that "damping" does not occur. If it does, once the balloon has been advanced across the stenosis, the guiding catheter should be withdrawn immediately to a more proximal or ostial position.

With the balloon in place across the stenosis, a 2 atm inflation is performed under fluoroscopy to identify balloon indentation. This confirms appropriate balloon position (see Fig. 15.6). Subsequently, the balloon is slowly inflated to higher pressures sufficient to provide full expansion of the balloon. However, full inflation may not be necessary on the first inflation and may be achieved with subsequent inflations to higher pressures. Some operators believe that excessively rapid, initial high-pressure inflations are associated with greater degrees of local dissection. Balloon inflations are usually maintained for 30 to 60 sec. Longer, frequently lower, pressure inflations have been utilized to attempt to "mold" lesions following acute closure or for major local dissection. Likewise, longer inflation periods have been employed in an attempt to prevent continued reclosure and/or reduce the incidence of restenosis (27). To date, convincing clinical evidence is not available to support the hypothesis that inflations of long duration are useful in preventing restenosis. There is some belief that longer inflations may be beneficial in terms of improving the acute angiographic and perhaps short-term clinical result. Furthermore, prolonged (>1 min) inflations frequently require special management to reduce or prevent severe ischemia. Intracoronary β-adrenergic blocker treatment may be effective to extend the length of inflation time in nontotal stenoses (28). Fluosol, an oxygen-carrying hydrocarbon, has been utilized experimentally to achieve longer, nonischemic inflations (29). Finally, a number of autoperfusion balloons are undergoing investigation in an attempt to extend the duration of inflation as blood flows through the balloon catheter to the distal vessel (30).

Balloon sizing is a very important consideration in dilatation. Regardless of the balloon size utilized to achieve initial lesion crossing, the final balloon diameter should be very

Figure 15.6.   Balloon indentation (*left panel*) associated with an initial low pressure inflation documenting excellent balloon position. Full balloon inflation (*right panel*) with no residual indentation at high pressure.

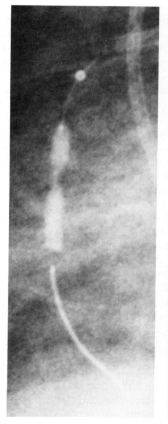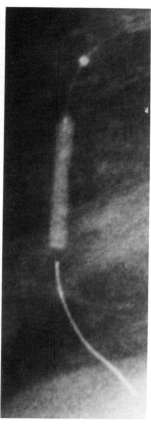

similar to the estimated diameter of the native coronary artery. Restenosis rates appear higher in lesions which had incomplete initial dilatation determined angiographically or by a final translesion gradient of ≥15 mm Hg (31). Conversely, intentionally oversizing balloons to create dissections and/or "overdilate" lesions is associated with higher initial complication rates that override any potential late effectiveness in reduced restenosis.

Because factors associated with restenosis are still largely unknown, absolute guidelines regarding adequacy of initial dilatation are philosophy more than truth. Operators utilizing a gradient system perform repeated inflations to subsequently higher balloon pressures and/or to full balloon expansion until the translesion gradient is ≤15 mm Hg. This has been suggested to be associated with a lower restenosis rate (31). Others rely on an angiographic assessment of the dilatation result, utilizing long wire techniques or

smaller catheters to assure excellent angiographic assessment. Finally, after removal of the balloon and guidewire system follow-up angiography is obtained, as outlined earlier in the chapter to identify lesion result and any indication of markers of early occlusion (see Fig. 15.7).

COMPLICATIONS

Major complications associated with coronary angioplasty include acute myocardial infarction, urgent bypass surgery, and/or death (see Chapter 3). The risk of major complications is 4 to 5%. Death occurs in 1% or less in most studies while acute myocardial infarction occurs in approximately one-half of the 3 to 4% of patients that require urgent bypass surgery (5, 32). In studies of patients undergoing multiple vessel coronary angioplasty the risk of serious complications is essentially the

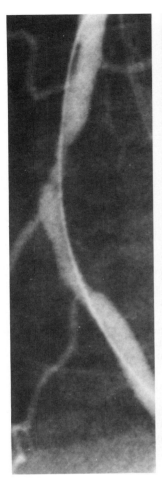 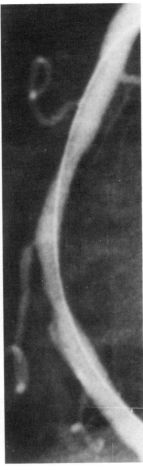

Figure 15.7. Utilization of a long guide-wire (*left panel*) allows excellent vessel opacification with continued access. There is marked irregularity and persistent stenosis despite the initial dilatation with a 3-mm balloon. Utilizing the long wire technique, the balloon was ex-changed for a 3.5-mm balloon. A much-improved angiographic result (*right panel*) follows dilatation with the larger balloon.

same as for patient populations not subcategorized for this more complex subgroup analysis (33). Thus, appropriate patient selection in multiple vessel disease provides an outcome that, from a risk standpoint, is not substantially different from coronary artery bypass surgery.

Acute Closure

Acute closure represents the major cause of urgent coronary artery bypass surgery. Major factors relate to lesion thrombus, perhaps in the setting of recent unstable ischemia or infarction and/or major vessel dissection (34) (Fig. 15.8, Table 15.10). As noted above, recognition of patients at risk, based on clinical and angiographic findings, allows acute closure to be anticipated and treated in the laboratory.

If acute closure is identified, most lesions can be recrossed with subsequent successful angioplasty. Factors relating to continued success after redilatation are unclear, although most operators tend to use longer-duration inflation periods and/or slightly larger balloons, often inflated to higher pressures to ensure adequate dilatation, as well as "molding." At the Medical College of Virginia, over 80% of patients with acute closure undergoing redilatation ultimately stabilized clinically with a patent lesion (23). Thus, if acute closure can be recognized early and managed by redilatation, the need for urgent bypass surgery may be reduced. Patients going to emergency bypass surgery today, directly from the catheterization laboratory, are frequently stabilized because of "bailout" or autoperfusion catheters placed across the stenotic lesion (30). In the future, the availability of stents may further reduce the need for urgent surgery (see Chapter 16).

Figure 15.8. A complex thrombus-associated lesion (*left panel*) identified in a patient with a recent non-Q-wave myocardial infarction and refractory un-stable angina. Despite excellent angiographic results seen immediately after dilatation (*right panel*), this patient was observed for 15 min in the catheterization laboratory because the predilatation clinical and angiographic profiles suggested high risk for acute closure.

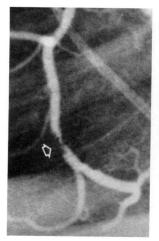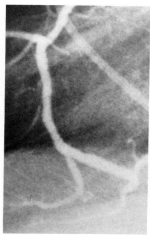

CLINICAL RESULTS

As noted earlier, the overall lesion success rate for coronary angioplasty ranges between 88 and 92% (4, 35). Clinical success, defined as symptomatic improvement with successful primary lesion dilatation although smaller branch lesions may be unsuccessfully dilated, is also greater than 90% in most studies (36). Interestingly, the incidence of success seems to be equally high for multiple vessel disease, as compared with that of single-vessel disease, suggesting appropriate selection of patients whose primary ischemic lesion and, probably, most secondary lesions are amenable to dilatation (37).

Several reports comparing outcomes of patient subgroups have demonstrated variable responses, but persistent differences in outcome have not surfaced. For instance, comparison of patients with stable vs. unstable angina and/or acute myocardial infarction has not repeatedly shown major differences in

Table 15.10.
Predictors of Acute Closure

Clinical
  Recent lesion-associated unstable ischemia
    or infarction
Angiographic
  Pre-PTCA
    Complex lesions, thrombus
  Post-PTCA
    Thrombus
    Large dissections, particularly with flow
      compromise

acute success rate (38, 39). Likewise, the clinical success rate for multivessel disease is comparable to that for single-vessel disease (33, 36). In contrast, lower success rates are reported for nonacute total occlusions and, as described earlier, the major difficulty relates to attempts to dilate chronic occlusion.

Restenosis

Restenosis remains the major unresolved issue in coronary angioplasty today. The incidence of restenosis is dependent upon the definition. Clinical restenosis occurs in approximately 20 to 25% of patients followed long-term (33). Angiographic restenosis may be as high as 30 to 40%, again partly dependent upon the extent of lesion recurrence that is defined as restenosis. The peak incidence of restenosis occurs in the first 6 months after angioplasty (40). After 6 months there appears to be a lower but continued incidence of late restenosis up to 1 year, particularly in patients with partial restenosis at 6 months (41). After 1 year most patients who develop recurrent angina are much more likely to have a new lesion in a previously undilated segment than to exhibit restenosis. Interestingly, this outcome parallels coronary artery bypass surgery in which, along with graft disease, there is a relatively high incidence of recurrent ischemic symptoms related to progression of native vessel disease.

The cause of restenosis is unknown, although there is increasing evidence that a proliferative intimal or medial reaction may play an important role (42). Thus, it is not surprising that many of the risk factors associated with development of atherosclerotic disease are not strong predictors of restenosis. Although a variety of individual risk factors have been identified in single studies of restenosis, only a limited number of factors seemed to be consistently related to restenosis (Table 15.11). These include proximal anterior descending coronary disease, unstable angina at the time of angioplasty, and nonacute total occlusions. These findings suggest that disease activity manifested by the onset of acute unstable clinical syndrome is as-sociated with a higher incidence of restenosis.

Prevention of restenosis remains problematic. Although antiplatelet agents appear effective during acute dilatation to reduce thrombotic complications (43), the longer-term efficacy of antiplatelet drugs is less clear. However, preliminary data from a multicenter study utilizing ciprostene, a prostacycline-like derivative, suggests that there may be some benefit from this potent antiplatelet agent (44). Other treatments have not been effective, including corticosteroids (45), calcium channel-blocking agents (46, 47) and coumadin (48), in affecting the course of restenosis. A recent unblinded study suggests that pretreatment with large doses of n-3 fatty acids in a fish oil preparation plus aspirin and dipyridamole may decrease the risk of restenosis in men (49). This study was limited to only 82 men, and the fish oil group restenosis rate was 16% compared with 36% for patients receiving only aspirin and dipyridamole. A very recent double-blind placebo-controlled study showed no protective effect (50).

Table 15.11.
Restenosis: Predictive Factors

Clinical
    Recent lesion-associated unstable ischemia
      or myocardial infarction
    Males
Angiographic
    Thrombus at lesion
    Long lesions
    "Incomplete" lesion dilatation
    ≥15 mm Hg final translesion gradient
Anatomic
    Proximal LAD lesions[a]
    Ostial RCA lesions

[a] LAD, left anterior descending; RCA, right coronary artery.

Thus, patients undergoing angioplasty must be followed closely to identify restenosis. In certain circumstances, particularly in high risk patients, routine repeat catheterization after 6 months is warranted to identify **asymptomatic recurrence** that occurs in approximately 25% of restenosis patients. If routine follow-up angiography is not planned, exercise testing with or without associated radionuclide studies soon after successful dilatation and again at 6 months is essential in an attempt to identify patients at risk for asymptomatic or "silent" restenosis. Based upon either symptoms or exercise test changes, repeat angiography is warranted for patients with suspected restenosis. Such angiography may be performed with surgical standby so that if recurrent disease is identified, a second dilatation can be performed. A patient undergoing an initially successful dilatation has an 85 to 90% chance of long-term success, although a second dilatation may be necessary to achieve this result. Recently, we have developed a multivariate model that seems to be helpful in predicting high (>55%) and low (<25%) risks of restenosis (51).

SUMMARY

Coronary angioplasty has produced a major impact in the management of coronary artery disease. The exponential increase in the number of procedures does not represent simply a substitution of angioplasty for coronary bypass surgery. Instead, it reflects the fact that many patients are now undergoing angioplasty who in the past would not have been considered candidates for bypass surgery as a primary treatment because of the limited nature of their disease. Coronary angioplasty in many cases with single-vessel disease is more likely to be an alternative to medical therapy than an alternative to surgical therapy. There is no doubt that for significantly symptomatic patients unresponsive to medical treatment, angioplasty is the treatment of choice for patients with single-vessel disease. Whereas, in selected patients with multivessel disease, angioplasty may also represent a reasonable alternative to bypass surgery. Conversely, for patients with left main disease and/or three-vessel disease, in whom some lesions are not amenable to angioplasty, surgery may

Table 15.12.
Potential Applications of New Devices

Stents
    Reduce/prevent acute closure
    Prevent restenosis
Atherectomy, laser, "hot" tips
    Enhance efficacy in total occlusions
    Decrease/prevent restenosis

represent the treatment of choice. Thus, arguments relative to angioplasty vs. bypass surgery or angioplasty vs. medical therapy seem unwarranted.

If patients with coronary artery disease are well-managed, they will have several management strategies that will vary according to the extent and complexity of disease. Throughout most of their course many patients will have some medical management while angioplasty will be utilized either before or following coronary bypass surgery for appropriate but somewhat less extensive disease. Conversely, coronary bypass surgery will remain the treatment of choice for patients with extensive disease not amenable to angioplasty. Newer devices and drugs may extend the safety and efficacy of coronary angioplasty. Some potential applications for new devices, which may advance the procedure, are outlined in Table 15.12. Coronary stents may reduce the risk of acute closure and/or restenosis. Laser and atherectomy devices may extend the usefulness in total or longer diffuse lesions and perhaps affect restenosis and acute closure.

Considering the major advances that have occurred in the decade since the first application of coronary angioplasty, it is certain that changes will continue to evolve extending the applicability and efficacy of angioplasty. For the present, cautious and thoughtful use of the technique, with careful scientific data collection, will continue to assure the quality and reliability of the procedure.

References

1. Meier B, Gruentzig AR. Learning curve for PTCA: skill, technology and patient selection. Am J Cardiol 1984; 53: 65C–66C.
2. Kelsey SF, Mullin SM, Detre KM, et al. Effects of investigator experience on PTCA. Am J Cardiol 1984; 53: 56C–64C.
3. Gruentzig AR, Senning A, Siegenthaler WE. Non–operative dilatation of coronary artery stenosis: percutaneous transluminal coronary angioplasty. N Engl J Med 1979; 301: 61–68.
4. Anderson HV, Roubin GS, Leimgruber PP, et al. Primary angiographic success rates of percutaneous transluminal coronary angioplasty. Am J Cardiol 1985; 56: 712–717.
5. Bredlau CE, Roubin GS, Leimgruber PP, et al. In–hospital morbidity and mortality in patients undergoing elective coronary angioplasty. Circulation 1985; 72: 1044–1052.
6. Vetrovec GW, Cowley MJ, Wolfgang TC, et al. Effects of percutaneous transluminal coronary angioplasty on lesion–associated branches. Am Heart J 1985; 109: 921–925.
7. Meier B, Gruentzig, AR, King SB, et al. Risk of side branch occlusion during coronary angioplasty. Am J Cardiol 1984; 53: 10–14.
8. Meier B. Kissing balloon coronary angioplasty. Am J Cardiol 1984; 54: 918–919.
9. George SB, Myler RK, Stertzer SH, et al. Balloon angioplasty of coronary bifurcation lesions: the kissing balloon technique. Cathet Cardiovasc Diagn 1986; 12: 124–138.
10. DiSciascio G, Vetrovec GW, Cowley MJ, et al. Early and late outcome of PTCA for subacute and chronic total coronary occlusion. Am Heart J 1986; 111: 833–839.
11. Holmes DR, Vliestra RE, Reeder GS, et al. Angioplasty in total coronary artery occlusion. J Am Coll Cardiol 1984; 3: 845–849.
12. Dorros G, Cowley MJ, Simpson J, et al. Percutaneous transluminal coronary angioplasty: report of complications from the National Heart, Lung and Blood Institute PTCA Registry. Circulation 1983; 67: 723–730.
13. Killip T, Passamani E, Davis K, et al. Coronary artery surgery study (CASS): a randomized trial of coronary bypass surgery. Eight years' follow–up and survival in patients with reduced ejection fraction. Circulation 1985; 72: V–102–109.
14. Dorros G, Johnson WD, Tector AJ, et al. Percutaneous transluminal coronary angioplasty in patients with prior coronary artery bypass grafting. J Thorac Cardiovasc Surg 1984; 87: 17–26.
15. Block PC, Cowley MJ, Kaltenbach M, et al. Percutaneous angioplasty of stenoses of bypass grafts or of bypass graft anastomotic sites. Am J Cardiol 1984; 53: 666–668.
16. Gamal EM, Bonnier H, Michels R, et al. Percutaneous transluminal angioplasty of stenosed aortocoronary bypass grafts. Br Heart J 1984; 52: 617–620.
17. Hartzler G, Rutherford BD, McConahay DR. Percutaneous transluminal coronary angioplasty: application for acute myocardial infarction. Am J Cardiol 1984; 53: 117C–121C.
18. Holmes DR, Smith HC, Vliestra RE, et al. Percutaneous transluminal coronary angioplasty, alone or in combination with streptokinase therapy during acute myocardial infarction. Mayo Clin Proc 1985; 60: 449–456.
19. Hospital Statistics. American Hospital Association. Survey of United States Hospital. American Hospital Association. Washington, D.C., 1986.
20. Topol EJ, Bates ER, Walton JA, et al. Community hospital administration of intravenous tissue plasminogen activator in acute myocardial infartion:

improved timing, thrombolytic efficacy and ventricular function. J Am Coll Cardiol 1987; 10: 1173–1177.

21. Pepine CJ, Prida X, Hill J, et al. Percutaneous transluminal coronary angioplasty in acute myocardial infarction. Am Heart J 1984; 107: 820–822.

22. Goldbaum TS, DiSciascio G, Cowley MJ, et al. The usefulness of the lateral projection in the assessment of the right coronary artery during percutaneous transluminal coronary angioplasty. Cathet Cardiovasc Diagn 1987; 13: 277–283.

23. Goldbaum TS, Cowley MJ, DiSciascio G, et al. Clinical & angiographic markings of early occlusion following successful PTCA. Cathet Cardiovasc Diagn, in press, 1988.

24. Kaltenbach M, Beyer J, Walter S, et al. Prolonged application of pressure in transluminal coronary angioplasty. Cathet Cardiovasc Diagn 1984; 10: 213–219.

25. Watson LE. Snare loop technique for removal of broken steerable PTCA wire. Cathet Cardiovasc Diagn 1987; 13: 44–49.

26. Kaltenbach M, Vallbracht C, Kober G. The long technique for coronary angioplasty. Cathet Cardiovasc Diagn 1986; 12: 337–340.

27. Kaltenbach M, Koberg G. Can prolonged application of pressure improve the results of coronary angioplasty (PTCA)? (abstr). Circulation 1982; 66: III–123.

28. Feldman RL, MacDonald RG, Hill, JA, et al. Effect of propranolol on myocardial ischemia occurring during acute coronary occlusion. Circulation 1986; 73: 727–733.

29. Bowman L, Cleman M, Cabin H, Hasselman S, Jaffe CC. Preservation of diastolic function and cardiac output during PTCA with distal coronary perfusion of fluosol–DA 20% (abstr). J Am Coll Cardiol 1988; 11: 133A.

30. Hinohara T, Simpson JB, Phillips HR, et al. Transluminal intracoronary reperfusion catheter: a device to maintain coronary perfusion between failed coronary angioplasty and emergency coronary bypass surgery. J Am Coll Cardiol 1988; 11: 977–982.

31. Hollman J, Gruentzig A, Meier B, Bradford J, Galan K. Factors affecting recurrence after successful coronary angioplasty (abstr). J Am Coll Cardiol 1983; 1: 644.

32. Dorros G, Cowley MJ, Janke L, et al. In–hospital mortality rate in NHLBI PTCA Registry. Am J Cardiol 1984; 53: 17C–21C.

33. Myler RK, Topol EJ, Shaw RE, et al. Multiple vessel coronary angioplasty: classification, results and patterns of restenosis in 494 consecutive patients. Cathet Cardiovasc Diagn 1987; 13: 1–15.

34. Kent KM, Bentivoglio LG, Block PC, et al. Percutaneous transluminal angioplasty: Registry of National Heart, Lung and Blood Institute. Am J Cardiol 1982; 49: 2011–2020.

35. Faxon DP, Kelsey SF, Ryan TJ, et al. Determinant of successful PTCA: report from the NHLBI Registry. Am Heart J 1984; 108: 1019–1023.

36. Cowley MJ, Vetrovec GW, DiSciascio G, et al. Coronary angioplasty of multivessels: short term outcome and long term results. Circulation 1985; 72: 1314–1320.

37. DiSciascio G, Cowley MJ, Vetrovec GW. Angiographic patterns of restenosis following coronary angioplasty of multiple vessels. Am J Cardiol 1986; 58: 922–925.

38. Faxon DP, Detre KM, McGabe CH, et al. Role of PTCA in the treatment of unstable angina: report from NHLBI PTCA and CASS Registries. Am J Cardiol 1984; 53: 131C–135C.

39. Simonton, CA, Mark DB, Hinohara T, et al. Late restenosis after emergent coronary angioplasty for acute myocardial infarction: comparison with elective coronary angioplasty. J Am Coll Cardiol 1988; 11: 698–705.

40. Holmes DR, Vliestra RE, Smith HC, et al. Restenosis after percutaneous transluminal coronary angioplasty (PTCA): a report from the PTCA Registry of National Heart, Lung and Blood Institute. Am J Cardiol 1984; 53: 77C–81C.

41. Robert EW, Ricks WB, Rossen RM, et al. Late recurrence of angina following coronary angioplasty: the role of new atherosclerotic disease (abstr). J Am Coll Cardiol 1986; 7: 21A.

42. Austin GE, Ratliff NB, Hallman J, et al. Intimal proliferation of smooth muscle cells as an explanation of recurrent coronary artery stenosis after percutaneous transluminal coronary angioplasty. J Am Coll Cardiol 1985; 6: 369–375.

43. Schwartz L, Bourassa MG, Lesperance J, et al. Aspirin and dipyridamole in the prevention of restenosis after percutaneous transluminal coronary angioplasty. N Engl J Med 1988;318:1714–1719.

44. Raizner A, Hollman J, Demke D, Wakefield L, and the Ciprostene Investigators. Beneficial effects of Ciprostene in PTCA: a multicenter, randomized, contolled trial (abstr). Circulation 1988;78:II–290. 1988.

45. Pepine CJ, Hirshfeld JW, Macdonald RG, et al. A controlled trial of corticosteroids to prevent restenosis following coronary angioplasty. (abstr.) Circulation 1988;78:II–291.

46. Whitworth HB, Roubin GS, Hollman J, et al. Effect of nifedipine on recurrent stenosis after percutaneous transluminal coronary angioplasty. J Am Coll Cardiol 1986; 8: 1271–1276.

47. Corcos T, David PR, Val PG, et al. Failure of diltiazem to prevent restenosis after percutaneous transluminal coronary angioplasty. Am Heart J 1985; 109: 926–931.

48. Thornton, MA, Gruentzig AR, Hollman J, et al. Coumadin and aspirin in prevention of recurrence after transluminal coronary angioplasty: a randomized study. Circulation 1984; 69: 721–727.

49. Dehmer GJ, Popma JJ, van den Berg EK, et al. Reduction in the rate of early restenosis after coronary angioplasty by a diet supplemented with n–3 fatty acids. N Engl J Med 1988; 319: 733–740.

50. Reis GS, Sipperly ME, Boucher TM, et al. Results of a randomized, double-blind placebo-controlled trial of fish oil for prevention of restenosis after PTCA (abstr). Circulation 1988;78:II–291.

51. Hirshfeld JW, Schwartz JS, Jugo R, et al. and the M-Heart Group. A multivariate model for predicting the risk of restenosis after PTCA (abstr). Circulation 1988;78:II–289.

16

Other Catheter-Based Techniques for Treatment of Coronary Artery Disease

George S. Abela, M.D.

INTRODUCTION

The advent of coronary artery balloon angioplasty and its clinical success have led to further investigation into catheter-based approaches for intervention in both the coronary and peripheral circulation. Although balloon angioplasty has gained wide acceptance, it still has certain shortcomings. Specifically, chronic totally occluded segments, diffuse long narrowings, coronary ostial stenosis, and some other lesions present important limitations. In the peripheral circulation long-term patency following balloon angioplasty has been less than that seen in the coronary circulation, a finding perhaps related in part to the length of the segment dilated. Some other shortcomings associated with balloon angioplasty relate to thrombus and occlusive dissections that result in sudden reocclusion, as well a high frequency of restenosis.

THE LASER

The laser was first built in 1960 and introduction quickly followed into dermatology, ophthalmology, and surgery. These medical applications did not require a delivery system to transmit the energy from remote sites to an internal target area. The advent of optical fibers to transmit this energy made application of lasers to the cardiovascular system feasible. Properties of laser light that make it potentially useful for treatment of arterial obstructions are numerous. The laser can vaporize

arterial plaque into its elemental components that consist mainly of water vapor, carbon dioxide, and other combustion by-products (1–8). Because laser light can be conducted through flexible optical fibers, ablation of plaque may be accomplished by passage of the light waves through these fibers from distant sites using catheterization techniques.

Laser Light

The laser is a coherent and monochromatic light source. These properties allow for either tissue vaporization or coagulation by conversion of light energy into heat. Most efficient tissue ablation depends greatly upon absorption properties of the tissue for the specific light waves. This is related to the efficacy for absorption of the specific tissue for the monochromatic light. Laser parameters that determine its effectiveness also include the power density (watts/cm^2) and exposure duration (seconds). The product of these two factors (watts-sec/cm^2) determines the actual amount of energy deposited at a given tissue site.

Experimental Studies

In Vitro Experiments

In the early 1980s reports first described the potential for lasers in the treatment of obstructive vascular disease (5, 8). These studies described the histopathology of laser vaporization of plaque. They demonstrated that the

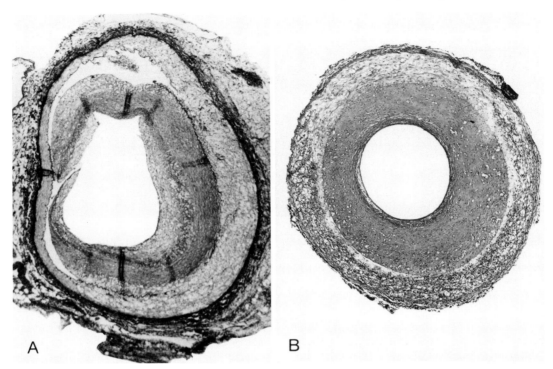

Figure 16.1. Cross-sections of atherosclerotic rabbit iliac arteries are demonstrated following balloon angioplasty *(A)* and laser recanalization *(B)*. Both vessels were demonstrated to have high-grade stenoses by angiography prior to treatment. *Panel A* shows plaque compression and dissection with intimal medial separation and tearing following balloon inflation. *B* illustrates the smooth-walled recanalized atheromatous plaque with the thermal laser vaporization. There is a thin layer of charring along the edges of the recanalized channel but no evidence of dissection. Hematoxylin and eosin stain, ×50.

site of laser impact resulted in a zone of vaporization surrounded by a zone of thermal charring and vacuolization. Variation in peak power and Hertz showed that pulsed laser systems could result in vaporization with less surrounding thermal damage.

In Vivo Experiments

In general, when large volumes of atheromatous plaque are obstructing a vessel, large amounts need to be removed to affect adequate revascularization (i.e., "debulking"). Here, tissue selectivity is greatly overwhelmed by the extensive thermal effects generated during this debulking process. Hence, true vaporization of plaque continues to require high energy densities, and this, of course, increases the risk of vessel wall perforation (9). When compared with standard balloon angioplasty, however, laser recanalization results in a smooth-walled lumen without dissection or distortion of vessel architecture. This result has the potential of reduced restenosis when using the laser approach (Fig. 16.1).

Fiber Optic Catheter Delivery Systems

The availability of small (≤0.5 mm in diameter) and flexible optical fibers that can be inserted via standard angiographic catheters makes percutaneous laser recanalization feasible. The configuration of the fiber system is perhaps the single most important factor in any laser delivery system. Several characteristics of the fiber make modifications necessary for its use in the vascular system. The bare fiber is composed of a silica core surrounded by a cladding and plastic jacket and is radiolucent. The core of the bare fiber is a sharp-edged piece of silica that can readily puncture the arterial wall. Furthermore, the bare fiber tip melts with the reflected heat generated during the lasing process (5).

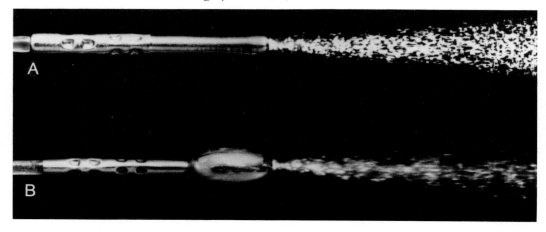

Figure 16.2. Two 300-μm core optical fibers with *(A)* a 1-mm metal sleeve and *(B)* a 2-mm elliptical metal sleeve at the tips. In both *A* and *B* the back of the sleeve is crimped onto the fiber cladding, and an argon laser beam (1 watt) is seen exiting from the tip at a 15° angle. The beam of the 2-mm probe in *B* has a narrower waist and is less intense than the 1-mm probe in *A*. (From Abela GS, Seeger JM, Barbieri E, et. al. Laser angioplasty with angioscopic guidance in humans. J Am Coll Cardiol 1986;8:184–192.)

The first modification of the optical fiber for recanalization was placement of a metal ring around the tip (10). This allowed radiographic visualization of the tip and prevented melting and destruction of the fiber (Fig. 16.2*A*). However, the tip still had a rough end that resulted in frequent perforation. Additionally, scattered laser light from the end of a bare fiber caused diffusion of power. A further fiber modification was complete encapsulation of the fiber tip with a metal cap. This resulted in a pure thermal probe system, or "hot tip" (11, 12). Further improvement of the fiber tip was made by introducing a window at the end of the metal probe. This allowed 20% of the laser beam power to exit. A sapphire lens was then placed behind the window that refocused the beam and reduced the forward light scatter (Fig. 16.2*B*). This system was mechanically less traumatic, as compared with the flat-ended, bare fiber. Also, laser beam scatter from the end of the fiber was eliminated and, thus fewer perforations occurred. Channel size, however, was limited by the size of the cap. Also, because the size of the free laser beam attenuated, the effect of the device was confined to the area of mechanical contact with the metal tip.

Other delivery systems have been developed that utilize a sapphire-tipped fiber. These systems can focus the beam and provide thermal contact with the tissue by the sapphire tip itself (13). Thus, both mechanisms for plaque vaporization may result (e.g., indirect heating and direct laser). Systems using multiple fibers receive fluorescence from the plaque that is excited by the laser light reflected from the tissue (14-17). Signals specific for plaque can then be analyzed, and this information can be utilized to select which fibers and laser wavelengths will discharge laser radiation at the target sites that are most likely to be absorbed by plaque only. Further refinement of this feedback system includes video enhancement techniques and excitation of plaque, with the use of ultraviolet and blue light sources. These approaches seem to enhance the process, but at present all these effects have only been demonstrated in vitro and their in vivo application is theoretical. Finally, the fluorescent signals become weaker following repeated laser irradiation of the tissue (18). Hence, the usefulness of this technique remains to be determined.

With all of these systems, adaptation of a **steerable guidewire,** like that currently available for balloon angioplasty techniques, has been shown to help prevent the frequent perforations seen when bare optical fibers are used (19).

The use of a **laser thermal balloon angioplasty** system has been proposed as a method for fusing torn endothelial flaps or, perhaps, for reducing restenosis rates following balloon angioplasty (20). This technique appears promising from preliminary animal studies and is in clinical trial at present. Whether this technique will emerge as "adjunctive" therapy for use with balloon angioplasty remains to be determined.

Other thermal mechanisms for dissolution of arterial plaque include **spark erosion**, **radiofrequency**, and **chemically activated catheter systems** (21-23). All of these systems have the potential for miniaturization to catheter sizes adaptable for the coronary circulation. However, as with the thermal systems used with laser activation, their interaction with tissue, specifically, the atheromatous plaque, is very similar. Thus, as seen with the earlier experiments using laser-activated hot-tip systems, heavily calcific lesions could not be adequately removed. Also, good surface contact is necessary between the plaque and the delivery system in order to achieve vaporization. Early experience in the coronary circulation demonstrated that in eccentric or calcific plaque poor contact with the probe system results in failure to recanalize or cross the lesion. Consequently, excessive thermal damage to the surrounding vessel with resulting perforation has occurred in this setting. Obviously, thermal monitoring with feedback control is necessary for such systems to avoid sticking of the probe tips to the arterial wall. The benefits of thermal monitoring have been shown to result in a potentially safer approach.

The spark erosion system vaporizes tissue as a result of discharge of sparks that vaporize the water in the tissue, creating steam. Thus, a steam pocket develops between the spark erosion catheter tip and the tissue, resulting in a miniexplosion. This has the tendency of creating tissue tearing, which is seen especially in plaque with high lipid content. As with other thermal systems, no effective vaporization was present in the calcific portions of plaque. Also because of the use of an electric current, the discharge is triggered only during the refractory period of the ventricular cycle. Finally, the hydration state of the tissue greatly influences the effectiveness of the vaporization, resulting in a variability in coagulation of tissue.

Chemically activated thermal systems have been used. These utilize a catalytic converter thermal tip. The principle of combustion energy from a stoichiometric reaction between oxygen and hydrogen gas catalyzed by a small piece of palladium sponge within the tip is used. Gas flow regulates the temperature, which is monitored by a thermocouple inside the tip. Temperatures reached have been greater than 350° C in less than 1 sec. In saline solution, a maximum temperature of 170° C has been achieved at 5-sec duration.

Radiofrequency catheter systems have also been reported to be successful in recanalization of peripheral arteries in humans. This device has the capacity for thermal angioplasty using a 5 Fr catheter shaft. The tip is composed of a gold-plated, completely encapsulated metal cap that can be heated in air up to 550° C. In total peripheral occlusion, perforation and lack of recanalization in heavily calcified plaque similar to that of the other thermally activated devices has also been noted. Once again, these devices rely heavily on adequate mechanical surface tissue contact for effective recanalization.

Clinical Investigations

Experience in Peripheral Arteries

Ginsburg et al. first reported a case of limb salvage using an argon laser and an open-ended bare fiber held in a coaxial position to a vessel lumen within a balloon catheter (24). Geshwind et al. reported on improvement of lumen diameter in three patients' peripheral arteries, using a bare fiber and an Nd-YAG laser (25).

In a group of 16 patients Ginsburg et al. described recanalization of occluded arteries using bare fibers as he had described earlier (26). Eight of the 16 patients were recanalized, but two were perforated. Those that were perforated did not have any major adverse reaction. In another group of six patients Geshwind et al. reported successful recanalization with a bare fiber and an Nd Yag laser, but on follow-up all patients reoccluded (27). Two went on to have amputation, and the vascular tissue that had received laser treatment was examined. This did not reveal evidence for the dissection typical of balloon angioplasty. No thrombosis of the artery segment was present in spite of charring and thermal necrosis. It was postulated that the small-sized channel was not of sufficient size to maintain flow.

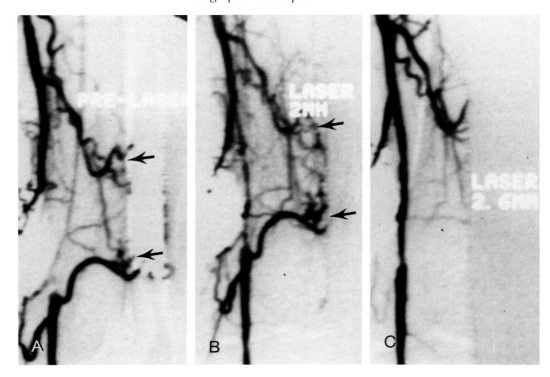

Figure 16.3. Digital angiograms of a left superficial femoral artery (SFA) in a 47-year-old male with a 12-day history of rest ischemia. Angiogram before laser recanalization *(A)* showed a totally occluded SFA segment measuring 12 cm in length. Distal portion of artery fills by collateral branches *(arrows)*. Angiogram after initial laser recanalization *(B)*, using a 2-mm hybrid probe shown in Figure 16.2. Several areas of residual focal stenosis can be seen. Collateral branches are still present *(arrows)*. Angiogram following laser irradiation *(C)* with a 2.6-mm hybrid probe. Further reduction in residual stenosis is noted. The collateral branches are no longer seen. (From Abela GS, Conti CR. Use of the laser in the treatment of coronary artery obstruction. In Hurst JW, ed. The Heart. ed 7. New York: McGraw Hill, in press, 1989.)

Using the laser thermal probe or hot-tip approach, Cumberland and colleagues demonstrated the feasibility of creating a channel in high-grade stenosis and total occlusions in the peripheral circulation (28). They reported 56 cases with a 75% success rate for recanalization of occluded segments. Because channel size was small, all of these patients also underwent balloon angioplasty. Using a laser-thermal probe combination or hybrid probe, Abela et al. reported initially on 11 arteries treated intraoperatively in patients with peripheral artery segments not amenable to balloon angioplasty (29). Subsequently, 51 arteries have been treated in a percutaneous fashion or via cutdown technique using a similar approach (Fig. 16.3). Recanalization was feasible in 78% with a 20% perforation rate (30). All segments treated were not amenable to balloon angioplasty as initial therapy. In this group of patients, none with perforation required urgent surgery or blood transfusion. Also, because of the larger channel size made by the hybrid probe system used, seven patients were treated with the laser as sole therapy. Long-term follow-up of these patients has demonstrated that the final outcome was not different from comparable historical studies done with balloon angioplasty alone. The advantage of this system, however, is that patients who were previously balloon angioplasty candidates could be treated in a less invasive fashion, avoiding or postponing the need for bypass surgery. Nordstrom utilized a defocusing lens system that allows a balloon catheter to be advanced into a small channel made by the optical fiber and subsequent balloon angioplasty to be

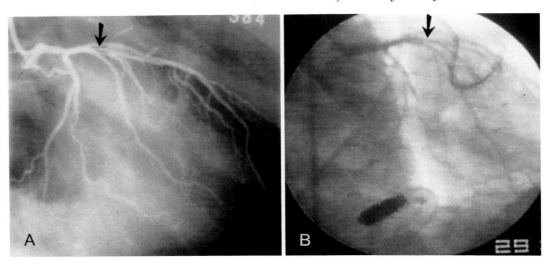

Figure 16.4. *A,* Cineangiogram of a patient with stable angina, showing severe left anterior descending artery stenosis *(arrow). B,* Angiogram of left coronary artery (obtained by recording the fluoroscopic image on videotape) immediately after the delivery of laser energy (132J). Reduction in severity of the left anterior descending artery stenosis is suggested *(arrow).* (From Crea F, Davies G, McKenna WJ, et al. Laser recanalization of coronary arteries by metal capped optical fiber: early clinical experience in patients with stable angina pectoris. Br Heart J 1988;59:168–174.)

performed (31). The procedure takes slightly longer to perform because of the slowly advancing process of 1-mm fiber movement followed by standard balloon angioplasty catheter.

Experiences in the Coronary Circulation

Numerous attempts have been made to evaluate laser recanalization in the coronary circulation. The first was conducted by Choy et al., using a bare optical fiber at the time of bypass surgery (32). A new vascular channel was made in four of the five vessels, but the longest patency noted was 25 days in one of the vessels. In a brief report Cumberland and colleagues demonstrated the results of percutaneous, hot-tip laser angioplasty (33) followed by balloon angioplasty in the coronary circulation. In two of these vessels it appears that reocclusion occurred as evidenced by an elevation in the cardiac enzymes and ECG changes. In another brief report Crea et al. used the same technique of percutaneous hot-tip angioplasty in the operative setting (34). Sanborn et al., using a hot-tip system, were able to recanalize only four of seven arteries (35). In six patients Crea et al. used a percutaneous hot-tip approach in the operating room and demonstrated improvement in lumen diameter in three of the six patients with two unchanged and one vessel perforated (36) (Figs. 16.4 and 16.5).

Remaining Problems for Laser Recanalization

Guiding the laser delivery systems has remained an important problem. Because angioscopes have generally been too large, have been relatively traumatic, and have required large volumes of fluid infusion to displace blood in the field, direct visualization has not been practical. Fluoroscopic guidance, using guiding catheters and guidewires, as with percutaneous transluminal coronary angioplasty (PTCA), at present is the method used by most operators, but these systems need to be refined for laser work. At present, ultrasound catheter systems are being evaluated to provide assessment of the wall and plaque thickness at a given site (37). Another technique for guiding laser recanalization is the fluorescent feedback system. Finally, the advent of microangioscopes, 0.5 mm in diameter, with a high resolution may provide for intraluminal diameter measurement and

Figure 16.5. *A*, Cineangiogram of a patient with stable angina, showing a proximal left anterior descending artery stenosis *(arrow)*. *B*, Fluoroscopic image obtained after delivery of laser energy that allowed passage of the optical fiber through the stenosis. The metal cap *(arrow)* is now distal to the stenosis. *C*, Angiogram of the left coronary artery (obtained by recording the fluoroscopic image on videotape) immediately after delivery of laser energy. There is improvement of severity of stenosis *(arrow)*. (From Crea F, Davies G, McKenna WJ, et al. Laser recanalization of coronary arteries by metal capped optical fiber: early clinical experience in patients with stable angina pectoris. Br Heart J 1988;59:168–174.)

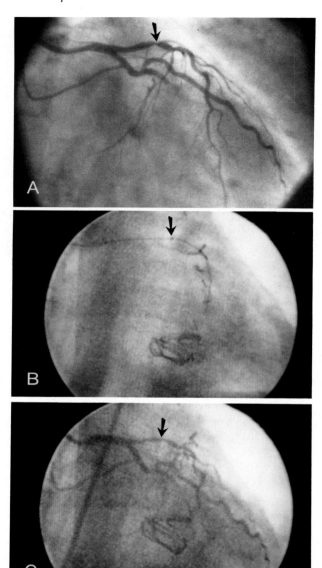

guidance that were not feasible with the previous angioscope designs (38).

SAFETY CONSIDERATIONS

Catheter-directed laser irradiation of vascular tissue must be used carefully and by experienced personnel according to the guidelines set by the American Society for Lasers in Medicine and Surgery. These guidelines require that personnel be trained in the use of lasers with hands-on experience as well as

some basic knowledge of laser technology. Lasers have been demonstrated to be hazardous to humans. They may cause damage to the retina by either direct or reflected laser beams. Irradiation of the skin may lead to thermal burns. Also, the use of lasers may be associated with electrical shock, fire, explosion of ignitable gases, and toxic fumes, as well as with exposure to the potential carcinogenic effects of ultraviolet light. It is strongly suggested that the operating team have hands-on experience with lasers and recognize the

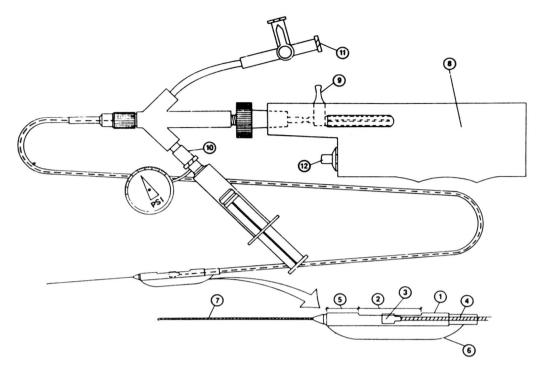

Figure 16.6. Atherectomy catheter system. Components of the catheter are as follows: *(1)* cylindrical housing, *(2)* longitudinal opening, *(3)* cutter, *(4)* cutter drive cable (to motor), *(5)* specimen collection area, *(6)* balloon support mechanism, *(7)* fixed guidewire, *(8)* motor, *(9)* cutter-advance lever, *(10)* balloon inflation port, *(11)* flush port, and *(12)* Touhy Borst opening for cable connector. (From Simpson JB, Selmon MR, Robertson GC, et al. Transluminal atherectomy for occlusive peripheral vascular disease. Am J Cardiol 1988;61:96G–101G. Reprinted with permission of the *American Journal of Cardiology.*)

limitations of the various laser systems available for use.

MECHANICAL DEVICES FOR ARTERIAL VASCULAR RECANALIZATION

Other techniques for the recanalization of occluded vessels have been proposed recently. These include several mechanical devices, such as the Kensey catheter, Simpson atherectomy catheter, and rotational atherectomy devices (39, 40). All of these systems have certain potential advantages. Like the laser, an advantage of atherectomy and rotational atherectomy devices is that the plaque is either removed or ablated, and thereby reduced in volume. Rotational atherectomy (Kensey catheter, Ritchie catheter) has been shown to create vascular channels by abrasive removal of atheromatous plaque. Preliminary reports

in coronary and peripheral circulation have appeared, demonstrating the feasibility of this abrasive system.

The Simpson atherectomy catheter is a technique that uses a miniature shaving device within a chamber to remove plaque. The sharp cutting edge is compressed against eccentric plaque by inflating a soft balloon on the opposite side of the opening that exposes the cutting edge (see Figs. 16.6 and 16.7). Atheromatous tissue has been successfully removed from both peripheral and coronary arteries, as well as coronary bypass grafts. In the peripheral circulation numerous passes are required in order to achieve removal of enough plaque material. One advantage of this approach is the ability to examine the histology of removed material. This is of special interest relative to lesions that have restenosed following balloon angioplasty. This approach seems to lend itself best to proximal lesions that are relatively short

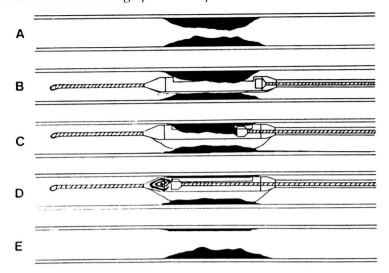

Figure 16.7. Diagram of atherectomy procedure. *A*, The lesion before atherectomy. *B*, atherectomy catheter in position across the lesion; *C*, the balloon support inflated; *D*, the cutter advanced and specimen trapped in the housing; *E*, the balloon deflated and the catheter removed. (From Simpson JB, Selmon MR, Robertson GC, et al. Transluminal atherectomy for occlusive peripheral vascular disease. Am J Cardiol 1988;61:96G–101G. Reprinted with permission of the *American Journal of Cardiology.*)

and recurrent occlusions following balloon angioplasty, but experience is limited. Critical evaluation with long-term follow-up is underway to define the role of this device.

Intravascular Stents

Currently, the most limiting disadvantage of balloon angioplasty is the restenosis rate, as well as the abrupt closure that is occasionally seen following balloon dilation. One other method, in addition to the various laser mechanical systems of plaque ablation, that could potentially solve the problems of balloon angioplasty is the use of intravascular stents. Initial studies in animal models, as well as in early experiences in human patients, have shown that stents can be successful in maintaining vascular patency following failed balloon angioplasty. At present, medical treatment with high dosages of calcium channel blockers, steroids, and other drug regimens has failed to solve these problems.

Animal studies in dog coronary and peripheral arteries have shown that both the steel stent and other types of stents may maintain vascular patency following several months of implantation. Soon after deployment the stent is covered by a thin thrombotic layer that eventually endothelializes.

Early clinical experience in coronary and peripheral arteries has shown success and maintenance of successful patency over a 6-month period (41). Thrombosis of the vessel seen on occasion following stent placement has been ascribed to either competitive flow or poor distal runoff in the vascular bed of the stented artery. One case report of possible induced vascular spasm following an exercise treadmill test 2 days after stent placement in the left anterior descending coronary vessel has been entertained. This patient went on to have bypass surgery and died from complications following surgery. In this vessel segments of thrombus were noted in the stented portion of the vessel; however, no distal embolization was noted.

Numerous stents have been developed. Many have different features that include elastic self-expanding spiral, a memory metal type that self-extends with heating in the body and balloon deformable-type models. Side branches appear to remain patent, with most of these systems resulting in endothelial lining covering the stent materials on long-term follow-up in various animal model studies. Obviously, the various alloys of metal, such as nickel and steel, used to make these stents could result in an endothelial reaction that could, over the long-term, result in early occlusion of the vessel. The perfect stent configuration that leads to minimal tissue reaction has yet to be developed.

Further follow-up, as well as improvement in these materials used to make the stents, will be needed to have a more predictable long-term outcome.

SUMMARY

Availability of laser techniques, as well as other devices for removal of arterial obstructions through percutaneous approaches, has markedly altered the future for nonoperative treatment of coronary and peripheral arterial obstruction. These devices have the potential for vaporization or removal of plaque, resulting in a clean incision performed via a percutaneous approach. It is likely that some or all of these devices in some form will play an important role in the treatment of occlusive vascular disease. Because the effects of these techniques are different and the type of lesion best suited for each technique seems to differ, the interventional catheter specialist will probably be able to approach a wide variety of lesions with a reasonable chance of success in the near future.

References

1. Gruntzig RA, Senning A, Siegenthaler WE. Nonoperative dilation of coronary artery stenosis: percutaneous transluminal coronary angioplasty. N Engl J Med 1979;301:61–68.
2. Holmes DR, Vleistra RE, Smith HC, et al. Restenosis after percutaneous transluminal coronary angioplasty (PTCA). A report from the PTCA registry of National Heart Lung and Blood Institute. Am J Cardiol 1984;53:77C–81C.
3. Leimgruber PP, Roubin GS, Hollman J, et al. Restenosis after successful coronary angioplasty in patients with single vessel disease. Circulation 1986;73:710–717.
4. Johnston WK, Rae M, Hogg-Johnston SA. 5-year results of a prospective study of percutaneous transluminal angioplasty. Ann Surgery 1987;206:403–412.
5. Abela GS, Normann S, Cohen D, et al. Effects of carbon dioxide, Nd:YAG and Argon laser radiation on coronary atheromatous plaque. Am J Cardiol 1982;50:1199–1205.
6. Choy DSJ, Stertzer S, Rotterdam HZ, Sharrock N, Kaminow IP. Laser coronary angioplasty: experience with nine cadaver hearts. Am J Cardiol 1982;50:1206–1208.
7. Lee G, Ikeda R, Herman I, et al. The qualitative effects of laser irradiation on human arteriosclerotic disease. Am Heart J 1983;105:885–889.
8. Isner JM, Clarke RH, Donaldson RF, Aharon A. Identification of photoproducts liberated in vitro argon laser irradiation of atherosclerotic plaque, calcific valves and myocardium. Am J Cardiol 1985;55:1192–1196.
9. Abela GS, Pepine CJ. Emerging applications of laser therapy for occlusive vascular disease. Cardiovasc Rev Rep 1985;6:269–278.
10. Abela GS, Normann SJ, Cohen DM, et al. Laser recanalization of occluded atherosclerotic arteries: an in vivo and in vitro study. Circulation 1985;71:403–411.
11. Abela GS, Fenech A, Crea F, Conti CR. "Hot-tip": another method of laser vascular recanalization. Lasers Surg Med 1985;5:327–335.
12. Sanborn TA, Faxon DP, Haudenschild CC, Ryan TJ. Experimental angioplasty: circumferential distribution of laser thermal energy with a laser probe. J Am Coll Cardiol 1985;5:934–938.
13. Fourrier JL, Marache P, Brunetaud JM, Mordon S, Lablanche JM, Bertrand ME. Laser recanalization of peripheral arteries by contact sapphire in man (abstr). Circulation 1986;74:II204.
14. Cothren RM, Hayes CB, Kramer JR, Sacks B, Kittrell C, Feld MS. A multifiber catheter with an optical shield for laser angiosurgery. Lasers Life Sci 1986;1:1–12.
15. Deckelbaum LI, Lam JK, Babin HS, Clubb KS, Long MB. Discrimination of normal and atherosclerotic aorta by laser-induced fluorescence. Lasers Surg Med 1987;7:330–335.
16. Leon MB, Prevosti LG, Smith PD, et al. Probe and fire laser angioplasty: fluorescence atheroma detection and selective atheroma ablation (abstr). Circulation 1987;76:IV–409.
17. Sartori M, Weilboecher D, Henry PD, Kubodera S, Tittel FK, Sauerbrey R. Autofluorescence maps of human arteries (abstr). Circulation 1987;76:IV–408.
18. Chaudhry H, Richards-Kortum R, Kolubayev T, Kittrell C, Ratliff N, Feld MS. Alteration of artery wall fluorescence due to excessive laser irradiation (abstr). J Am Coll Cardiol 1988;11:49A.
19. Abela GS, Barbieri E, Roxey T, Conti CR. Guided laser thermal angioplasty in coronary arteries of live dogs without perforation (abstr). Circulation 1986;74:II–457.
20. Spears JR. Percutaneous transluminal coronary angioplasty restenosis: potential prevention with laser balloon angioplasty. Am J Cardiol 1987;60:61B–64B.
21. Slager CJ, Essed CE, Schuurbiers JCH, Bom N, Serruys PW, Meester GT. Vaporization of atherosclerotic plaques by spark erosion. J Am Coll Cardiol 1985;5:1382–1386.
22. Litvack F, Grundfest W, Mohr F, et al. Percutaneous "hot-tip" angioplasty in man by a radio frequency catheter system (abstr). J Am Coll Cardiol 1988;11:108A.
23. Lu DY, Leon MG, Bowman RL. A prototype catalytic thermal tip catheter: design parameters and in vitro tissue studies (abstr). Lasers Surg Med 1987;7:101.
24. Ginsburg R, Kirr DS, Guthaner P, Tolh J, Mitchell RS. Salvage of an ischemic limb by laser

angioplasty: description of a new technique. Clin Cardiol 1984;7:54–58.

25. Geshwind H, Boussignac G, Teisseire B. Percutaneous transluminal laser angioplasty in man [letter]. Lancet 1984;2:844.

26. Ginsburg R, Wexler L, Mitchell RS, Profitt D. Percutaneous transluminal laser angioplasty for treatment of peripheral vascular disease: clinical experience with 16 patients. Radiology 1985; 156:619–624.

27. Geshwind HJ, Boussignac G, Teisseire B, Benhaiem N, Bittoun R, Laurent D. Conditions for effective Nd:YAG laser angioplasty. Br Heart J 1984;52:484–489.

28. Cumberland DC, Tayler DI, Welsh CL, et al. Percutaneous laser thermal angioplasty: initial clinical results with a laser probe in total peripheral artery occlusions. Lancet 1986;28:1457–1459.

29. Abela GS, Seeger JM, Barbieri E, et al. Laser angioplasty with angioscopic guidance in man. J Am Coll Cardiol 1986;8:184–192.

30. Abela GS, Seeger JM, Pry RS. Percutaneous laser recanalization of totally occulated peripheral arteries: a technical approach. Dynamic Cardiovascular Imaging, 1988;1:302–308.

31. Nordstrom L. Laser enhanced angioplasty: the use of direct argon exposure as an alternative to contact probe plaque ablation (abstr). Lasers Surg Med 1988;8:151.

32. Choy DS, Stertzer SH, Myler RK, Marco J, Fourinal G. Human coronary laser recanalization. Clin Cardiol 1984;7:377–381.

33. Cumberland DC, Oakley GDG, Smith GH, et al. Percutaneous laser–assisted coronary angioplasty [letter]. Lancet 1986;2:214.

34. Crea F, Davies C, McKenna W, Pashazade M, Taylor K, Maseri A. Percutaneous laser recanalization of coronary arteries [letter]. Lancet 1986;2:214–215.

35. Sanborn TA, Faxon DP, Kellett MA, Ryan TJ. Percutaneous coronary laser thermal angioplasty. J Am Coll Cardiol 1986;8:1437–1440.

36. Crea F, Davies G, McKenna WJ, et al. Laser recanalization of coronary arteries by a metal capped optical fiber: early clinical experience in patients with stable angina pectoris. Br Heart J 1988;59:168–174.

37. Yock PG, Linker DT, Thapliyal HV, et al. Real time, two–dimensional catheter ultrasound: a new technique for high resolution intravascular imaging (abstr). J Am Coll Cardiol 1988;11:130A.

38. Seeger JM, Abela GS. Angioscopy as an adjunct to arterial reconstructive surgery: a preliminary report. J Vasc Surg 1986;4:315–320.

39. Simpson JB, Selmon MR, Robertson GC, et al. Transluminal atherectomy for occlusive peripheral vascular disease. Am J Cardiol 1988;61:96G–101G.

40. Zacca NM, Raizner AE, Noon GP, et al. Short term follow up of patients treated with a recently developed rotational atherectomy device and in vivo assessment of the particles generated (abstr). J Am Coll Cardiol 1988;11:109A.

41. Sigwart U, Puel J, Mirkovitch V, Joffre F, Kappenberger L. Intravascular stents to prevent occlusion and restenosis after transluminal angioplasty. N Engl J Med 1987;316:701–706.

17

Valvuloplasty

James A. Hill, M.D.
J. Patrick Kleaveland, M.D.

INTRODUCTION

Corrective, nonexcisional valve procedures have been used since the first closed mitral commissurotomy was performed for mitral stenosis. Cardiac surgeons have performed a variety of different operations with the goal of palliating symptoms while preserving both native valve tissue and function. These have included open aortic valvuloplasty, closed and open mitral commissurotomy, and pulmonary valvotomy for stenotic valve lesions as well as mitral and aortic valve repair for regurgitant lesions. In children, there is frequently a need to delay valve replacement because of prolonged life expectancy and growth. As a result, nonexcisional corrective valve surgery has been applied for many years for aortic and mitral stenosis in young patients. In the elderly, the problems are different. Often the patients have an increased risk for cardiac surgery or a probability that the life-prolonging benefits of such an operation will not be realized because of advanced age or other life-limiting disease. With the interest in balloon technology stimulated by coronary angioplasty, the use of balloons to perform nonoperative opening of stenotic cardiac valves has grown.

HISTORY

The modern era of balloon valvuloplasty was begun when it was first reported as successful therapy for pulmonic stenosis in children in 1982 (1). Also in 1982, the first adult patient to undergo pulmonic valvuloplasty was reported by Pepine et al. (2). Lababidi et al. (3)

began to apply the procedure to the aortic valve in children, and in 1984, Inoue et al. (4), using a unique balloon design, reported on six patients undergoing successful mitral valvuloplasty. In 1985, Locke and colleagues (5) reported a series of children undergoing mitral valvuloplasty for rheumatic mitral stenosis, and the procedure became more well-known. Widespread application of the procedure to left-sided valvular stenoses in adults was understandably delayed. There were multiple reasons for this, including the fear of systemic emboli or of excessive damage, resulting in valvular insufficiency, and the excellent short- and long-term results obtained with aortic and mitral valve replacement and repair. In 1986, Cribier et al. (6) reported on three elderly patients with calcific aortic stenosis who underwent balloon aortic valvuloplasty because of either severe symptoms and reluctance to undergo surgery or high surgical risk. All had short-term improvement, both hemodynamically and clinically, and the procedure began to be applied in a more widespread fashion.

MECHANISMS OF EFFECT

The mechanism by which balloon dilatation increases effective valve area varies, depending on the pathology of the specific valve dilated, individual characteristics of the valve, and the technique utilized. Potential mechanisms include separation of fused commissures, leaflet tearing, fracture of calcific nodules, annular fracture, annular and leaflet stretching, and increasing leaflet mobility by a combination of these mechanisms.

Unfortunately, many of these mechanisms also may lead to the complications of the procedure.

Dilatation of the **pulmonic valve** is almost certainly due primarily to commissural separation, leaflet tearing, and cusp avulsion (7). Most stenotic pulmonic valves are not calcified in younger patients, but the presence of calcium in adults does not seem to affect the ability to effectively dilate the valve (2). The results of successful dilatation may be expected to be long-term from a hemodynamic standpoint, but long-term follow-up has yet to verify this. Because the stenotic lesion is based on leaflet margin shortening rather than commissural fusion, the severely dysplastic valve is much less likely to permit successful balloon dilatation (8, 9).

The stenotic **mitral valve**, generally rheumatic in origin, also has commissural fusion as a prominent part of the stenotic process. Other aspects of the pathologic process, such as subvalvular apparatus thickening, shortening, and fibrosis, probably are not amenable to balloon dilatation by current techniques. When the valve does calcify, fracture of calcific areas probably contributes to improved leaflet mobility, but the primary therapeutic mechanism appears to be commissural separation, much like that which occurs with a surgical commissurotomy. In vitro data (10) suggest that, even with calcium in the valve only, commissural separation occurs and that progressive separation occurs with progressively larger balloon sizes. Other in vitro studies (11) confirm these data and suggest that fracture of nodular calcium also occurs. Studies on patients undergoing mitral valve dilatation support commissural separation as the primary mechanism of beneficial effect but suggest that severe calcification may limit beneficial results (12).

Dilatation of congenital **aortic stenosis** improves valve function by either tearing the valve or separating the commissures, depending on the underlying pathoanatomy. The mechanism for relief of calcific aortic stenosis by balloon dilatation seems to be different. Several reports suggest that multiple mechanisms are responsible for improving valve opening (13, 14). The most prominent mechanism in elderly patients with senile calcific aortic stenosis appears to be fracture of nodular calcification and improvement of leaflet mobil-ity. In selected cases, particularly those with a history of rheumatic fever, commissural separation may occur, but this does not seem to occur in those patients with congenital fusion. As commissural fusion is not a prominent feature of degenerative aortic stenosis, commissural separation does not appear to be a significant factor in the improvement noted in these patients. Likewise, in the elderly group, leaflet tearing appears to be a rare occurrence. Unfortunately, some of the immediate improvement noted may only be due to leaflet stretching which may not result in long-term benefit. The specific mechanism responsible for dilatation in any individual, such as calcium nodule fracture, may influence selection criteria.

INDICATIONS

As with many procedures undergoing active development, indications for valvuloplasty are changing. It is generally accepted that balloon dilatation should be the primary treatment of choice in most pediatric and adult patients with pulmonic stenosis. Patients with pulmonic stenosis and others with associated lesions requiring heart surgery and those with dysplastic valves represent the exceptions. Indications for dilatation of the left-sided valvular lesions are less clearly defined.

The most prevalent lesion for which balloon valvuloplasty is applied is acquired aortic stenosis in elderly patients. While valvuloplasty has not been shown to prolong life, there are several situations where balloon valvuloplasty may be indicated. These include: (*a*) increased risk for aortic valve replacement for cardiac reasons (severe coronary heart disease, pulmonary hypertension, or extremely poor left ventricular function); (*b*) high surgical risk because of other medical illness, such as renal failure, hepatic disease, obstructive lung disease, and/or advanced age; (*c*) expectation that the life-prolonging benefits of aortic valve replacement are limited, as in the case of a malignancy or other severe debilitating disease; (*d*) to lessen the risk of an urgent non-cardiac procedure; (*e*) to temporarily improve aortic valve obstruction to stabilize an unstable state; (*f*) to reduce the risks associated with aortic valve replacement in a patient with severe left ventricular dysfunction and congestive heart failure; and (*g*) where surgical therapy is neither available nor economically feasible, as in some third world countries.

Reasons for performing mitral valvuloplasty are similar to those of aortic valvuloplasty, but differ in that a larger proportion of potential candidates are young. In this circumstance, mitral valve surgery should be delayed whenever possible because of the longer life expectancy of the patients, and mitral dilatation may be appropriate. This younger group, however, includes patients who are excellent candidates for surgical mitral commissurotomy, but it is not clear when one procedure should be performed instead of the other. Balloon valvuloplasty probably should not be performed in the presence of left atrial thrombus demonstrated by echocardiography or any other condition which prohibits transseptal catheterization or severe subvalvular disease. To date, experience with balloon mit-ral valvuloplasty is limited, and direct comparisons with surgical commissurotomy have not been reported.

Balloon dilatation of the tricuspid valve or prosthetic valves has been so limited that indications for the procedure in these areas must be individualized using some of the same guidelines as for other valve dilatation.

EQUIPMENT

Balloon Catheters

At present, catheters available for percutaneous balloon valvuloplasty have been approved by the Food and Drug Administration (FDA) only for treatment of pulmonic valve stenosis. Use of these catheters for balloon valvuloplasty in patients with aortic, mitral, or tricuspid valve stenosis is not FDA approved. The technique is, however, in widespread use under research protocols approved by individual institutions and hospital investigational review boards.

Balloon valvuloplasty catheters (Mansfield) (Fig. 17.1) have a shaft diameter that is 8, 9, or 10 Fr, but even with the deflated balloon, they are effectively larger in profile for insertion because the deflated balloon is bulky. They are available with fully inflated balloon diameters of 8, 10, 12, 15, 18, 20, 23, and 25 mm. The balloons come in 3- and 5.5-cm lengths but may be obtained up to 8 cm in length. The balloon

length describes the effective working length of the parallel surfaces available for dilatation. There is a radiopaque marker at either end of the balloon where it is attached to the catheter. Because of tapering of the balloon at either end, the 1 to 1.5 cm portions at each end of the balloon are not useful for dilatation.

Currently, the balloon itself is made of polyethylene and inflates to a fixed diameter at inflation pressures up to 3.5 atm, the maximum recommended by the manufacturer. At higher inflation pressures, the balloon may increase in size, become oval-shaped, and eventually rupture. Most balloons will rupture between 3.5 and 5 atm, usually tearing in a linear fashion along the long axis of the balloon.

There are a number of modifications of these catheters that are being evaluated that may increase their ease of use, safety, and general clinical applicability. Lower profile balloons with smaller shaft size that will fit through smaller sheaths are a major development. Balloon catheters with stepped 15- and 20-mm or 18- and 23-mm balloons mounted on one catheter would allow sequential dilatation without the need to change catheters. In another modification, a curved, pigtail-type loop is placed on the end of the catheter to guard against trauma to the ventricle and vascular structures. This catheter also has two separate pressure ports that can be positioned on both sides of a stenotic valve, which allow pressure measurements without removing the balloon. Other designs include two or three balloons that inflate separately side by side on the same shaft (15, 16).

Guidewires

Theoretically, any guidewire could be used for valvuloplasty, but the balloon catheters are quite stiff, and a certain amount of rigidity in a guidewire is helpful for balloon insertion and stabilization. Generally, an 0.038-inch guidewire is necessary, as an 0.035-inch guidewire is too flexible. The 260-cm exchange length should be used. Teflon-coated guidewires with three different degrees of stiffness are available from several manufacturers, but all have a flexible tip. The "extra stiff" wire is recommended for aortic valvuloplasty, but the standard stiffness is adequate for mitral and pulmonic dilatation. The extra stiffness is due to a heavy-duty mandril that is tapered and

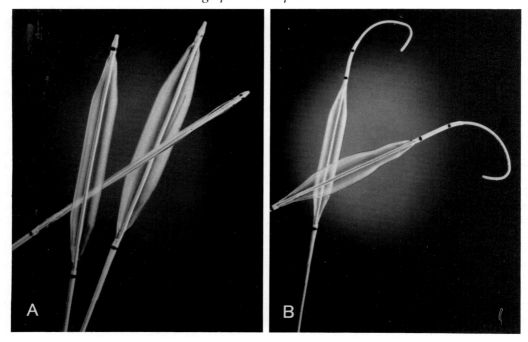

Figure 17.1. **A,** Standard valvuloplasty balloon catheters of two different sizes inflated, and one size deflated. **B,** Cribier-Letac balloon with graduated balloon size on the same balloon. Pigtail end on this catheter provides for less trauma in the ventricle and for the measurement of distal pressure without removing the balloon. A proximal port (not shown) also allows for measurement of aortic pressure. (Courtesy of Mansfield Scientific).

welded to a thin mandril wire at one end to provide the soft flexible tip.

Sheaths

Large lumen introducer sheaths with check-flow valves have been developed for insertion of balloon dilatation catheters into both the arterial and venous systems. They are available in 10, 12, 13, and 14 Fr sizes. The currently available balloon catheters (Mansfield) fit in 12 and 14 Fr size sheaths, but the size necessary for each individual balloon varies and should be checked prior to insertion. The check-flow valve will prevent back-bleeding when the dilating catheter has been inserted or when the diagnostic catheter is placed through the sheath. Catheter exchanges through this sheath should be rapid because, when only the guidewire is in the sheath, excessive bleeding can occur. The sheaths come in a variety of lengths. The longest has a Mullins curve and is designed to fit across the atrial septum to allow better stabilization of the balloon across the mitral valve.

Special Equipment

Because of the occasional need to place two balloon systems across the atrial septum, a catheter has been developed that has two lumens and will accept two large 0.038-inch guidewires. This double-lumen catheter is size 10 Fr with two side by side lumina of 0.042-inch diameter. These catheters are used after an initial guidewire has been placed. The double-lumen catheter is then placed over the first guidewire, a second guidewire is advanced through the other lumen, and the catheter is removed, leaving both wires in place. Balloon catheters can then be placed over both wires.

MEDICATIONS

Medication use during valvuloplasty is variable. Mild sedation along with adequate local anesthesia, rarely general anesthesia, is necessary in the uncooperative patient. Drugs that should be available for immediate administration include vasopressors (phenylephrine, dopamine, epinephrine), atropine, and other drugs used for resuscitation. Most operators use full heparinization, which may or may not be reversed with protamine at the end of the procedure. Adequate blood and fluid replacement are essential, and some routinely use plasma expanders instead of saline.

TECHNIQUES

The most effective techniques for performing balloon valvuloplasty are not yet known. As new equipment is developed and greater experience is gained, the optimal techniques will become clearer. This section will provide the operator with a reasonable base on which to develop a practice of balloon valvuloplasty but is not meant to be inclusive of all the possible nuances of the technical aspects of these procedures.

There are several general measures that should be employed in any valvuloplasty procedure, especially those of the mitral and aortic valves. Right heart catheterization will be necessary to determine cardiac output and should be used to monitor pulmonary artery pressure during the procedure. Special attention should be given to maintaining adequate fluid volume, as blood loss can occur rapidly and vagal reactions can be prolonged and much more poorly tolerated when the patient is hypovolemic. In addition, in patients with conduction abnormalities such as right bundle branch block, temporary pacing should be immediately available because bradycardia, left bundle branch block, and complete heart block are common during catheter manipulation and balloon inflation. Temporary pacing can usually be achieved by using a pulmonary artery catheter with pacing capabilities. Systemic pressure monitoring is also necessary and may be done from the femoral, radial, or brachial artery. It is the authors' preference to use a catheter in the contralateral femoral artery to monitor either aortic pressure during aortic valvuloplasty or left ventricular pressure during mitral valvuloplasty.

Aortic Valvuloplasty

Retrograde Technique

While results from retrograde and antegrade aortic valvuloplasty seem similar (17), the retrograde technique (Fig. 17.2) is the most commonly utilized approach for aortic valvuloplasty at the present time. Insertion of the balloon catheters can be performed via the femoral or brachial route, but the femoral approach is favored because of the size of the balloons relative to the vessel. The artery can be entered either by direct surgical cutdown or percutaneously. Since a femoral cutdown is more involved and generally performed by vascular surgeons, the percutaneous approach is used by most operators. Whichever approach is used, a sheath with a check-flow valve may be inserted to aid in balloon catheter stability and limit blood loss. Although a sheath may make removing the balloon catheters difficult, particularly if the balloon has burst, the balloons can generally be removed with slow gentle pressure and rotation. If the balloon cannot be removed using this technique, the balloon and sheath should be removed together, leaving the guidewire in place. With the percutaneous technique, if a sheath is not used, manual pressure must be maintained on the insertion site at all times to limit blood loss. A J-tip guidewire should be used for all manipulations of either sheaths or catheters to help prevent arterial damage.

After arterial access is obtained, any end-hole catheter can be utilized to cross the aortic valve, using standard techniques (See Chapter 6). After the aortic valve is crossed and hemodynamic measurements made, an exchange-length 0.038-inch extra stiff guidewire (260 cm) is inserted, and the catheter is removed leaving the exchange wire in the ventricle. This larger, stiff guidewire will allow for easier balloon catheter manipulation and stability. The tip should be further enlarged to an exaggerated pigtail loop configuration prior to insertion to cushion the catheter tip end to help avoid ventricular perforation.

With the guidewire in the left ventricle, the balloon catheter is advanced over it and across the aortic valve under fluoroscopic guidance. Negative pressure should be exerted on the balloon to make it as small as possible as it is advanced through the skin, using a twisting motion. It should be kept in mind that extra pressure on the femoral artery at the time of insertion and removal of the balloons can provoke pain and vagal reactions, which are poorly tolerated in patients with aortic stenosis; therefore, adequate local

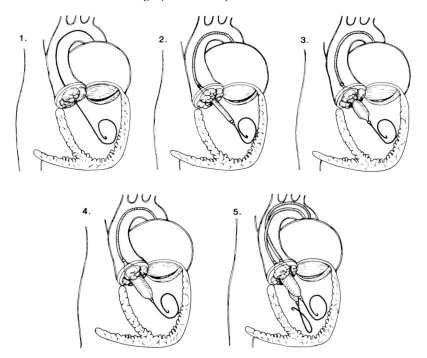

Figure 17.2. Schematic representation of the retrograde technique for aortic valvuloplasty. See text for details.

anesthesia is important. While advancing the balloon, the guidewire should be kept taut to maintain position in the left ventricle. When the radiopaque markers marking the ends of the balloon are straddling the valve, the balloon is in proper position for inflation. The guidewire should be kept in the balloon at all times to keep the catheter from perforating vascular structures.

The dilating balloons may be inflated with a 60-cc syringe attached directly to the balloon. This syringe can be used to provide a large vacuum for rapid balloon deflation. However, it is often difficult to control balloon inflation and fixation across the aortic valve or to generate sufficient inflation pressure with a 60-cc syringe. For an optimum result, the balloon must not only be fixed across the valve, but must also be inflated to sufficient hardness, generally to approximately 3 atm. Most operators use a setup that will allow partial inflation with a larger syringe and final inflation with a smaller syringe. This allows more rapid full inflation at the higher pressures and easier fixation across the valve. Other devices

are being developed which allow for easier inflation (18).

The selection of the appropriate balloon size for aortic stenosis is important. Small balloons will tend to slide back and forth across the aortic valve without fixation, and there is little change in aortic pressure with full balloon inflation. As the balloon size approaches the size of the aortic annulus, there is a rapid fall in aortic pressure with balloon inflation often to 40 to 50 mm Hg systolic. If the dilating balloon is too large for the aortic annulus, there is a risk of rupture of the aorta, avulsion of aortic valve leaflets, or rupture of the left ventricular myocardium just below the valve. An estimate of aortic annulus size by two-dimensional echocardiography or aortogram is helpful in determining the appropriate balloon size. The size of balloon initially inserted is dependent on the size of the aortic root and severity of the aortic stenosis but will generally be either 18 or 20 mm. In general, a 23-mm balloon is the maximum size for most men and a 20-mm balloon, for most women. A 5.5-cm length balloon appears to be the

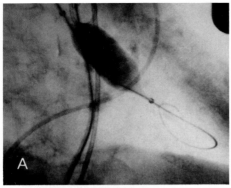

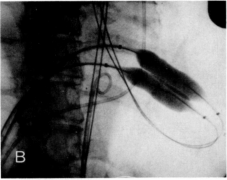

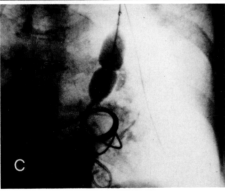

Figure 17.3. **A,** 20-mm balloon inflated in the aortic valve using the retrograde technique. Notice the guidewire coiled in the left ventricular apex. **B,** Two 15-mm balloons inflated in the mitral valve using the antegrade technique across the atrial septum. There is slight indentation of both balloons in the area of the valve annulus. Notice the guidewires are passed out of the ventricle and into the descending aorta. **C,** 20-mm balloon inflated in the pulmonic valve. Notice the characteristic "waisting" of the balloon, which usually occurs immediately prior to dilatation.

optimal length for aortic valvuloplasty. This longer length allows the balloon to be more easily stabilized across the valve and helps to prevent squeezing of the balloon forward into the left ventricle during inflation, so-called "pumpkin seeding," which limits the potential for ventricular trauma.

Inflations must be performed in such a way as to fix the balloon across the valve (Fig. 17.3A). It is frequently helpful to exert forward pressure on the balloon catheter and guidewire as well as provide rapid balloon inflation in order to accomplish this. The amount of time the balloon is inflated across the valve will be determined somewhat by how well it is tolerated. Occasionally, in patients with severe aortic stenosis, merely passing the balloon across the valve will cause a significant drop in blood pressure. With balloon inflation, the blood pressure frequently drops precipitously, and if this is not tolerated, the inflations should be brief, lasting for only a few seconds. Between inflations the balloon should be removed from the valve into the ascending aorta, and the blood pressure and heart rate allowed to recover. It is important that the balloon be fully inflated to sufficient hardness. Some operators feel better results are gained with longer inflations, but there are no data to indicate how long is optimal for balloon inflation. Likewise, there are no data to indicate how many inflations should be performed. If a balloon can not be passed across the valve because the orifice is too small or it is wedged in the commissure, an inflation immediately above the valve will move the catheter and sometimes allow passage or a smaller balloon should be tried.

After three to four inflations or elimination of the "waist" in the inflated balloon, it should be removed. This is best achieved by maintaining negative pressure on the balloon and rotating it as it is removed through the skin. The guidewire should remain in the ventricle to facilitate recrossing the valve. A catheter to measure left ventricular pressure is then reinserted over the wire, and the hemodynamics reassessed. Based on these measurements, a larger balloon or two balloons may be inserted and the process repeated until the desired results are achieved. The goal with each size utilized is to eliminate any waist that is apparent in the balloon when fully inflated and fixed in the valve. If significant blood pressure decline occurs with a 20-mm balloon, it is probably not prudent to go to a larger balloon, as the balloon size is probably approaching the size of the aortic annulus.

Use of the double-balloon technique with two 15-, two 18-, or combinations of 15-, 18-, and 20-mm balloons has several potential advantages. Smaller balloons are easier to inflate and deflate and have a lower profile, resulting in easier vascular access, especially in patients with peripheral vascular disease. The use of two balloons allows space on either side for blood to be ejected, and there will not be as great a drop in aortic pressure with full balloon inflation. However, there is still the risk of oversizing the aortic annulus with two balloons and the potential for aortic or ventricular rupture or severe valve damage. From preliminary studies, the double-balloon technique does not appear to produce larger final aortic valve areas or result in fewer complications. The double-balloon technique requires two arterial access sites, crossing the aortic valve twice, and inflation of both balloons simultaneously unless the femoral/cutdown technique is used. With the open technique, a double-lumen or large-lumen catheter can be placed into the ventricle over the existing guidewire and a second guidewire passed through it, thus eliminating crossing the valve twice, which can be time-consuming. Then both balloons are advanced across the valve through the same artery and simultaneously inflated. The procedure is then the same for assessing results.

Antegrade Technique

The antegrade technique for aortic valvuloplasty is considerably different in that it necessitates transseptal catheterization. The transseptal catheterization is performed in a standard manner using a Brockenbrough needle and Mullins sheath as described in Chapter 6. Once the Mullins sheath is in the left atrium, a 7 Fr end-hole, balloon flotation catheter (Berman type) is advanced into the left atrium, through the mitral valve, and out into the ascending aorta. The balloon should be inflated when it traverses the mitral valve to assure that the catheter does not pass through the chords of the mitral valve apparatus. A curved end of a stiff guidewire is sometimes necessary to help direct the catheter up toward the aortic valve. A 260-cm, 0.038-inch guidewire should then be advanced out of the catheter and into the descending aorta. The catheter is then removed, leaving the wire in place. An 8-mm balloon dilatation catheter is then advanced over the wire and positioned across the atrial septum where several short dilatations are performed to enlarge the hole in the atrial septum. The balloon for aortic valve dilatation is then advanced across the atrial septum, across the mitral valve and into the aortic valve over the guidewire, and the valvular dilatations are performed. After the dilatation procedure is complete and the catheters removed from across the atrial septum, an assessment of possible left to right shunting across the atrial septum should be performed. Care and handling of the balloons and other aspects of the technique are similar to the retrograde approach.

Mitral Valvuloplasty

The mitral valve is generally approached for dilatation via the antegrade or transseptal route (Fig. 17.4). The techniques for transseptal puncture and catheter and guidewire placement are identical to those utilized for the antegrade aortic technique, but several points regarding differences are worth mention. First, crossing the mitral valve can be considerably more difficult in the presence of mitral stenosis, but in general this can be achieved using either balloon-tipped catheters, as with aortic valvuloplasty, or pigtail catheters with various angles and guidewires. Using a balloon-tipped catheter and crossing the valve with the balloon inflated will assure that the guidewire and dilatation balloon system is in a relatively large area of the mitral valve apparatus, thus limiting trauma to the subvalvular structures with dilatation. Second, the need to cross the aortic valve antegrade with the guidewire and keep it across the aortic valve with mitral valvuloplasty is not absolutely essential as it is in aortic valvuloplasty. However, most catheterizing physicians feel that keeping the wire in the aorta offers a margin of safety in that the balloons are more likely to remain stable across the valve and not bounce back and forth into the ventricle. By restricting the balloon movement and directing the tip away from the left ventricular apex, the catheter is less likely to perforate the ventricle. Some catheterizing

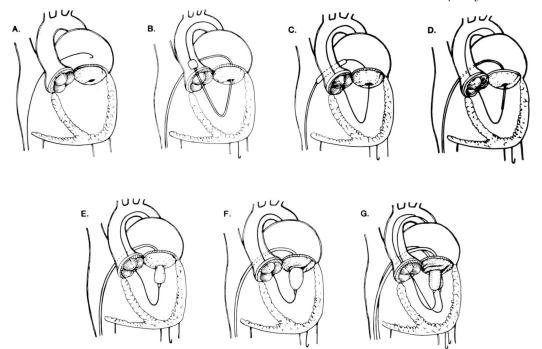

Figure 17.4.   Schematic representation of the antegrade technique for mitral valvuloplasty. See text for details.

physicians advocate snaring the guidewire in the aorta and holding it in position in the descending aorta for balloon stabilization. Third, the passage of multiple balloons across the atrial septum can be achieved via several methods. A second transseptal puncture can be performed or a second guidewire can be placed via a large lumen guiding catheter or double-lumen exchange catheter, as previously discussed. This latter method seems preferable.

Balloon size for mitral dilatation is generally larger than for aortic valvuloplasty, and two balloons are used much more frequently (Fig. 17.3B). As with aortic and pulmonic valvuloplasty, the balloon should be 5.5 cm in length to allow better fixation. With small ventricular chambers, this can be a problem, in which case a shorter 3-cm balloon should be used. Again, squeezing of the balloon into the left ventricle can cause considerable damage, and ventricular rupture can occur.

Pulmonic Valvuloplasty

For pulmonic valvuloplasty the basics of technique remain the same. A catheter and long guidewire are placed across the pulmonary valve, positioned distally in the left pulmonary artery, and used to guide the balloon catheter into position across the valve (Fig. 17.3C). The technique is generally performed via a femoral vein, but in neonates occasionally it is necessary to use the femoral artery and cross the valve in a retrograde fashion via a patent ductus arteriosus. Balloon sizing is somewhat more precise however, in that the literature suggests that balloons approximately 20% (19) larger than the pulmonic annulus produce better long-term results, although short-term results may be similar. A major difference also exists in pulmonic stenosis in that there is frequent infundibular stenosis present which will influence results (2). Data suggest that the long-term improvement is influenced by the degree of improvement in any infundibular gradient as the right ventricular hypertrophy improves over time (20).

Dilatation of Other Valves

Balloon dilatation has been applied to both the stenotic tricuspid valve (21) as well as stenotic bioprosthetic valves in a variety of positions (22–25). The techniques that have been described for these valvular lesions are similar to those of other valves previously described. Leaflet dehiscence does not appear to be a problem, but experience with these techniques is limited.

Balloon Preparation

The balloon catheter is prepared in much the same way that angioplasty balloons are prepared. Through the inflation port, the balloon is filled with a solution containing no more than 60% radiographic contrast material. Only 20 to 30% is necessary for visualization. Full strength contrast has a high viscosity and will not allow for rapid balloon inflation and deflation. The nonionic low-osmolar contrast agents should not be used here because of their higher viscosity than the conventional contrast agents (see Chapter 10). As the balloon is filled with the contrast mixture, it should be held with the tip down to allow for the removal of residual air by aspiration. Because of the possibility of rupture, either accidentally or intentionally, care should be taken to evacuate all air from the balloon with either carbon dioxide or the contrast and saline mixture.

After the balloon is filled, negative pressure should be exerted on the inflation port and the packaging sleeve replaced over the balloon to maintain it as small as possible until insertion.

Balloon Sizing

Balloon sizing for aortic valvuloplasty will depend primarily on the size of the valve orifice and the aortic annulus. The specific geometry of the valve in each case will determine how well any balloon will fit and dilate, so it is best to start with a balloon that will easily cross the valve and provide a reasonable initial dilatation based on measurements from the echocardiogram or aortogram. Most stenotic aortic valves will take an 18-mm diameter balloon initially and many will accommodate a 20-mm. Likewise, with mitral valvuloplasty, initial balloon size should be determined based on mitral annulus size. Most mitral valves, except in the young, should accommodate a 20-mm balloon or larger without difficulty. There is no particular reason to start with a small balloon and replace it with a larger balloon after a series of dilatations. As newer balloons become available with several sizes on the same catheter,

initial balloon selection will become less important. It is also not clear whether larger single balloons or smaller multiple balloons will provide better results in any valve lesion.

NONVALVULAR DILATATION TECHNIQUES

There has been a substantial experience with peripheral angioplasty in virtually all vessels, most prominently the renal and iliofemoral systems. More cardiologists are becoming proficient with these techniques, particularly as adjunctive laser therapy is being applied, but a complete discussion of these procedures is beyond the scope of this chapter.

Coarctation of the aorta is a potential site for dilatation and is one vascular stenosis where the cardiologist, particularly one with a large pediatric population, will be influential in management. Dilatation of coarctation may be successfully performed in patients who have never had operation and in those who have restenosis after operation (26, 27). It is not clear when this procedure should be performed instead of surgery but it is generally safe, and although there are limited follow-up data, short-term results appear good. However, some patients do develop aneurysms at the site that may necessitate repair (26). There are other similar lesions where balloon dilatation has been reported to be successful, such as subaortic membranes, peripheral pulmonic stenosis, and postoperative vascular stenoses from repairs of various congenital lesions of the great vessels. The general techniques utilized are the same as for valvular balloon dilatation.

PREVALVULOPLASTY ASSESSMENT AND PERIOPERATIVE CARE

Presently, the assessment and management of patients undergoing valvuloplasty differ among institutions. Some do nothing more than a clinical assessment prior to catheterization and make all the decisions regarding valvuloplasty at the time of cardiac catheterization. Others perform lengthy evaluation prior to catheterization and make all the decisions regarding valvuloplasty at the time of cardiac catheterization. Others perform lengthy evaluation prior to considering balloon dilatation. In the authors' opinion, some degree of precatheterization assessment other than clinical examination is generally warranted. This evaluation should include two-dimensional echocardiography with Doppler interrogation of the severity of valvular stenosis and preliminary sizing of the valve annulus for choosing balloon size. This is helpful for assessing left ventricular function and size and providing a baseline for follow-up. Some cardiologists prefer radionuclide angiography for ventricular function evaluation and determination of regurgitant fraction when regurgitation is present with stenosis. If the femoral artery is to be utilized for catheterization, it may be helpful to perform a peripheral Doppler examination to determine patency of arteries, especially if the pulses are diminished. Other standard testing such as hemoglobin, clotting profile, renal function, ECG, and chest x-ray should also be performed as for any catheterization.

At the current time, most patients undergoing valvuloplasty are managed in much the same way that the coronary angioplasty patients are managed in the perioperative period. As with any catheterization, patients are premedicated as the operator chooses, generally given mild sedation, given nothing by mouth for several hours prior, and urged to empty the bladder prior to arriving in the laboratory. All patients should be typed and crossed for several units of packed red blood cells (usually 4 units are sufficient), as blood loss can be substantial. Antibiotic prophylaxis for endocarditis is used by some but is not uniform. Unlike coronary angioplasty, valvuloplasty patients are generally not given antiplatelet agents. Surgical back-up is not standard but may be arranged in select circumstances. After the procedure, it is our practice to place patients in an intensive care unit for monitoring for at least several hours after the procedure. After 24 hours, patients may be discharged if there are no further reasons for hospitalization.

RESULTS

Balloon valvuloplasty has not been performed long enough to appropriately analyze results, especially with long-term follow-up. The technique and equipment continue to evolve but some discussion of the available data is appropriate. As noted, pulmonic stenosis responds well to balloon dilatation and is felt by many to be the procedure of choice for this condition. Both immediate results and results over months of follow-up suggest sustained benefit if a good initial result is achieved.

Because aortic stenosis is much more common than other valvular stenoses in developed nations, experience with aortic dilatation is the most extensive. Lababidi et al. (3) were the first to report the technique. All of their 23 patients were children with congenital aortic stenosis. In this initial series, the average gradient went from 113 ± 48 to 32 ± 15 mm Hg. Six of the 23 patients underwent repeat catheterization 3 to 9 months later, which revealed no significant change from the immediate postvalvuloplasty results. Choy et al. (28) have reported similar results in children. In adults with calcific aortic stenosis, numerous reports of using balloon dilatation suggest a modest short-term improvement in valve gradient and area (14, 29-31). The general range of acute improvement is an increase in valve area of approximately 0.4 to 0.5 cm^2. In addition, clinical and left ventricular function improvement also occur over time. The results are remarkably similar in most reported series, but despite the improvement, there continues to be significant mortality. Variables that affect results are not known, but the degree of calcium and the type of valve anatomy probably play as important a role as any technical consideration.

Follow-up of patients after aortic valve dilation has recently become available. Safian et al. (32) have reported the experience from the Beth Israel Hospital in Boston, which included 170 consecutive patients treated with balloon aortic valvuloplasty. Of these, 168 had successful valvuloplasty and of these, 5 had aortic valve replacement and 6 died during the initial hospitalization. The 157 patients discharged after successful valvuloplasty were followed for 9.1 (mean) months (range 1 to 23). Of these 157 patients, 25 (16%) died 6.4 ± 5.3 (mean) months after valvuloplasty. In 44 (28%) of the patients, there was recurrence of symptoms 7.5 ± 5.7 (mean) months after valvuloplasty. These patients were treated by valve replacement (17 patients), medical therapy (11 patients), or repeat valvuloplasty (16 patients). At the last follow-up contact, 66% of the patients, including 15 patients who had a repeat valvuloplasty, were symptomatically improved. Safian et al. estimated the restenosis rate to be approximately 50%, but catheterization was not uniformly performed. The probability for survival at 1 year was 74%, but event-free survival (events defined as recurrent symptoms or death) was only 50%.

Block (33) reported equally discouraging results with 56% of the patients having a recurrence of symptoms, hemodynamic restenosis, or death, occurring 5.6 (mean) months after valvuloplasty. In the M-HEART Balloon Valvuloplasty Registry, during an average of 7 ± 5 month follow-up, 16.3% of 166 patients died in addition to a 4.2% in-hospital mortality. Eighteen percent had aortic valve replacement. Of 99 surviving patients, 49% remained in New York Heart Association (NYHA) functional class 1 or 2 at follow-up (34).

Letac and colleagues in Rouen have reported the results (35) in 218 patients, with clinical follow-up for 8 (mean) months in 144 patients. There were 24 deaths (17%) in the follow-up period with a total mortality of 34 for the 218 (16%) patients. In the remaining 120 patients, clinical improvement was considered "good" in 101 (84%) with only 14 in NYHA class 3 or 4 at follow-up. These data are consistent with other reports.

Data on results of balloon mitral valvuloplasty are also limited. Existing reports (36, 37) suggest that valve area can be improved by 0.7 to 1.0 cm^2 on average, and better results may be achievable in selected cases (38). It seems that results from mitral valvuloplasty are somewhat more uniform and are influenced by the balloon size, use of multiple balloons, and other factors. However, like aortic valvuloplasty, specific factors that influence success are not completely understood.

Herrmann and colleagues (39) have identified various factors influencing mitral valvuloplasty success. They analyzed 60 consecutive mitral dilation procedures and found that in 21 of the 60 patients (35%) a suboptimal result (a postprocedure valve area ≤1.0 cm^2, an increase in valve area of ≤25%, or a final gradient of ≥10 mm Hg) was obtained. Those with severe valve leaflet thickening or immobility and an extreme amount of subvalvular thickening and calcification by echocardiogram were more likely to have such a result. Too small a balloon dilating area and atrial fibrillation also predicted a poorer result (40). Based on these results, Block and coworkers have developed an echocardiographic score that seems to help predict outcome (39, 41). Leaflet mobility, leaflet thickening, subvalvular thickening, and calcification are each rated on a scale of 1 to 4 with the last two factors being the most important. A good candidate is defined as having a total echo score ≤8, young age, and normal sinus rhythm. A poor candidate is one who is >70 years of age, has long-standing atrial fibrillation, and an echo score ≥11. Other patients are considered at intermediate risk for a good result. Long-term studies on the effect of mitral balloon valvuloplasty are generally incomplete or lacking. Most studies reflect less than a year of follow-up, and most do not have catheterization as an endpoint.

COMPLICATIONS

There are a number of complications that can occur as a result of balloon valvuloplasty. These include adverse events that occur with catheterization itself as well as some that are more common with valvuloplasty. The nature of the procedure with its brief intermittent occlusion of valves tends to create transient instability of blood pressure and rhythm, including ventricular arrhythmias and heart block. These may require therapy acutely, and occasionally heart block may be permanent. Bleeding in excess of what occurs with catheterization is common, depending on the technique used, and transfusion may be necessary. Vascular damage because of the large size of the balloon catheters may occur, especially in elderly patients with peripheral vascular disease. The incidence may be as high as 10 to 12%. Cerebrovascular accidents, either transient or permanent, occur in approximately 2%. Death, usually from ventricular perforation or annulus rupture, occurs with an incidence of 1 to 2% in left-sided lesions. However, the incidence of complications due strictly to the procedure itself is hard to discern because valvuloplasty, particularly for calcific aortic stenosis, is frequently performed in critically ill patients who are at high risk with any intervention. It would seem that as long as valvuloplasty is performed as a palliative procedure in high-risk patients, a high rate of complication is likely to continue despite improvement in technique and increase in experience.

FUTURE OF BALLOON VALVULOPLASTY

The creativity of cardiologists and radiologists performing therapeutic techniques and the technological advances that have allowed for the current success of nonsurgical interventions provide an environment that encourages refinements of existing techniques and new advances (42). With the application of lasers to the cardiovascular system, smaller catheters, and more durable balloon materials, major modifications of how we approach patients with stenotic cardiac valves will likely continue over the next several years. While a number of authors have supported the use of balloon valvuloplasty in selected individuals, numerous questions about and problems with the technique remain. What is the long-term benefit? How does valvuloplasty compare with valve surgery in similar groups of patients? How often does restenosis occur and how is it best dealt with? Who are appropriate candidates? What is the appropriate technique? What is the course of valvular insufficiency after valvuloplasty? What is the course of the atrial septal defects often created after mitral and antegrade aortic valvuloplasty? How these questions are approached and answered will determine the appropriate role of balloon valvuloplasty as a therapeutic technique in the catheterization laboratory.

References

1. Kan JS, White RI Jr, Mitchell SE, Gardner TJ. Percutaneous balloon valvuloplasty: a new method for treating congenital pulmonary-valve stenosis. N Engl J Med 1982;307:540–542.
2. Pepine CJ, Gessner IH, Feldman RL. Percutaneous balloon valvuloplasty for pulmonic valve stenosis in the adult. Am J Cardiol 1982;50:1442–1445.
3. Lababidi Z, Wu JR, Walls JT. Percutaneous balloon aortic valvuloplasty: results in 23 patients. Am J Cardiol 1984;53:194–197.
4. Inoue K, Owaki T, Nakamura T, Kitamura F, Miyamoto N. Clinical application of transvenous mitral commissurotomy by a new balloon catheter. J Thorac Cardiovasc Surg 1984;87:394–402.
5. Lock JE, Khalilullah M, Shrivastava S, Bahl V, Keane JF. Percutaneous catheter commissurotomy in rheumatic mitral stenosis. N Engl J Med 1985;313:1515–1518.
6. Cribier A, Saoudi N, Berland J, Savin T, Rocha P, Letac B. Percutaneous transluminal valvuloplasty

7. of acquired aortic stenosis in elderly patients: an alternative to valve replacement? Lancet 1986;1:63–67.
7. Block PC, Palacios IF, Jacobs ML, Fallon JT. Mechanism of percutaneous mitral valvotomy. Am J Cardiol 1987;59:178–179.
8. Sullivan ID, Robinson PJ, Macartney FJ, et al. Percutaneous balloon valvuloplasty for pulmonary valve stenosis in infants and children. Br Heart J 1985;54:435–441.
9. Kan JS, White RI, Mitchell SE, Anderson JH, Gardner TJ. Percutaneous transluminal balloon valvuloplasty for pulmonary valve stenosis. Circulation 1984;69:554–560.
10. Kaplan JD, Isner JM, Karas RH, et al. In vitro analysis of mechanisms of balloon valvuloplasty of stenotic mitral valves. Am J Cardiol 1987;59:318–323.
11. McKay RG, Lock JE, Safian RD, et al. Balloon dilation of mitral stenosis in adult patients: postmortem and percutaneous mitral valvuloplasty studies. J Am Coll Cardiol 1987;9:723–731.
12. Reid CL, McKay CR, Chandraratna PAN, Kawanishi DT, Rahimtoola SH. Mechanisms of increase in mitral valve area and influence of anatomic features in double-balloon, catheter balloon valvuloplasty in adults with rheumatic mitral stenosis: a Doppler and two-dimensional echocardiographis study. Circulation 1987;76:628–636.
13. Safian RD, Mandell VS, Thurer RE, et al. Postmortem and intraoperative balloon valvuloplasty of calcific aortic stenosis in elderly patients: mechanisms of successful dilation. J Am Coll Cardiol 1987;9:655–660.
14. McKay RG, Safian RD, Lock JE, et al. Balloon dilatation of calcific aortic stenosis in elderly patients: postmortem, intraoperative, and percutaneous valvuloplasty studies. Circulation 1986;74:119–125.
15. Meier B, Friedli B, Oberhaensli I, Belenger J, Finci L. Trefoil balloon for percutaneous valvuloplasty. Cathet Cardiovasc Diagn 1986;12:277–281.
16. van den Berg EJM, Niemeyer MG, Plokker TWM, Ernst SMPG, de Korte J. New triple-lumen balloon catheter for percutaneous (pulmonary) valvuloplasty. Cathet Cardiovasc Diagn 1986;12:352–356.
17. Block, PC, Palacios IF. Comparison of hemodynamic results of anterograde versus retrograde percutaneous balloon aortic valvuloplasty. Am J Cardiol 1987;60:659–662.
18. Hill JA, Martin DB, Carr AM. A new device for balloon inflation during valvuloplasty: a preliminary report. Clin Cardiol 1989, in press.
19. Ring JC, Kulik TJ, Burke BA, Lock JE. Morphologic changes induced by dilation of the pulmonary valve anulus with overlarge balloons in normal newborn lambs. Am J Cardiol 1985;55:210–214.
20. Kveselis DA, Rocchini AP, Snider R, Rosenthal A, Crowley DC, Dick M II. Results of balloon valvuloplasty in the treatment of congenital valvar pulmonary stenosis in children. Am J Cardiol 1985;56:527–532.
21. Zaibag MA, Ribeiro P, Kasab SA. Percutaneous balloon valvotomy in tricuspid stenosis. Br Heart J 1987;57:51–53.
22. Waldman JD, Schoen FJ, Kirkpatrick SE, Mathewson JW, George L, Lamberti JJ. Balloon dilatation of

porcine bioprosthetic valves in the pulmonary position. Circulation 1987;76:109–114.

23. Lloyd TR, Marvin WJ, Mahoney LT, Lauer RM. Balloon dilation valvuloplasty of bioprosthetic valves in extracardiac conduits. Am Heart J 1987;114:268–273.

24. Feit F, Stecy PJ, Nachamie MS. Percutaneous balloon valvuloplasty for stenosis of a porcine bioprosthesis in the tricuspid valve position. Am J Cardiol 1986;58:363–364.

25. Calvo OL, Sobrino N, Gamallo C, Oliver J, Dominguez F, Iglesias A. Balloon percutaneous valvuloplasty for stenotic bioprosthetic valves in the mitral position. Am J Cardiol 1987;60:736–737.

26. Saul JP, Keane JF, Fellows KE, Lock JE. Balloon dilation angioplasty of postoperative aortic obstructions. Am J Cardiol 1987;59:943–948.

27. Cooper RS, Ritter SB, Rothe WB, Chen CK, Griepp R, Golinko RJ. Angioplasty for coarctation of the aorta: long-term results. Circulation 1987;75:600–604.

28. Choy M, Beekman RH, Rocchini AP, et al. Percutaneous balloon valvuloplasty for valvar aortic stenosis in infants and children. Am J Cardiol 1987;59:1010–1013.

29. Cribier A, Savin T, Berland J, et al. Percutaneous transluminal balloon valvuloplasty of adult aortic stenosis: report of 92 cases. J Am Coll Cardiol 1987;9:381–386.

30. Isner JM, Salem DN, Desnoyers MR, et al. Treatment of calcific aortic stenosis by balloon valvuloplasty. Am J Cardiol 1987;59:313–317.

31. McKay RG, Safian RD, Lock JE, et al. Assessment of left ventricular and aortic valve function after aortic balloon valvuloplasty in adult patients with critical aortic stenosis. Circulation 1987;75:192–203.

32. Safian RD, Berman AD, Diver KJ, et al. Balloon aortic valvuloplasty in 170 consecutive patients. N Engl J Med 1988;319:125–130.

33. Block PC. Aortic valvuloplasty—A valid alternative? N Engl J Med 1988;319:169–171.

34. Kleaveland JP, Hill J, Margolis J, et al. M–HEART registry for percutaneous transluminal aortic valvuloplasty: followup report (abstr). Circulation 1988;78:II–533.

35. Letac B, Cribier A, Koning R, Bellefleur J–P. Results of percutaneous transluminal valvuloplasty in 218 adults with valvular aortic stenosis. Am J Cardiol 1988;62:598–605.

36. Palacios I, Block PC, Brandi S, et al. Percutaneous balloon valvotomy for patients with severe mitral stenosis. Circulation 1987;75:778–784.

37. Pandian NG, Isner JM, Hougen TJ, Desnoyers MR, McInerney K, Salem DN. Percutaneous balloon valvuloplasty of mitral stenosis aided by cardiac ultrasound. Am J Cardiol 1987;59:380–381.

38. Palacios IF, Lock JE, Keane JF, Block PC. Percutaneous transvenous balloon valvotomy in a patient severe calcific mitral stenosis. J Am Coll Cardiol 1985;7:1416–1419.

39. Herrmann HC, Wilkins GT, Abascal VM, Weyman AE, Block PC, Palacios IF. Percutaneous balloon mitral valvotomy for patients with mitral stenosis. J Thorac Cardiovasc Surg 1988;96:33–38.

40. Herrmann HC, Kleaveland JP, Hill JA, et al. for the M-Heart Study Group. Results and follow-up of a multicenter registry for balloon mitral valvuloplasty (abstr). J Am Coll Cardiol 1989, in press.

41. Block PC. Who is suitable for percutaneous balloon mitral valvotomy? Int J Cardiol 1988;20:9–14.

42. Isner JM. Aortic valvuloplasty: Are balloon–dilated valves all they are "cracked" up to be? (Editorial). Mayo Clin Proc 1988;63:830–834.

18

Pressure Measurement

Charles R. Lambert, M.D., Ph.D.
Carl J. Pepine, M.D.
Wilmer W. Nichols, Ph.D.

INTRODUCTION

Ventricular systole produces systemic and pulmonary blood flow secondary to generation of pulsatile pressure that is transmitted throughout the vascular tree. It follows that measurement of pressure waveforms is a key element in evaluation of normal and abnormal cardiovascular physiology. Indeed, with current technology, pressure should be the most accurate determination of all hemodynamic measurements made during cardiac catheterization. In this chapter the principles and application of pressure measurement in the cardiac catheterization laboratory will be addressed.

THEORETICAL CONSIDERATIONS

By definition pressure is force per unit area. The International System of Units defines the standard unit for pressure measurement as the Pascal (Pa). A Pascal is the pressure, acting uniformly on an area of 1 m^2, which exerts a vertical force of 1 Newton. In cardiovascular physiology, noncoherent technical units of pressure are used most commonly. Such units include the centimeter of water and millimeter of mercury. The millimeter of mercury (mm Hg) is defined in accordance with the International Barometric Conventions of the World Meteorological Organization as the pressure exerted by a column of liquid 1 mm in height with a density of 13.5951 gm/cm^3 under standard acceleration due to gravity. In practice this definition is realized by a column of mercury 1 mm in height at 0° C and standard atmospheric pressure. Conversions for some other commonly used units of pressure are given in Table 18.1. In clinical catheterization practice, pressures are often measured in reference to a point at midchest level in the supine position and thus are relative, not absolute, values. Other choices include relating zero to the sternal angle or 10 cm above tabletop, but these levels have no reference to the patient's size. Some attempt should be made to identify the center of the heart, using a lateral x-ray done with the patient standing, and relate zero to this point. This is very time-consuming and has no relation to the position of the heart when the patient is supine. In addition, pressures are usually measured without consideration to possible conversion of kinetic energy in flowing blood to pressure energy. This conversion may be measurable when using an end-hole vs. a side-hole fluid-filled system. The blood impinging upon the end hole facing the stream loses some kinetic energy when the velocity of the blood near this point falls secondary to catheter obstruction. This gives rise to a small difference in "lateral" vs. "end" or "impact" pressure in such systems. In vivo this difference is usually no more than 1 mm Hg or so and thus is of limited clinical importance.

PRESSURE TRANSDUCERS

Blood pressure has been measured using an enormous number of devices reviewed in an interesting monograph by Geddes (1). Perhaps the simplest direct writing blood pressure transduction system was that described

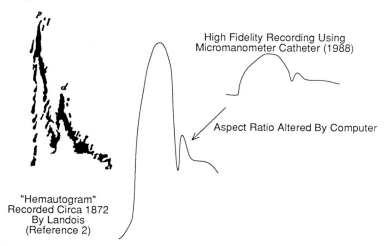

High Fidelity Recording Using
Micromanometer Catheter (1988)

Aspect Ratio Altered By Computer

"Hemautogram"
Recorded Circa 1872
By Landois
(Reference 2)

Figure 18.1. Comparison between the "Hemautogram" recorded in the 1800s by spraying blood from a dog artery onto a drum with a high-fidelity catheter-tip micromanometer recording of arterial pressure. Altering the aspect ratio (vertical and horizontal gain) by computer, shows that the records are strikingly similar in morphology. Thus, it appears that Landois made the first high-fidelity pressure recordings in the 19th century (see Ref. 2).

by Landois in 1872 (2), who used a needle in an artery to direct spraying blood onto a moving paper surface (Fig. 18.1). This "hemautogram" yielded information of surprising accuracy regarding the amplitude and contour of the arterial pulse, including existence of the dicrotic notch. Many transducers have been developed subsequently using various methods to convert pressure into electrical signals for recording and processing. Transduction devices used for pressure measurement have included variable resistance, variable capacitance, variable inductance, and piezoelectric types. The most commonly used of these is the variable resistance transducer, which usually consists of a metal diaphragm, upon which is applied a full or partial resistive bridge. This is connected to a pressure preamplifier or bridge amplifier in a configuration similar to that of a classical Wheatstone bridge. An AC or DC excitation voltage is applied to the bridge from the preamplifier through appropriate patient isolation transformers. A change in pressure of the fluid in the system causes a small movement of the diaphragm, which in turn changes the resistance of the bridge. This change is amplified, filtered, and recorded as a pressure waveform with respect to time. Components of such a system are illustrated in Figure 18.2. Details concerning pressure preamplifiers and recorders are given in Chapter 21.

The key to proper application of instrumentation to pressure recording is an understanding of the dynamic frequency response characteristics of the recording system and what factors modify these characteristics. For a given pressure measurement system the input signal is the true pressure being measured, and the output signal is the analog signal usually recorded on paper to be analyzed. For this discussion we will assume that the recorder, or the portion of the system beyond the pressure transducer in Figure 18.2, has perfect response characteristics. Thus, our concerns are in regard to the catheter-connector-transducer (or manometer) apparatus and its response characteristics. If a system is perfect in this regard, both the frequency and the amplitude of the input signal will be reproduced exactly at the output without distortion. In reality, most commonly used catheterization laboratory pressure-measuring systems distort the intravascular pressure waveform with respect to both amplitude and phase of the signal. The magnitude of this distortion is

Table 18.1.
Pressure Conversions

1 mm Hg = 1.00000014 torr
1 mm Hg = 133.3 Pa
1 mm Hg = 1.36 cm H_2O
1 mm Hg = 1334 dyn/cm^2

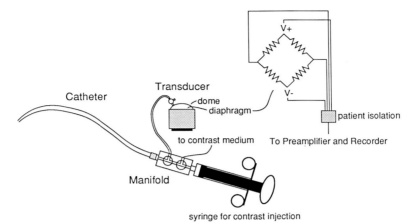

Figure 18.2. Components of a typical pressure measurement system used in clinical catheterization for a left heart study. A catheter is attached via Luer connectors to a manifold which, in turn, is connected to contrast medium and pressure transducer. The transducer may be attached directly to the manifold or via extension pressure tubing, as illustrated. The active element of the pressure transducer is a resistive bridge deposited on, or attached to, the diaphragm and connected, via isolation amplifiers, to the recording system.

generally dependent upon the frequency being considered (i.e., the higher the frequency, the greater the distortion).

Neglecting phase shift distortion, which is usually not of significant magnitude to be of clinical importance, a transducer system must be evaluated with regard to linearity and frequency characteristics of amplitude response. In this context linearity simply means that input plotted against output gives a straight line, as demonstrated in Figure 18.3. For real systems, however, as the frequency of a given alternating signal increases, a point is reached when the amplitude of the output signal is no longer equal to the amplitude of the input signal, as illustrated in Figure 18.3. This latter phenomenon defines the frequency response of the system (with respect to signal amplitude) and can be graphically demonstrated by plotting output amplitude vs. frequency, as illustrated in Figure 18.3. Real pressure-measuring systems usually exhibit a "flat" or constant frequency response curve to a certain level, at which point output either "falls off" toward zero or shows a second rise in amplitude at higher frequencies if the system is "underdamped" or resonates. The origin of these characteristics resides in mechanical properties, such as mass, inertia, and frictional resistance and also electronic characteristics of the system. The dynamic behavior of most transducer systems can be described by

a second order differential equation as $F(t) = M(d^2y/dt^2) + R(dy/dt) + Sy$.

By this relation, the response of the system (y) to the force exerted on the transducer by the pressure ($F(t)$) is governed by the mass of the moving liquid (M), frictional resistance (R), and stiffness or elastance (S) of the system. The frequency response of such a system can be predicted if the damping constant (β_0) and undamped natural frequency (ω_0) are known. In terms of the physical properties of the system, these parameters are defined as

$$\omega_0 = (S/M)^{1/2} = (\pi r^2 E/\rho L)^{1/2}$$

and

$$\beta_0 = R/(2M) = 4\mu/\rho r^2.$$

$E = \Delta P/\Delta V$ is the volume elasticity, where P is pressure, V is volume, and L and r, respectively, are the length and internal radius of the catheters. ρ and μ are the density and viscosity of the liquid.

These equations may be applied to experimentally evaluate the frequency characteristics of a transducer system by the transient or "pop" method. Although currently the frequency response characteristics of modern measurement systems are most often determined by use of special pressure generators designed for this purpose, the transient method is still useful and is presented here to illustrate the principles involved (3, 4).

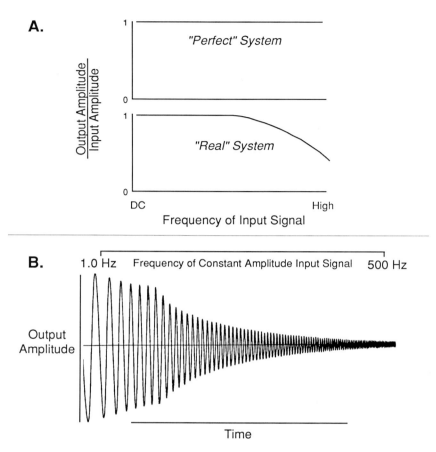

Figure 18.3. *A*, Ratio of output to input amplitude of a periodic signal for a theoretically *"perfect"* pressure measurement system would be 1.0 for all input frequencies while *"real"* systems show a drop off in output signal amplitude that may also be associated with a resonant effect at certain frequencies (not shown). The latter may cause the ratio of output to input to transiently exceed 1.0, as described in the text. *B*, Output waveform from a real pressure measurement system as a constant amplitude sine wave input is applied and swept from low to high frequencies. As shown in the *"real"* system of *A*, as frequency increases, output signal amplitude decreases.

Using degassed (or boiled) saline, an apparatus, as illustrated in Figure 18.4, is constructed consisting of a pressurized chamber closed with a thin rubber membrane (a surgical glove is satisfactory). After all connections are tightened, the pressure in the chamber is increased to distend the membrane. The recording system is started at rapid speed, and the membrane is ruptured suddenly with a very sharp, pointed instrument or lighted match. This drops the pressure essentially to 0 (atmospheric), and a typical underdamped system will undergo several oscillations of decreasing amplitude before reaching a steady level, as illustrated in the recording shown in Figure 18.4. After transient excitement such as

this, the system oscillates at its damped natural frequency (ω_D) defined by $\omega_D = (\omega_0^2 - \beta_0^2)^{1/2}$.

The record is analyzed to determine the damped natural frequency (ω_D) by means of the following relationship, where T is the time interval (seconds) between the peaks of the oscillation, i.e. $\omega_D = 2\pi f_D = 2\pi/T$.

The exponential rate at which the oscillations decrease in amplitude is defined by a logarithmic decrement Λ, defined as $\Lambda = \log_e(y_{n+1}/y_n)$, where y_1, y_2, etc. represent successive peak-to-peak amplitudes of oscillation, as illustrated in Figure 18.4.

It follows then that $\beta_0 = \Lambda/T$ and $\omega_0 = \sqrt{(4\pi^2 + \Lambda^2)}/T$.

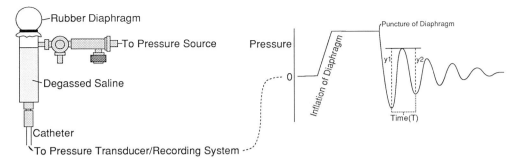

Figure 18.4. A system for the "pop test" to define the frequency response characteristics of a system, as described in the text. A closed chamber filled with degassed saline and capped with a rubber diaphragm is connected to a pressure source. The system is pressurized, and the diaphragm is ruptured with a sharp instrument. The resulting pressure waveform is recorded at high speed for analysis of time (*T*) and pressure oscillations *y1* and *y2* for analysis, as given in the text.

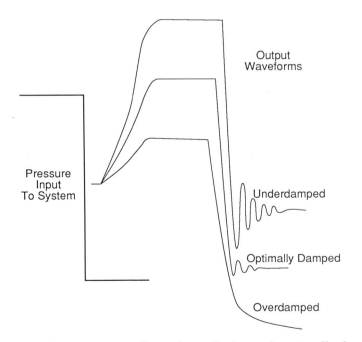

Figure 18.5. Representative output waveforms for underdamped, optimally damped, and overdamped pressure measurement systems to application of a stepped pressure change as input.

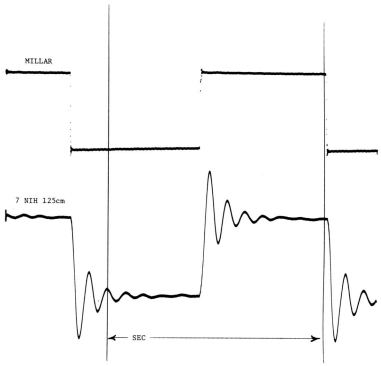

MILLAR

7 NIH 125cm

SEC

Figure 18.6. Example of simultaneously obtained pressure recordings in response to a step pressure input for a high-fidelity (Millar) catheter–tip micromanometer and a standard fluid-filled NIH-Statham resistive bridge pressure measurement system.

The damping coefficient (or factor) β is then defined as $\beta = \beta_0/\omega_0 = \Lambda/\sqrt{(4\pi^2 + \Lambda^2)} = (4\mu/r^3)(L/\rho\pi E)^{1/2}$

In general, an "optimal" damping coefficient is around 0.64, where there is minimal resonant peak, and the response of the system remains constant $\pm 2\%$ to about 67% of the undamped, natural frequency (4–6). Phase lag is also relatively inert at a damping ratio of 0.64. The adequacy of a catheter-manometer system for recording certain events can be judged by determination of the frequency response and damping coefficient. These parameters can also be used to correct data retrospectively to those that would have been recorded with a system having perfect frequency characteristics (3). Examples of a step pressure response for an underdamped, optimally damped, and overdamped system are illustrated in Figure 18.5.

In practice, if high-fidelity pressure data are critical in patient evaluation or for research purposes, catheter-tip micromanometer catheters are used (7). These catheters have a semi-conductor strain gauge built into the catheter-tip with frequency characteristics that will enable not only precise measurements of pressure waveforms but also intravascular recording of sounds. Responses to a step change in pressure of a catheter-tip micromanometer and a standard fluid-filled NIH catheter-transducer system are compared in Figure 18.6. Using a catheter-tip micromanometer as a reference standard, it is useful to document the effects of altering frequency response characteristics using a typical clinical catheter-transducer system. Barring the presence of air or contrast medium in a system, errors in balancing or calibration, and inaccurate zero reference determination, the most common causes of pressure distortion clinically are addition of extensions and stopcocks between the catheter and transducer and catheter whip artifact. Such distortion is illustrated in Figure 18.7 for left ventricular pressure. Distortion is amplified with such a system when catheters are moved, such as during a pullback recording from left ventricle to aorta (Fig. 18.8).

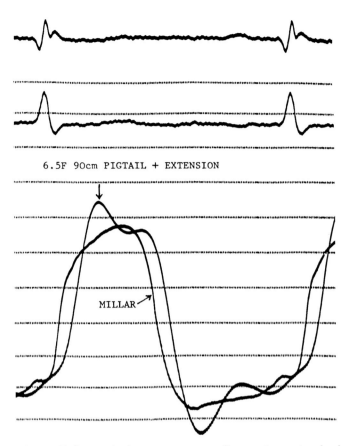

6.5F 90cm PIGTAIL + EXTENSION

MILLAR

Figure 18.7. Comparison of left ventricular pressure recordings using a standard clinical fluid-filled catheter system and a high-fidelity catheter-tip micromanometer (Millar) that were calibrated to respond in an equisensitive manner to the same static pressure using a mercury manometer. Note inaccuracy in peak systolic and early diastolic pressures.

The frequency response needed to accurately record pressure waveforms in man can be estimated by Fourier analysis, which breaks a complex periodic wave into a series of component sine waves of increasing frequency (see Chapter 21). When the harmonic contents of left ventricular and aortic pressure waves are examined in this manner, most of the signal content (>99%) is contained in the first 10 harmonics (4, 8, 9), as shown in Table 18.2. For a fundamental frequency or heart rate of 120 bpm, the frequency of the 10th harmonic would be 20 cycles/sec (Hz). Experimental work has verified that a system with a frequency response range that is flat to 20 Hz is necessary for accurate pressure reproduction (Chapter 21), although many systems routinely used in clinical catheterization studies usually have lower frequency response

characteristics, as illustrated in Table 18.3. If recorded pressure data are to be used for further calculations such as first or second time derivative computation, the transducer systems must have correspondingly better frequency characteristics (flat to 60 Hz) (10). Such applications usually employ catheter-tip micromanometers.

NORMAL PRESSURE WAVEFORMS

Normal pressure waveforms for the cardiac chambers and great vessels are illustrated in Figure 18.9 as recorded using a standard clinical fluid-filled system. Normal values for the phasic and mean components of these waveforms are listed in Table 18.4. In order to properly perform diagnostic cardiac catheteri-

Table 18.2.
Harmonic Content of Pressure Waves in Humans [a, b]

Harmonic No.	Left Ventricle		Aorta	
	mm Hg	Vs/Vt[c]	mm Hg	Vs/Vt
1	59	73.0%	15	66.0%
2	37	86.0%	6	89.0%
3	17	91.0%	2	93.0%
4	10	94.0%	1	95.0%
5	7	95.0%	1	96.0%
6	6	97.0%	1	97.0%
7	5	97.0%	1	98.0%
8	4	98.0%	0	99.0%
9	3	99.0%	0	99.6%
10	2	99.3%	0	99.7%

[a] Nichols WW, Pepine CJ. Unpublished data.
[b] Heart rate, 76 beats/min (1.3 Hz).
[c] Vs, series variance representing the component contribution of a given harmonic; Vt, total variance representing the relative proportion contributed to the total pressure signal by a given harmonic (expressed as a percentage).

Table 18.3.
Frequency Response Characteristics of Some Catheter-Manometer Systems [a, b]

Catheter	Flat Frequency Cutoff (Hz)	Resonant Frequency (Hz)	Damping Coefficient
Sones 8F			
80 cm	20	30	0.15
Dome			
with membrane	19	28	0.15
Renografin			
in system	19	22	0.31
NIH[c] 7F			
80 cm	13	20	0.19
NIH 8F			
125 cm	14	22	0.19
NIH 8F			
125 cm direct to transducer	30	39	0.17
NIH 8F			
125 cm + 140 cm ext	2	7	0.24
Pigtail 6.5 F			
90 cm + 40 cm ext	5	11	0.21
Swan-Ganz 7F	7	12	0.33
Cournand 7F			
125 cm	11	17	0.20

[a] Nichols WW, Pepine CJ. Unpublished data.
[b] Values determined using Statham P23ID transducer, disposable dome, and three-way stopcock.
[c] ext, extension tubing; NIH, National Institutes of Health.

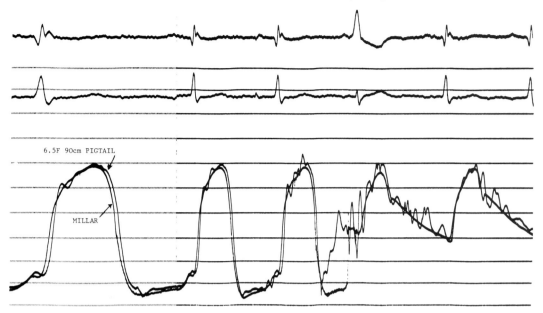

Figure 18.8. Example of artifact imposed during left ventricle to aorta pullback on recordings made with a standard fluid-filled catheter system compared with a high-fidelity catheter-tip micromanometer (Millar).

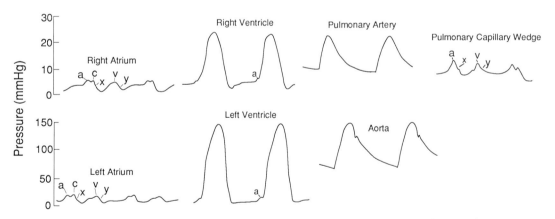

Figure 18.9. Supine right and left heart pressures recorded from standard fluid-filled catheter systems in humans.

zation it is important to have a thorough knowledge of normal pressure waveform morphology. As a basis for understanding alterations of pressures in pathologic states, pertinent facts regarding normal pressures will be addressed with reference to Figure 18.9.

A normal right atrial pressure waveform begins with the *a* wave which follows the P wave of the electrocardiogram and has its origin from right atrial systole. Fall of pressure from this point proceeds along the *x* descent, to be interrupted by a small upward inflection, the *c* wave, which is coincident with closure of the tricuspid valve. The *x* descent continues during atrial relaxation, to be followed by a slow rise in pressure due to atrial filling from the venous circulation until inscription of the *v* wave, which is coincident with right ventricular systole. The tricuspid

Table 18.4.
Normal Supine Resting Pressure Values in Humans[a]

	RA[b]	RV	PA	PCW	LA	LV	Ao
Systolic		15–30	15–30			100–140	100–140
End-diastolic		0–8	3–12			3–12	60–90
Mean	0–8		9–16	1–10	1–10		70–105
a Wave	2–10			3–15	3–15		
v Wave	2–10			3–12	3–12		

[a]All values are in mm Hg.
[b]Ao, aorta; LA, left atrium; LV, left ventricle; PA, pulmonary artery; PCW, pulmonary-capillary wedge; RA, right atrium; RV, right ventricle.

valve then opens and pressure falls as the atrium empties into the right ventricle along the *y* descent. Following the *y* descent, right atrial and right ventricular diastolic pressures equilibrate before the next cardiac cycle. Data usually reported include mean right atrial pressure, as well as the peak value for the *a* and *v* waves. In the normal right atrium, the *a* wave is usually the highest wave recorded.

A normal right ventricular pressure waveform consists of a small rapid-filling wave, a slow-filling wave, the *a* wave coincident with right atrial systole, and then systolic pressure generation. The shape is somewhat "triangular" with respect to the rise and fall of pressure during systole. Pressures usually reported include end-diastolic pressure, which is measured just after the *a* wave, and peak systolic pressure. With atrial fibrillation, when no *a* wave is present, end-diastolic pressure is usually measured 0.04 seconds after the peak of the R wave on the electrocardiogram. There is no reason to measure the initial diastolic pressure when fluid-filled catheters are used.

A normal pulmonary artery pressure waveform consists of a systolic pulse coincident with right ventricular emptying. As right ventricular ejection ends, pulmonary pressure begins to fall, and the incisura occurs as right ventricular pressure falls below that in the pulmonary artery and the pulmonic valve closes. Pulmonary artery pressure continues to fall as blood "runs off" into the pulmonary venous circulation. The nadir of this phase is measured as pulmonary end-diastolic pressure and is usually reported along with peak systolic and mean pressures. The pulmonary-capillary wedge pressure has a configuration similar to that of left atrial pressure, with the added effects of delay with respect to time and damping of pressure waves due to transmission through the pulmonary-capillary and venous beds. Similar to right atrial pressure discussed above, *a* and *v* waves should be present corresponding to left atrial systole and left atrial filling from the pulmonary venous system. In most cases distinct *x* and *y* descents are seen, however, a *c* wave is usually not apparent. Values reported should include mean pulmonary-capillary wedge pressure, as well as peak values for the *a* and *v* waves. Normally pulmonary artery end-diastolic pressure is equal to mean pulmonary-capillary wedge pressure since the pulmonary circulation has low intrinsic resistance.

A normal left atrial pressure waveform is similar in morphology to that of the right atrium with *a*, *c*, and *v* waves and corresponding *x* and *y* descents. The *v* wave, however, is usually the highest wave in the normal left atrium. Unless transseptal catheterization is done, this pressure will not usually be measured, and the pulmonary-capillary wedge pressure will be used as an estimate of left atrial pressure. In most cases this is adequate; however, error may be introduced unless care is taken to avoid overdamping and correct positioning is confirmed by fluoroscopy and, if necessary, determination of oxygen saturation in blood drawn from the catheter in wedge position is made. The pulmonary-capillary wedge pressure will not reflect left atrial pressure in the occasional case with pulmonary venous obstruction or mechanically related anomalies such as an obstructive left atrial myxoma. One should remember that although the mean pulmonary wedge pressure correlates closely with left ventricular end-diastolic pressure in the absence of mitral valve obstruction, these two pressures may not necessarily be equivalent. The mean pulmonary wedge pressure will relate most closely with the mean diastolic left ventricular pressure.

Normal left ventricular pressure is similar in contour to that of the right ventricle described above. The left ventricular pressure, however, is usually somewhat less "triangular" with more rapid upstroke and descent than the right ventricular pressure pulse. The early filling wave is followed by late filling, the *a* wave of left atrial contraction, and systole. As ventricular pressure rises, the mitral valve closes, and isovolumic contraction ensues until the aortic valve opens. The course of isovolumic pressure rise may be used as an index of left ventricular contractile state and is usually studied in this context as its first derivative or a function thereof. Following ventricular ejection, as ventricular pressure falls below aortic pressure, the aortic valve closes. The period between aortic valve closure and mitral valve opening is termed isovolumic relaxation, and the fall of pressure during this period has been shown to follow a monoexponential course although other mathematical models have been used as well. The time constant describing the decay of left ventricular isovolumic pressure is sensitive to processes affecting myocardial relaxation and thus may be one of the earliest indicators of ischemia. Values reported include end-diastolic, which is measured at the end of the *a* wave or "z" point, and peak systolic left ventricular pressure. In atrial fibrillation it is customary to report end-diastolic pressure 0.04 sec after peak of the *R* wave. There is little meaning in the initial diastolic pressure when fluid catheters are used, as this point is highly variable (see Fig. 18.7).

Normal central aortic pressure is comprised of a rapidly rising systolic pulse, an incisura, and a subsequent decay of pressure similar to that described above for the pulmonary artery. Values usually reported include peak systolic, end-diastolic, and mean pressures. The composition of the central aortic pressure in man has been studied in detail using harmonic analysis and related techniques useful in describing pulse transmission (11, 12). These studies have shown that the measured aortic pressure waveform is comprised of both forward and antegrade pressure waves and reflected or retrograde pressure waves. The measured central aortic pressure wave is a conjugate of these forward and reflected waves. The component forward and reflected waves may vary with disease and with pharmacologic manipulation, as

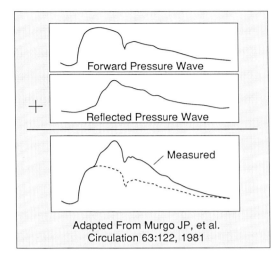

Adapted From Murgo JP, et al.
Circulation 63:122, 1981

Figure 18.10. A representative high-fidelity recording of central aortic pressure in man and the component forward and reflected waves as described in the text. (Adapted from Murgo JP, Westerhof N, Giolma JP, Altobelli SA. Manipulation of ascending aortic pressure and flow wave reflections with the Valsalva maneuver: relationship to input impedance. Circulation 1981;63:122–132.)

well as with the functional status of the left ventricle. These changes will be reflected in the morphology of the central aortic pressure tracing, as illustrated in Figure 18.10.

Peripheral arterial pressure waveforms, usually from the brachial or femoral arteries, are also commonly recorded in the catheterization laboratory. In general, the contours of these waveforms are similar to those of the aortic pressure with a slightly higher peak pressure and greater pulse pressure in the periphery. This phenomenon is due to a slight amplification resulting from wave reflection from the periphery, and it may be marked with the decreased arterial compliance and increased pulse wave velocity seen in older individuals. The mean peripheral and aortic pressures are usually equal, or there may be a slight decrease apparent in the periphery; however, this is rarely of clinical importance from a diagnostic standpoint (3, 4, 13)

ABNORMAL PRESSURE WAVEFORMS

Virtually every cardiovascular disease entity may be associated with abnormalities in

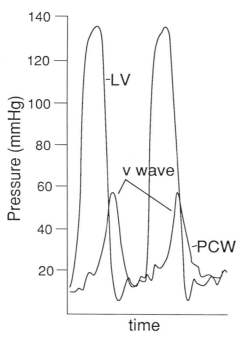

Figure 18.11. Left ventricular (*LV*) and pulmonary-capillary wedge pressure (*PCW*) tracings recorded during and with relief of angina pectoris in a patient with severe three-vessel coronary artery disease with nitroglycerin (0.4 mg sl). Although afterload reduction is seen with a fall in systolic *LV* pressure, marked improvement in the degree of mitral insufficiency is apparent with reduction in the *v* wave of the *PCW* pressure. Left ventricular end-diastolic pressure is also improved.

systemic or pulmonary pressures. Many of these conditions and their associated pressure abnormalities are illustrated elsewhere in this volume. In the section below specific pathophysiologic entities are considered that have characteristic pressure abnormalities and are common in the routine practice of diagnostic cardiac catheterization.

Atrioventricular Valve Insufficiency

Pressure waveform alterations are similar in morphology for both mitral and tricuspid insufficiency. The primary abnormality in recorded pressure waveforms is secondary to abnormal transmission of ventricular pressure to the corresponding atrial chamber via the incompetent valve. The right atrial pressure or left atrial pressure (pulmonary-capil-

lary wedge pressure) will contain an accentuated *and early v* wave that may obscure other components of the normal waveform, as illustrated in Figure 18.11. The magnitude of the *v* wave is dependent primarily upon the degree of atrioventricular valve incompetence, the compliance of the receiving chamber, and ventricular function. With long-standing moderate mitral insufficiency and a dilated, compliant left atrium, one will record a less prominent *v* wave than in acute mitral insufficiency related to papillary muscle rupture, in which a similar volume of regurgitant blood ejected into a normal atrium produces a large *v* wave. In patients with large *v* waves in the pulmonary-capillary wedge pressure recording it may be difficult to estimate left ventricular filling pressure in the ICU setting using a balloon flotation catheter. It has recently been shown that the trough of the *x* descent is the best indicator of true left ventricular end-diastolic pressure in these cases (14). The absence of a large *v* wave does not rule out significant atrioventricular valve insufficiency. This may be the usual finding in patients with long-standing mitral insufficiency, dilated cardiomyopathy, and large left atrial volumes. In general, angiographically severe mitral insufficiency is present when the height of the left atrial or pulmonary-capillary wedge *v* wave is 3 to 5 times that of the mean left atrial or pulmonary-capillary wedge pressure. Associated pressure abnormalities may include pulmonary or systemic venous hypertension and

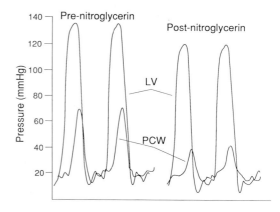

Figure 18.12. Effects of intravenous nitroglycerin on left ventricular (*LV*) and pulmonary-capillary wedge (*PCW*) pressures in a patient with ischemia-related mitral insufficiency related to severe right coronary artery stenosis.

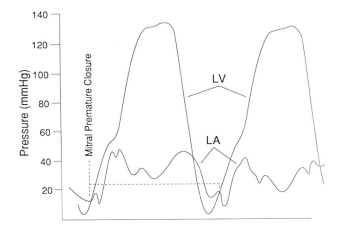

Figure 18.13. Left ventricular (*LV*) and left atrial (*LA*) pressure recordings in a patient with acute aortic insufficiency due to prosthetic valve dysfunction. *LV* end-diastolic pressure is markedly increased to approximately 50 mm Hg, causing early closure of the mitral valve, as indicated.

systemic hypotension with severe mitral insufficiency. In many cases with large *v* waves in the pulmonary wedge pressure, the *v* waves will also be seen in the pulmonary artery pressure waveform. In most patients with severe mitral insufficiency the magnitude of the regurgitant blood volume and corresponding *v* wave can be reduced with afterload reduction using sodium nitroprusside. If mitral insufficiency is due to myocardial ischemia affecting ventricular geometry, administration of nitroglycerin may produce dramatic relief, as illustrated in Figure 18.12. Further discussion of hemodynamic abnormalities with atrioventricular valve incompetence may be found in Chapters 24 and 27.

Aortic Insufficiency

The principle pressure abnormality in isolated aortic insufficiency is directly related to regurgitant blood volume and systemic vascular impedance. This is manifested primarily by a widened systemic pulse pressure. This widening is due principally to decreased diastolic pressure with maintenance of systolic pressure unless cardiac failure intervenes. Associated with regurgitation of blood from the aorta into the left ventricle in diastole is rapid ventricular filling and premature closure of the mitral valve as the rising ventricular diastolic pressure quickly exceeds that in the left atrium. This is particularly common with acute aortic insufficiency when compen-

satory ventricular enlargement has not taken place as in the chronic setting. An example of pressure tracings with acute aortic insufficiency is given in Figure 18.13. Again, other associated pressure abnormalities may include pulmonary hypertension and systemic hypotension.

Aortic Stenosis

In valvular aortic stenosis the left ventricular pressure is altered in keeping with the changes of chronic pressure overload and hypertrophy. These include primarily diastolic abnormalities due to diminished distensibility, such as elevated end-diastolic pressure, and an accentuated filling wave. The systolic ventricular pressure pulse depends upon the state of left ventricular function but is generally normal in contour and increased in amplitude until cardiac failure intervenes. The stenotic aortic valve alters the characteristics of the aortic pressure contour by delaying the rate of pressure rise during systole and decreasing the absolute amplitude of peak systolic pressure achieved. Such abnormalities are illustrated in Figure 18.14. Associated pressure abnormalities may include elevated pulmonary pressures and systemic hypotension. In patients with critical aortic stenosis simply having a catheter across the stenotic valve may increase the measured pressure gradient. The hemodynamics of aortic stenosis are further discussed in Chapters 24 and 27.

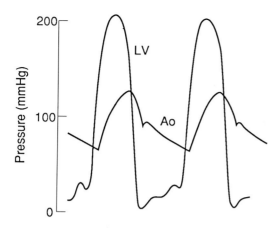

Figure 18.14. Left ventricular (*LV*) and aortic (*Ao*) pressure tracings in a patient with severe aortic stenosis.

Mitral Stenosis

As with any of the valvular abnormalities noted above, the pressure findings in mitral stenosis may vary, depending on the state of the disease and compensation in the individual patient. This is particularly true of mitral stenosis since the status of the pulmonary vasculature may undergo marked change in the course of this disease, as discussed in Chapters 24 and 27. In general, mitral stenosis is evaluated by recording the diastolic pressure difference between the pulmonary-capillary wedge catheter and a left ventricular catheter with simultaneously obtained cardiac

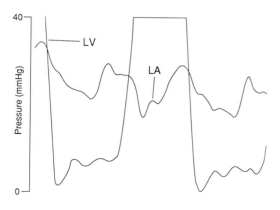

Figure 18.15. Simultaneous left atrial (*LA*) and left ventricular (*LV*) pressures in a patient with severe mitral stenosis.

output. Without intervening pulmonary venous disease or left atrial obstructive abnormalities this is generally valid, however, transseptal catheterization may be required to obtain accurate measurements in some patients. With significant mitral stenosis some degree of pulmonary hypertension is present with associated increases in right ventricular pressures. As pulmonary vascular resistance increases with time, pulmonary hypertension may become severe, and vasodilator administration may be necessary in the catheterization laboratory to determine how much of this increase is reversible and to increase the safety of angiography. Concomitant mitral insufficiency or aortic insufficiency may further alter recorded pressure data in mitral stenosis. An example of recordings in a case of mitral stenosis is given in Figure 18.15.

Idiopathic Hypertrophic Subaortic Stenosis

Pressure measurements have been of particular interest in this spectrum of disorders from a pathophysiologic and technical standpoint. The pressure finding of interest is a systolic left intraventricular gradient that may occur between the outflow tract and the apex or between other locations within the cavity. In some patients this gradient may be associated with asymmetric septal hypertrophy alone, and in others it appears to be primarily associated with obstruction of ventricular outflow

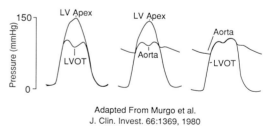

Adapted From Murgo et al.
J. Clin. Invest. 66:1369, 1980

Figure 18.16. Pressure measurements in a patient with idiopathic hypertrophic subaortic stenosis at the left ventricular apex (*LV apex*), left ventricular outflow tract below the aortic valve (*LVOT*), and in the ascending aorta revealing an intracavitary gradient. (Adapted from Murgo JP, Alter BR, Dorethy JF, Altobelli SA, McGranahan GM. Dynamics of left ventricular ejection in obstructive and nonobstructive hypertrophic cardiomyopathy. J Clin Invest 1980;66:1369–1382.)

by the mitral valve apparatus. The pathophysiology of this disorder has been addressed in several recent reviews (15–17) and in Chapter 24. From a technical standpoint this disorder presents several interesting problems with respect to pressure measurement. First, it is desirable to measure the intraventricular pressure gradient continuously in such patients for good documentation and also to assess the effects of interventions. In order to do this a micromanometer catheter with two pressure sensors is generally utilized in our laboratories. The distance between the sensors may range from 2 to 4 cm or so. Extreme care must be exercised when making such measurements to ensure that the catheter is free-floating within the ventricular cavity. If this is not done, entrapment of the pressure sensors may occur within trabeculations, and a false gradient may be recorded. Entrapment can usually be detected with the combination of fluoroscopic visualization and observation of the diastolic pressure contour. The latter is altered when the catheter is entrapped such that both sensors read different pressures during diastasis. The contour of the usual diastolic filling wave is also usually distorted. In some patients it may be impossible to make such recordings due to ventricular irritability or geometric considerations. In such cases a pullback recording can be made from the ventricular apex to the outflow tract and across the aortic valve using a pigtail catheter. It is very difficult to entrap a pigtail, however, localization of the gradient may be less precise, and measurements are not continuous with this method. A representative recording from a patient with idiopathic hypertrophic subaortic stenosis is given in Figure 18.16.

CONCLUSIONS

Of all hemodynamic measurements performed in the modern cardiac catheterization laboratory, pressure determination should be the most accurate and precise. This depends, however, on meticulous attention to detail and knowledge concerning catheters, transducers, recording systems, and the characteristics thereof. Accurate pressure measurement is extremely important in assessing the severity and functional significance of many pathophysiologic states, as discussed elsewhere in this volume. Invasive cardiologists should be especially aware of proper technique for pressure measurement and pitfalls involved therein.

References

1. Geddes LA. The direct measurement of blood pressure. Chicago: Year Book Medical Publishers, 1970.
2. Luciani L. Human physiology (trans by FA Welby). London: Macmillan, 1911;1:592.
3. Milnor WR. Hemodynamics. Baltimore: Williams & Wilkins, 1982.
4. McDonald DA. Blood flow in arteries. London: Edward Arnold, 1974.
5. Geddes LE, Baker LE. Principles of applied biomedical instrumentation. New York: John Wiley & Sons, 1975.
6. Gabe IT. Pressure measurement in experimental physiology. In: Bergel DH, ed. Cardiovascular fluid dynamics. London: Academic Press, 1972;1:11-50.
7. Miller HD, Baker LE. A stable ultraminiature catheter tip pressure transducer. Med Biol Eng 1973;11:86-89.
8. Patel DJ, Mason OT, Ross J, Braunwald E. Harmonic analysis of pressure pulses obtained from the heart and great vessels of man. Am Heart J 1965;69:785-794.
9. Nichols WW, Pepine CJ, Conti CR. Catheter tip manometer system: pressure and velocity system. In: Ghista DN, ed. Advances in cardiovascular physics. New York: S. Karger, 1983;5:144-176.
10. Gersch BJ, Hahn CEW, Prys-Roberts C. Physical criteria for measurement of left ventricular pressure and its first derivative. Cardiovasc Res 1971;5:32-40.
11. Murgo JP, Westerhof N, Giolma JP, Altobelli SA. Aortic input impedance in normal man: relationship to pressure wave forms. Circulation 1980;62:105-116.
12. Murgo JP, Westerhof N, Giolma JP, Altobelli SA. Manipulation of ascending aortic pressure and flow wave reflections with the Valsalva maneuver: relationship to input impedance. Circulation 1981;63:122-132.
13. O'Rourke MF. Arterial function in health and disease. New York: Churchill Livingstone, 1982.
14. Haskell RJ, French WJ. Accuracy of left atrial and pulmonary artery wedge pressure in pure mitral regurgitation in predicting left ventricular end-diastolic pressure. Am J Cardiol 1988;61:136-141.
15. Maron BJ, Bonow RO, Cannon RO, Leon MB, Epstein SE. Hypertrophic cardiomyopathy: interrelations of clinical manifestations, pathophysiology, and therapy (part 1). N Engl J Med 1987;316:780-789.
16. Maron BJ, Bonow RO, Cannon RO, Leon MB, Epstein SE. Hypertrophic cardiomyopathy: interrelations of clinical manifestations, pathophysiology, and therapy (part 2). N Engl J Med 1987;316:844-852.
17. Murgo JP, Alter BR, Dorethy JF, Altobelli SA, McGranahan GM. Dynamics of left ventricular ejection in obstructive and nonobstructive hypertrophic cardiomyopathy. J Clin Invest 1980;66:1369-1382.

19

Blood Flow Measurement

Michael D. Winniford, M.D.
Charles R. Lambert, M.D., Ph.D.

INTRODUCTION

The determination of blood flow complements that of pressure in formulating a rigorous description of cardiovascular hemodynamics in health and disease. Flow measurements performed in the modern cardiac catheterization laboratory vary from standard thermodilution determination of cardiac output to subselective coronary blood flow velocity derived from Doppler catheter methodology. Although the technology involved in making such measurements has evolved greatly, the basic physiologic principles applied for measurement of blood flow have been modified very little since their original descriptions. The purpose of this chapter is to review the basic physiologic principles involved in measurement of blood flow, to outline the limitations of currently available methodology, and to describe the general application of blood flow determination to description of pathophysiologic states in the cardiac catheterization laboratory. Blood flow alterations unique to specific disease states are covered in their respective chapters.

CARDIAC OUTPUT

Cardiac output is the most frequent blood flow measurement performed in the cardiac catheterization laboratory. Cardiac output, determined at rest and in some cases during exercise, is an extremely useful parameter in the overall assessment of cardiovascular function and is essential for the calculation of vascular resistances, valve orifice areas

and regurgitant fractions. The two most common methods used clinically to measure cardiac output are the Fick and indicator dilution techniques.

Fick Method

Theory

The Fick principle is based on the simple concept of conservation of mass. This principle, first postulated by Adolph Fick in 1870, states that in a steady state the rate at which an indicator leaves a system (e.g., an organ) must equal the rate at which it is introduced. Consider the model shown in Figure 19.1. Fluid containing a known concentration of an indicator (C_{in}) enters a chamber at a flow rate of Q. If additional indicator is added to the fluid in the chamber at a constant rate ($\dot{V}$), the concentration of indicator at the outflow will increase to C_{out}. In a steady state, the rate at which the indicator leaves the chamber must equal the rate at which it enters plus the rate at which it is added: rate of indicator out = rate in + rate added.

$$QC_{out} = QC_{in} + \dot{V} \qquad (1)$$

Solving equation 1 for Q:

$$Q = \dot{V}/(C_{out} - C_{in}) \qquad (2)$$

When the Fick principle is applied to measurement of cardiac output, oxygen is used as the indicator, and flow is determined by

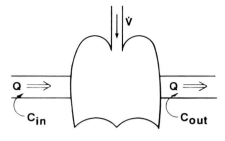

Rate of indicator out =
Rate in + Rate added

$$Q \times C_{out} = Q \times C_{in} + \dot{V}$$

$$Q = \frac{\dot{V}}{(C_{out} - C_{in})}$$

When O_2 is used as indicator:

$$Q = \frac{\dot{V}O_2}{C_A O_2 - C_V O_2}$$

Figure 19.1. Schematic illustration of flow measurement using the Fick principle. Fluid containing a known concentration of an indicator (C_{in}) enters a system at flow rate, Q. As the fluid passes through the system, indicator is continuously added at rate $\dot{V}$, raising the concentration in the outflow to C_{out}. In a steady state, the rate of indicator leaving the system (QC_{out}) must equal the rate at which it enters (QC_{in}) plus the rate at which it is added ($\dot{V}$). When oxygen is used as the indicator, cardiac output can be determined by measuring oxygen consumption ($\dot{V}O_2$), arterial oxygen content ($C_A O_2$), and mixed venous oxygen content ($C_v O_2$).

measuring arterial-mixed venous oxygen content difference and rate of oxygen consumption. Other indicators, including carbon dioxide and nitrous oxide, are rarely used clinically (1, 2). It is important to emphasize that the Fick principle is only valid in a steady state when both cardiac output and oxygen consumption are constant.

Oxygen Consumption

Accurate measurement of cardiac output using the Fick principle requires that both oxygen uptake by the lungs and oxygen content in arterial and mixed venous blood be carefully determined. In some laboratories, oxygen uptake is estimated from a formula, table, or nomogram. There are major limitations with this approach. Many factors which can influence oxygen consumption, such as level of sedation, medications, body temperature, and posture, are not accounted for when assuming an empiric value. In a study by Dehmer and associates (3), oxygen consumption was calculated from cardiac output (measured by thermodilution or green dye) and arterial-mixed venous oxygen content difference in 108 patients undergoing cardiac catheterization. While average oxygen uptake was 126 ± 26 cc/min/m^2 (mean ± standard deviation), there was wide variability (65 to 250 cc/min/m^2). Thus, any estimate of oxygen consumption in an individual patient may be grossly

inaccurate. When oxygen consumption cannot be measured, the use of tables based on the patient's age, sex, heart rate, and body weight is probably more accurate than an empiric formula based on body weight alone (4).

The traditional method of measuring oxygen consumption involves the timed collection of expired air in a Douglas bag. Typically, the patient's expired air is collected over a 3- to 4-minute period using a 60-liter Douglas bag and a two-way valved mouthpiece. A nose clamp is used to prevent breathing through the nostrils, and care is taken to avoid air leakage around the mouthpiece. The volume of air collected is measured with a spirometer and corrected for standard temperature and pressure. A sample of expired air is withdrawn from the bag, and oxygen concentration is determined using a gas analyzer. The difference in oxygen content (cubic centimeters of O_2/liter) between inspired (room) air and expired air is multiplied by minute ventilation (liters/minute) to obtain oxygen consumption (cubic centimeters of O_2/minute). A more detailed description of this method is provided by Slonim et al. (5).

Determination of oxygen consumption using the Douglas bag method is time-consuming, and incomplete collection of expired air is a common problem leading to important error. Oxygen consumption can be measured more simply by a metabolic rate meter (MRM-2, Waters Instruments, Rochester, MN). This device gives a time-averaged oxygen consumption rate without the calculations or temperature and pressure corrections required with the Douglas bag method. A clear plastic hood is placed over the subject's head so that air may enter only from around the loose seal at the patient's neck. A blower in the MRM-2 unit is connected by a hose to the top of the hood and draws room air through the hood at a rate rapid enough to assure that all of the patient's expired air is collected. The oxygen concentration of this room and expired air mixture (C_M) is determined by the MRM-2's polarographic oxygen sensor. Assuming that the patient's inspired and expired minute volumes are identical (i.e., respiratory quotient = 1), the average rate at which room air enters the hood ($\dot{V}_H$) is the same as the rate at which the expired and room air mixture is drawn into the MRM-2 unit ($\dot{V}_M$). The patient's rate of oxygen consumption ($\dot{V}_{O_2}$) is then simply the difference between the rate of oxygen entering and leaving the hood:

$$\dot{V}_{O_2} = 0.21(\dot{V}_H) - C_M(\dot{V}_M) \qquad (3)$$

Since $\dot{V}_H = \dot{V}_M$ when the respiratory quotient is 1, equation 3 can be rewritten:

$$\dot{V}_{O_2} = \dot{V}_M(0.21 - C_M)$$

where $\dot{V}_M$ is determined by the MRM-2's blower speed. Every 20 sec, the time-averaged oxygen consumption, in cubic centimeters of O_2/minute, is displayed digitally. After a 1-min equilibration period, oxygen consumption is determined from the mean of consecutive readings obtained over 2 to 4 min. The MRM-2 unit accurately measures oxygen consumption rates up to 1000 cc of O_2/min. For exercise studies, a metabolic rate meter that can measure oxygen consumption values up to 5000 cc of O_2/min is available (MRM-1).

The metabolic rate meter has several advantages over the Douglas bag method. Patients are more comfortable since the nose is not clamped and a mouthpiece is not used. Patient cooperation is not required to insure adequate air collection. Finally, errors in analyzing the Douglas bag volume and oxygen content are avoided. The polarographic oxygen cell in the MRM-2 deteriorates during use and must be calibrated periodically to maintain accuracy.

Sources of Error

Determination of oxygen consumption is usually the least precise component of the Fick measurement of cardiac output. One of the most common sources of error is incomplete collection or inaccurate analysis of expired air when the Douglas bag is used. In addition, air may diffuse from the bag if there is a long delay before it is analyzed. Although the respiratory quotient can be determined by analyzing the CO_2 content of the Douglas bag (5), this is not usually done in clinical laboratories, and a value between 0.8 and 1.0 is assumed. A small error (usually less than 5%) will be introduced when the respiratory quotient is greater or less than the assumed value. Patients may become anxious and hyperventilate when the Douglas bag collection is started or the MRM-2 hood is placed over their head. A significant change in functional residual capacity due to hyperventilation or hypoventilation during the period when oxygen consumption is being measured will produce an erroneous result. For example, if lung volume progressively increases during the measurement period, the amount of oxygen entering the lungs will also increase, but this additional oxygen is not taken up by the pulmonary-capillary blood (6). Oxygen consumption measured with either the metabolic rate meter or Douglas bag will be overestimated. Overall, the average error of carefully performed oxygen consumption measurements has been estimated to be about 6% (7).

Arterial-Venous Oxygen Content Difference

The second step in calculation of cardiac output by the Fick principle is determination of arterial and mixed venous oxygen contents. Systemic arterial and mixed venous blood samples are obtained simultaneously midway through the oxygen consumption determination. Because of incomplete mixing of inferior and superior vena cavae and coronary sinus drainage in the right atrium and right ventricle, the mixed venous blood sample should be obtained from the pulmonary artery. Oxygen content is determined directly using an oxygen-sensitive fuel cell (Lex-O_2-Con) or is calculated from a spectrophotometric measurement of oxygen saturation and hemoglobin concentration. Since the oxygen-carrying capacity of fully saturated hemoglobin is 1.36 cc of O_2/gm, oxygen content (volume %) equals oxygen saturation $\times$ 1.36 (cc of O_2/gm) $\times$ hemoglobin (gm %). (This ignores the small amount of oxygen dissolved in plasma). For example, assume arterial and mixed venous oxygen saturations are 95 and 70%, respectively, and hemoglobin concentration is 14 gm %:

$$C_{O_{2}art} = 0.95 \times 1.36 \text{ (cc of } O_2/\text{gm)}$$
$$\times 14 \text{ (gm/100 cc)}$$
$$= 18.1 \text{ cc of } O_2/100 \text{ cc}$$

$$C_{O_{2}MV} = 0.70 \times 1.36 \text{ (cc of } O_2/\text{gm)}$$
$$\times 14 \text{ (gm/100 cc)}$$
$$= 13.3 \text{ cc of } O_2/100 \text{ cc}$$

where $C_{O_{2}art}$ = arterial oxygen content, and $C_{O_{2}MV}$ = mixed venous oxygen content. If oxygen consumption is 240 cc of O_2/min, cardiac output (Q) can be calculated using equation 2:

$$Q = \dot{V}_{O_2}/(C_{O_{2}art} - C_{O_{2}MV})$$
$$= 240 \text{ (cc of } O_2/\text{min)}/[(18.1 - 13.3)$$
$$\text{(cc of } O_2/100 \text{ cc)} \times 10 \text{ (100 cc/liter)]}$$
$$= 5.0 \text{ (liter/min)}$$

Sources of Error

The arterial-mixed venous oxygen content difference can usually be determined with greater accuracy than oxygen consumption, especially when an oxygen-sensitive fuel cell is used. Errors can occur if blood samples are diluted with excess heparin, contain large air bubbles, or are allowed to sit at room temperature for several minutes before being analyzed. Indocyanine green dye has a maximum spectral absorbance at about 800 nm and can significantly interfere with oxygen saturation measurements made with spectrophotometers operating at wavelengths near 800 nm. Indocyanine green dye does not interfere with spectrophotometers that operate in the 530 to 630 nm range (e.g., IL-282 CO-Oximeter, Instrumentation Laboratory) (8). Abnormal hemoglobins (methemoglobin, sulfhemoglobin) and markedly lipemic samples will also interfere with spectrophotometric determination of oxygen saturation. Falsely elevated pulmonary arterial oxygen content values may be obtained if the tip of the pulmonary artery catheter is being intermittently thrust into the wedge position by cardiac or respiratory motion. Finally, the Fick method assumes that the measured oxygen contents of the arterial and mixed venous blood samples are representative of average oxygen concentrations during the measurement period. An error could be caused by phasic changes in pulmonary or systemic arterial oxygen saturation during the cardiac or respiratory cycle. During normal respiration, phasic changes in arterial-mixed venous oxygen content difference are negligible (9).

Errors in measurement of arterial or mixed venous oxygen content will have a greater impact on the accuracy of cardiac output, determined by the Fick technique, when arterial-mixed venous oxygen content difference is very small. Therefore, the Fick method is generally regarded as being most accurate when cardiac output is low and arterialvenous oxygen content difference is large (7). The average error in the arterial-mixed venous oxygen content difference determination is about 5%, and overall error in the Fick cardiac output measurement by the Fick method is about 10% (7).

Indicator Dilution Methods

Like the Fick method, indicator dilution techniques are based on the conservation of mass principle (10). The two most common indicator dilution techniques used in the cardiac catheterization laboratory are the dye dilution and thermodilution methods. The indicator dilution principle can be applied when the indicator is infused continuously or given as a bolus. Since the continuous infusion method is rarely used clinically (11), only the bolus technique will be discussed. (Actually, the Fick technique is a form of continuous infusion indicator dilution method with oxygen being the indicator.)

Theory

A schematic illustration of the indicator dilution principle is shown in Figure 19.2. When a bolus containing a known mass of indicator (M) is suddenly introduced into the flow entering a chamber, the concentration of indicator in the fluid exiting the chamber (C_{out}) increases in a curvilinear fashion. After reaching a peak, the concentration of indicator falls

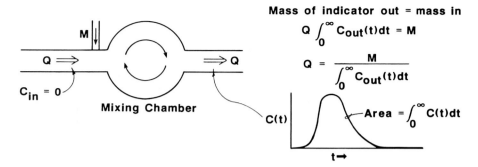

Figure 19.2. Schematic illustration of the bolus indicator dilution method of determining flow. A known quantity of indicator (M) is added to blood entering a mixing chamber at flow rate Q. The concentration of indicator in blood leaving the mixing chamber is continuously recorded and plotted as a function of time, $C(t)$. The total amount of indicator leaving the system is the product of flow and the integrated area under the concentration-time curve. By the principle of conservation of mass, the total mass of indicator which leaves the chamber must equal the amount which enters. C_{in}, fluid containing a known concentration of an indicator entering chamber; C_{out}, concentration of indicator at the outflow.

until all of the indicator has left the system. At any given moment in time, the rate at which indicator leaves the system is the product of flow (Q), and the concentration of indicator at that time, $C(t)$. If there is no indicator present before the bolus ($C_{in} = 0$), the total amount of indicator which leaves the system is given by the formula:

$$Q = {_0}\!\int^{\infty} C_{out}(t)dt$$

Assuming all of the indicator which was added to the system eventually leaves:

$$M = Q \, {_0}\!\int^{\infty} C_{out}(t)dt$$

and

$$Q = M/[{_0}\!\int^{\infty} C_{out}(t)dt] \qquad (4)$$

The integral term $C(t)dt$ is the product of concentration and time and, thus, represents the area beneath the concentration curve.

Dye Dilution Method

Of the numerous dyes used as indicators, the only one in common use today is indocyanine green dye. It is nontoxic, rapidly metabolized and excreted by the liver (half-life approximately 10 min), and easily measured by spectrophotometry. A known amount of green dye, usually 5 mg, is rapidly injected proximal to a mixing chamber. Blood from a site distal to the mixing chamber is withdrawn at a constant rate through a densitometer, a simple photoelectric device, and the concentration of

dye is continuously recorded until recirculation is detected. The injection site is chosen as close to the sampling point as possible, as long as adequate mixing of the dye and blood can be assured. Most commonly, the pulmonary artery is chosen as the injection site, mixing occurs in the left atrium and left ventricle, and the concentration of dye is sampled in the aorta, femoral or brachial artery. By injecting into the left ventricle and sampling from the femoral or brachial artery, the green dye output can be determined without a right heart catheterization (12). According to equation 4, cardiac output is equal to the mass of green dye injected divided by the area under the concentration-time curve (Fig. 19.3). In practice, the area under the concentration curve cannot be measured directly because recirculation of dye occurs before the concentration falls to zero. However, since the downslope of the curve before recirculation occurs follows an exponential decline, the curve can be extrapolated to the baseline. There are several ways to manually eliminate the effect of recirculation and obtain the area under the concentration curve, but they require replotting the curve on a semilogarithmic scale and are time-consuming (13). Small, analog cardiac output computers are commercially available which rapidly extrapolate the dye curve to the baseline, measure the area under the curve, and digitally display the cardiac output. These devices must be calibrated periodically to assure accuracy.

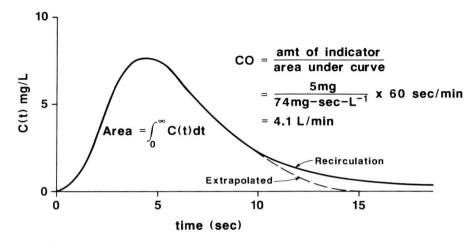

Figure 19.3. Determination of cardiac output by the dye dilution method. Five milligrams of indocyanine green dye are given as a bolus into the pulmonary artery. Systemic arterial blood is continuously withdrawn through a densitometer, and the concentration of green dye is recorded over time [$C(t)$]. The effect of recirculation is eliminated by extrapolating the exponential portion of downslope of the concentration-time curve to zero. Cardiac output (CO) is equal to the amount of dye injected divided by the area under the concentration-time curve (74 mg-sec/L), where L = length of the base of curve on time axis.

Sources of Error

Errors in the green dye method occur if the exact amount of dye delivered to the blood is inaccurately measured, there is incomplete mixing of dye and blood, the concentration-time curve is distorted, or the area under the curve is imprecisely determined. Since indocyanine green dye deteriorates with exposure to light, it should be used within one hour of preparation. Rate of blood withdrawal through the densitometer must be constant, and the length of tubing between sampling site and densitometer should be kept as short as possible to avoid distorting the concentration curve (14). When an analog output computer is used, the downslope of the dye concentration curve between approximately 85 and 50% of the peak concentration must be exponential since this is the portion of the curve usually used to calculate the decay constant needed to extrapolate the curve to baseline. A careful analysis of the dye curve will often indicate the cause of erroneous outputs.

Several reports have shown that Fick and green dye measurements of cardiac output agree within 20% of each other in the majority of patients (15, 16). There is a greater disparity between Fick and dye outputs in patients with low cardiac output (less than 2 liters/min/m^2)

and in those with significant mitral or aortic regurgitation (Fig. 19.4) (15, 17). In these individuals, the downslope of the concentration curve is prolonged, and recirculation distorts the curve before an accurate area can be calculated (18). In these cases one may correct the error by moving the injection and sampling sites closer together. If this does not correct the error, a nonrecirculated indicator (e.g., thermal) should be used. As discussed in Chapter 20, the downslope of the curve is also distorted by early recirculation of dye in patients with a left to right intracardiac shunt.

Thermodilution

The thermodilution technique is based on the same principle as the dye dilution method described above (19, 20). In this case, the indicator is "cold" and the "concentration" of indicator is temperature. A thermistor-tipped, triple-lumen balloon catheter is positioned in the pulmonary artery. A carefully measured volume of iced or room temperature saline or 5% dextrose is injected as a bolus into the right atrium, and the temperature of the blood-injectate mixture in the pulmonary artery is continuously recorded. The cardiac output (Q) is inversely proportional to the area under the

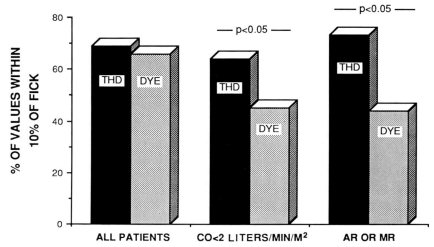

Figure 19.4. Comparison of thermodilution and dye dilution cardiac output determinations. Cardiac output (*CO*) was measured by Fick and either thermodilution (*THD*) (242 patients) or dye dilution (556 patients) techniques. Overall, the difference between the Fick and the *THD* or dye output was less than 10% in approximately 70% of patients. However, the dye output was within 10% of the Fick output in only about 45% of patients with low cardiac output, aortic regurgitation (*AR*), or mitral regurgitation (*MR*). (From data in Hillis LD, Firth BG, Winniford, MD. Analysis of factors affecting the variability of Fick versus indicator dilution measurements of cardiac output. Am J Cardiol 1985;56:764-768.)

temperature-time curve and can be calculated using the following formula:

$$Q = 60V_IS_IC_ICF(T_B - T_I)/[S_BC_B \cdot {_0}{\int^\propto} \Delta T_B(t)dt],$$

$$= 60(V_IS_IC_ICF/S_BC_B) \cdot (T_B - T_I)/[{_0}{\int^\propto} \Delta T_B(t)dt] \quad (5)$$

where V_I = volume of injectate, S_I = specific gravity of injectate, C_I = specific heat of injectate, CF = correction factor accounting for warming of indicator during passage through the catheter, S_B = specific gravity of blood, C_B = specific heat of blood, T_B = blood temperature, T_I = injectate temperature, and ${_0}{\int^\propto} \Delta T_B(t)dt$ = area under the temperature-time curve. In practice, analog cardiac output computers are routinely used to integrate the temperature-time curve and calculate cardiac output using equation 5 (21).

The thermodilution method has several advantages over Fick and dye dilution. It is the easiest and quickest of the three techniques to perform. No arterial blood samples are required. Since there is negligible recirculation of indicator in the absence of an intracardiac shunt, calculation of the area under the temperature-time curve is simplified. There is close agreement between the thermodilution and Fick methods over a wide range of cardiac outputs (19, 22, 23). Unlike dye dilution techniques, accuracy of the thermodilution method is not reduced in patients with aortic or mitral regurgitation or moderately depressed cardiac output (Fig. 19.4) (15, 17). At extremely low outputs (less than 2.5 liters/min), the thermodilution method appears to overestimate cardiac output, presumably due to loss of thermal indicator between the injection site and pulmonary artery (24). The Fick method would be preferable to either of the indicator dilution techniques in these individuals.

Sources of Error

Accurate measurement of cardiac output by the thermodilution technique requires attention to several details. If ice-cold injectate is used, syringes should be prepared and placed in an ice bath at least one hour prior to use. Excessive handling of the syringe after removal from the ice bath will warm the injectate (loss of indicator), resulting in overestimation of true cardiac output. This problem can be minimized if injectate temperature is measured by a thermistor placed in-line between the injection syringe and the hub of the thermodilution catheter (Model 93-500, CO-Set, American Edwards) (25). Patients who are tachypneic or require mechanical ventilation-may have large fluctuations in pulmonary artery blood temperature which increase the variability of thermodilution output measurements (26, 27). Reproducibility will be improved in these patients if injection is timed to begin at end-expiration and ice-cold injectate is used. Although use of ice-cold indicator is frequently cited as having a greater signal-to-noise ratio, there is no clear difference in accuracy and reproducibility of ice-cold vs. room temperature (20 to 25°C) injectate in most clinical settings (25, 28, 29). It is possible that the advantage of a greater signal-to-noise ratio is offset by increased uncertainty as to the amount of indicator (cold) lost during passage through the catheter. Ice-cold injectate is required in hypothermic patients and when room temperature exceeds 25°C. Ice-cold injectate may also be preferable when cardiac output is very high (e.g., during exercise), where the area under the temperature-time curve is small, and when there are large fluctuations in pulmonary artery blood temperature (30). The thermodilution technique may be inaccurate in patients with intracardiac shunts, where recirculation of indicator distorts the temperature-time curve (31, 32), and in those with tricuspid regurgitation (23). Thermodilution cardiac output should always be based on the average of at least three individual measurements. The reproducibility of triplicate determinations is usually about 5%.

Velocity Catheter Techniques (Noncoronary)

Both Doppler (33) and electromagnetic (34–38) techniques have been adapted to catheter measurement of blood velocity in the pulmonary artery and aorta. As noted in the section on coronary velocity catheters, volumetric flow is measured with these techniques only when vessel cross-sectional area is known or independent calibration is done. The latter is most frequently performed in human studies with use of cardiac output measurement by thermodilution or other indicator dilution techniques. The aortic or pulmonary artery velocity signal can be electronically meaned and normalized in this manner. Alternatively, in vitro calibration can be done. Recordings made in the great vessels using these techniques should resemble those seen using cuff-type electromagnetic flow probes. When used in combination with high-fidelity, catheter-tip micromanometers, vascular impedance spectra and wave reflections can be studied (37, 38). Other uses include quantitation of valvular regurgitation (39). Effects of pharmacologic agents and oscillatory components of afterload can be quantified using these techniques.

The primary practical problem with use of velocity catheters in the great vessels is a function of catheter placement and stabilization. Since blood flow velocity profiles in the great vessels in vivo are not flat, catheter sampling from one location may not represent an average of true blood velocity. Catheter placement should be adjusted such that the velocity profile approximates that seen with a cuff flow probe. This is usually accomplished by placing the proximal (pulmonary artery) or distal (aorta) stabilizing portion of the catheter through the valve and positioning the velocity sensor just distal to the valve. If serial measurements are to be taken, great care must be exercised to prevent catheter movement. Present use of catheter-tip velocity transducers is mainly in the research setting.

Cardiac Output Determination

It should be evident from the preceding discussion that each of the most commonly used methods for measuring cardiac output has important limitations. All require that the patient be in a steady state with a constant cardiac output during the measurement period. Traditionally, the Fick method has been used as the reference standard against which other techniques are compared. From a practical standpoint, the accuracy of the Fick method is dependent upon the care taken in measuring oxygen consumption and arterial and mixed venous oxygen contents especially in patients with high cardiac outputs. The thermodilution technique is subject to error in patients with tricuspid regurgitation, intracardiac shunts, or extremely low cardiac outputs. The dye dilution method is not well-suited for patients with significant mitral or aortic regurgitation or low cardiac outputs. In many laboratories, it is common practice to determine cardiac output by both the Fick method and an indicator dilution technique, especially when calculating a valve orifice area or regurgitant fraction. In the future, newer techniques that can provide a continuous record of cardiac output, such as electrical impedance determination of ventricular stroke volume (40), may become clinically useful.

CORONARY BLOOD FLOW

Because of the lack of a reliable, clinically practical method for measuring regional coronary blood flow during routine cardiac catheterization, information about coronary flow is usually inferred from the coronary anatomy defined by angiography. In patients with coronary artery disease (CAD), an assessment of the degree of impairment of coronary flow at rest or during exercise is usually made based on the angiographic severity of the coronary stenosis. There are significant limitations with this approach. Visual interpretation of the coronary angiogram is plagued by so much marked intraobserver and interobserver variability that attempts to determine the functional significance of a coronary stenosis are severely limited. Quantitative coronary angiography provides a more accurate and objective measurement of arterial geometry, but cannot overcome the limitations imposed by the complex relationship between stenosis geometry and coronary flow, inability to quantitate diffuse atherosclerotic narrowing in angiographically normal appearing coronary segments, and the inability to determine the effect of myocardial factors on coronary flow (see Chapter 23). By combining anatomic information provided by the coronary angiogram with physiologic information obtained from measurement of resting and peak coronary blood flow, a much more complete assessment of the effect of pathologic states on the coronary circulation can be made (41). While gas clearance and coronary sinus thermodilution techniques have been important research tools, these methods have a limited ability to provide clinically useful information about the physiologic severity of coronary lesions in any given patient. As experience grows with several new approaches, including Doppler flow probes, digital videodensitometry, and positron emission tomography, sophisticated measurement of coronary flow and flow reserve may assume a more important role in the clinical evaluation of patients with suspected ischemic heart disease (42).

Gas Clearance Methods

Gas clearance methods are used to measure the average left ventricular blood flow per unit weight and represent adaptations of the Kety-Schmidt nitrous oxide technique originally applied to the quantitation of cerebral blood flow (43–45). Gas clearance methods are based on the same concept of conservation of mass described by the Fick principle (45, 46). A diffusible inert gas which is not metabolized by the myocardium is added to the systemic circulation, usually by inhalation. The most commonly used nonradioactive inert gases are nitrous oxide, helium, hydrogen, and argon. As saturation of the myocardium with the gas is achieved, the coronary arterial and venous blood concentrations of gas are periodically recorded. According to the Fick principle, flow is equal to the myocardial gas uptake divided by the mean arterial-venous gas content difference. The mean arterial-venous gas content difference is found by integrating the instantaneous arterial-venous gas content differences over the time period required to achieve saturation. Since myocardial uptake of inert gas cannot be measured directly, it is expressed as the product of myocardial mass (W) and the change in tissue inert gas concentration (ΔC_t). Therefore, the equation for flow (F) becomes

$$F = (W \Delta C_t)/{_0\!\int^t} (C_a - C_v)dt \qquad (6)$$

where C_a and C_v are coronary arterial and venous gas contents, respectively, and t is the time required to reach saturation. Solving equation 6 for flow/unit weight (W) of myocardium:

$$F/W = \Delta C_t/{_0\!\int^t} (C_a - C_v)dt.$$

Since the tissue concentration of inert gas (C_t) also cannot be measured directly, it is expressed as the product of the change in gas concentration in coronary venous blood (ΔCv) and the tissue-blood partition coefficient (λ):

$$F/W = \lambda \Delta C_v/{_0\!\int^t} (C_a - C_v)dt \qquad (7)$$

An example of the inert gas measurement of myocardial blood flow using nitrous oxide is shown in Figure 19.5. Equation 7 is equally valid when the coronary arterial and venous gas contents are measured during the

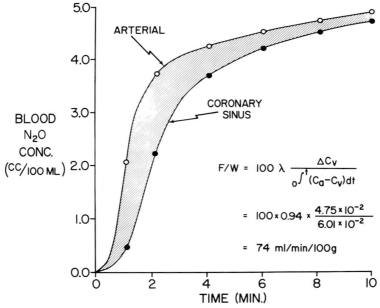

The figure shows a graph with axes: y-axis labeled "BLOOD N$_2$O CONC. (CC/100 ML)" ranging 0.0 to 5.0, x-axis labeled "TIME (MIN.)" ranging 0 to 10. Two curves labeled ARTERIAL and CORONARY SINUS.

$$F/W = 100\ \lambda\ \frac{\Delta C_v}{\int_0^t (C_a - C_v)\,dt}$$

$$= 100 \times 0.94 \times \frac{4.75 \times 10^{-2}}{6.01 \times 10^{-2}}$$

$$= 74\ ml/min/100g$$

Figure 19.5. Illustration of inert gas measurement of left ventricular flow per unit weight (*F/W*) using nitrous oxide (N$_2$O). Arterial and coronary sinus blood samples are obtained periodically during a 10-minute period in which the subject breathes a gas mixture containing 15% N$_2$O. Arterial and coronary venous N$_2$O saturation curves are drawn through the individual points, and equation 7 in the text is applied. The tissue-blood partition coefficient (λ) is 0.94 cc/gm (assuming a hematocrit of 40%). Since the initial venous N$_2$O concentration (*CONC*) is zero, C_v is simply the final venous N$_2$O concentration (4.75 $\times$ 10-2 cc/cc). The mean arterial-venous N$_2$O difference (6.01 $\times$ 10-2 cc/cc/min) is obtained by planimetry of the area between the arterial and venous saturation curves. (From Klocke FJ. Coronary blood flow in man. Prog Cardiovasc Dis 1976;19:117–166.)

desaturation phase as the systemic gas concentration falls to zero.

The inert gas clearance technique can also be used to measure average left ventricular flow following the bolus intracoronary injection of a radioactive tracer such as xenon-133 (43, 47–49). The xenon-133 washout curve is analyzed by precordial counting of radioactivity using a scintillation camera. When a multicrystal camera is used, washout from specific regions of the heart can be recorded and regional blood flow estimated (50).

Limitations of Gas Clearance Methods

Several assumptions are made when the Kety-Schmidt approach is applied to measurement of coronary blood flow. First, there must be a steady state of coronary flow during the measurement period. This requires that flow remain unchanged for the 5 to 20 min required to reach saturation or desaturation.

Thus, rapid changes in flow cannot be assessed. Second, the venous blood being sampled must be representative of venous drainage from the area under study. The accuracy of the technique is reduced when the sampled blood contains venous drainage from structures other than the left ventricle or when venous drainage from certain regions of the left ventricle do not drain into the coronary sinus. In humans, up to 17% of all veins that enter the coronary sinus arise from structures other than the left ventricle (51). Drainage from regions of the left ventricle supplied by the posterior descending artery enters the coronary sinus near the ostium and is usually not represented in blood obtained from a catheter positioned 2 or 3 cm within the sinus (52). Third, the measured flow per unit weight represents the average flow in the entire myocardial region draining into the coronary sinus upstream from the sampling catheter. At best, an attempt can be made to measure regional flow in the territory of the left anterior descending artery by sampling from the great cardiac vein. Using a modification of the inert gas clearance method, Grines et al. (53) measured regional myocardial perfusion by subselective intracoronary hydrogen infusion while monitoring the hydrogen washout curve in the pulmonary artery with a platinum electrode. In dogs, there was a good correlation between regional perfusion measured by this technique and by radiolabeled microspheres at flow rates below 2 cc/min/gm. At higher flow rates, the hydrogen washout method underestimated flow. While this method would allow assessment of regional perfusion without the limitations imposed by coronary sinus sampling, additional validation studies are needed before it can be applied clinically. Fourth, a uniform gas concentration must be achieved throughout the region under study. This requirement is satisfied when there is homogeneous perfusion of normal myocardial tissue. It may not be valid when there is marked heterogeneity of perfusion and when several tissue components are present in the region, including muscle, scar, and fat (54, 55). Therefore, the gas clearance methods are best suited for patients with normal coronary arteries and homogeneous left ventricular perfusion. In patients with CAD who have heterogeneous perfusion and, in some case, myocardial scar, meticulous techniques must be used to avoid overestimating flow, including prolonged gas administration, the use of highly sensitive analytic techniques, and prolonged measurement of arterial and venous gas concentrations during the desaturation phase (46, 56). Finally, the inert gas indicator must not be metabolized by the myocardium and should be free of recirculation. This requirement is met by most of the inhaled inert gas tracers.

The xenon-133 precordial counting method is technically demanding and suffers from several limitations (46, 48). Because xenon-133 is highly fat-soluble, adipose tissue contributes a large fraction of the total radioactivity detected by precordial counting during the later portion of the washout curve. The high fat solubility also limits the number of measurements that can be made during each study. Recirculation of about 5% of an injected dose of xenon-133 complicates interpretation of the washout curve. The accuracy of xenon-133 measurements of average left ventricular

blood flow, especially at high flow rates, remains controversial.

The nonradioactive and radioactive inert gas clearance techniques are time-consuming, require special equipment for sample analysis, and may not be accurate at high coronary flow rates. While not practical for clinical use, they continue to be utilized in a small number of laboratories for research studies examining physiologic regulation of coronary flow and the effect of pathologic conditions or pharmacologic agents on myocardial perfusion.

Coronary Sinus Thermodilution

In 1971, Ganz and associates (57) described a method for measuring coronary sinus blood flow using the thermodilution technique. Room temperature injectate (5% dextrose solution or saline) is injected at a rate of 35 to 55 cc/min into the coronary sinus through a 7 or 8 Fr thermodilution catheter. The injectate mixes with the coronary sinus blood, and the temperature of the injectate-blood mixture is recorded by a thermistor placed on the external surface of the catheter 10 to 45 mm proximal to the injectate orifice. Assuming there is adequate mixing of injectate with coronary sinus blood, heat gained by injectate = heat lost by blood:

$$M_I S_I (T_M - T_I) = M_B S_B (T_B - T_M)$$

where M_I = mass of injectate, S_I = specific heat of injectate, T_M = temperature of injectate-blood mixture, T_I = temperature of injectate, M_B = mass of blood, S_B = specific heat of blood, and T_B = temperature of blood. Since mass equals volume (V) times density (D):

$$V_I D_I S_I (T_M - T_I) = V_B D_B S_B (T_B - T_M)$$

and

$$V_B = [(V_I D_I S_I)(T_M - T_I)]/[D_B S_B (T_B - T_M)]$$

Expressed as volume flow:

$$
\begin{aligned}
Q_{CS} &= F_I [D_I S_I / D_B S_B][T_M - T_I/T_B - T_M] \\
&= F_I [D_I S_I / D_B S_B][(T_B - T_I) \\
&\quad /(T_B - T_M) - 1]
\end{aligned}
\tag{8}
$$

where Q_{cs} = coronary sinus flow and F_I = flow rate of indicator. The constant term ($D_I S_I / D_B S_B$) = 1.08 for 5% dextrose solution and 1.10 for normal saline.

If the catheter is advanced into the great cardiac vein, venous flow from the anterior region of the left ventricle can be recorded. Catheters with two external thermistors (Regional Pepine 2, Webster Laboratories, Baldwin Park, CA; Baim, Electro-Catheter Corp., Rahway, NJ) permit simultaneous measurement of great cardiac vein and coronary sinus flow (58, 59). Pacing electrodes placed near the tip of the thermodilution catheter can be used to control atrial rate during flow measurements. Coronary venous blood samples can usually be obtained from the injectate lumen, although this may be difficult when the catheter tip is placed in the great cardiac vein. When blood sampling is required, a thermodilution catheter with a larger lumen or a separate catheter for blood sampling can be used.

The validity of the thermodilution technique using equation 8 has been convincingly demonstrated in models of the coronary sinus and in animal studies which have secured the catheter within the coronary sinus. A poorer relationship between flow measured by thermodilution and krypton-85 washout was found when the catheter was placed in intact dogs (60). Few studies have compared the coronary sinus thermodilution technique with other methods of measuring coronary flow in humans (59).

The coronary sinus thermodilution technique has several advantages. First, the method is relatively simple and inexpensive. With experience, adequate flow signals from both great cardiac vein and coronary sinus can be obtained in over 90% of patients studied. Second, since there is no significant accumulation of indicator cold, multiple measurements can be made over a relatively short period of time. A steady injectate-blood mixture temperature is usually achieved within 10 to 15 sec after the start of injectate infusion; flow measurements can usually be completed within 30 sec. Third, the time constant of the method is rapid enough to permit detection of flow changes which occur in 2 to 3 sec. Fourth, the thermodilution method is safer than those techniques that require cannulation of a coronary artery. Transient atrial arrhythmias may occur during manipulation of the catheter in the right atrium. Perforation of the atrium or coronary sinus is extremely rare. Finally, volumetric flow in cubic centimeters/minute is measured, rather than flow/unit weight or flow velocity.

Limitations of Coronary Sinus Thermodilution

As with all methods of measuring coronary flow in humans, the thermodilution technique has several limitations. First, like the gas clearance methods, the portion of left ventricular flow measured depends on the precise position of the catheter within the coronary sinus and the origin of venous blood entering the sinus proximal to the catheter. In normal subjects, there is some variability in the entry site of veins draining the lateral and inferior regions of the left ventricle. In addition, extensive venous anastomoses may occur in human hearts (52). In the presence of severe coronary disease, the pattern of venous drainage may be further distorted by venous collaterals. Therefore, it may be difficult in some cases to attribute coronary sinus flow to any specific portion of the left ventricle.

This limitation can be partially overcome by measuring great cardiac vein flow, as noted above, since the majority of resting great cardiac vein flow arises from the anterior region and, conversely, the majority of anterior region flow drains into the great cardiac vein. Validation studies in animals (61–63) have shown excellent regionalization of coronary flow signals from the great cardiac vein to the anterior descending coronary artery perfusion bed. Pepine and co-workers have also validated the regionalization of thermodilution coronary blood flow determinations in patients at the time of surgery (59). Using an electromagnetic flow probe in the operating room, a close relationship was demonstrated between thermodilution great cardiac vein flow and left anterior descending bypass graft flow in patients with occluded or subtotally occluded left anterior descending arteries (Fig. 19.6). Great cardiac vein flows in this study were all below 130 cc/min. At higher flow rates, the thermodilution technique may underestimate anterior region flow. Using Doppler or videodensitometric techniques, coronary flow in normal subjects has been shown to increase fourfold to sixfold above resting flow during maximal pharmacologic vasodilation. With the thermodilution technique, great cardiac vein and coronary sinus flow rarely rise above three times the resting value (64-67). Therefore, coronary flow reserve (*CFR*), the ratio of peak to resting

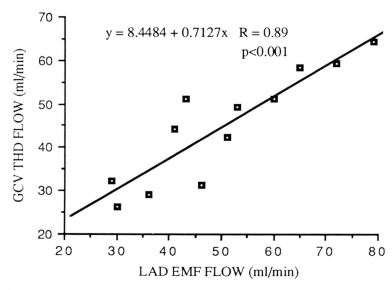

Figure 19.6. Relationship between great cardiac vein thermodilution (*GCV THD*) flow and left anterior descending (*LAD*) artery bypass graft flow measured simultaneously with an electromagnetic flow (*EMF*) probe. There is a close correlation between anterior regional blood flow measurements obtained by these two techniques. (Modified from Pepine CJ, Mehta J, Webster WW Jr, Nichols WW. In vivo validation of a thermodilution method to determine regional left ventricular blood flow in patients with coronary disease. Circulation 1978;58:795-802.)

blood flow, may be underestimated by the thermodilution technique (Fig. 19.7). Second, thermodilution flow measurements are affected by changes in catheter position within the coronary sinus, although excellent reproducibility of such measurements may be obtained (68). While the location of the catheter should be frequently checked radiographically, it may not be possible to detect small changes in position caused by catheter softening, patient movement, coughing, etc. An unrecognized change in catheter position may also occur if an intervention, such as rapid atrial pacing, produces a change in heart size or shape. The reliability of the coronary sinus thermodilution technique during exercise in patients with CAD may be variable (69). Third, reflux of right atrial blood into the coronary sinus when right atrial pressure is increased may cause an overestimation of coronary sinus thermodilution flow (70). In the authors' experience, coronary sinus reflux is rarely observed when the proximal thermistor is advanced at least 2 cm beyond the ostium. This possibility can be detected simply by injecting room temperature saline into the low right atrium

while recording from the coronary venous thermistors.

Despite the limitations of the coronary sinus thermodilution technique, it has provided valuable information about the pathophysiology of angina pectoris in patients with and without CAD (65, 71–74), the mechanism of action of antianginal drugs (75), and the effect of myocardial revascularization on coronary blood flow (76, 77). Like the gas clearance technique, the thermodilution method is best suited for patients with homogeneous perfusion and normal coronary arteries. When used in patients with CAD, the measurement of resting great cardiac vein flow has been best validated. By careful selection of control measurements, positioning the catheter within the great cardiac vein, avoiding changes in catheter position or heart size, and restricting the use of flow measurements to a comparison of changes in flow in individual subjects, the limitations of the thermodilution technique in patients with CAD can be minimized. The thermodilution technique has not emerged as a clinically useful method for quantitating coronary flow reserve in individual patients with CAD.

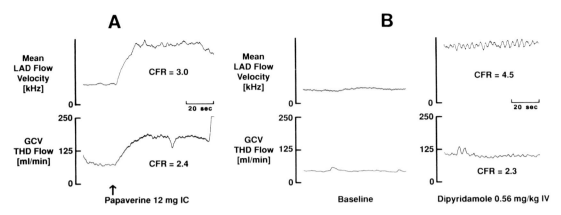

Figure 19.7. Comparison of simultaneous measurements of coronary flow reserve (*CFR*) in the anterior region of the left ventricle by Doppler and coronary sinus thermodilution methods. A Doppler catheter is positioned in the left anterior descending (*LAD*) artery and a thermodilution catheter in the great cardiac vein (*GCV THD*). In *A*, flow velocity (in kilohertz phase shift) is recorded before and after a maximally vasodilating dose of intracoronary (*IC*) papaverine in a patient with marked left ventricular hypertrophy and normal coronary arteries. Flow reserve, the ratio of peak to resting flow (or flow velocity) is lower with the thermodilution technique. In *B*, flows are measured before and after intravenous (*IV*) dipyridamole in a patient with atypical chest pain and normal coronary arteries. There is an even larger discrepancy between flow reserve measurements made with these two methods.

Doppler Techniques

The Doppler technique has been used to measure phasic coronary blood flow velocity in animals for many years and has been applied to the surface of epicardial coronary arteries of patients undergoing coronary artery bypass surgery (78). Initial attempts to measure coronary flow velocity during cardiac catheterization were made with a Doppler crystal mounted on the tip of a Sones catheter (79). This device could not be advanced selectively into a coronary artery. More recently, the development of a small intracoronary Doppler catheter has made it possible to record changes in phasic flow velocity in individual coronary arteries in awake humans during cardiac catheterization (80). In the version developed at the University of Iowa, a 20-MHz Doppler crystal is mounted at a 30 to 45° angle 5 mm from the tip of a 3 Fr polyurethane or polyethylene catheter (NuVEL, NuMED, Inc., Hopkinton, NY) (Fig. 19.8). A catheter with the Doppler crystal mounted on the tip is also available (DC-101, Millar Instruments, Houston, TX) (81). The Doppler catheter is passed through an angioplasty guiding catheter and positioned in the proximal portion of a coronary artery over an 0.014-inch steerable angioplasty guidewire. Mean and resting flow

velocity (kilohertz phase shift) can be continuously recorded on a strip-chart recorder. Coronary flow reserve can be determined by measuring mean flow velocity before and after maximal coronary vasodilation with intracoronary papaverine or intravenous dipyridamole (Fig. 19.9). Intracoronary of papaverine is preferable because the duration of coronary vasodilation is brief (less than 3 min), allowing multiple measurements of flow reserve over a short period of time (67, 82). A maximal vasodilator effect is usually produced by 12 mg of papaverine in the left coronary artery and 8 mg in the right coronary artery. The standard intravenous dose of dipyridamole (0.56 mg/kg) does not always produce maximal vasodilation (83). In addition, its prolonged duration of action makes repetitive measurements of flow reserve impossible.

The Doppler technique has been extensively validated in animal studies (80, 81). As shown in Figure 19.10, changes in coronary blood flow velocity correlate closely with timed venous collection of coronary sinus blood over a wide range of coronary flows. Peak coronary flow velocity, measured with an epicardial Doppler crystal, is similar to the intracoronary Doppler catheter present or absent from the vessel, confirming that the

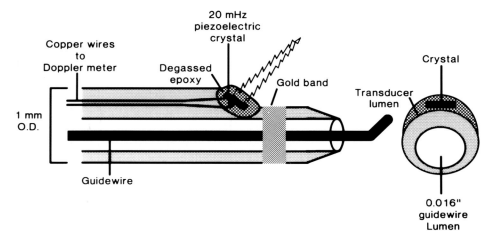

Figure 19.8. Schematic diagram of the distal portion of the intracoronary Doppler catheter. The copper wires attached to the piezoelectric crystal exit from the proximal end of the catheter and are connected to a pulsed Doppler meter. The catheter is advanced into the coronary artery over an 0.014-inch angioplasty guidewire. *O.D.*, outside diameter. (Modified with permission from Wilson RF, Laughlin DE, Ackell PH, et al. Transluminal, subselective measurement of coronary artery blood flow velocity and vasodilator reserve in man. Circulation 1985;72:82–92.)

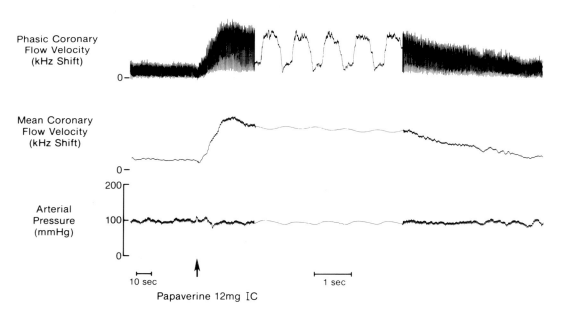

Figure 19.9. The effect of intracoronary papaverine on phasic and mean coronary blood flow velocity measured with a 3 Fr Doppler catheter positioned in the proximal portion of the left anterior descending artery. Flow velocity rises rapidly to a peak value approximately five times resting flow velocity. Thus, coronary flow reserve, the ratio of peak to resting flow velocity, is 5:1 in this patient with atypical chest pain and angiographically normal coronary arteries. Intracoronary papaverine causes only a slight, transient fall in arterial pressure.

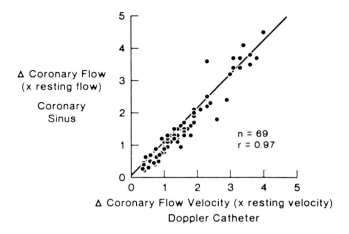

Figure 19.10. Validation of the coronary Doppler catheter in vivo with timed-volume collection of coronary sinus flow. Changes (Δ) in coronary blood flow velocity were highly correlated with simultaneously measured changes in coronary sinus flow over a wide range of flows. (From Wilson RF, Laughlin DE, Ackell PH, et al. Transluminal, subselective measurement of coronary artery blood flow velocity and vasodilator reserve in man. Circulation 1985;72:82-92.)

catheter itself does not significantly obstruct flow in normal vessels. No endothelial damage is caused by the placement of the catheter in animals (80).

Studies in humans have shown that placement of the Doppler catheter is a relatively safe procedure. Careful patient selection, full systemic heparinization and use by individuals skilled in coronary angioplasty should minimize the risks of the procedure. Coronary artery dissection, thrombosis, and spasm are obvious potential complications. Intracoronary papaverine is generally well-tolerated, but can cause marked QT-interval prolongation and, rarely, ventricular tachycardia. This has occurred in two patients at the University of Iowa; both were women with normal coronary arteries. Dipyridamole may cause hypotension, headache, or angina in patients with CAD. These adverse effects are usually promptly relieved by intravenous aminophylline.

There are several advantages to the intracoronary Doppler technique. First, a continuous record of flow velocity is provided. With the thermodilution technique, flow can be recorded continuously for only about 1 min, and the effect of interventions on coronary flow usually must be assessed by repetitive flow measurements. Second, the rapid time constant (milliseconds) permits measurement of nearly instantaneous changes in blood flow velocity. Third, the technique is accurate over a

wide range of flow velocities, including those found during maximal coronary blood flow. Finally, the Doppler catheter technique of measuring flow velocity is relatively simple to perform, making it one of the most clinically practical methods for the assessment of coronary flow reserve.

Limitations of the Doppler Technique

In addition to its advantages, the intracoronary Doppler method has significant limitations. First, Doppler techniques assess flow velocity; **volumetric** blood flow is not directly measured. Changes in flow velocity are proportional to changes in volumetric flow only when there is no change in vessel cross-sectional area at the site of the crystal. This is not a major limitation to the determination of coronary flow reserve, since papaverine exerts little effect on large coronary arteries. When the effect of other interventions on coronary flow velocity is being assessed, measurement of vessel cross-sectional area at the site of probe with quantitative coronary angiography is necessary to properly interpret changes in flow velocity. It must be assumed that this site does not change as the heart beats or over longer periods of time. Second, the need for intracoronary placement means that there will always be a risk associated with this technique. Third, the presence of very proximal coronary obstructions or severe, diffuse disease may make safe placement of the

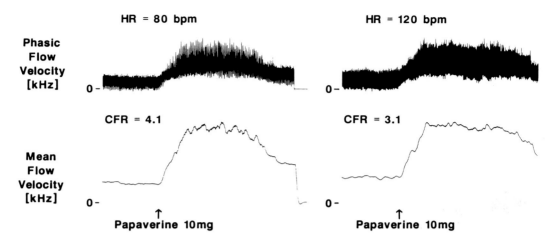

Figure 19.11. Effect of heart rate (*HR*) on coronary flow reserve (*CFR*). Peak and resting blood flow velocity (in kilohertz shift) are measured with a Doppler catheter in the left circumflex artery of a patient with normal coronary arteries. At resting heart rate of 80 bpm, coronary flow reserve is 4.1. During atrial pacing at a rate of 120 bpm, resting flow increases, and therefore, measured coronary flow reserve falls to 3.1. Baseline hemodynamics must be carefully considered when interpreting coronary flow reserve values.

catheter impossible. Although nonobstructive in normal arterial segments, the catheter may become obstructive when placed in very small vessels or across coronary lesions. Finally, damping or partial obstruction of the coronary ostium by the guiding catheter may restrict peak coronary flow. This may not be evident from the pressure waveform recorded from the tip of the guiding catheter. Gentle withdrawal of the guide from the ostium during maximal flow will help insure that the guide is not obstructive.

As a research device, the intracoronary Doppler catheter can be used to examine basic mechanisms of coronary flow regulation, the relationship between left ventricular hypertrophy and coronary flow reserve, neural control of the coronary circulation (84), the effect of pharmacologic agents on the coronary circulation (82,83), and the utility of noninvasive diagnostic tests in patients with CAD. Clinically, the device is probably most useful in assessing the physiologic significance of coronary lesions (85) and the function of coronary artery bypass grafts (86). The Doppler catheter may help provide insight into the cause of chest pain in patients with angiographically normal coronary arteries. Finally, the ability of Doppler flow velocity measurements to evaluate the efficacy of coronary angioplasty is being assessed.

Because there are many factors independent of coronary anatomy which can influence coronary flow reserve, including heart rate, blood pressure, contractility, hypertrophy, previous infarction, and coronary collaterals, an abnormal flow reserve in an individual patient must be interpreted cautiously (42). For example, consider the patient who is anxious and tachycardic when flow reserve is measured. As shown in Figure 19.11, tachycardia produces a metabolically mediated rise in resting coronary flow velocity. If peak flow velocity remains unchanged, calculated flow reserve, the ratio of peak to resting flow velocity, will be lower than it would have been had it been measured at the patient's baseline heart rate.

Videodensitometry

The first successful radiographic method to measure coronary blood flow was developed by Rutishauser et al. (87, 88) and Smith et al. (89) (see Chapter 23). These investigators measured the density of injected contrast material at two locations in a proximal coronary vessel to determine the transit time of the contrast bolus between the two points. If the distance between the two points is known, the flow velocity can be calculated. Volumetric flow is obtained by multiplying the cross-sectional area of the vessel times the blood flow velocity. Limitations of this technique include the short distance between regions of interest, the pulsatile nature of coronary flow, and artifacts caused by cardiac and respiratory motion. Using modern technology, Spiller et al. (90) reported a good correlation between flow measured by a videodensitometric technique and electromagnetic flow probes. These videodensitometric techniques work especially well in bypass grafts, which are long, straight, free of branches, and large in diameter. However, this method has not gained wide acceptance. Foerster et al. (91) described a method to measure reactive hyperemia by means of comparative densitometric analysis of a known amount of injected contrast medium as it traversed a region of interest over a coronary artery. This technique did not require measurement of either coronary artery diameter or segment length. More recently, determination of contrast appearance time with digital subtraction angiography has been applied to the measurement of regional coronary blood flow (92). Vogel and associates (93, 94) have used color and intensity coded parametric images to depict the timing and density of contrast medium as it transits the coronary circulation. Regional flow reserve is calculated by quantitatively comparing appearance time and maximum contrast concentration at baseline and during hyperemia.

Limitations of Videodensitometric Techniques

The digital subtraction videodensitometric techniques have several limitations. First, most of these techniques provide an estimate of flow reserve; absolute coronary blood flow is not measured. Using an analysis of time-density after intracoronary contrast injection, recent attempts have been made to assess regional myocardial blood flow in a manner similar to the xenon-133 washout technique (95, 96). Second, the time constant of the videodensitometric techniques is slow; rapid changes in flow cannot be measured. Third, the use of atrial pacing to control heart rate and electrocardiographically triggered power injection of contrast into the coronary artery increase the complexity of these methods. Fourth, artifacts due to patient motion are common. Finally, coronary flow reserve in initial studies was usually underestimated, especially when contrast medium was used to produce hyperemia (97–99). More recent studies using intracoronary papaverine or adenosine as the vasodilator have reported higher flow reserve values in the range of 4:1 to 5:1 (100–103). As further developments in digital imaging technology are made, refinements in these methods for measuring regional coronary blood flow and flow reserve will undoubtedly be made.

Newer Imaging Techniques

The ability of three new noninvasive imaging techniques, positron emission tomography, ultrafast computed tomography, and magnetic resonance imaging (MRI) to quantitate regional myocardial perfusion is being actively investigated. Of these new modalities, positron emission tomography has proven most useful for perfusion imaging (104–107). A positron-emitting radionuclide suitable for perfusion imaging, such as rubidium-82, $[N^{13}]$ammonia, or $[O^{15}]$water, is injected intravenously and accumulates in the myocardium. As the isotope decays, the masses of a positron and an electron annihilate to form two 511–keV photons that are emitted 180° apart. These photons are detected by a circumferential array of external radiation detectors, and tomographic images are mathematically reconstructed. The resultant tomographic image represents the cross-sectional distribution of the tissue radioisotope concentration. Regional myocardial perfusion can then be quantitated by analyzing the kinetics of the tissue concentration of the isotope. By using other positron-emitting tracers, such as $[C^{11}]$palmitate or $[F^{18}]$ 2-fluoro-2-deoxyglucose, regional myocardial metabolism can also be determined (60). Animal studies have confirmed the ability of positron emission tomography to accurately measure myocardial perfusion, and initial human studies suggest that this technique can be extremely useful clinically (108, 109). Unfortunately, a positron emission tomography facility is tremendously expensive. An on-site cyclotron is necessary when imaging with tracers other than rubidium-82, which can be produced by an inexpensive generator (109). Other limitations of this technique include underestimation of high perfusion rates with some tracers, limited resolution of positron cameras, and imaging motion artifacts. Although preliminary studies have been reported, much less is known about the ability of ultrafast computed tomography (110) and MRI (111) to measure myocardial perfusion.

SUMMARY

In summary, measurements of blood flow are an essential part of diagnostic cardiac catheterization. Cardiac output or systemic blood flow is one of the single most useful flow measurements made and carries the least error, provided flow is not greatly reduced. Regional blood flow measurements are largely for investigational use at present. Rapid changes in technology can be expected to make some regional blood flow methods clinically useful tools in the near future.

References

1. Clausen JP, Larsen OA, Trap–Jensen J. Cardiac output in middle–aged patients determined with CO_2 rebreathing method. J Appl Physiol 1970;28:337–342.

2. Ayotte B, Seymour J, McIlroy MB. A new method for measurement of cardiac output with nitrous oxide. J Appl Physiol 1970;28:863–866.

3. Dehmer GJ, Firth BG, Hillis LD. Oxygen consumption in adult patients during cardiac catheterization. Clin Cardiol 1982;5:436–440.

4. Crocker RH Jr, Ockene IS, Alpert JS, Pape LA, Dalen JE. Determinants of total body oxygen consumption in adults undergoing cardiac catheterization. Cathet Cardiovasc Diagn 1982;8:363–372.

5. Slonim NB, Bell BP, Christensen SE. Cardiopulmonary Laboratory Basic Methods and Calculations. Springfield, IL: Charles C Thomas, 1967.

6. Wessel HU, Stout RL, Bastanier CK, et al. Breath-by-breath variation of FRC: effect on VO_2 and VCO_2 measured at the mouth. J Appl Physiol 1979;46:1122–1126.

7. Selzer A, Sudrann RB. Reliability of the determination of cardiac output in man by means of the Fick principle. Circ Res 1958;6:485–490.

8. Mook GA, Buursma A, Gerding A, Kwant G, Zijlstra WG. Spectrophotometric determination of oxygen saturation of blood independent of the presence of indocyanine green. Cardiovasc Res 1979;13:233–237.

9. Wood EH, Bowers D, Shepherd JT, Fox IJ. O_2 content of mixed venous blood in man during various phases of the respiratory and cardiac cycles in relation to possible errors in measurement of cardiac output by conventional application of the Fick method. J Appl Physiol 1955;7:621–628.

10. Meier P, Zierler KL. On the theory of the indicator dilution method for measurement of blood flow and volume. J Appl Physiol 1954;6:731–744.

11. Hamilton AR, Hamilton WF, Dow P. Limitations of the continuous method for measuring cardiac output by dye dilution. Am J Physiol 1953;175:173–177.

12. van den Berg E Jr, Pacifico A, Lange RA, Wheelan KR, Winniford MD, Hillis LD. Measurement of cardiac output without right heart catheterization: reliability, advantages, and limitations of a left-sided indicator dilution technique. Cathet Cardiovasc Diagn 1986;12:205–208.

13. Hamilton WF, Moore JW, Kinsman JM, et al. Studies on the circulation: further analysis of the injection method and of changes in hemodynamics under physiological and pathological conditions. Am J Physiol 1931;99:534–551.

14. Glassman E, Blesser W, Mitzner W. Correction of distortion in dye dilution curves due to sampling systems. Cardiovasc Res 1969;3:92–99.

15. Hillis LD, Firth BG, Winniford, MD. Analysis of factors affecting the variability of Fick versus indicator dilution measurements of cardiac output. Am J Cardiol 1985;56:764–768.

16. Reddy PS, Curtiss EI, Bell B, et al. Determinants of variation between Fick and indicator dilution estimates of cardiac output during diagnostic catheterization. Fick vs. dye cardiac outputs. J Lab Clin Med 1976;87:568–576.

17. Hillis LD, Firth BG, Winniford, MD. Comparison of thermodilution and indocyanine green dye in low cardiac output or left-sided regurgitation. Am J Cardiol 1986;57:1201–1202.

18. Maramba LC, Javier RP, Hildner FJ, Samet P. A reappraisal of the abnormal indicator dye dilution curves in valvular incompetence and low output states. Recognition of a diagnostic pitfall and a possible preventive measure with specific reference to left to right shunt. Am J Med 1971;50:20–23.

19. Branthwaite MA, Bradley RD. Measurement of cardiac output by thermal dilution in man. J Appl Physiol 1968;24:434–438.

20. Weisel RD, Berger RL, Hechtman HB. Measurement of cardiac output by thermodilution. N Engl J Med 1975;292:682–684.

21. Mackenzie JD, Haites NE, Rawles JM. Method of assessing the reproducibility of blood flow measurement: factors influencing the performance of thermodilution cardiac output computers. Br Heart J 1986;55:14–24.

22. Enghoff E, Michaelsson M, Pavek K, Sjogren S. A comparison between the thermal dilution method and the direct Fick and the dye dilution methods for cardiac output measurements in man. Acta Soc Med Ups 1970;75:157–170.

23. Lipkin DP, Poole–Wilson PA. Measurement of cardiac output during exercise by the thermodilution and direct Fick techniques in patients with chronic congestive heart failure. Am J Cardiol 1985;56:321–324.

24. van Grondelle A, Ditchey RV, Groves BM, Wagner WW Jr, Reeves JT. Thermodilution method overestimates low cardiac output in humans. Am J Physiol 1983;245:H690–H692.

25. Barcelona M, Patague L, Bunoy M, Gloriani M, Justice B, Robinson L. Cardiac output determination by the thermodilution method: compar-

ison of ice-temperature injectate versus room-temperature injectate contained in prefilled syringes or a closed injectate delivery system. Heart Lung 1985;14:232–235.

26. Okamoto K, Komastsu T, Kumar V, et al. Effects of intermittent positive-pressure ventilation on cardiac output measurements by thermodilution. Crit Care Med 1986;14:977–980.

27. Stevens JH, Raffin TA, Mihm FG, Rosenthal MH, Stetz CW. Thermodilution cardiac output measurement. Effects of the respiratory cycle on its reproducibility. JAMA 1985;253:2240–2242.

28. Daily EK, Mersch J. Thermodilution cardiac outputs using room and ice temperature injectate: comparison with the Fick method. Heart Lung 1987;16:294–300.

29. Elkayam U, Berkley R, Azen S, Weber L, Geva B, Henry WL. Cardiac output by thermodilution technique. Effect of injectate's volume and temperature on accuracy and reproducibility in the critically ill patient. Chest 1983;84:418–422.

30. Wessel HU, Paul MH, James GW, et al. Limitations of thermal dilution curves for cardiac output determinations. J Appl Physiol 1971;30:643–652.

31. Alpert BS, Eubig C. Thermodilution Qp/Qs: an indicator dilution method. Pediatr Cardiol 1983;4:13–17.

32. Morady F, Brundage BH, Gelberg HJ. Rapid method for determination of shunt ratio using a thermodilution technique. Am Heart J 1983;106:369–373.

33. Benchimol A, Desser KB, Gartlan JL Jr. Bidirectional blood flow velocity in the cardiac chambers and great vessels studied with the Doppler ultrasonic flowmeter. Am J Med 1972;52:467–473.

34. Gabe IT, Gault JH, Ross J Jr, et al. Measurement of instantaneous blood flow velocity and pressure in conscious man with a catheter tip velocity probe. Circulation 1969;40:603–614.

35. Jewitt D, Gabe I, Mills C, Maurer B, Thomas M, Shillingford J. Aortic velocity and acceleration measurements in the assessment of coronary heart disease. Eur J Cardiol 1974;1:299–305.

36. Uther JB, Peterson KL, Shabetai R, Braunwald E. Measurement of force-velocity-length relationships in man using an electromagnetic flowmeter catheter. Adv Cardiol 1974;12:198–209.

37. Pepine CJ, Nichols WW, Curry RC, Conti CR. Aortic input impedance during nitroprusside infusion. J Clin Invest 1979;64:643–654.

38. Nichols WW, Conti CR, Walker WE, Milnor WR. Input impedance of the systemic circulation in man. Circ Res 1977;40:451–458.

39. Nichols WW, Pepine CJ, Conti CR, Christie LG, Feldman RL. Quantitation of aortic insufficiency using a catheter-tip velocity transducer. Circulation 1981;61:375–380.

40. McKay RG, Spears JR, Aroesty JM, et al. Instantaneous measurement of left and right ventricular stroke volume and pressure-volume relationships with an impedance catheter. Circulation 1984;69:703–710.

41. Hoffman JIE. Maximal coronary flow and the concept of coronary vascular reserve. Circulation 1984;70:153–159.

42. Klocke FJ. Measurements of coronary flow reserve: defining pathophysiology versus making decisions about patient care. Circulation 1987;76:1183–1189.

43. Cannon PJ, Weiss MB, Sciacca RR. Myocardial blood flow in coronary artery disease: studies at rest and during stress with inert gas washout techniques. Prog Cardiovasc Dis 1977;20:95–120.

44. Eckenhoff JE, Hafkenschiel JH, Harmel MH, et al. Measurement of coronary blood flow by the nitrous oxide method. Am J Physiol 1948;152:356–364.

45. Kety SS. The theory and applications of the exchange of inert gas at the lungs and tissues. Pharmacol Rev 1951;3:1–41.

46. Klocke FJ. Coronary blood flow in man. Prog Cardiovasc Dis 1976;19:117–166.

47. Cannon PJ, Dell RB, Dwyer EM Jr. Measurement of regional myocardial perfusion in man with [133]Xenon and a scintillation camera. J Clin Invest 1972;51:964–977.

48. Cannon PJ, Sciacca RR, Fowler DL, et al. Measurement of regional myocardial blood flow in man: description and critique of the method using xenon-133 and a scintillation camera. Am J Cardiol 1975;36:783–792.

49. Ross RS, Ueda K, Lichtlen PR, Rees JR. Measurement of myocardial blood flow in animals and man by selective injection of radioactive inert gas into the coronary arteries. Circ Res 1964;15:28–41.

50. Lichtlen PR, Engel HJ, Hundeshagen H. Clinical application and results of the assessment of coronary blood flow by the regional precordial xenon residue detection technique. Nucl Med 1978;17:161–171.

51. Hood WB Jr. Regional venous drainage of the human heart. Br Heart J 1968;30:105–109.

52. Gregg DE, Shipley RE. Studies of the venous drainage of the heart. Am J Physiol 1947;151:13–25.

53. Grines CL, Mancini J, McGillem MJ, Gallagher KP, Vogel RA. Measurement of regional myocardial perfusion and mass by subselective hydrogen infusion and washout techniques: a validation study. Circulation 1987;76:1373–1379.

54. Klocke FJ, Koberstein RC, Pittman DE, Bunnell IL, Greene DG, Rosing DR. Effects of heterogeneous myocardial perfusion on coronary venous H2 desaturation curves and calculations of coronary flow. J Clin Invest 1968;47:2711–2724.

55. Schanzenbacher P, Klocke FJ. Inert gas measurements of myocardial perfusion in the presence of heterogeneous flow documented by microspheres. Circulation 1980;61:590–595.

56. Klocke FJ, Bunnell IL, Greene DG, Wittenberg SM, Visco JP. Average coronary blood flow per unit weight of left ventricle in patients with and without coronary artery disease. Circulation 1974;50:547–559.

57. Ganz W, Tamura K, Marcus HS, Donoso R, Yoshida S, Swan HJ. Measurement of coronary sinus blood flow by continuous thermodilution in man. Circulation 1971;44:181–195.

58. Baim DS, Rothman MT, Harrison DC. Simultaneous measurement of coronary venous blood flow and oxygen saturation during transient

alterations in myocardial oxygen supply and demand. Am J Cardiol 1982;49:743–752.

59. Pepine CJ, Mehta J, Webster WW Jr, Nichols WW. In vivo validation of a thermodilution method to determine regional left ventricular blood flow in patients with coronary disease. Circulation 1978;58:795–802.

60. Weisse AB, Regan TJ. A comparison of thermodilution coronary sinus blood flows and krypton myocardial blood flows in the intact dog. Cardiovasc Res 1974;8:526–533.

61. Kurita A, Azorin J, Granier A, Bourassa MG. Estimation of coronary reserve in left anterior descending and circumflex coronary arteries by regional thermodilution technique. Jpn Circ J 1982;46:964–973.

62. Roberts DL, Nakazawa HK, Klocke FJ. Origin of great cardiac vein and coronary sinus drainage within the left ventricle. Am J Physiol 1976;230:486–492.

63. Nakazawa HK, Roberts DL, Klocke FJ. Quantitation of anterior descending vs. circumflex venous drainage in the canine great cardiac vein and coronary sinus. Am J Physiol 1978;234:H163–H166.

64. Brown BG, Josephson MA, Peterson RB, et al. Intravenous dipyridamole combined with isometric handgrip for near maximal acute increase in coronary flow in patients with coronary artery disease. Am J Cardiol 1981;48:1077–1085.

65. Cannon RO, Schenke WH, Leon MB, Rosing DR, Urqhart J, Epstein SE. Limited coronary flow reserve after dipyridamole in patients with ergonovine–induced coronary vasoconstriction. Circulation 1987;75:163–174.

66. Picano E, Simonetti I, Masini M, et al. Transient myocardial dysfunction during pharmacologic vasodilation as an index of reduced coronary reserve: a coronary hemodynamic and echocardiographic study. J Am Coll Cardiol 1986;8:84–90.

67. Zijlstra F, Serruys PW, Hugenholtz PG. Papaverine: the ideal coronary vasodilator for investigating coronary flow reserve? A study of timing, magnitude, reproducibility, and safety of the coronary hyperemic response after intracoronary papaverine. Cathet Cardiovasc Diagn 1986;12:298–303.

68. Bagger JP. Coronary sinus blood flow determination by the thermodilution technique: influence of catheter position and respiration. Cardiovasc Res 1985;19:27–31.

69. Magorien RD, Frederick J, Leier CV, Unverferth DV. Influence of exercise on coronary sinus blood flow determinations. Am J Cardiol 1987;59:659–661.

70. Mathey DG, Chatterjee K, Tyberg JV, Lekven J, Brudage B, Parmley WW. Coronary sinus reflux. A source of error in the measurement of thermodilution coronary sinus flow. Circulation 1978;57:778–786.

71. Cannon RO, Cunnion RE, Parrillo JE, et al. Dynamic limitation of coronary vasodilator reserve in patients with dilated cardiomyopathy and chest pain. J Am Coll Cardiol 1987;10:1190–1200.

72. Mudge GH Jr, Grossman W, Mills RM Jr, Lesch M, Braunwald E. Reflex increase in coronary vascular resistance in patients with ischemic heart disease. N Engl J Med 1976;295:1333–1337.

73. Pichard AD, Smith H, Holt J, Meller J, Gorlin R. Coronary vascular reserve in left ventricular hypertrophy secondary to chronic aortic regurgitation. Am J Cardiol 1983;51:315–320.

74. Winniford MD, Wheelan K, Kremers MS, et al. Smoking–induced coronary vasoconstriction in patients with atherosclerotic coronary artery disease: Evidence for adrenergically mediated alterations in coronary artery tone. Circulation 1986;73:662–667.

75. Mehta J, Pepine CJ. Effect of sublingual nitroglycerin on regional flow in patients with and without coronary disease. Circulation 1978;58:803–807.

76. Nicklas JM, Diltz EA, O'Neill WW, Bourdillon PDV, Walton JA Jr, Pitt B. Quantitative measurement of coronary flow during medical revascularization (thrombolysis or angioplasty) in patients with acute infarction. J Am Coll Cardiol 1987;10:284–289.

77. Serruys PW, Wijns W, van den Brand M, et al. Left ventricular performance, regional blood flow, wall motion, and lactate metabolism during transluminal angioplasty. Circulation 1984;70:25–63.

78. Marcus ML, Wright C, Doty D, et al. Measurement of coronary velocity and reactive hyperemia in the coronary circulation of humans. Circ Res 1981;49:877–891.

79. Cole JS, Hartley CJ. The pulsed Doppler coronary artery catheter: preliminary report of a new technique for measuring rapid changes in coronary artery flow velocity in man. Circulation 977;56:18–25.

80. Wilson RF, Laughlin DE, Ackell PH, et al. Transluminal, subselective measurement of coronary artery blood flow velocity and vasodilator reserve in man. Circulation 1985;72:82–92.

81. Sibley DH, Millar HD, Hartley CJ, Whitlow PL. Subselective measurement of coronary blood flow velocity using a steerable Doppler catheter. J Am Coll Cardiol 1986;8:1332–1340.

82. Wilson RJ, White CW. Intracoronary papaverine: an ideal coronary vasodilator for studies of the coronary circulation in conscious humans. Circulation 1986;73:444–451.

83. Rossen JD, Simonetti I, Winniford MD. Coronary dilation with dipyridamole and dipyridamole combined with handgrip (abstr). Circulation 1987;76:IV–65.

84. Nabel EG, Ganz P, Gordon JB, Alexander RW, Selwyn AP. Dilation of normal and constriction of atherosclerotic coronary arteries by the cold pressor test. Circulation 1988;77:43–52.

85. Wilson RF, Marcus ML, White CW. Prediction of the physiologic significance of coronary arterial lesions by quantitative lesion geometry in patients with limited coronary artery disease. Circulation 1987;75:723–732.

86. Wilson RF, White CW. Does coronary artery bypass surgery restore normal maximal coronary flow reserve? The effect of diffuse atherosclerosis and focal obstructive lesions. Circulation 1987;76:563–571.

87. Rutishauser W, Bussmann W, Noseda G, Meier W, Wellauer J. Blood flow measurement through

single coronary arteries by roentgen densitometry. Part I: A comparison of flow measured by a radiologic technique applicable in the intact organism and by electromagnetic flowmeter. AJR 1970;109:12–20.

88. Rutishauser W, Noseda G, Bussmann W, Preter B. Blood flow measurement through single coronary arteries by roentgen densitometry. Part II: Right coronary artery flow in conscious man. AJR 1970;109:21–24.

89. Smith HC, Frye RL, Donald DE, Davis GD, et al. Roentgen videodensitometric measurement of coronary blood flow. Determination from simultaneous indicator-dilution curves at selected sites in the coronary circulation and in coronary artery saphenous vein grafts. Mayo Clin Proc 1971;46:800–806.

90. Spiller P, Schmiel FK, Politz B, et al. Measurement of systolic and diastolic flow rates in the coronary artery system by x–ray densitometry. Circulation 1983;68:337–347.

91. Foerster J, Link DP, Lantz BMT, Lee G, Holcroft JW, Mason DT. Measurement of coronary reactive hyperemia during clinical angiography by video dilution technique. Acta Radiol 1981;22:209–216.

92. Mancini GBJ, Higgins CB: Digital subtraction angiography: a review of cardiac applications. Prog Cardiovasc Dis 1985;28:111–141.

93. Vogel RA. The radiographic assessment of coronary blood flow parameters. Circulation 1985;72:460–465.

94. Vogel R, LeFree M, Bates E, et al. Application of digital techniques to selective coronary arteriography: use of myocardial contrast appearance time to measure coronary flow reserve. Am Heart J 1984;107:153–164.

95. Ikeda H, Koga Y, Utsu F, Toshima H. Quantitative evaluation of regional myocardial blood flow by videodensitometric analysis of digital subtraction coronary arteriography in humans. J Am Coll Cardiol 1986;8:809–816.

96. Whiting JS, Drury JK, Pfaff JM, et al. Digital angiographic measurement of radiographic contrast material kinetics for estimation of myocardial perfusion. Circulation 1986;73:789–798.

97. Bates BR, Aueron FM, Legrand V, et al. Comparative long-term effects of coronary artery bypass graft surgery and percutaneous transluminal coronary angioplasty on regional coronary flow reserve. Circulation 1985;72:833–839.

98. Hodgson JM, LeGrand V, Bates ER, et al. Validation in dogs of a rapid digital angiographic technique to measure relative coronary blood flow during routine cardiac catheterization. Am J Cardiol 1985;55:188–193.

99. Nissen SE, Elion JL, Booth DC, Evans J, DeMaria AN. Value and limitations of computer analysis of digital subtraction angiography in the assessment of coronary flow reserve. Circulation 1986;73:562–571.

100. Cohen MD, Fields WR, Hodgson JM. Correlation of digital angiographic with Doppler estimation of coronary flow reserve (abstr). J Am Coll Cardiol 1987;9:A161.

101. Cusma JT, Toggart EJ, Folts JD, et al. Digital subtraction angiographic imaging of coronary flow reserve. Circulation 1987;75:461–472.

102. Hodgson JM, Riley RS, Most AS, Williams DO. Assessment of coronary flow reserve using digital angiography before and after successful percutaneous transluminal coronary angioplasty. Am J Cardiol 1987;60:61–65.

113. Zijlstra F, van Ommeren J, Reiber JH, Serruys PW. Does the quantitative assessment of coronary artery dimensions predict the physiologic significance of a coronary stenosis? Circulation 1987;75:1154–1161.

104. Bergmann SR, Fox KAA, Geltman EM, Sobel BE. Positron emission tomography of the heart. Prog Cardiovasc Dis 1985;28:165–194.

105. Goldstein RA, Mullani NA, Marani SK, Fisher DJ, Gould KL, O'Brien HA Jr. Myocardial perfusion with rubidium-82. II. Effects of metabolic and pharmacologic interventions. J Nucl Med 1983;24:907–915.

106. Mullani NA, Goldstein RA, Gould KL. Myocardial perfusion with rubidium-82. I. Measurement of extraction fraction and flow with external detectors. J Nucl Med 1983;24:898–906.

107. Wisenberg G, Schelbert HR, Hoffman EJ, et al. In vivo quantitation of regional myocardial blood flow by positron-emission computed tomography. Circulation 1981;63:1248–1258.

108. Goldstein RA, Kirkeeide RL, Demer LL, et al. Relation between geometric dimensions of coronary artery stenoses and myocardial perfusion reserve in man. J Clin Invest 1987;79:1473–1478.

109. Gould KL, Goldstein RA, Mullani NA, et al. Noninvasive assessment of coronary stenoses by myocardial perfusion imaging during pharmacologic coronary vasodilation. VIII. Clinical feasibility of positron cardiac imaging without a cyclotron using generator-produced rubidium-82. J Am Coll Cardiol 1986;7:775–789.

110. Rumberger JA, Feiring AJ, Lipton MJ, Higgins CB, Ell SR, Marcus ML. Use of ultrafast computed tomography to quantitate regional myocardial perfusion: a preliminary report. J Am Coll Cardiol 1987;9:59–69.

111. Peshock RM, Malloy CR, Buja LM, Nunnally RL, Parkey RW, Willerson JT. Magnetic resonance imaging of acute myocardial infarction: gadolinium diethylenetriamine pentaacetic acid as a marker of reperfusion. Circulation 1986;74:1434–1440.

20

Shunt Detection and Quantification

Ira H. Gessner, M.D.
Benjamin E. Victorica, M.D.

INTRODUCTION

Intracardiac and central vascular shunts can be detected and quantified during cardiac catheterization by several techniques. For example, a left-to-right shunt can be identified and quantified by assessing the increase that occurs in oxygen content of blood as systemic venous blood from the body is mixed with pulmonary venous blood that traverses the defect. Similarly, an agent such as indocyanine green (Cardiogreen) can be introduced into the circulation in such a manner as to allow identification and measurement of a shunt by means of the indicator-dilution technique. Actually, oxygen is also an indicator, albeit a natural one. In fact, all forms of shunt detection and measurement, i.e., oximetry, dye curves, radioisotopes, and angiography, can be considered variations of indicator-dilution methodology.

Seldom does the operator begin cardiac catheterization without nearly complete knowledge regarding the presence of central shunting. Clinical evaluation, including non-invasive assessment, is relatively precise. Cardiac catheterization, therefore, is primarily concerned with accuracy of shunt measurement so that the patient's hemodynamic status and the contribution of any associated lesions can be determined.

This chapter will focus on common techniques of evaluation by cardiac catheterization of a patient with a central shunt. Oximetry and dye curves will be emphasized since these techniques are readily available in most, if not all, catheterization laboratories.

OXIMETRY

Use of oxygen sampling for shunt evaluation requires accurate and reproducible methods for measuring blood oxygen. It is possible to measure **oxygen content** directly (ml O_2/volume of blood), **oxygen saturation** (% of hemoglobin to which O_2 is bound), and **oxygen tension** (partial pressure of O_2 in blood expressed in mm Hg). Each of these values is useful, and sometimes crucial, to proper patient evaluation.

The earliest method used during cardiac catheterization was measurement of oxygen content, that is the total amount of oxygen in blood, including that dissolved in plasma and that bound to hemoglobin. The manometric technique of Van Slyke and Neill (1) requires substantial volumes of blood and is time-consuming. It is seldom used now. Modern, semi-automated equipment currently used in cardiac catheterization laboratories utilizes a spectrophotometric method to measure oxygen saturation directly. This method can be used in whole blood by reflectance spectrophotometry, which is independent of the number of red blood cells. At a wave length of 600 mμm, light transmission is a function of oxyhemoglobin concentration, and at a wave length of 506.5 mμm, it is a function of reduced hemoglobin concentration. The spectrophotometer calculates the two concentrations from Beer's law and thereby obtains percent saturation as follows:

$$\% \text{ oxygen saturation} = \frac{\text{oxyhemoglobin}}{\text{oxyhemoglobin} + \text{reduced hemoglobin}} \times 100.$$

It is important to keep in mind that oxygen saturation does not give information about oxygen content. It is necessary to know oxygen capacity in order to determine the absolute amount of oxygen contained in a sample of blood. Capacity can be estimated by measuring hemoglobin and multiplying by 1.39 (2), as each gram of hemoglobin can hold 1.39 ml O_2. It is useful to consider, in the example that follows, that an individual with an elevated hemoglobin due to cyanotic heart disease does not necessarily have a low oxygen content. A normal person with a hemoglobin concentration of 15 gm/100 ml of blood has a capacity of $15 \times 1.39 \times 10 = 208$ ml O_2/liter blood. If saturation is 97%, content is $0.97 \times 208 = 202$ ml O_2/liter. A cyanotic individual with a hemoglobin of 18 gm/100 ml has a capacity of 250 ml O_2/liter. If saturation is 81%, content is again 202 ml O_2/liter. Oxygen content may also be measured directly using fuel cell type devices (LexO$_2$ Con).

Oxygen content does not control oxygen delivery to the tissues, however, as this is a function of the relationship between oxygen saturation and oxygen tension, that is, the oxygen-hemoglobin dissociation curve and blood flow. It is also important to appreciate that oxygen content calculated in this manner does not take into account dissolved oxygen, which is a function of oxygen tension or partial pressure. Oxygen is dissolved in plasma at a rate of 0.3 ml O_2/100 ml blood/100 mm Hg O_2 tension. Breathing room air, a normal individual has an arterial pO_2 of 100 mm Hg and, therefore, a normal individual in the example just mentioned would add 3 ml O_2/liter to the 202 ml O_2/liter attached to hemoglobin, obviously an insignificant amount of oxygen at 1.5% (i.e., $3/(3 + 202)$). If the individual were breathing 100% oxygen, and arterial pO_2 increased to 600 mm Hg, 18 ml/liter would be added, or 8.2% (i.e., $18/(18 + 202)$) of oxygen content. If the individual were anemic, however, with a hemoglobin of 8 gm/100 ml, note the effect of dissolved oxygen. Oxygen capacity for this person is $8 \times 1.39 \times 10 = 111$ ml/liter. Breathing 100% oxygen with an arterial pO_2 of 600 mm Hg, 18 ml O_2/liter is dissolved, or 14% (i.e., $18/(18 + 111)$) of the total oxygen content. Dissolved oxygen must be taken into account when shunts are calculated during oxygen inhalation, as will be discussed later in this chapter.

Oxygen tension can be measured directly by a blood gas apparatus. Availability of this equipment is considered essential to a cardiac catheterization laboratory. This measurement is accomplished by placing blood in contact with a polarographic pO_2 electrode. Usually this equipment also is capable of measuring directly blood pH and pCO_2. If one has these data, and also can measure hemoglobin, oxygen saturation and, therefore, oxygen content can be calculated. Modern blood gas equipment will make all of these measurements and calculations rapidly and accurately on samples of blood as small as 0.5 ml.

NORMAL BLOOD OXYGEN LEVELS

In order to quantify central shunts it is necessary to determine **mixed venous oxygen saturation,** or the average of all systemic venous return. In the absence of a shunt, pulmonary artery oxygen saturation is mixed venous oxygen saturation. In the presence of a left-to-right shunt, however, problems arise. Three streams of blood enter the right atrium. The superior vena cava oxygen saturation is approximately 70% in the normal resting individual, inferior vena cava saturation generally is 5 to 7% higher (because of highly saturated renal vein blood entering the inferior vena cava); and coronary sinus saturation is approximately 45%. It is not possible, therefore, to obtain a reliably mixed sample in the right atrium, although some authors (3) have suggested that a sample from the lateral wall of the right atrium reasonably approximates mixed venous saturation. If the left-to-right shunt is at the great vessel level (a patent ductus arteriosus (PDA), for example), the right ventricle is adequate for mixed venous saturation. In other types of left-to-right shunts, fully mixed venous blood cannot be obtained. It is fortunate, however, that superior vena cava saturation closely approximates mixed venous saturation. Large series of catheterization data in patients without cardiac shunting have shown that superior vena cava and pulmonary artery saturations are nearly identical (3, 4). Our own data are similar. Our usual practice, therefore, is to use superior vena cava saturation for mixed venous saturation. One must be careful, however, to be sure that there are no abnormalities, such as partial anomalous pulmonary venous return, that could affect superior vena cava saturation.

TECHNIQUES OF BLOOD SAMPLING

Great care must be taken when blood is sampled for oxygen determination, or serious errors are likely to occur. Samples must be obtained from a catheter that provides relatively rapid withdrawal. If it is difficult to withdraw blood, miniature air bubbles are more likely to be obtained, and sampling will take too long when multiple sites need to be assessed. One must use caution when an angiographic catheter with a large number of holes, arranged over a long distance (e.g., pigtail), is used for blood sampling. It is not possible to localize the sampling site with these catheters. Only minimal volumes of heparin should be used, and any saline or blood from a previous sample must be completely washed out before the actual sample is obtained. Hubs of needles and stopcocks have a tendency to retain blood or saline from previous sampling or flushing. Some laboratories measure hematocrits on each sample, and only use samples without hematocrit differences. Sampling problems are most likely to go unrecognized during rapid sequential sampling.

It is also important that all sampling of blood for oxygen saturation determinations for calculation of shunts be accomplished under unchanging patient conditions. A minimal amount of time should elapse between obtaining all the samples necessary for these calculations, and the operator should be sure that the patient's status in terms of activity, respiration, rhythm, etc., has not changed. Ideally, multiple catheters can be used to obtain these measurements simultaneously. In clinical practice, however, this is seldom done.

SHUNT DETECTION BY OXIMETRY

Left-to-Right Shunt Detection

Modern equipment should allow oxygen saturation measurement with an accuracy of ±2%. An increase of 3% in oxygen saturation between the superior vena cava and a downstream right heart chamber should raise suspicion of abnormality, and an increase of 5% should be considered indicative of a left-to-right shunt.

If samples are obtained simultaneously from the superior vena cava and pulmonary artery, a difference of 3% can be considered significant. Note that as mixed venous saturation becomes higher, a shunt must be larger in order to be detected by oxygen saturation. This is demonstrated in the following example. If a volume of pulmonary venous blood at a saturation of 100% mixes with an equal quantity of mixed venous blood at a saturation of 60%, the final saturation will be 80%, an increase of 20% above mixed venous saturation. If mixed venous saturation is 80%, however, the final saturation will be 90%, or only 10% above mixed venous saturation. The relative flows in each of these situations are the same, that is, pulmonary flow is twice systemic flow. It should be apparent that small shunts may be masked totally by this phenomenon. Similarly, multiple levels of left-to-right shunting increase the difficulty of detecting the downstream shunt. Another example demonstrates this.

In the example just cited, assume that the first shunt is atrial. Let us assume that systemic blood flow is 5 liters/min. In the example, 5 liters/min would be shunted left to right at the atrial septal defect to mix with 5 liters/min of systemic venous return. Now let us assume that there is also a patent ductus arteriosus, again with a left-to-right shunt flow of 5 liters/min (actually, a rather large shunt for a patent ductus arteriosus). Mixing one part (5 liters/min) of PDA flow at 100% saturation with two parts (10 liters/min) of right ventricular flow at 90% saturation would produce three parts (15 liters/min) of pulmonary artery flow at a saturation of 93.3% (assuming complete mixing). This increase in saturation of 3.3% is of borderline significance. Figure 20.1 illustrates this example. Reliability of oxygen saturation differences at lower limits of significance can be enhanced by multiple sets of samples, with each set obtained as close together in time as possible.

Right-to-Left Shunt Detection

An intracardiac or great vessel right-to-left shunt will decrease oxygen saturation in left heart chambers and vessels downstream from

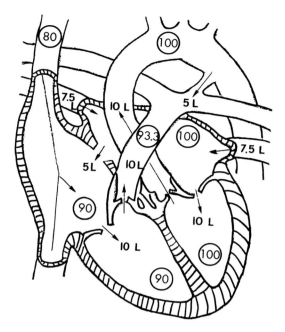

Figure 20.1. Oxygen saturations (*circled*) and flows in the presence of an atrial septal defect and a patent ductus arteriosus. Shunt flows are equal at 5 liters/min, but the distal shunt (*PDA*) results in a much smaller percentage step-up in oxygenation.

the shunt site. The decrease in saturation will be in proportion to the magnitude of the shunt, analogous with the increase in saturation that occurs in the right heart due to a left-to-right shunt. Ideally, pulmonary venous saturation should be compared with systemic arterial saturation, again with samples obtained as closely in time as possible and with steady patient conditions. If the atrial septum (foramen ovale) can be traversed, as it can be in many individuals with congenital heart disease when the catheterization approach is from the femoral vein, proper sampling for right-to-left shunt detection is relatively easy. An oxygen saturation decrease of 2 to 3% from pulmonary vein to left heart should be considered significant. Oxygen tension measurement, however, is a much more sensitive method of detecting right-to-left shunting. Pulmonary vein oxygen tension normally is 100 to 110 mm Hg in a resting individual at sea level. The oxygen dissociation curve is flat at high pO_2 levels, so that above 70 mm Hg pO_2, saturation remains above 95%. Therefore, small right-to-left

shunts will decrease oxygen tension well before saturation is decreased.

If pulmonary vein or left atrial samples cannot be obtained, detection of a small right-to-left shunt by oximetry may be difficult. In the absence of evidence of pulmonary disease that by itself would lower pulmonary vein oxygen levels, systemic arterial saturation of less than 95% or systemic arterial pO_2 under 90 mm Hg in younger patients should be considered suspicious for right-to-left shunting. Keep in mind, however, that alveolar hypoventilation, as can occur in a well sedated patient, may cause a decrease in pulmonary venous pO_2 to levels as low as 70 to 80 mm Hg. The normal value for pulmonary venous pO_2 decreases with age, so in elderly patients these may represent normal values. The four pulmonary veins also may not be equal in oxygen tension, particularly if there is lung disease, congestive heart failure, etc. Therefore, if a low volume is obtained at one site another should be sampled.

If the operator believes that it is essential to determine whether a small intracardiac right-to-left shunt exists in such a circumstance, the patient should be given 100% oxygen to breath for 5 to 10 min. If the low pO_2 is due to a ventilation perfusion abnormality, it will be overcome by oxygen inhalation, and systemic arterial pO_2 will rise to 400 to 600 mm Hg. If a true cardiac right-to-left shunt exists, however, systemic arterial pO_2 will not rise to normal levels. It should be apparent that oxygen saturation measurements cannot be used to make this distinction because once pO_2 reaches 80 to 90 mm Hg, oxygen saturation approaches 100% and can go no higher.

SHUNT CALCULATION BY OXIMETRY

Introduction

Quantitation of intracardiac shunts is often essential to proper patient management. If a patient has evidence of increased pulmonary vascular resistance, decisions regarding surgical management may depend on accurate assessment of blood flows since resistance cannot be measured directly.

All forms of shunt measurement commonly used in the catheterization laboratory are based on the indicator-dilution technique. This technique is quite simple, as the following example illustrates. Assume a bucket of water and a substance whose concentration can be measured. If a known quantity of indicator is added to the bucket and the solution is thoroughly mixed, measuring the concentration of substance will allow calculation of the volume of water in the bucket. For example, if 1 mg of substance *a* is added to the bucket, and the final concentration is 0.5 mg/liter of substance *a*, then the bucket contains 2 liters. Assume that instead of a bucket, there is a fluid flowing through a pipe. Again, a known volume of indicator is added to the pipe. Thorough mixing of indicator with the flowing solution must take place. An instrument is placed downstream to constantly record concentration of the indicator. Following the time course of substance concentration from appearance to disappearance will allow calculation of volume per unit time or, in hemodynamic terms, cardiac output. Similarly, instead of measuring the addition of a substance to the fluid, one can measure removal of a substance. This is the basis for the Fick method (see Chapter 19).

The method uses oxygen as the indicator, and instead of measuring oxygen added to the circulation, oxygen removed, that is oxygen consumption, is measured (5). If one knows the amount of oxygen in arterial blood, the amount in mixed venous blood, and the rate at which oxygen is removed, cardiac output (CO) is easily calculated as:

$$CO = \frac{O_2 \text{ consumption (ml/min)}}{\text{arterial } O_2 \text{ content (ml/liter)} - \text{mixed venous } O_2 \text{ content (ml/liter)}}.$$

Oxygen consumption can be measured easily and accurately with modern equipment (6). A polarographic oxygen sensor constantly measures the oxygen content of air to which it is exposed. The apparatus is zeroed by drawing room air through it. The patient's expired air is captured by placing a plastic hood loosely over the patient's head. All expired air mixed with room air is drawn through the apparatus at a known, constant speed. The drop in concentration of oxygen is directly proportionate to oxygen consumption. The equipment assumes a respiratory exchange ratio of 1.0 between oxygen and carbon dioxide. If this ratio is not 1, as often happens, a small error occurs. For example, for a respiratory ratio of 0.8, oxygen consumption error

would be 3.2%. In practice, most patients have respiratory ratio values between 0.85 and 1.1, thus the percent error is acceptably small (see Chapter 19).

In patients with no shunts, mixed venous blood is obtained from the pulmonary artery and arterial blood from any systemic artery.

Left-to-Right Shunt Calculation

The presence of a left-to-right shunt adds oxygenated blood from the left heart to systemic venous blood in the right heart. Quantification of shunt volume depends upon ability to obtain a thoroughly mixed sample distal to the shunt. In patients with either an atrial septal defect or a ventricular septal defect, a sample from the pulmonary artery (PA) is usually satisfactory. Sampling from both pulmonary arteries will improve accuracy. Superior vena cava (SVC) saturation can be used for a mixed venous oxygen saturation, as described previously. All samples should be obtained under steady state conditions and again as close in time as possible. Consider the following example (Ao, aorta; PV, pulmonary vein):

Site	Saturation	Content (Capacity = 200 ml/liter)
SVC	70%	140 ml/liter
PA	88%	176 ml/liter
PV	97%	194 ml/liter
Ao	97%	194 ml/liter

If oxygen consumption is measured at 216 ml/min, then:

$$\text{systemic blood flow (SBF)} =$$

$$\frac{O_2 \text{ consumption}}{(\text{Ao } O_2 \text{ content} - \text{SVC } O_2 \text{ content})} =$$

$$\frac{216}{(194 - 140)} = 4.0$$

and

$$\text{pulmonary blood flow (PBF)} =$$

$$\frac{O_2 \text{ consumption}}{(\text{PV } O_2 \text{ content} - \text{PA } O_2 \text{ content})} =$$

$$\frac{216}{(194 - 176)} = 12.0.$$

Shunts are usually expressed either as a pulmonary-to-systemic flow ratio (QP/QS) or as the percentage of pulmonary blood flow contributed by the shunt. In this example,

Table 20.1.
Conversion of Percent Shunt to
Pulmonary/Systemic Flow Ratio

% Shunt	QP/QS
33⅓	1.5
50	2
66⅔	3
75	4
80	5

QP/QS = 3.0. The percentage shunt is calculated by $\frac{PBF - SBF}{PBF} \times 100 = 67\%$. The absolute shunt is QP – QS, or 8.0 liters/min.

If oxygen consumption cannot be measured, shunt percentage still can be calculated directly from oxygen saturation measurements as:

$$\% \text{ left-to-right shunting} = \frac{PA - SVC}{PV - SVC}$$

In the above example:

$$\% \text{ left-to-right shunting} = \frac{88 - 70}{97 - 70}$$
$$= 67\% \text{ of PBF.}$$

Similarly, QP/QS can be calculated as:

$$\frac{Ao - SVC}{PV - PA} = \frac{97 - 90}{97 - 88} = 3.0$$

Keep in mind that calculating a shunt in this manner gives an estimate of only relative flows. Pulmonary blood flow is three times systemic blood flow, but absolute flows are not known. It is useful to convert from percentage shunt to QP/QS. Table 20.1 gives these values.

Right-to-Left Shunt Measurement

It should be apparent that right-to-left shunt measurement is analogous to that for left-to-right shunt. It is necessary to measure oxygen content on the left side proximal to the shunt. For example, if the shunt is at the atrial level, a pulmonary vein sample is required. If entry into the left atrium is not possible, one can assume pulmonary vein saturation to be 97%, provided there is no reason to suspect a pulmonary ventilatory abnormality. Samples may also be drawn from a catheter in the pulmonary wedge position confirmed by pressure and fluoroscopy.

Another example will illustrate this:

Site	Saturation	Content (Capacity = 200 ml/liter)
SVC	70%	140 ml/liter
PA	70%	140 ml/liter
PV	100%	200 ml/liter
Ao	90%	180 ml/liter

If oxygen consumption is 200 ml/min, then:

$$SBF = \frac{200}{180 - 140} = 5.0 \text{ liters/min}$$

$$PBF = \frac{200}{200 - 140} = 3.3 \text{ liters/min}$$

$$QP/QS = 0.67 \text{ and } \% \text{ right-to-left shunt}$$
$$= \frac{100 - 90}{100 - 70}$$
$$= 33\,1/3\%.$$

This means that one-third of systemic blood flow is contributed by the right-to-left shunt.

Effective Pulmonary Blood Flow

One further concept should be kept in mind when considering intracardiac shunts, that is, effective PBF. Effective PBF (which is equal to effective systemic blood flow) is the volume of systemic venous blood returned to the heart that traverses the pulmonary capillary bed and becomes oxygenated. In any situation:

$$\text{Effective PBF} = \frac{O_2 \text{ consumption}}{PV\ O_2 \text{ content} - SVC\ O_2 \text{ content.}}$$

The concept of effective PBF is particularly important when multiple levels of shunts are present, or when bidirectional shunting is encountered, as is always the case when dealing with admixture lesions, such as various types of single ventricle. Calculation of effective pulmonary blood flow is also useful in patients with transposition of the great vessels. In this abnormality, pulmonary blood flow and systemic blood flow are independent of each other and, therefore, unequal. Effective pulmonary blood flow represents the volume of blood exchanged between the two circulations.

Measurement of Flow during Oxygen Inhalation

It is sometimes necessary to provide supplemental oxygen in order to fully evaluate a patient, particularly one with pulmonary venous hypoxemia. This is especially important if the patient has elevated pulmonary vascular resistance while breathing room air. In this circumstance, it is essential to take into account dissolved oxygen, therefore, saturation measurement alone will not suffice. Consider this example:

Assume oxygen consumption = 150 ml/min, capacity = 200 ml/liter, and the patient is breathing room air, then:

Site	Saturation	Content
SVC	65%	130 ml/liter
PA	80%	160 ml/liter
PV	95%	190 ml/liter
PBF = 150/(190 − 160) = 5.0 liters/min		
SBF = 150/(190 − 130) = 2.5 liters/min		

Under conditions of 100% oxygen inhalation, assuming no change in oxygen consumption, and if dissolved oxygen is ignored, then

Site	Saturation	Content
SVC	70%	140 ml/liter
PA	95%	190 ml/liter
PV	100%	200 ml/liter
PBF = 150/(200 − 190) = 15 liters/min		
SBF = 150/(200 − 140) = 2.5 liters/min		

If pO_2 is measured, dissolved oxygen can be calculated at 3 ml O_2/liter/100 mm Hg pO_2. Adding dissolved oxygen to the content derived by saturation results in the following:

Site	Saturation	pO_2	Content
SVC	70%	40	140 + (3 × 0.4) = 141.2
PA	95%	80	190 + (3 × 0.8) = 192.4
PV	100%	550	200 + (5.5 × 3) = 216.5
PBF = 150/(216.5 − 192.4) = 6.2 liters/min			
SBF = 150/(216.5 − 141.2) = 2.0 liters/min			

As can be seen, QP/QS, ignoring dissolved oxygen, is 6, whereas it is 3.1 when dissolved oxygen is properly taken into account. It is obvious that serious errors can occur in calculation of flow if dissolved oxygen is overlooked when the patient is breathing

oxygen. This, in turn, will introduce substantial errors in calculation of pulmonary arteriolar resistance.

Shunt Calculation with Multiple Shunt Levels

In most instances, the presence of multiple levels of shunting is important more from an anatomic than a physiologic standpoint. It is usually sufficient to measure total shunt as long as the operator is aware that more than one shunt is present. In fact, it may be difficult to accurately characterize each shunt level. The following example illustrates this:

Assume O_2 consumption = 150 ml/min and capacity = 200 ml/liter, then:

Site	Saturation	Content
SVC	70%	140 ml/liter
RA	85%	170 ml/liter
RV	90%	180 ml/liter
PA	90%	180 ml/liter
PV	100%	200 ml/liter
SBF = 150/(200 − 140) = 2.5 liters/min		
Atrial Flow = 150/(200 − 170) = 5 liters/min		
PBF = 150/(200 − 180) = 7.5 liters/min.		

The step-up of 15% from SVC to right atrium (RA) reflects an atrial level shunt flow of 2.5 liters/min. The step-up of 5% from right atrium to right ventricle (RV) is caused by a ventricular level shunt also equal to 2.5 liters/min. This example also illustrates that a seemingly small oxygen saturation step-up may be due to a substantial left-to-right shunt.

INDICATOR-DILUTION CURVES

Introduction

Indicator-dilution curves provide a reproducible and accurate means of assessing circulatory pathways and volumetric rates of blood flow. Indocyanine green (Cardiogreen) is the most commonly accepted indicator for use in the cardiac catheterization laboratory, as it has a number of characteristics that make it close to being an ideal indicator. Indocyanine green is easily detectable, nontoxic, stable, rapidly cleared from the circulation, unaffected by oxygen content or concentration in blood, and independent of hemoglobin concentration.

This section will give examples of how indicator dilution curves are used to detect and localize shunts and will review methods of quantification of cardiac output and shunt flow. Detailed discussion of indicator-dilution theory and practice can be found in comprehensive reviews such as the monograph edited by Bloomfield (7).

Cardiac Output

Cardiac output can be measured by injecting dye into the central venous circulation (e.g., pulmonary artery) and sampling in a systemic artery (see also Chapter 19). Calculation accuracy depends upon recording an undistorted curve, therefore, the method is most reliable when no left-to-right shunt is present. A right-to-left shunt generally invalidates this technique unless one can make the injection beyond the shunt. For example, in the case of an atrial septal defect one can inject directly into the left ventricle and sample from the femoral artery to obtain systemic blood flow or cardiac output. Similarly, valvular regurgitation creates distortion that can be overcome only by special methods.

Figure 20.2 illustrates a normal dye curve. The time from injection (*arrow*) to onset of the curve is the appearance time. The observed appearance time can be corrected for catheter length and blood withdrawal speed, although this is not necessary for measurement of cardiac output. Time from onset of the curve to the point of peak concentration (PC) is termed buildup time (BT). Note that because of recirculation, the downslope (disappearance) of the curve does not reach baseline. The rate of disappearance is logarithmic, however, allowing the downslope to be extrapolated to near zero concentration by replotting concentrations on semilogarithmic graph paper.

Cardiac output is calculated by the following formula initially derived by Stewart and Hamilton (8):

$$\frac{CO = I\,(mg) \times (60)}{C\,(mg/liter) \times (unit\ time)} = \text{liters per minute}$$

where I = mg dye injected, C = average concentration during one circulation period, and unit time = duration (in seconds) of one circulation period.

Several techniques can be used to calculate average concentration during one circulation

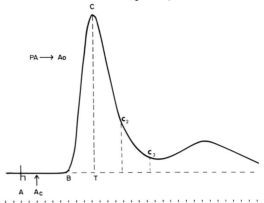

Figure 20.2. Normal dye curve recorded in the aorta (*Ao*) after injection into the pulmonary artery (*PA*). Note that because of recirculation the downslope does not reach the baseline. $A - B$, actual appearance time; $Ac - B$, corrected appearance time; $B - T$, buildup time; C, peak concentration; C_2, concentration at 2 BT; C_3, concentration at 3 BT.

period. The method most commonly used is: Measure concentration at regular time intervals, sum these individual time intervals, and then divide by the number of time intervals. In order to do this it is necessary to construct a calibration curve so that centimeters of deflection of the curve above baseline can be converted to milligrams per liter. A quantity of patient blood is removed before any dye is injected and used as a zero reference. With the use of 5- or 10-ml volumetric flasks, several known concentrations of indocyanine green are made, for example, 2.5, 5, and 10 mg/liter. Together with undyed blood (zero concentration), each sample is drawn through the detecting instrument (densitometer), resulting in a specific deflection for each concentration. The magnitude of these deflections is plotted on graph paper and connected to construct a calibration curve. Most currently used densitometers are designed to be linear, so the calibration curve should be almost a straight line.

Figure 20.3 illustrates transfer of the dye curve in Figure 20.2 to semilogarithmic graph paper with extrapolation of the downslope to eliminate recirculation. As long as the densitometer is linear it is not necessary to convert centimeters of deflection to concentration until the average deflection is calculated. Magnitude of deflection is measured each second

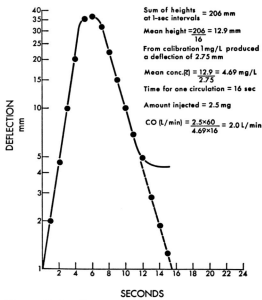

Sum of heights at 1-sec intervals = 206 mm

Mean height = $\frac{206}{16}$ = 12.9 mm

From calibration 1 mg/L produced a deflection of 2.75 mm

Mean conc.(c̄) = $\frac{12.9}{2.75}$ = 4.69 mg/L

Time for one circulation = 16 sec

Amount injected = 2.5 mg

CO (L/min) = $\frac{2.5 \times 60}{4.69 \times 16}$ = 2.0 L/min

Figure 20.3. Stewart-Hamilton method for calculating cardiac output from a standard indicator dilution curve. (From Rudolph AM. Congenital diseases of the heart. Chicago: Year Book Medical Publishers, 1974.)

and plotted. These values are summed, and the calculated downslope points are added. The total is divided by the number of points, and this average measurement is then converted to concentration by use of the calibration curve. Cardiac output can then be calculated by the formula given above. The calculation is multiplied by 60 in order to convert it from seconds to minutes so that the result can be expressed in liters per minute. This method is time-consuming, but it is also accurate.

Simpler methods of analyzing dye curves have been devised. The most widely accepted is the forward triangle method of Benchimol et al. (9), which is based on the previous work of Hetzel et al. (10). These workers observed that the area of the initial portion of a dye curve bears a constant relation to the entire curve. This initial portion can be thought of as a triangle, with the base being the time from onset of the curve to the point of peak deflection, i.e., buildup time (in seconds), and the height being the maximal deflection or peak concentration (in milligrams per liter). This is illustrated in Figure 20.4. A constant, 0.34, derived by Benchimol et al., is applied. The formula for cardiac output is:

$$CO = \frac{I \, (mg) \times 60 \, (sec/min) \times 0.34}{\frac{1}{2} \, BT \times PC}$$

In addition to its simplicity, the forward triangle method has the advantage of being unaffected by distortion of the downslope. It, therefore, may be more accurate than the Stewart-Hamilton method when a left-to-right shunt is present.

Measurement of cardiac output by indicator-dilution curve techniques presents special problems in patients with significant mitral or aortic regurgitation because each of these abnormalities will distort the downslope of a dye curve in direct proportion to the magnitude of the volume of regurgitation. Use of the forward triangle method for calculation of cardiac output may allow accurate determination since this method does not require use of the downslope. In individuals with severe regurgitation, however, even the initial portion of an indicator-dilution curve accomplished by right heart injection and systemic arterial sampling may be distorted. In these special circumstances, we have found that placing two catheters on the right side of the heart permits recording of indicator injection into the superior vena cava and sampling in the pulmonary artery (11). Adequate mixing of indicator is a concern, but our data suggest that this technique is valid, provided there is no right-sided valvular regurgitation and no right-to-left shunt.

SHUNT DETECTION AND QUANTIFICATION BY INDICATOR-DILUTION TECHNIQUES

Left-to-Right Shunts

Left-to-right shunts result in earlier than usual recirculation because flow through the shunt and lungs is more rapid than is recirculation through the body. In steady state conditions, distortion of the downslope is predictable. Carter et al. (12) observed that in normal curves, points on the curve that occur at times equal to two and three times the buildup time show a constant relation to peak concentration. They analyzed curves by injecting indocyanine green into the right heart with radial artery sampling. Their derived equations are as follows:

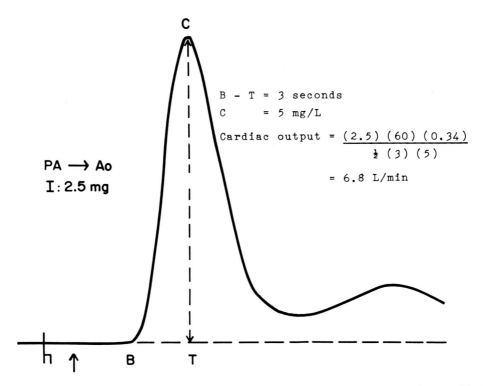

Figure 20.4. Forward triangle method for calculation of cardiac output from an indicator-dilution curve. *B - T,* buildup time in seconds; *C,* peak concentration in milligrams per liter; *I,* amount of dye injected; *arrow,* corrected injection time.

Left-to-right shunt (% of PBF) = 142
$\times \dfrac{\text{concentration at 2 BT}}{\text{peak concentration}} - 42$

Left-to-right shunt (% of PBF) = 135
$\times \dfrac{\text{concentration at 3 BT}}{\text{peak concentration}} - 14.$

If the calibration curve is a straight line, it is not necessary to convert centimeters of deflection to milligrams per liter, as the ratio of concentrations in the formula will be the same.

The two values obtained, which should be close, are averaged. The method assumes an undistorted peak concentration. If shunt recirculation occurs before peak concentration is reached, this method is not valid. The method is also based upon curves whose downslope is relatively smooth. In certain circumstances, shunt recirculation may be so discrete as to create a distinct peak of its own. This is particularly true when injection and sampling sites are close together (e.g., injection into pul-

monary artery, sampling in ascending aorta) or in smaller subjects such as young children in whom circulation times are faster. In these circumstances a curve of the type illustrated in Figure 20.5 might be recorded. The Carter formula has been found to be unreliable in this situation. We have analyzed curves of this type and found that a simple ratio of shunt peak concentration to primary curve peak concentration gives an accurate estimation of percent shunt, as follows (13):

Left-to-right shunt (% PBF) =

$$\dfrac{P_2 \text{ concentration}}{P_1 \text{ concentration}} \times 100.$$

Certain other limitations should be kept in mind. Valvular regurgitation distorts the downslope of an indicator-dilution curve and, therefore, invalidates shunt calculation. Shunt calculation is reasonably accurate with shunts greater than 25% of pulmonary blood flow. Smaller shunts may be apparent by means of inspection of the curve, but accuracy of shunt calculation is questionable.

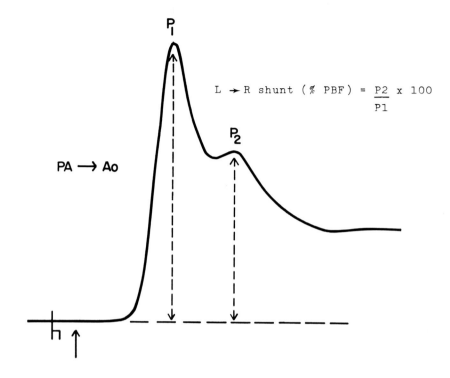

Figure 20.5. Victorica-Gessner formula for calculation of left-to-right shunt in the presence of rapid shunt recirculation. $P1$, concentration of primary peak; $P2$, concentration of shunt peak; *Ao*, aorta; *PA*, pulmonary artery .

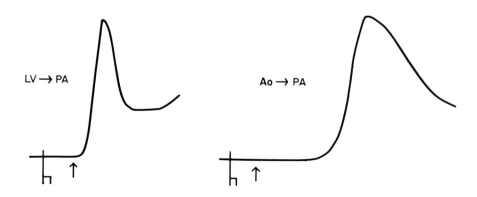

Figure 20.6. Reverse indicator-dilution curves injecting left ventricle (*left*) and aorta (*right*) sampling pulmonary artery. *Arrow* indicates corrected injection time. Early appearance of ventricular septal defect is evident.

Small shunts can be detected and localized by special techniques that do not involve calculation of volume. These methods use the indicator-dilution technique to detect flow pathways. For example, a tiny ventricular septal defect or patent ductus arteriosus can be detected by injecting dye into the left ventricle and sampling in the pulmonary artery, a method sometimes referred to as a reverse curve. As illustrated in Figure 20.6, dye appears rapidly at the sampling site, creating an early peak that is proportionate to shunt size. Shunts of less than 5% of pulmonary blood flow can be detected in this manner. Localization of shunt site can be achieved by varying injection and sampling sites. For example, positive left ventricle to pulmonary artery curve, together with a negative ascending aorta to pulmonary artery curve, establishes that the early peak is due to a ventricular septal defect. (The astute reader can argue that the curve recorded in the pulmonary artery after left ventricular injection in a patient with a small ventricular septal defect can be mimicked by mitral regurgitation, together with an atrial septal defect. If an operator is truly concerned about this possibility, the sampling site can be moved back to the right atrium.)

Small left-to-right shunts can also be detected by the double venous technique. Two venous catheters are placed, one for injection and one for sampling. In the patient with a small ventricular septal defect, dye can be injected into the distal right pulmonary artery and sampled in the left pulmonary artery. Early appearance of dye in the left pulmonary artery, as illustrated in Figure 20.7, may establish the presence of a left-to-right shunt. Localization requires recording curves from other, more proximal sampling sites, until the early appearance of dye is no longer recorded.

Modern noninvasive procedures and angiography have substantially reduced the use of these indicator-dilution techniques. They can be very helpful at times, however. We believe, therefore, that physicians performing cardiac catheterizations, particularly in patients with congenital heart disease, should be familiar with this methodology.

Right-to-Left Shunt

Right-to-left shunts in the central circulation can be detected easily and with great sensitiv-

ity provided the injection times are accurately recorded. Injecting indocyanine green into the right atrium with sampling in a systemic artery of a patient with cyanotic tetralogy of Fallot will result in a curve, such as that illustrated in Figure 20.8. The primary features of this curve caused by the right-to-left shunt are the early appearance of dye and the small initial peak. Detection of a right-to-left shunt requires only that early appearance of dye be identified. Right-to-left shunts of less than 2% of systemic blood flow can be identified in this manner. The shunt can be localized by moving the injection site distally. For example, in a patient with a right-to-left atrial level shunt, early appearance will be recorded in a systemic artery after injection into either the superior vena cava or inferior vena cava. If the injection catheter tip is advanced into the right ventricle, however, no early appearance will occur (unless the patient has tricuspid regurgitation as well).

Several similar methods exist for evaluating the volume of a right-to-left shunt. The method described by Thorburn (14), depicted in Figure 20.8, is based upon the forward triangle principle. It is simple and reasonably accurate. The area of the forward triangle of the shunt curve is compared with the forward triangle area of the primary curve. It is necessary to extrapolate the upslope of the primary curve back to the baseline in order to obtain the base of the primary curve forward triangle. This introduces an error, but it is acceptably small. The formula is as follows:

$$\text{Right-to-left-shunt (\%SBF)} = \frac{1/2 \, (CP_1 \times BT_1)}{\frac{1}{2} \, (CP_1 \times BT_1) + \frac{1}{2} \, (CP_2 \times BT_2)} \times 100.$$

In practice, it is rarely necessary to make clinical decisions based upon the magnitude of a right-to-left shunt, so that detection of a shunt, together with a reasonably accurate estimation of its magnitude, is usually adequate for clinical purposes.

Bidirectional Shunts

The combination of a left-to-right and right-to-left shunt creates significant distortion of indicator-dilution curves invalidating all volumetric estimates. Recording circulation times and circulation pathways, however,

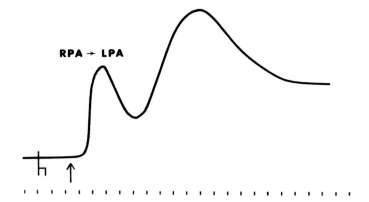

Figure 20.7. Double venous indicator-dilution curve. Injection is into the right pulmonary artery with sampling in the left pulmonary artery. *Arrow* indicates corrected injection time. The small initial peak suggests a left-to-right shunt. Confirmation that the initial peak is early, and due to a left-to-right-shunt as well as localization of shunt site, requires recording curves from other more proximal sites until the early appearance is no longer recorded.

Figure 20.8. Indicator-dilution curve recorded in the aorta (Ao) after injection into the right atrium (RA) in a patient with a small right-to-left shunt. Ac, corrected time of injection; $B_1 - T_1$, buildup time of shunt curve; CP_1, peak concentration of shunt curve; $B_2 - T_2$, buildup time of primary curve; CP_2, peak concentration of primary curve; right to left shunt (%SRF) =

$$\frac{^{1}/_2 [CP_1 \times (B_1 - T_1)]}{^{1}/_2[CP_1 \times (B_1 - T_1)] \times ^{1}/_2 [CP_2 \times (B_2 - T_2)]}.$$

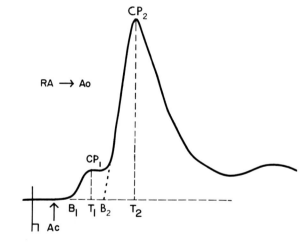

can provide qualitative information that can be useful.

Special Indicator-Dilution Methods

Indicator-dilution techniques can be used in a variety of ways for evaluating the central circulation. Several of these methods, such as reverse curves and double venous curves, have already been discussed in this chapter. Another example may serve to stimulate the reader's interest further. In a patient with an atrial septal defect, it is sometimes valuable to determine whether a pulmonary vein returns

anomalously. This can be done by a combination of curves, as illustrated in Figure 20.9. Curves are recorded from a systemic artery after injection of dye into the superior vena cava and into the pulmonary vein in question. If there is no significant right-to-left shunt as determined by superior vena cava injection (curve A in Fig. 20.9), the curve recorded after injection into the pulmonary vein identifies its drainage. If the pulmonary vein is connected to the left atrium some dye will proceed normally to the systemic artery, producing at least a small rapid appearance, even

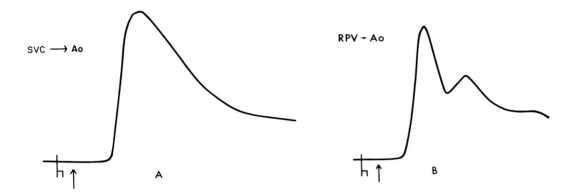

Figure 20.9. Indicator-dilution curves recorded in aorta (*Ao*) after injection into superior vena cava (*SVC*, curve *A*), and right pulmonary vein (*RPV*, curve *B*). Normal appearance time in curve *A* confirms absence of a right-to-left shunt. Rapid appearance of the initial peak in curve *B* establishes that the pulmonary vein injected drains into the left atrium. If it had drained anomalously into the right atrium, appearance time would not have been rapid and would have been equal to that of curve *A*.

though most of the dye crosses the atrial septal defect, resulting in a larger but later peak. This is illustrated by curve *B* in Figure 20.9. If the injected pulmonary vein is connected to the right atrium, the recorded curve will have an appearance time and shape equivalent to that recorded after injection into the superior vena cava, as illustrated in curve *A*.

References

1. Van Slyke DD, Neill JM. Blood gases 1. J Biol Chem 1924;61:523–573.
2. Eilers RJ. Notification of final adoption of an international method and standard solution for hemoglobinometry. Specification for preparation of standard solution. Am J Clin Pathol 1967;47:212–214.
3. Freed MD, Miettinen 0, Nadas AS. Oximetric detection of intra-cardiac left-to-right shunts. Br Heart J 1979;42:690-694.
4. Barratt-Boyes BG, Wood EH. The oxygen saturation of blood in the venae cavae, right-heart chambers, and pulmonary vessels of healthy subjects. J Lab Clin Med 1957;50:93–106.
5. Fick A. Uber die Messung des Blutquantums in den Herzventrikeln. Phys-Med ges Wurzberg, July 9, 1870:16.
6. Lister G, Hoffman JIE, Rudolph AM. Oxygen uptake in infants and children: a simple method for measurement. Pediatrics 1974;53:656–662.
7. DA Bloomfield, ed. Dye curves. In: The theory and practice of indicator dilution. Baltimore; University Park Press, 1974.
8. Hamilton WF, Moore JW, Kinsman JM, Spurling RG. Studies on the circulation. IV. Am J Physiol 1932;99:534–551.
9. Benchimol A, Dimond EG, Carvalho FR, Roberts M. New method: the forward triangle formula for calculations of cardiac output, the indicator-dilution technic. Am J Cardiol 1963;12:119–125.
10. Hetzel PS, Swan HJC, Ramirez-DeArellano A, Wood EH. Estimation of cardiac output from first part of arterial dye dilution curves. J Appl Physiol 1958;13:92–96.
11. Victorica BE. Right heart double venous dye curves for estimation of cardiac output. Personal communication, 1987.
12. Carter SA, Bajec SF, Yannicelli E, Wood EH. Estimation of left to right shunts from arterial dilution curves. J Lab Clin Med 1960;55:77–88.
13. Victorica BE, Gessner IH. A simplified method for quantitating left to right shunts from arterial dilution curves. Circulation 1975;51:530–534.
14. Thorburn GD. Estimates of cardiac output from forward part of indicator dilution curves. J Appl Physiol 1961;16:891–895.

21

Recorders and Other Instrumentation

Wilmer W. Nichols, Ph.D.
Charles R. Lambert, M.D., Ph.D.
Carl J. Pepine, M.D.

INTRODUCTION

Physiological waveforms (or cardiovascular variables) recorded in the cardiac catheterization laboratory are usually time-varying periodic functions, such as the electrocardiogram, blood pressure, and blood flow. Various transducers are used to convert these physiologic events to electrical signals that are amplified, monitored, recorded, processed, and stored (Fig. 21.1). A large amount of information can be obtained from simple inspection of the wave contours (1–3), but more specific quantified data are even more valuable, for example, the reduced rate of rise of aortic and left ventricular pressures in aortic stenosis and myocardial disease, respectively. Recording of cardiovascular variables at the time of cardiac catheterization is therefore only a first step to be followed by quantitative analysis. The goal of the analysis is to put the observations in a numerical form for easy tabulation and understanding.

The objective of physiological recording in the diagnostic catheterization laboratory is to obtain a faithful reproduction of the cardiovascular variable of interest. If this is not totally achieved, a measuring error must exist (4). Measuring errors may arise in any part of the recording system (e.g., the transducer, amplifier, recorder, or any other component). Therefore, when testing for accuracy, the entire system should be evaluated.

Transducers, the instruments used to convert force, motion, or other cardiovascular variables into electrical signals, have already been discussed in Chapters 18 and 19. This chapter, therefore, is concerned with amplifying, recording, displaying, processing, and storing these signals. Any system designed for faithful reproduction of an event or variable must meet the following criteria: (*a*) amplitude linearity, (*b*) adequate frequency response, and (*c*) phase linearity (5).

AMPLITUDE LINEARITY

Amplitude **linearity** refers to the ability of the transducer-processor-reproducer system to produce an output signal that is directly proportional in magnitude to the input signal amplitude. This condition must be satisfied for measurements both above and below the zero baseline and should include the entire range of measurement (Fig. 21.2). Thus, before calibration and linearity testing, the range of the variable to be measured should be known. This can usually be obtained from the literature or a few preliminary measurements. In Figure 21.2, linearity of the electrical output of an electromagnetic flowmeter-catheter tip velocity transducer system was tested in a bidirectional hydraulic pump model (6). The velocity of the fluid detected by the electromagnetic velocity transducer, amplified by the flowmeter, and transmitted to the chart

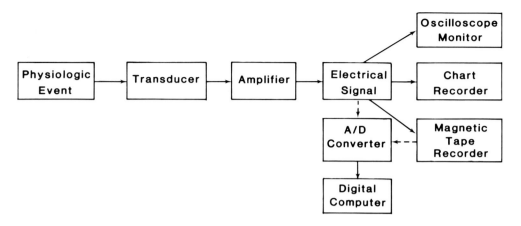

Figure 21.1. Diagrammatic representation of data handling schema for a cardiac catheterization laboratory. The physiologic waveform (or cardiovascular variable) being recorded may be blood pressure, blood flow, electrocardiogram, or other events that vary with time. The event detected by the transducer is amplified and transmitted to an oscilloscope monitor, a strip chart recorder, and a magnetic tape recorder. If desired, the analogue signals may be converted to digital form and analyzed by a digital computer. The digitized signals may be stored on cards, tapes, or disks.

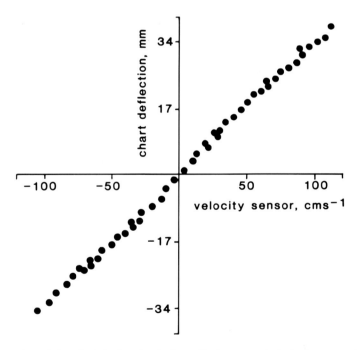

Figure 21.2. Linearity of the electrical output of a catheter-mounted electromagnetic velocity transducer-flowmeter system over the range of velocities recorded in normal humans. Linearity was determined in a bidirectional hydraulic pump model filled with physiologic saline. Reverse flow is indicated by a *minus sign*. The correlation coefficient was 0.996. (From Nichols WW, Paley DM, Thompson LV, Lambert CR. Experimental evaluation of a multisensor velocity-pressure catheter. Med Biol Eng Comput 1985;23:79–83.)

recorder was linear over the range -103 to $+110$ cm/sec, which covers the range of blood flow velocity measurements reported in the literature for normal humans (2, 7–9). Although the input-output characteristics of a system may be represented as a straight line, careful testing with accurate inputs usually reveals a small deviation from linearity (see Fig. 21.2). Under these conditions, regression analysis should be performed to obtain the line of best fit and this relation used in calibration.

Hysteresis

Another quality related to system linearity is **hysteresis** (i.e., lagging behind), which is a measure of the ability of the system to produce an output that follows the input independent of the direction or change in magnitude of the input. When hysteresis is present in a system, an open curve (or Lissajou loop) results from linearity testing (Fig. 21.3). The amount of hysteresis is usually expressed in terms of the percentage of full-scale value. In the exaggerated example shown in Figure 21.3, the hysteresis error is approximately 20%. With most modern recording systems, this error must be less than 1%.

Noise

Another potential problem in recording systems is the addition of unwanted **noise** superimposed on the measured variable. The frequency of this noise is usually much higher than the variable being measured. It is part of the output of an instrument not related to the variable itself. Sometimes, it is generated within the instrument; at other times, it is caused by external interference. In any recording system, it is necessary to distinguish the signal from the unwanted noise. This can be done by measuring the signal-to-noise ratio and calculating the noise figure (10). The amount of noise in the output signal depends on the amount of noise presented to the input and the amount of noise amplified by the amplifier and presented to the output. The signal-to-noise ratio at the input divided by the signal-to-noise ratio at the output is the noise figure and ideally should equal unity.

Since the patient tends to act as an antenna, a spectral analysis of the noise (the amount of noise concentrated at each fre-

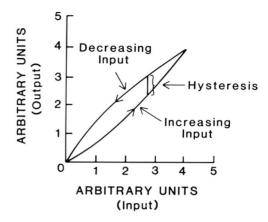

Figure 21.3. Example of a hysteresis (or Lissajou) loop showing deviation from linearity during increases and decreases in system input and the corresponding variation in output.

quency) would show a rather large 60 Hz component. This is because most electrical appliances in the United States use 60-Hz current, and this 60-Hz noise is radiated from a variety of wires and devices.

The best approach to handling unwanted noise is to identify its source and then eliminate it. In most cases this can be accomplished by proper grounding. Every cardiac catheterization laboratory should be provided with a good reference ground. This means that electrostatic shields must be provided with an extremely low resistance path to the earth. In this way, excess electrons can travel to and from the earth, which acts like an infinitely large source of electrons and also an infinitely large sink into which electrons can flow (10). All electronic instruments in the laboratory should be grounded to this reference ground point, care being taken to avoid an excessive number of ground leads. In some cases it may be necessary to ground the patient. However, the patient table and the particular instrument must not be grounded to the reference point and the table then grounded to the instrument. If this is done, a ground loop would be established and the noise would increase considerably. All ground wires should be arranged as symmetrically as possible and should be at least 12-gauge insulated wire.

High-frequency noise can also be eliminated or minimized by introducing a low-frequency bandpass electronic filter into the circuit. However, when adding electronic filters, care must be taken not to filter the cardiovascular variable itself (see below). Another approach to removal of noise from periodic signals is digital signal averaging. This technique is seldom used for routine clinical studies but is useful in the research setting.

Drift

The tendency for recording systems to **drift** or gradually change their output can complicate a catheterization procedure. In most cases, instrumentation drift affects only the baseline calibration. If baseline drift does occur, then the calibration (or linearity) curve (see Fig. 21.2) moves vertically up or down without a change in slope. If the calibration factor (or step) is affected, then the slope of the calibration curve changes. Baseline drift in a fluid-filled pressure recording system can be detected and corrected by frequent checks of the "zero baseline" by opening a stopcock and exposing the pressure transducer to atmospheric pressure. When measuring blood flow velocity in the main pulmonary artery or ascending aorta, one assumes that the flat portion of the velocity curve in late diastole represents zero baseline; electronic zero, especially of electromagnetic flowmeters, cannot always be trusted (4). Changes in the calibration factor can only be detected by recalibration. No matter how carefully a system was calibrated initially, erroneous measurements will be obtained if changes occur in either the zero baseline or the calibration factor. Fortunately, the recording systems used in modern cardiac catheterization laboratories are designed to minimize instrumentation drift and maintain constant calibration, but it is still unwise to assume system stability, and catheterization procedures should allow for periodic checking and readjustment if necessary. Some transducers, especially those used to measure pressure, are particularly sensitive to environmental temperature; therefore, the recording system should be turned on well in advance of any measurement. In a busy laboratory, it may be desirable to leave the recorder on during the week days.

Calibration

Calibration must be carried out over the range of input amplitudes to be measured (see above). Calibration involves determination of the response of the entire system including the recording apparatus and any other devices, such as strip chart recorders, oscilloscope monitors, and magnetic tape recorders. Fluid-filled catheter-manometer systems, those most commonly used in the cardiac catheterization laboratory for measuring pressure, are usually calibrated against a column of mercury. Calibration for every catheterization procedure is essential. Incremental increases in mm Hg (input) are applied to the pressure transducer, and the resulting output signals are measured (Fig. 21.4). A plot of the input-output values results in a linear calibration relationship. Using the relationships of Figures 21.2 and 21.4, one obtains calibrated scales for the chart recording of ascending aortic pressure and blood flow velocity signals (Fig. 21.5). The velocity signal can be calibrated in volumetric flow units by multiplying by the cross-sectional area of the ascending aorta (or main pulmonary artery) or by comparison of the mean velocity to a simultaneous measurement of cardiac output (7).

ADEQUATE FREQUENCY RESPONSE AND PHASE LINEARITY

The dynamic frequency response and phase linearity refer to the ability of the recording system to provide a signal that is identical (except in amplitude) to the event presented to it. The dynamic frequency response of a recording system must be great enough to detect the highest harmonic of the event being recorded. Before the frequency response of such a system can be adequately discussed, it is necessary first to establish the relationship between sine waves and waves of nonsinusoidal form. All periodic waves of nonsinusoidal form are designated complex waves (2, 4, 11). By use of Fourier series analysis, it is possible to show that any periodic complex wave can be dissected into a series of sine and cosine waves, which when added, will produce the original complex wave. Although this type of analysis was little used in cardiovascular physiology until it was introduced by Womersley (12) and McDonald (13), it had been used theoretically by Frank (14) in addition to the emphasis on transient phenomena in the Windkessel analysis. Since Fourier series analysis is unfamiliar to most cardiolo-

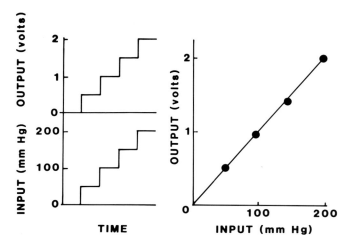

Figure 21.4. Calibration of a fluid-filled catheter-manometer system. Incremental increases in pressure are applied to the manometer, and the resulting output voltage signal recorded (*left*). These input-output values are plotted as a linear relationship (*right*). (From Milnor WR. Hemodynamics. Baltimore: Williams & Wilkins, 1982.)

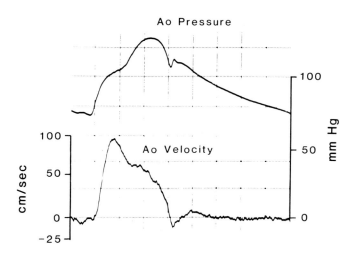

Figure 21.5. Calibrated ascending aortic (*Ao*) pressure and blood flow velocity waves recorded in a normal human subject using a Millar multisensor pressure-velocity catheter.

gists, a general account of the nature and application of the series is given here. We will not attempt to be mathematically rigorous, especially in relation to the type of curves under concern since they cannot be defined as a function of an algebraic variable on which the processes of integration can be performed. Instead, these curves have to be dealt with as a finite sum of measured values.

A periodic function, $F(t)$ is defined as one which repeats itself after a given time period,

T. This may be expressed as $F(t) = F(t + T)$. This is familiar in the definition of a sinusoidal wave, which repeats after 2π radians so that $\sin x = \sin(x + n2\pi)$, as the frequency f is $1/T$, and then the angular frequency, ω, in radians/second, is given by $\omega = 2\pi/T = 2\pi f$. The Fourier theorem may be stated: if $y = F(t)$ is any continuous function of the variable, t, which repeats with a period, T, then $F(t) = A_0 + A_1 \cos \omega t + A_2 \cos 2\omega t + A_3 \cos 3\omega t + \ldots + A_n \cos n\omega t + B_1 \sin \omega t + B_2 \sin 2\omega t +$

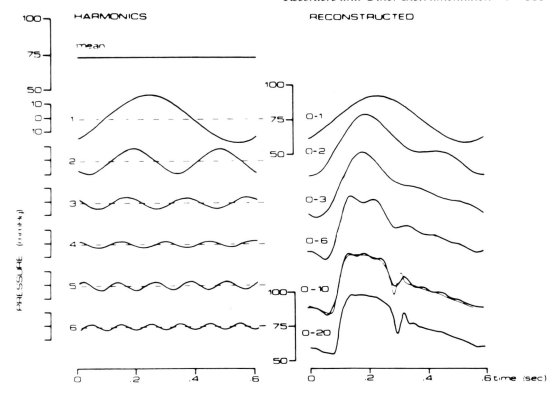

HARMONICS

RECONSTRUCTED

Figure 21.6. Example of Fourier series representation of a periodic wave. *Left,* The mean term and first six harmonics of a pressure wave, recorded in the ascending aorta of a dog. *Right,* Individual harmonics are added to reproduce (or resynthesize) the original (measured) wave. Agreement is relatively close with the first six harmonics (0–6) summed, and better with the first 10 harmonics (0–10), while the resynthesized wave is almost identical to the original wave (*thin line*) with the summation of the first 20 harmonics (0–20). (From Westerhof N, Sipkema P, Elzinga G, Murgo JP, Giolma JP. Arterial impedance. In: Hwang HC, Gross DR, Patel DJ, eds. Quantitative cardiovascular studies. Baltimore: University Park Press, 1979.)

$B_3 \sin 3\omega t + \dots + B_n \sin n\omega t$, where n is an integer. A_0 is the mean value of the function over the period T, or from 0 to 2π. The sinusoidal components are called harmonics with $n = 1$ being the first or fundamental harmonic. The frequency of the fundamental is that of a composite wave.

The Fourier coefficients A and B can be calculated from the following equations:

$$A_n = (1/\pi)\int_0^{2\pi} F(t) \cos n\omega t \,(dt)$$

and

$$B_n = (1/\pi)\int_0^{2\pi} F(t) \sin n\omega t \,(dt).$$

The Fourier coefficients can be converted to modulus (M) and phase (ϕ) by:

$$M_n = \sqrt{(A_n^2 + B_n^2)}$$

and

$$\tan \phi_n = B_n/A_n.$$

This is the mathematical method for determining the Fourier series of a periodic function.

The actual calculation of the Fourier series of a curve (e.g., a cardiovascular variable) is performed by drawing a number, $2r$, of equally spaced ordinates that will each have the value y_r. Then we may write

$$A_0 = \frac{1}{2}r \sum_{(r=1)}^{(2r-1)} y_r$$

and

$$A_n = \frac{1}{r} \sum_{(r=1)}^{(2r-1)} y_r \cos(n\pi/r)$$

$$B_n = \frac{1}{r} \sum_{(r=1)}^{(2r-1)} y_r \sin(n\pi/r)$$

LV PRESSURE $f_0 = 1.3$ Hz

COMPARISON OF TOTAL VARIANCE TO SERIES VARIANCE

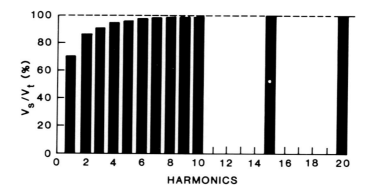

Ao PRESSURE $f_0 = 1.3$ Hz   **Ao VELOCITY** $f_0 = 1.3$ Hz

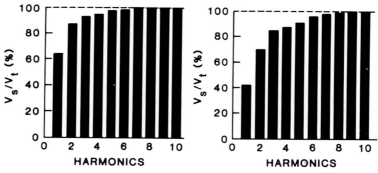

Figure 21.7. Histograms representing the cumulative variance of the Fourier series (V_s) to the total variance (V_t) of left ventricular (*LV*) pressure (*top*) and ascending aortic (*Ao*) pressure (*bottom left*) and blood flow velocity (*bottom right*) waveforms. More than 99% of the variance of each waveform is included in the first 10 harmonics.

The values of y_r are now given by the finite series.

$$y_r = A_0 + \sum_{(n=1)}^{r} (A_n \cos n\pi/r + B_n \sin n\pi/r)$$

A digital computer program is used to carry out this operation (see below).

The arterial pressure pulse is a good example of the application of Fourier series analysis to a periodic wave. Westerhof et al. (15), using a high-fidelity catheter-tip pressure transducer, recorded the arterial pressure in the ascending aorta of a dog and subjected the wave to Fourier series analysis. Their results (Fig. 21.6) show the degree of fidelity obtain-

able by summing various harmonics. Individual harmonics are shown at the *left* and the reconstructed (or resynthesized) curves are shown at the *right*. Reconstruction of the curve using the first six harmonics leads to a curve similar to the original arterial pressure wave; however, this is much improved by adding higher harmonics (up to 20 Hz).

Reproduction of the original curve from a given number of harmonic terms can, by inspection, give a qualitative check on the adequacy of the analysis. For a more quantitative measure, the variance of the curve and of the Fourier series is compared (4, 11). The variance of a curve is the square of the standard

INPUT

OUTPUT

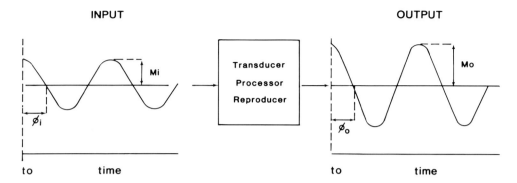

Figure 21.8. Diagrammatic representation of sine wave input and output of a recording system. ϕ_i is the phase of the sine wave and M is the modulus or amplitude. Phase of the output should be identical to that of the input.

deviation. Thus, for a curve delineated by m ordinates with a mean value of $\bar{y}$, we have

$$\text{Variance} = (1/m) \sum_{i=1}^{m} (y_i - \bar{y})^2$$

or, more usually, calculated as

$$\text{Variance} = (1/m) \sum_{i=1}^{m} y_i^2 - (1/m \sum_{i=1}^{m} y_i)^2.$$

The variance of a Fourier series is given from the following equation resulting from Parseval's theorem

$$\text{Variance (series)} = (1/2) \sum_{n=1}^{k} M_n^2$$

(i.e., half the sum of the squares of the moduli (M_n) of the harmonic terms used). The graphs shown in Figure 21.7 give the progressive sum of the variance of series representing typical aortic and left ventricular pressure and aortic blood flow velocity waveforms as a percentage of the variance of the original curves. Numerical values for the aortic and left ventricular pressure waves are given in Table 18.2. It can be seen that more than 99% of the variance of each curve is reached by the 9th or 10th harmonic. No appreciable improvement is achieved by going to 20 harmonics and the residual loss appears to consist mostly of noise in the recording system and the low energy content of cardiovascular sounds (4). It is evident from these results and those of others

(16) that no significant propagated wave in relation to blood flow exists above 30 Hz (harmonic number × heart frequency) in humans and those above 20 Hz are extremely small. Therefore, the system used to record pressure and flow waves should have a dynamic frequency response that is flat ±5% to at least 20 Hz. A system capable of recording the pressure amplitude without distortion up to 60 Hz is mandatory for accurate peak left ventricular dP/dt determination (17). For electrocardiographic recordings, the bandwidth of the system should be 0.05 to 100 Hz (5), and for His' bundle recordings the bandwidth should be 30 to 500 Hz.

The dynamic frequency characteristics of a recording system can be tested using a sine wave forcing function as input and observing the output (Fig. 21.8). The output of the system should also be a sine wave of similar frequency and phase but not amplitude. If the phase of the output differs from that of the input, it must be linear with frequency (see below) so that a correction factor can be introduced in analysis (4). The use of a sine wave generator to determine the frequency response of a fluid-filled catheter-manometer system is illustrated in Figure 21.9. The catheter-manometer system was then used to measure left ventricular pressure, and this signal was compared with that measured with a high-fidelity, catheter-tip pressure manometer (18). It is evident that pressure measured with the low-frequency response fluid-filled, catheter-manometer system is much distorted

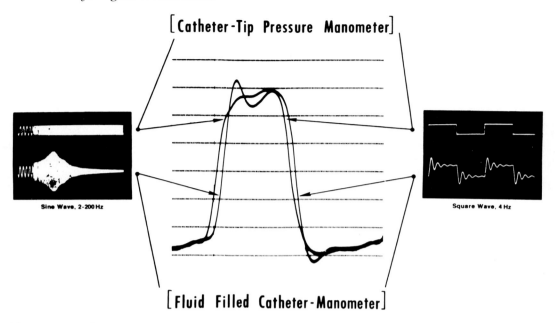

Figure 21.9. Illustration to demonstrate the testing of the dynamic frequency response of an under-damped, fluid-filled catheter-manometer system. Left ventricular pressure recorded with the low-frequency response, fluid-filled system is compared with the pressure recorded with a high-fidelity catheter-tip pressure manometer. (From Nichols WW, Pepine CJ, Miller HD, Christie LG, Conti CR. Percutaneous left ventricular catheterization with an ultraminiature catheter-tip pressure transducer. Cardiovasc Res 1978;7:566–568.)

in both phase and contour. In this example, the error is introduced in the fluid-filled, catheter-manometer system (see Chapter 18); however, the event can be distorted by any component of the recording system. Therefore, before recording a cardiovascular variable, the entire recording system must be tested for amplitude linearity, adequate frequency response, and phase linearity. As mentioned above, dynamic frequency response and phase linearity of a system can be tested using a sine wave forcing function as input and recording the output. The frequency of the sine wave generator is increased in increments, and the relative amplitude (output/input) and phase lag (output − input) are recorded and plotted vs. frequency (see Fig. 21.10). Relative amplitude and phase lag are both influenced by the degree of damping in the system (see Chapter 18). With optimal damping, amplitude and phase distortion are minimal. In the example given in Figure 21.10, the frequency response of the system is almost flat to approximately 35 Hz and the phase lag is relatively linear over this fre-

quency range. Therefore, accurate recordings of pulsatile hemodynamic variables could be obtained with this system; however, recordings of the electrocardiogram would be in error.

Graphic Records

Recorders used to record cardiovascular variables in the cardiac catheterization laboratory are generally of two types, mechanical or optical (11). The first type includes ink writing pens or heated styluses that write on thermosensitive paper. The second type uses photographic methods to record a beam of light reflected from a mirror galvanometer or the spot on a cathode ray tube. Optical recorders, especially the commonly used oscillographic type, offer better dynamic frequency characteristics, but some modern pen writing recorders are quite capable of reproducing arterial pressure, blood flow velocity, and electrocardiographic waveforms adequately as stated earlier. The frequency characteristics of any recording system are no better than their weakest link, which may be amplifier, recorder, transducer, or any other component. The frequency characteristics needed for faithful reproduction of physiologic events depends on the variable being recorded (see above).

Amplifiers of many graphic recorders have a panel control knob labeled "filter," which allows the operator to filter out unwanted noise at the output. "Noisy" records can be made to look better in this way, but one must make certain that the cardiovascular variable itself is not being distorted at the same time. The frequency contents of several variables are given above. The "nominal" frequencies indicated on an instrument dial or in the manufacturer's operational manual are not always defined in the same way. Therefore, it is always wise to test the dynamic frequency response of a system under the experimental conditions in which it is to be used, plotting a frequency response curve like that in Figure 21.10. Usually, the nominal frequency is that frequency at which the relative amplitude is reduced by approximately 30%.

The quantitative analysis of data in a finished graphic record begins with translation of selected points on the tracings into numbers (or digits), a form of analogue-to-digital (A/D) conversion. Measurement with a good millimeter scale (and small calculator) is the simplest method, but a higher degree of accuracy can be obtained with manually operated instruments designed for that purpose. The accuracy to be sought depends on the precision of the record itself, and it is rarely possible to resolve the measurements into units any smaller than a distance of 0.3 mm on the recording paper (11). The measurements obtained with the millimeter scale are calibrated by comparison with the recorded response to a known signal (see Fig. 21.2 and 21.4).

Magnetic Records

Two types of magnetic data storage, analogue and digital, are available. The analogue form is essentially a continuous magnetic tape record of input voltage, its intensity varying with time in the same way as the original physiological signal (see Fig. 21.1). Reel-to-reel (or cassette) tape recorders are used for this purpose, and are similar in design to those for

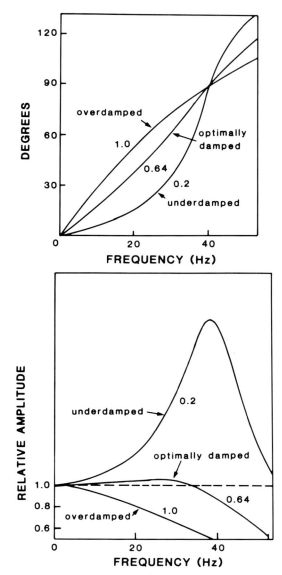

Figure 21.10. Dynamic frequency response of a recording system, with different degrees of damping when driven by a sine wave forcing function. *Top,* Relative amplitude (output/input) vs. frequency of the sine wave. When the system is underdamped, the amplitude tends to be augmented as the frequency approaches the resonant frequency of the system. With optimal damping the relative amplitude remains almost flat to a certain frequency and then declines. Overdamping limits the response to lower frequencies. *Bottom,* Phase lag (output/input) vs. frequency of the sine wave. When the system is optimally damped the phase lag is relatively linear with frequency; however, with overdamping and underdamping, the relation deviates from linearity.

recording and reproduction of sound. Because it is technically difficult to transform the direct current (D.C.) components of the physiological signal directly into magnetic code, the signal placed on the magnetic tape is usually a frequency modulated version of the input voltage (11). The upper limit of the dynamic frequency response in such recordings depends on the tape speed; the faster the speed, the higher the frequency response. Relatively slow speeds are accurate for magnetic tape recording of most cardiovascular variables. Many magnetic tape recorders are available that give a flat frequency response from 0 to 200 Hz at a tape speed of $15/16$ inches/sec. A faster speed is necessary for His' bundle recordings.

In digital systems, the analogue voltage input is sampled at specified intervals of time, and each sample is converted into a number proportional to that voltage. The sampling rate is controlled by an internal clock, and a wide choice of time intervals is usually available to the programmer. Magnetic patterns represent digits in this method, and a series of coded numbers is stored on the recording medium (magnetic card, tape, or disk). Although the continuously changing input voltage is changed into a series of discrete readings, this list of numbers can represent almost any waveform adequately if the sampling interval is made sufficiently small. The highest frequencies that can be recorded are related to the sampling interval; a sampling interval of 5 or 10 msec is adequate for most hemodynamic variables (4, 11). Calibration signals are recorded and used to translate the digital data into the proper units at a later time.

DIGITAL COMPUTERS

The last step in the processing of cardiovascular variables (or events) obtained during cardiac catheterization is the calculation of desired variables (e.g., impedance spectra, ventricular wall stress). The amplified variable (or electrical analogue signal) from the patient can be recorded on magnetic tape in analogue form and analyzed later, after analogue/digital conversion, using a digital computer, or the signal can be converted to digital form and analyzed

on-line during the catheterization procedure (see Fig. 21.1).

Before a calculation can be performed by the computer, the analogue signal must be converted or translated into a set of numbers (or digits). Mathematical operations and other manipulations are performed by the computer using a step-by-step sequence of instructions called a program. In recent years computer programming has become relatively simple, and application packages to process routine clinical hemodynamic variables are commercially available from several sources. Despite the outward simplicity of such programs, it behooves the invasive cardiologist to use such applications critically to ensure quality control and measurement accuracy. As digital applications for the cardiac catheterization laboratory continue to expand, computer literacy on the part of the cardiologist will become a necessity.

References

1. Murgo JP, Westerhof N, Giolma JP, Altobelli SA. Aortic input impedance in normal man: relationship to pressure wave shape. Circulation 1980;62:105–116.
2. O'Rourke MF. Arterial function in health and disease. London: Churchill Livingstone, 1982.
3. Wiggers CJ. The pressure pulses in the cardiovascular system. London: Longmans, 1928.
4. McDonald DA. Blood flow in arteries. 2nd ed. Baltimore: Williams & Wilkins, 1974.
5. Geddes LA, Baker LE. Principles of applied biomedical instrumentation. 2nd ed. New York: John Wiley & Sons, 1975.
6. Nichols WW, Paley DM, Thompson LV, Lambert CR. Experimental evaluation of a multisensor velocity–pressure catheter. Med Biol Eng Comput 1985;23:79–83.
7. Nichols WW, Conti CR, Walker WE, Milnor WR. Input impedance of the systemic circulation in man. Circ Res 1977;40:451–458.
8. Laskey WK, Kussmaul WG, Martin JL, Kleaveland JP, Hirshfeld JW, Shroll S. Characteristics of vascular hydraulic load in patients with heart failure. Circulation 1985;72:61–71.
9. Nichols WW, O'Rourke MF, Avolio AP, et al. Effects of age on ventricular–vascular coupling. Am J Cardiol 1985;55:1179–1184.
10. Yanof HM. Biomedical electronics. 2nd ed. Philadelphia: FA Davis, 1972.
11. Milnor WR. Hemodynamics. Baltimore: Williams & Wilkins, 1982.
12. Womersley JR. Method for the calculation of velocity, rate of flow and viscous drag in arteries when the pressure gradient is known. J Physiol (Lond) 1955;127:553–563.
13. McDonald DA. The relation of pulsatile pressure to

flow in arteries. J Physiol (Lond) 1955;127:533–552.

14. Frank O. Die Theorie der Pulswellen. A Biol 1927;85:91–130.
15. Westerhof N, Sipkema P, Elzinga G, Murgo JP, Giolma JP. Arterial impedance. In: Hwang HC, Gross DR, Patel DJ, eds. Quantitative cardiovascular studies. Baltimore: University Park Press, 1979.
16. Patel DJ, Mason DT, Ross J, Braunwald E. Harmonic analysis of pressure pulses obtained from the heart and great vessels in man. Am Heart J 1965;69:785–794.
17. Gersh BJ, Hahn CEW, Prys–Roberts C. Physical criteria for measurement of left ventricular pressure and its first derivative. Cardiovasc Res 1971;5:32–40.
18. Nichols WW, Pepine CJ, Millar HD, Christie LG, Conti CR. Percutaneous left ventricular catheterization with an ultraminiature catheter–tip pressure transducer. Cardiovasc Res 1978;7:566–568.

22

Assessment of Cardiovascular Function

Richard A. Lange, M.D.
L. David Hillis, M.D.

INTRODUCTION

A complete evaluation of the cardiovascular system entails an assessment of both anatomic and functional cardiac abnormalities. With physiologic testing, one may (*a*) assess the functional significance of an anatomic abnormality and (*b*) obtain prognostic and therapeutic information. Such a functional assessment may be performed during exercise (dynamic or isometric), rapid atrial pacing, a variety of hemodynamic maneuvers, and several pharmacologic interventions. The proper selection of each method and interpretation of the results require knowledge of the normal responses to each, as well as of the alterations produced by various kinds of cardiac disease.

PHYSIOLOGIC STRESS

Dynamic Exercise

Responses in Normal Subjects

In the cardiac catheterization laboratory, dynamic exercise is usually performed by bicycle ergometry with the subject in the supine position. In the exercise laboratory, it is performed by bicycle ergometry with the subject in the upright position or, more commonly, by having the subject walk or jog on a treadmill. During stepwise increases in the intensity of exertion, oxygen consumption, cardiac output, and intracardiac pressures may be measured, and the electrocardiogram

may be observed. From these variables, one may assess the cardiac response to exercise.

Dynamic exercise increases oxygen demand. The primary function of the cardiovascular system is to ensure that oxygen supply rises commensurately with the increase in oxygen demand. The relation between oxygen consumption and workload is linear until the maximal oxygen consumption is reached (Fig. 22.1) (1), at which time continued exercise is not accompanied by a further increase in oxygen consumption. As a result, lactic acid accumulates (2–4); minute ventilation increases disproportionately in comparison to cardiac output; and exercise endurance declines (5). This is known as the anaerobic threshold. Although such anaerobic metabolism may provide adequate energy for a brief period of exercise, it cannot sustain prolonged activity. Oxygen consumption is determined by the cardiac output and the arteriovenous oxygen difference. Thus, if pulmonary function and the oxygen concentration of ambient air are normal, the maximal oxygen consumption is an index of maximal cardiovascular function. It is usually 1 to 2 liters/min in patients with coronary artery disease and left ventricular dysfunction, about 3 liters/min in normal sedentary individuals, and as much as 6 liters/min in endurance athletes. The maximal arteriovenous oxygen difference is similar in these various individuals, so that the differences in maximal oxygen consumption are due to differences in cardiac output.

The linear relation between cardiac output

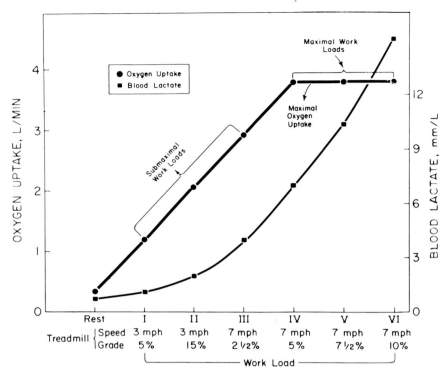

Figure 22.1. Oxygen consumption (uptake), in liters/minute (*L/MIN*), at increasing workloads. Note that this relation is linear until the maximal oxygen uptake is reached. Changes in blood lactate concentration are also shown. (From Mitchell JH, Blomqvist G. Maximal oxygen uptake. N Engl J Med 1971;284:1018–1022.)

and oxygen consumption is illustrated in Figure 22.2. This relation, termed the exercise index, may be used to assess whether or not cardiac output during exercise is appropriate for a given oxygen consumption. A measured cardiac output <80% of that predicted (based on oxygen consumption) is considered abnormal. Similarly, cardiac output should increase by at least 600 ml/min for every 100 ml/min increase in O_2 consumption (the so-called exercise factor)(6). An exercise factor less than this indicates that the subject cannot respond to exercise by increasing cardiac output appropriately.

The hemodynamic responses to dynamic exercise are the result of a complex interplay of central and reflex neural mechanisms (7), local metabolic influences (8), and postural changes. In general, the response of the cardiovascular system is related to the intensity of physiologic stress. Heart rate increases early during exercise and rises linearly with increased exertion. During mild exercise,

vagal withdrawal accounts for most of this chronotropic effect, whereas sympathetic activity predominates during intense exertion (9). Through complex humoral and neural interactions, blood flow is redistributed predominantly to working muscles, with a resultant decrease in systemic vascular resistance. Despite this fall in systemic vascular resistance, systolic and mean arterial pressures rise modestly due to a marked increase in cardiac output (10). Diastolic arterial pressure is usually unchanged or rises slightly, as do pulmonary arterial and pulmonary-capillary wedge pressures.

The hemodynamic responses to supine and upright exercise differ in certain respects. Resting left ventricular volumes are larger in the supine than in the standing position (11, 12), since venous return is diminished in the upright position. In comparison to the supine position, the upright position at rest is accompanied by a higher heart rate and diastolic arterial pressure but a lower pulmonary-capil-

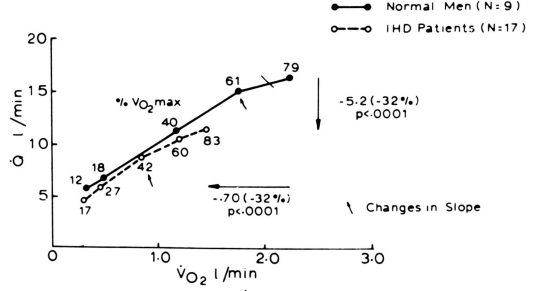

Figure 22.2. The relation of cardiac output ($\dot{Q}$), in liters per minute (vertical axis), and oxygen consumption ($\dot{V}O_2$), in liters/minute (horizontal axis), in normal men (*solid line*) and in patients with ischemic heart disease (*IHD*) (*dashed line*). Note that the normal subjects achieve a higher cardiac output and oxygen consumption than those with ischemic heart disease. (From Bruce RA, Petersen JL, Kusumi F. Hemodynamic responses to exercise in the upright posture in patients with ischemic heart disease. In: Dhalla HS, ed. Myocardial metabolism. Baltimore: University Park Press, 1973:849–865.)

lary wedge pressure, stroke volume, and cardiac output (10). With a comparable amount of exercise in the two positions, heart rate is higher in the upright position; pulmonary and intracardiac filling pressures are lower; and cardiac output is similar.

The increase in cardiac output that occurs with exercise is caused by an increase in both heart rate and stroke volume, but the contribution of each depends on the patient's position (13). Although stroke volume at maximal exercise is independent of position, the absolute and relative increases in stroke volume during exercise are greater in the upright position, since the initial stroke volume is lower in this position. Specifically, stroke volume increases by 20 to 50% with maximal exercise in the supine position (10, 14–16) and by approximately 100% in the upright position (13). Therefore, the increase in cardiac output in the supine position is primarily the result of an increased heart rate, whereas an increase in stroke volume contributes substantially to the increased cardiac output in the upright position.

The exercise-induced increase in stroke volume is due to an increase in left ventricular

contractility, which is caused by sympathetic nervous stimulation (17) and the Frank-Starling mechanism. The changes in left ventricular volumes that occur with exercise are shown in Figure 22.3. Both supine and upright exercise are accompanied by an increase in left ventricular end-diastolic volume and a decrease in end-systolic volume (14, 15, 18-21); thus, ejection fraction increases. In normals, left ventricular end-diastolic pressure is unchanged or falls slightly during exercise in young adults (22), whereas it usually rises modestly (by 6 to 8 mm Hg) in older adults (10, 23, 24). The diastolic pressure-volume relation is unchanged or shifted downward during exercise (Fig. 22.4)(25), indicating increased left ventricular compliance.

Responses in Subjects with Cardiac Disease

Abnormalities in hemodynamic variables and left ventricular function may be noted in patients with **coronary artery disease.** During submaximal exercise, these individuals often have a normal oxygen consumption (26, 27)

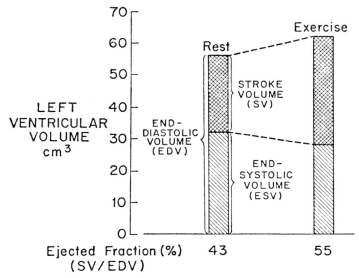

Figure 22.3. Changes in left ventricular volumes during dynamic exercise in normal subjects with exercise, end-diastolic volume increases, and end-systolic volume decreases; as a result, stroke volume and ejection fraction increase. (From Mitchell JH, Wildenthal K. Left ventricular function during exercise. In: Larsen OA, Malmborg RO, eds. Coronary heart disease and physical fitness. Copenhagen: Munksgaard, 1970:93-96.)

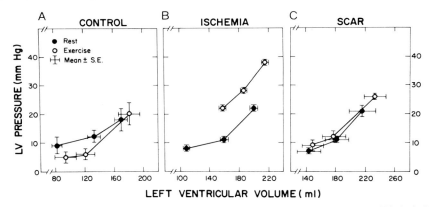

Figure 22.4. Left ventricular (*LV*) diastolic pressure-volume relations at rest (*solid circles*) and during exercise (*open circles*) in normal subjects (*control, A*), in patients with coronary artery disease (*ischemia, B*) and in patients with coronary artery disease who have old scar due to myocardial infarction (*scar, C*). With exercise, the pressure-volume curve shifts downward in the normal subjects (i.e., left ventricular compliance increases) (*A*). In patients with exercise-induced ischemia (*B*), the pressure volume curve shifts upward, indicating reduced left ventricular compliance. The patients with scar have similar ventricular diastolic pressure-volume relations at rest and during exercise. (From Carroll JD, Hess OM, Hirzel HO, Krayenbuehl HP. Dynamics of left ventricular filling at rest and during exercise. Circulation 1983;68:59-67. By permission of the American Heart Association, Inc.)

and maximal arteriovenous oxygen difference (i.e., a normal exercise index). During maximal exercise, however, cardiac output is reduced, due primarily to a diminished stroke volume. Figure 22.5 displays the pathogenesis of this diminution in stroke volume. As in normal subjects, left ventricular end-diastolic volume increases with exercise, but end-systolic volume is unchanged or increases. Therefore, stroke volume is unchanged, and ejection fraction falls (15, 18, 25, 28-30). An increase in ejection fraction of <5 to 7% during exercise is considered abnormal, regardless of the subject's position (supine or upright) (18, 21, 31).

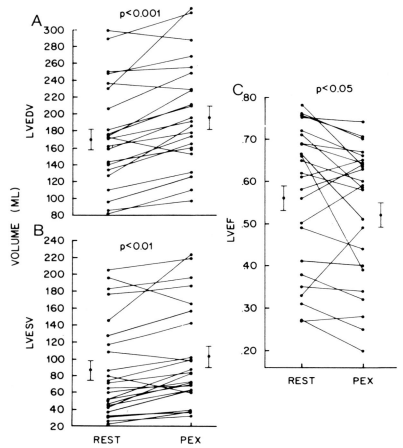

Figure 22.5. Left ventricular volumes at rest and at peak dynamic exercise (*PEX*) in patients with coronary artery disease. Each *line* represents the data from one patient, and the mean ± 1 SE is displayed on either side of each set of lines. At peak exercise, left ventricular end-diastolic volume (*LVEDV, A*) and left ventricular end-systolic volume (*LVESV, B*) increase, while ejection fraction (*LVEF, C*) declines.(From Dehmer GJ, Lewis SE, Hillis LD, Corbett J, Parkey RW, Willerson JT. Exercise-induced alterations in left ventricular volumes and the pressure-volume relationship: a sensitive indicator of left ventricular dysfunction in patients with coronary artery disease. Circulation 1981;63:1008–1018. By permission of the American Heart Association, Inc.)

In patients with coronary artery disease, the changes in ejection fraction are often accompanied by segmental wall motion abnormalities (demonstrable by echocardiography (32), radionuclide ventriculography, or contrast ventriculography (14, 18, 21, 29, 33-35)).

Left ventricular diastolic function may be impaired in patients with coronary artery disease and may be manifested by impaired left ventricular filling (25, 29), an elevated left ventricular end diastolic pressure (30), and an altered pressure-volume relation (15, 21, 25). In many patients, evidence of reduced left ventricular compliance precedes clinical and electrocardiographic evidence of ischemia.

Figure 22.4 displays a diastolic pressure-volume relation at rest and during exercise-induced ischemia. During exercise, the curve is shifted upward so that a given end-diastolic volume is associated with an increased end-diastolic pressure. In turn, pulmonary-capillary wedge and pulmonary arterial pressures may rise markedly during exercise in patients with exercise-induced ischemia (30, 36).

The specificity and sensitivity of routine exercise testing in identifying patients with coronary artery disease are improved if these exercise-induced abnormalities of left ventricular systolic and diastolic function are added to standard clinical and electrocardiographic variables (28, 37, 38). Although some authors report a sensitivity of 93 to 95% (33, 34), the specificity of such testing is lower since several kinds of cardiac disease other than coronary artery disease (i.e., dilated cardiomyopathy, hypertensive heart disease) may affect left ventricular performance during dynamic exercise (39).

The use of dynamic exercise testing in patients with **congestive heart failure** has only recently gained acceptance. Although some authors have considered congestive heart failure a relative contraindication to exercise testing (40) because of concerns for patient safety, a recent report of almost 3000 bicycle exercise tests in >600 patients with congestive heart failure demonstrated no major complications (death, pulmonary edema, or myocardial infarction), and <2% of the patients terminated the test prematurely because of arrhythmias or hypotension (41). Thus, exercise testing can be performed safely in patients with cardiac failure.

The hemodynamic alterations that accompany physiologic stress in patients with congestive heart failure are well characterized. At rest, these patients usually have reduced right and left ventricular ejection fractions. The pulmonary-capillary wedge and pulmonary arterial pressures are elevated, as are the pulmonary and systemic vascular resistances. The severity of these resting hemodynamic derangements is reflective of the severity of heart failure (42, 43). With dynamic exercise, systemic vascular resistance falls, and pulmonary vascular resistance is unchanged (42, 44, 45). Oxygen consumption, systemic arterial pressure, cardiac output, heart rate, and stroke volume rise (42-45), but the magnitude of their increase is inadequate to meet oxygen demands, so that exercise tolerance and maximal oxygen consumption are diminished, and anaerobic metabolism occurs at a low workload. In comparison to normal subjects, patients with congestive heart failure cannot manifest an appropriate increase in heart rate at an equivalent intensity of dynamic exercise (Fig. 22.6A) (46); in essence, they have "chronotropic incompetence" in response to stress. Similarly, these patients are unable to manifest an appropriate increase in systemic arterial pressure during exercise. As shown in Figure 22.6B, their maximal arterial pressure during upright bicycle exercise is reduced, in comparison with that of normal subjects, and

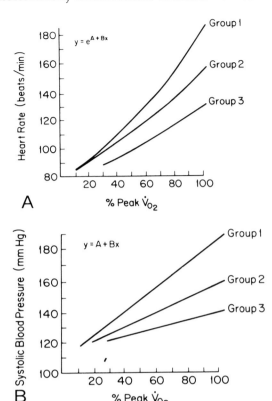

A

B

Figure 22.6. The relation of heart rate (*A*) and systolic blood pressure (*B*) (*vertical axes*) to the percent maximal oxygen consumption (*V*$_{O_2}$, *horizontal axes*) in normal subjects (*Group 1*) and in patients with mild (*Group 2*) or severe (*Group 3*) congestive heart failure. Those with congestive heart failure cannot raise their heart rates or blood pressures to the same magnitude as normal subjects at similar relative work intensities. (Reprinted with permission from Francis GS, Goldsmith SR, Ziesche S, Nakajima H, Cohn JN. Relative attenuation of sympathetic drive during exercise in patients with congestive heart failure. J Am Coll Cardiol 1985;5:832–839.)

the magnitude of its reduction is related to the severity of heart disease. These attenuated responses of heart rate and systemic arterial pressure during exercise in patients with congestive heart failure are caused by an abnormal response to exercise of the sympathetic nervous system. In support of this, the changes that occur in plasma norepinephrine concentrations during exercise are diminished in patients with heart failure (46).

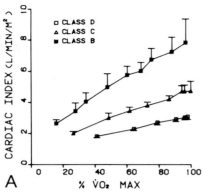
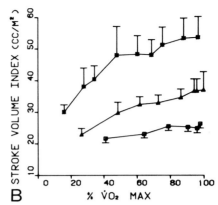

Figure 22.7. The relation of cardiac index (*A*) and stroke volume index (*B*) (*vertical axes*) to the percent maximal oxygen consumption (V_{O_2}, *horizontal axes*) in patients with mild (*class B*), moderate (*class C*), and severe (*class D*) congestive heart failure. With worsening heart failure, the increases in cardiac output and stroke volume that occur during dynamic exercise are attenuated. (From Weber KT, Kinasewitz GT, Janicki JS, Fishman AP. Oxygen utilization and ventilation during exercise in patients with chronic cardiac failure. Circulation 1982;65:1213–1223. By permission of the American Heart Association, Inc.)

In subjects with congestive heart failure, cardiac output rises during exercise, and the absolute change is determined by the severity of heart failure (Fig. 22.7) (43). As the magnitude of failure worsens, the exercise-induced increase in stroke volume declines because left ventricular end-diastolic and end-systolic volumes increase; in those with severe heart failure, the exercise-induced rise in cardiac output is almost entirely due to an increase in heart rate (Fig. 22.7) (43). In these individuals, pulmonary-capillary wedge and pulmonary arterial pressures increase during exercise, so that at peak exercise the wedge pressure may rise to 35 to 45 mm Hg, and the mean pulmonary arterial pressure may be 50 to 60 mm Hg (42–45, 47). Despite these marked exercise-induced increases in pulmonary-capillary wedge and pulmonary arterial pressures in patients with congestive heart failure, their diminished exercise tolerance is not due to the ventilatory consequences of pulmonary congestion, since exercise in these patients induces no decline in arterial oxygen tension or saturation and no increase in carbon dioxide tension (45). There is no difference in pulmonary-capillary wedge pressures between those who terminate exercise because of dyspnea and those who stop because of fatigue (45). In addition, neither rest nor exercise pulmonary-capillary wedge pressures correlate with exercise tolerance (48). In short, in patients with congestive heart failure, exercise

capacity is not limited by the pulmonary system, but rather by the inability of the cardiac system to increase cardiac output and oxygen delivery in response to increased demands.

Dynamic exercise testing may be used in patients with congestive heart failure (*a*) to grade the severity of heart failure objectively (49), (*b*) to measure cardiac reserve (43), (*c*) to quantitate the magnitude of improvement induced by a therapeutic intervention (50), and (*d*) to provide information on prognosis (42). Historically, the severity of chronic congestive heart failure has been assessed subjectively, according to information provided by the patient (New York Heart Association (NYHA) classification). In contrast to this, a measurement of oxygen utilization during stress helps to provide a reproducible and objective assessment of the patient's cardiac status, and the quantitation of maximal oxygen consumption and anaerobic threshold provides an accurate reflection of functional capacity and cardiac reserve (Table 22.1). Such

Table 22.1
Functional Classification Based on Maximal Oxygen Consumption

Class	Maximal Oxygen Consumption (ml/kg/min)
A	>20
B	16–20
C	10–15
D	<10

a functional classification offers valuable information concerning the severity of heart failure and the degree of cardiac reserve, and it is substantially more useful than resting hemodynamic variables (42, 43).

Resting indices of left ventricular function correlate poorly with exercise capacity (49–55), and pharmacologic agents that may improve resting left ventricular performance do not increase exercise capacity (56, 57). In contrast, maximal oxygen consumption and cardiac output during exercise correlate well with exercise capacity (42, 43). Thus, functional classification of patients with congestive heart failure is best performed by dynamic exercise testing, rather than by assessment of resting hemodynamic variables.

Exercise capacity may provide information on prognosis, since short-term survival is improved in patients who achieve a high maximal oxygen consumption during exercise (Fig. 22.8). However, long-term survival cannot be predicted by exercise capacity (58, 59). Although the efficacy of new pharmacologic agents for congestive heart failure is often assessed by measuring exercise capacity (60–64), the significance of this variable in assessing a drug response is not established.

In patients with **valvular heart disease,** dynamic exercise is used to help in assigning prognosis and to evaluate the efficacy of medical or surgical therapy. In addition, it may be used to evaluate the patient who has symptoms in the setting of normal resting hemodynamics. In the patient with mitral stenosis, exercise is usually accompanied by a slight increase in cardiac output and a substantial increase in left atrial and pulmonary arterial pressures (65, 66). In fact, the patient with elevated pressures at rest may develop pulmonary edema with only mild exercise. A transvalvular gradient that may be small at rest becomes larger with exercise, due to an increased cardiac output and a tachycardia-induced decrease in diastolic filling time (67, 68). In the patient with mitral stenosis whose cardiac output is low and whose transvalvular pressure gradient is small, exercise increases both variables, allowing a more reliable assessment of the severity of stenosis.

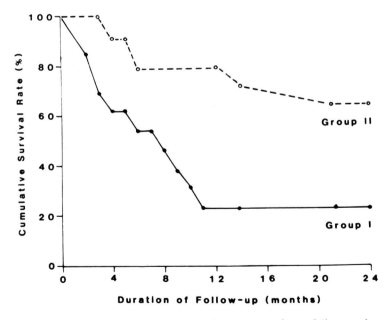

Figure 22.8. Cumulative survival rate for patients with congestive heart failure and severely (Group I) or mildly (Group II) impaired exercise tolerance over a 24-month period of observation. Those with severely impaired exercise tolerance (Group I) had a significantly higher mortality than those with only mildly impaired exercise tolerance (Group II). (From Szlachcic J, Massie BM, Kramer BL, Topic N, Tubau J. Correlates and prognostic implication of exercise capacity in chronic congestive heart failure. Am J Cardiol 1985;55:1037–1042.)

In most patients with aortic stenosis, an accurate measurement of the transvalvular gradient at rest allows one to calculate the valve area, even when the cardiac output is low; thus, dynamic exercise is rarely helpful in these individuals. The risk of exercise-induced sudden death in these patients (due to peripheral vasodilation) provides a relative contraindication to dynamic exercise testing (40, 69). If the patient with aortic stenosis performs dynamic exercise, cardiac output increases; the transvalvular gradient increases; and both left atrial and pulmonary arterial pressures rise (70-72). The calculated valve area may increase modestly with exercise due, in all probability, to improved leaflet movement with a higher flow across the valve (72).

Dynamic exercise may be of help in assessing the cardiovascular status of patients with chronic mitral regurgitation, particularly those whose symptoms are minimal and whose cardiac output, intracardiac filling pressures, and left ventricular function are reasonably normal at rest. The patient with mitral regurgitation whose cardiac reserve is adequate responds to dynamic exercise with an appropriate increase in forward output, little change in intracardiac filling pressures, a fall in regurgitant fraction, and a modest decrease in left ventricular ejection fraction (73). In contrast, the individual whose cardiac reserve is limited often demonstrates a blunted increase in forward cardiac output, a rise in intracardiac filling pressures, and a marked fall in left ventricular ejection fraction. In short, dynamic exercise in the patient with mitral regurgitation and minimal symptoms may help to identify those whose response to chronic volume overload is no longer normal, that is, those whose cardiac reserve is limited.

Because of uncertainty as to when to proceed with valve replacement in patients with asymptomatic aortic regurgitation, several studies have investigated the response to dynamic exercise in patients with this valvular abnormality. Symptomatic patients consistently demonstrate a fall in left ventricular ejection fraction with exercise, whereas asymptomatic subjects demonstrate a heterogeneous response (i.e., ejection fraction may rise, fall, or be unchanged) (13, 74-78). Although a fall in left ventricular ejection fraction during exercise in the asymptomatic patient is thought to identify those who may require valve replacement in the near future, this finding alone is not an indication for surgery. In fact, only 25 to 30% of asymptomatic patients with aortic regurgitation and an abnormal exercise response require surgery for worsening symptoms over an average follow-up period of 4 years (79). Since operative and postoperative survival is not diminished if surgery is delayed until symptoms appear, valve replacement is generally delayed until the patient has symptoms (79).

In short, dynamic exercise testing in the cardiac catheterization laboratory or the exercise laboratory may be used in patients with valvular heart disease, but its utility is substantially greater in those with valvular regurgitation than in those with predominant stenosis. In the patient with mitral or aortic stenosis, dynamic exercise provides the opportunity to calculate a valve area both at rest and during exercise, at a time when cardiac output and heart rate are augmented. This may be especially important in the patient with mitral stenosis and a cardiac output at rest that is low, with a resultant small transvalvular gradient. In this individual, dynamic exercise may be used to increase the transvalvular gradient, thereby allowing a second calculation of the valve area. In the patient with mitral or aortic regurgitation who is asymptomatic or only minimally symptomatic, dynamic exercise provides the opportunity to assess cardiac reserve. Thus, the patient with adequate reserve responds to exercise with an appropriate increase in forward output, little or no change in intracardiac filling pressures (left ventricular end-diastolic and pulmonary capillary wedge pressures), a decrease in left ventricular end-systolic volume, and an increase in left ventricular ejection fraction. In contrast, the patient with inadequate reserve responds to exercise with a blunted increase in forward output (i.e., a depressed exercise factor), a distinct rise in intracardiac filling pressures, no change or an increase in left ventricular end-systolic volume, and a decrease in ejection fraction. The patient whose cardiac reserve is inadequate should be observed frequently and closely, since he or she may require valve replacement in the near future.

The alterations in cardiac function that occur during dynamic exercise with **aging** in the absence of cardiovascular disease should be recognized, so as not to confuse them with changes that are caused by cardiac disease. First, the elderly patient responds to sympathetic stimulation with only a modest increase in heart rate; similarly, in comparison with younger subjects, these individuals manifest a blunted increase in heart rate with vigorous exercise (80, 81). Since plasma catecholamine levels are markedly increased during exercise in the elderly, the mechanism of this diminished chronotropic response appears to be a diminished end organ responsiveness to circulating catecholamines. Second, even though cardiac output rises appropriately during exercise in elderly patients, this is due to a greater reliance on the Frank-Starling mechanism, with a resultant increase in stroke volume, rather than to a marked increase in heart rate (82). These elderly patients often have a markedly increased end-diastolic and a modestly increased end-systolic volume. Third, maximal oxygen consumption is known to decrease with age, but this may be due to factors other than cardiovascular limitations, including sedentary life-style, motivation, orthopaedic considerations, and a decreased muscle mass. Thus, certain noncardiac factors may limit maximal oxygen consumption in the elderly population.

Isometric Exercise

Exercise in which skeletal muscle contraction causes primarily a change in tension with little change in length is termed isometric or static exercise. Isometric activities include lifting or pushing heavy objects and contracting muscles against immovable objects. In clinical practice, this is usually accomplished by having the subject perform handgrip, most often with a graded, hand dynamometer. The subject is asked to compress the dynamometer maximally several times, from which the maximal voluntary contraction is determined. Subsequently, measurements of hemodynamic variables and ventricular function are accomplished while the patient performs sustained handgrip at a percentage (usually 15 to 50%) of maximal contraction.

As with dynamic exercise, the magnitude of effort expended during isometric exercise is an important determinant of the cardio-vascular alterations that ensue. However, it is not the absolute tension developed during isometric exercise that is important but rather the percentage of maximal voluntary contraction that is developed (83). Furthermore, the size of the involved muscle group is unimportant in determining the cardiovascular response. Thus, a 30% maximal voluntary contraction during handgrip requires an actual tension of 20 kg, whereas a 30% contraction of the leg requires a tension of 70 kg. Despite this difference in absolute tensions, muscle group masses, and energy expenditures, the same hemodynamic response is elicited in both situations (83) and, as a result, the same cardiovascular effects occur. The magnitude of the cardiovascular response to isometric exercise also depends on the duration of sustained tension (83). At 15% of maximal voluntary contraction, hemodynamic responses reach a steady state within 2 to 3 min. At tensions >15% maximal voluntary contraction, these hemodynamic variables do not reach a steady state but continue to increase until fatigue intervenes. The duration of exercise varies with the tension exerted. At 50% maximal voluntary contraction, most subjects can sustain contraction for 2 to 3 min, whereas 3 to 5 min of sustained contraction are possible at 30% maximal voluntary contraction.

Since isometric exercise requires little equipment, it is simple and inexpensive. It is easily performed and easily repeated in the same subject. Handgrip does not involve body motion that may distort or interfere with the monitoring of hemodynamic variables or left ventricular function. Despite some concerns that isometric exercise might promote arrhythmias (84) numerous studies have been performed in normal subjects and in those with cardiac disease without serious arrhythmias (83, 85-100). As with any type of exercise, static exercise requires patient participation and cooperation that may limit its usefulness in some. In particular, one must ensure that isometric exercise is not confounded by the Valsalva maneuver, a frequent occurrence during unsupervised sustained static exertion. Careful monitoring of respiration, as well as persistent coaxing and engagement of the subject in conversation during the procedure, minimize the chance that this will occur.

Responses in Normal Subjects

The hemodynamic responses to isometric and dynamic exercise differ substantially from one another. With isometric exercise, systolic, diastolic, and mean arterial pressures rise markedly (by 25 to 50 mm Hg), whereas heart rate increases only modestly (by 20 to 30 bpm) (85, 88, 89, 91). In contrast, dynamic exercise induces little change in diastolic arterial pressure, a modest rise in systolic and mean arterial pressures, and a considerable increase in heart rate. With isometric exercise, cardiac output increases modestly, and systemic vascular resistance is unchanged (83, 97). The increase in cardiac output is due to an increase in heart rate, since stroke volume is unchanged (85, 87-89). There is no significant change in pulmonary arterial pressure or resistance during isometric exercise in normal subjects (88).

During dynamic exercise, stroke volume increases, and there is only a modest change in mean arterial pressure; thus, dynamic exercise causes primarily a volume load of the left ventricle. In contrast, isometric exercise induces no change in stroke volume and a substantial rise in systemic arterial pressure, resulting primarily in a pressure load of the left ventricle. Left ventricular end-diastolic volume decreases or is unchanged, and end-diastolic pressure is unchanged. The maintenance of stroke volume against an increased aortic impedance is accomplished by an increase in the inotropic state of the left ventricle; left ventricular preload is unchanged (11, 89, 95, 97, 100). In support of this, both invasively (92-94) and noninvasively measured (97, 99, 100) indices of left ventricular function (max dP/dt, dP/dt/P, V_{max}, fractional shortening, and shortening velocity) increase during isometric exercise.

Responses in Subjects with Cardiac Disease

In patients with **coronary artery disease,** isometric exercise rarely precipitates symptoms or electrocardiographic signs of ischemia (86, 89, 92, 101). Nevertheless, it may induce left ventricular wall motion abnormalities (86, 90, 95, 101), as well as a fall in left ventricular ejection fraction. The latter is caused by an increase in end-systolic volume; end-diastolic volume is unchanged (89, 99). Stroke volume

and cardiac output may decline during isometric exercise.

In patients with **congestive heart failure,** isometric exercise may be used to evaluate left ventricular function and cardiac reserve. During isometric exertion, those with heart failure cannot adequately increase left ventricular contractile function in response to the increased aortic impedance. Heart rate and systemic arterial pressure rise appropriately (102, 103), but cardiac output and stroke volume may fall, and left ventricular end-diastolic and pulmonary arterial pressures may rise. Patients with mild heart failure often have normal hemodynamics at rest, but their response to isometric stress is abnormal, in that an increased stroke work is accomplished at the expense of a high left ventricular end-diastolic pressure (Fig.22.9) (85, 89–93, 96).

Rapid Atrial Pacing

Although dynamic or isometric exercise may be performed in most individuals, alternative forms of stress are sometimes required. Exercise testing may be difficult in patients who are elderly, debilitated, poorly conditioned or motivated, or who have concomitant illnesses that preclude adequate exertion (i.e., chronic lung disease, peripheral vascular disease,

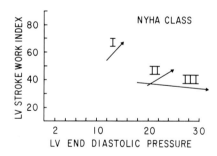

Figure 22.9. The relation between left ventricular stroke work index (vertical axis) and end-diastolic pressure (horizontal axis) in patients with coronary artery disease at rest and during isometric exercise (*arrowhead*). Patients are segregated according to NYHA classification. In class II and III patients, isometric exercise is associated with a marked rise in left ventricular end-diastolic pressure and little, if any, change in stroke work index. (From Kivowitz C, Parmley WW, Donoso R, Marcus H, Ganz W, Swan HJC. Effects of isometric exercise on cardiac performance. The grip test. Circulation 1971;44:994–1002. By permission of the American Heart Association, Inc.)

arthritis, or neuromuscular disorders). In these subjects, rapid atrial pacing may serve as an alternative to exercise. Although atrial pacing may be of use in assessing left ventricular function, its use in identifying those with coronary artery disease is somewhat limited.

Pacing is usually performed with the subject in the supine position. A pacing catheter is placed in the right atrium or coronary sinus, after which heart rate is increased incrementally (by 10 to 20 bpm) every 2 to 3 min until (*a*) chest pain occurs, (*b*)a heart rate of 160 bpm is achieved, or (*c*) atrioventricular block occurs. If 1:1 atrioventricular conduction does not occur at lower heart rates, 0.5 to 1.0 mg of atropine is given intravenously to enhance atrioventricular conduction.

Responses in Normal Subjects

Oxygen consumption increases slightly with rapid atrial pacing, but the magnitude of this increase is considerably less than that observed with exercise. Myocardial oxygen consumption increases due to the increase in heart rate and the augmented inotropic state that accompanies a tachycardia (termed the Treppe phenomenon or Bowditch effect) (104, 105). This increase in myocardial oxygen consumption is met by an appropriate increase in coronary blood flow, since the arteriovenous oxygen difference across the heart is unchanged (106, 107). Although myocardial oxygen consumption rises during rapid atrial pacing, the magnitude of its rise is less than that observed with exercise. During rapid atrial pacing, systolic, diastolic, and mean arterial pressures are unchanged. Cardiac output is unchanged despite a marked increase in heart rate; thus, stroke volume declines incrementally as heart rate increases. Pulmonary arterial and right atrial pressures are unchanged (107-117).

During incremental atrial pacing, left ventricular end-diastolic volume falls precipitously, and end-systolic volume declines as well, although the magnitude of the fall in end-diastolic volume may be greater than that of end-systolic volume. As a result, the changes in ejection fraction caused by atrial pacing may vary from one individual to another, with some studies reporting an increase (118, 119) and others reporting no significant change in this variable (108, 110).

This pacing-induced decline in left ventricular end-diastolic volume is accompanied by a decrease in left ventricular end-diastolic pressure; in normal subjects, end-diastolic pressure declines linearly as heart rate increases (115). Left ventricular contraction and relaxation, as reflected by positive and negative dP/dt (108, 109, 114, 120), peak diastolic filling rate (121), stroke volume to left ventricular end-diastolic pressure ratio (111, 112, 115, 116), time constant of left ventricular pressure fall (τ) (122), and fiber shortening velocity (123) are enhanced during rapid atrial pacing (i.e., contractility and compliance are increased).

Responses in Subjects with Cardiac Disease

In early reports, angina induced by rapid atrial pacing was thought to be a sensitive and specific marker of **coronary artery disease** (124, 125). Accordingly, in some studies, symptoms served as the standard to which other markers of ischemia (i.e., lactate production, changes in left ventricular end-diastolic pressure, and electrocardiographic ST segment alterations) were compared. However, subsequent investigations have shown that chest pain is neither a sensitive nor specific indicator of myocardial ischemia (118, 119, 126-131), since many patients cannot differentiate between ischemic chest pain and the palpitations associated with rapid atrial pacing. This may be particularly true at high pacing rates (>140 bpm). On the one extreme, several studies of patients with angiographically normal coronary arteries reported angina-like chest pain in many of the subjects at high pacing rates (125, 126, 131). On the other extreme, patients with known coronary artery disease and metabolic evidence of pacing-induced ischemia (i.e., lactate production) may not have chest pain. In short, chest pain during rapid atrial pacing is unreliable in assessing the presence of coronary artery disease.

If angina occurs during atrial pacing in the setting of coronary artery disease, it usually resolves 30 sec to 2 min after pacing is terminated (107), and it is reproducibly induced if pacing is performed again at the same rate. As a rule, angina that is induced by atrial pacing requires a higher heart rate (20 to 30 bpm) than that induced by dynamic exercise, since systemic arterial pressure is not affected substantially by pacing (107, 109, 115, 116, 124, 132). The heart rate at which angina occurs is unrelated to the severity of coronary artery disease (112, 124, 127).

The electrocardiographic changes that occur **during** pacing are difficult to interpret and are neither sensitive nor specific in the identification of ischemia. A substantial frequency of false-negative and false-positive results are noted, especially at paced heart rates >160 bpm (125). Several factors may render the interpretation of electrocardiographic changes during pacing difficult (130). Alterations in the P-R segment baseline may influence the assessment of ST segment changes (since the ST segment is compared with the P-R segment), and placement of the pacing lead may influence the P-R segment. Abnormal atrial repolarization may cause P-R segment elevation, which may confuse the interpretation of ST segment depression. Prolongation of the P-R interval occurs commonly at higher

paced heart rates (>140 bpm), and this may place the pacemaker spike on the T wave, ST segment, or J junction of the preceding QRS. Finally, a reentrant P wave induced by pacing is often located on the ST segment, making its interpretation difficult.

In an effort to improve the reliability of ECG alterations with pacing, some investigators have examined these changes immediately **after** pacing, and they have shown that ST segment alterations on a postpacing electrocardiogram offer excellent specificity and an acceptable sensitivity in the identification of subjects with coronary artery disease (118). In fact, if electrocardiographic alterations after pacing are utilized, the reliability of pacing in identifying patients with coronary artery disease approaches, but does not equal, that of standard exercise testing (133).

With rapid atrial pacing in patients with coronary artery disease, total oxygen consumption increases and is higher than in normal subjects at similar paced heart rates (107). This has been attributed to the anxiety and

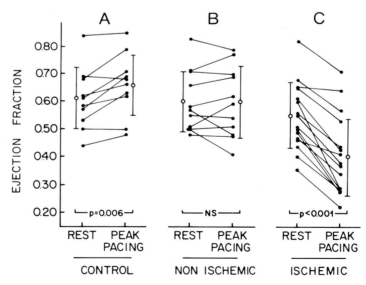

Figure 22.10. Left ventricular ejection fraction at rest and during peak atrial pacing in normal subjects (control, *A*) patients with coronary artery disease but without evidence of ischemia (nonischemic, *B*), and patients with coronary artery disease and pacing-induced ischemia (ischemic, *C*). Each *line* represents the data from 1 patient, and the mean ± 1 SD is displayed on either side of each set of lines. With pacing, ejection fraction increases in the normal individuals, does not change in patients in the nonischemic group and declines in those with ischemia. (From Dehmer GJ, Firth BG, Nicod P, Lewis SE, Hillis LD. Alterations in left ventricular volumes and ejection fraction during atrial pacing in patients with coronary artery disease: assessment with radionuclide ventriculography. Am Heart J 1983;106:114–124.)

increased ventilation associated with angina. Mean arterial pressure and cardiac output increase little, if any, and stroke volume falls. Pulmonary arterial pressure is frequently elevated if there is evidence of ischemia with pacing.

The alterations in left ventricular volumes that occur during atrial pacing-induced ischemia are similar in many respects to those noted during dynamic exercise. With an incremental increase in heart rate, left ventricular end-diastolic volume decreases; at the same time, left ventricular end-systolic volume does not change or may even increase. As a result, ejection fraction remains the same or may actually fall during rapid atrial pacing (Fig. 22.10). Contrast left ventriculography at peak pacing may demonstrate a worsening of existing segmental wall motion abnormalities as well as the appearance of new wall motion alterations (108, 110, 118, 134-136).

The changes in left ventricular end-diastolic pressure that occur with rapid atrial pacing can be interpreted only in the context of the changes in left ventricular volumes described previously. During pacing, end-diastolic pressure usually falls (since end-diastolic volume falls), but in an occasional patient it may be unchanged from baseline. Although left ventricular end-diastolic pressure is not markedly elevated during pacing, a careful comparison with that of normal subjects shows that left ventricular end-diastolic pressure is higher at each level of pacing in subjects with ischemia than in normals (Fig. 22.11). When pacing is abruptly terminated in patients with pacing-induced ischemia, left ventricular end-diastolic volume returns to its prepacing level, and left ventricular end-diastolic pressure rises markedly and remains elevated for 30 sec to 5 min (Fig. 22.12). In contrast, patients without coronary artery disease, as well as those with coronary disease but without ischemia, demonstrate no change or a minimal increase in end-diastolic pressure (in comparison to the prepacing values) after the abrupt termination of pacing. Although the etiology of pacing-induced diastolic dysfunction has been investigated extensively, a pacing-induced reduction in peak negative dP/dt and an increase in the time constant of left ventricular pressure fall (τ) support the hypothesis that it is due to a reduction in left ventricular compliance (122).

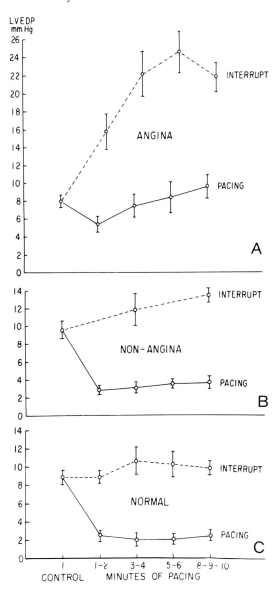

Figure 22.11. Left ventricular end-diastolic pressure (*LVEDP, vertical axes*) at rest (control), during rapid atrial pacing, and at points of interruption in normal subjects (*C*) and in patients with coronary artery disease with (*A*) or without (*B*) pacing-induced angina. In comparison to normals, *LVEDP* is elevated in the patients with pacing-induced ischemia (angina group) during pacing and with interruption of pacing. (From Parker JO, Ledwich JR, West RO, Case RB. Reversible cardiac failure during angina pectoris. Hemodynamic effects of atrial pacing in coronary artery disease. Circulation 1969;39:745–757. By permission of the American Heart Association, Inc.)

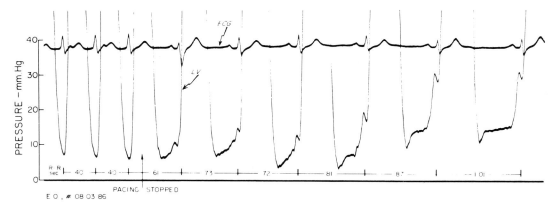

Figure 22.12. Left ventricular (LV) end-diastolic pressure (*vertical axis*) in a patient with ischemia induced by rapid atrial pacing. The LV end-diastolic pressure is normal during pacing but rapidly increases when pacing is terminated. (From O'Brien KP, Higgs LM, Glancy DL, Epstein SE. Hemodynamic accompaniments of angina. A comparison during angina induced by exercise and by atrial pacing. Circulation 1969;39:735–743. By permission of the American Heart Association, Inc.)

HEMODYNAMIC MANEUVERS

Valsalva Maneuver

With the Valsalva maneuver, the subject forcibly expires against a closed glottis. Its magnitude is quantitated by having the subject expire into a mouthpiece connected in parallel to a graduated manometer and pressure transducer. For most studies, a pressure of 30 to 50 mm Hg sustained for 10 to 15 sec is sufficient to produce the characteristic hemodynamic changes. The Valsalva maneuver has been performed safely and without complications in numerous studies (137-144).

Responses in Normal Subjects

The hemodynamic alterations induced by the Valsalva maneuver are displayed in Figure 22.13 (145) and are divided into four phases. Phase 1 begins with the onset of straining and is marked by a transient increase in intrathoracic pressure, which causes a transient increase in systemic arterial pressure. During phase 2, straining continues; venous return and cardiac output diminish; and peripheral vascular resistance increases. As a result of diminished cardiac output, systemic arterial pressure falls, and the pulse pressure narrows. The heart rate increases in response to the decline in arterial pressure. With the initial release of straining (phase 3), intrathoracic pressure decreases abruptly, and systemic arterial pressure transiently falls further as a result of pooling of blood in the expanded pulmonary vascular bed. Phase 4 quickly follows, with an overshoot of the arterial pressure caused by increased venous return and sympathetic activity. This overshoot of the pulse pressure and mean arterial pressure causes a reflex bradycardia, which is mediated by the parasympathetic nervous system.

During active straining, left ventricular end-diastolic and end-systolic volumes decrease by 45 to 50%, and stroke volume is diminished by 35 to 50%. During recovery from straining, left ventricular end-diastolic volume returns to baseline, but end-systolic volume remains low because of increased sympathetic activity. As a result, stroke volume is increased in the recovery phase of the Valsalva maneuver.

During straining, right atrial, pulmonary arterial, and pulmonary-capillary wedge pressures rise markedly, but this is due primarily to the increased intrathoracic pressure generated by the maneuver. In fact, the transmural intracardiac pressures (intracavitary minus intrapleural) actually fall during the active straining phase of the Valsalva maneuver.

Responses in Subjects with Cardiac Disease

Rapid changes in intracardiac volumes induced by the Valsalva maneuver reflexly

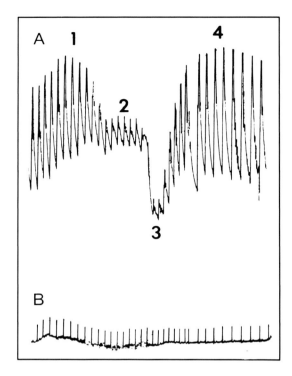

depressed baroreceptor response (147), and patients with diabetes mellitus and autonomic dysfunction display a blunted heart rate response during phase 4 (148). In subjects with idiopathic orthostatic hypotension, the overshoot of arterial pressure in phase 4 may be absent (149).

In patients with **congestive heart failure,** the behavior of heart rate in all phases of the Valsalva maneuver is abnormal, in that it neither rises nor falls substantially (140, 142). During the straining phase (phase 2), arterial pressure does not fall as it does in normal subjects; rather, it remains the same or may even increase. When the release phase is reached, there is no overshoot of arterial pressure. This is known as the "square wave response" and is shown in Figure 22.14. (138, 145, 150). This absence of marked changes in systemic arterial pressure and heart rate is believed to be due to increased pulmonary blood volume in

Figure 22.13. Systemic arterial pressure (*A*) and an electrocardiogram (*B*) during a Valsalva maneuver in a normal individual. With the onset of straining (phase *1*), arterial pressure transiently increases. With continued straining (phase *2*), systolic arterial pressure and pulse pressure decline, and heart rate increases reflexly. A further transient decrease in arterial pressure occurs in phase 3 with release of straining and is followed by a characteristic pressure overshoot and bradycardia in phase 4. (From Nishimura RA, Tajik AJ. The Valsalva maneuver and response revisited. Mayo Clin Proc 1986;61:211–217.)

stimulate compensatory mechanisms via the autonomic nervous system, such that the changes in heart rate and arterial pressure that occur with this maneuver may provide insight into the integrity of the autonomic system. For example, the release of straining in phase 4, with its associated overshoot of arterial pressure, causes bradycardia by stimulating the carotid body receptor. The assessment of the heart rate response during phase 4 has been used as a noninvasive indicator of baroreceptor function (146). The magnitude of the change in heart rate during phase 4 diminishes with advanced age because of a

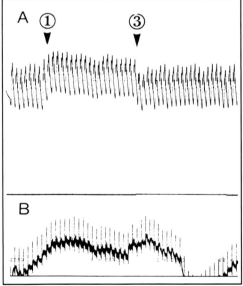

Figure 22.14. Systemic arterial pressure (*A*) and an electrocardiogram (*B*) during a Valsalva maneuver in a patient with congestive heart failure. Phases 1 and 3 are marked as in Figure 22.13. Absence of a decreased arterial pressure in phase 2 and an overshoot of arterial pressure in phase 4 characterize the "square wave response" observed in these patients. Likewise, heart rate does not change during the Valsalva maneuver. (From Nishimura RA, Tajik AJ. The Valsalva maneuver and response revisited. Mayo Clin Proc 1986;61:211-217.)

these patients, with continued left heart filling for a sustained period of time, even during active straining. As a result, left ventricular volumes and stroke volume are not diminished (140). Hence, systemic arterial pressure does not fall, and heart rate does not reflexly change. Interestingly, one study has reported that effective therapy of heart failure resulted in normalization of the hemodynamic response to the Valsalva maneuver (138).

Some patients with **coronary artery disease** may manifest an abnormal hemodynamic response to the Valsalva maneuver that is similar to that of subjects with congestive heart failure. These individuals have an attenuated response of heart rate and systolic arterial pressure during phases 2 and 4 of the Valsalva maneuver. This blunted hemodynamic response may be observed even in the absence of active ischemia (151).

In some patients with coronary artery disease, the Valsalva maneuver may help to alleviate episodes of myocardial ischemia (152). This occurs during the latter part of phase 2 (active straining) and is manifested as an abrupt reduction in left ventricular end-diastolic pressure, which is typically elevated during ischemia. Myocardial oxygen demand is decreased, due to diminished left ventricular volumes, and coronary blood flow (and myocardial oxygen supply) also is diminished during the Valsalva maneuver (153). This decrease in left ventricular volumes and pressures that occurs during the Valsalva maneuver may also favorably affect the oxygen supply-demand relation in asynergic segments of the left ventricle, leading to augmentation of reversibly injured segments (139). No untoward effects are observed when a Valsalva maneuver is performed during an episode of ischemia (151, 152). The Valsalva maneuver has been used in the recognition of patients with **obstructive hypertrophic cardiomyopathy** and to help in **differentiating right- and left-sided murmurs** (154). During forced expiration, the outflow tract gradient in patients with obstructive hypertrophic cardiomyopathy increases as peripheral pulse pressure and left ventricular volumes decline. As a result, the murmur increases in intensity (155, 156), whereas other systolic murmurs (i.e., aortic stenosis, mitral regurgitation) decrease or do not change with the Valsalva maneuver (157, 158). In an occasional patient

with obstructive hypertrophic cardiomyopathy, the murmur may paradoxically decrease in intensity during the Valsalva maneuver despite an increase in the gradient (159). This is thought to be due to a severe reduction in stroke volume and transaortic flow caused by the Valsalva maneuver. After release of the Valsalva maneuver, the intensity of a left-sided murmur usually returns to baseline in 4 to 11 cardiac cycles, whereas the intensity of a right-sided murmur returns to baseline in 1 to 2 cycles. This difference may be used to differentiate left- and right-sided murmurs (160).

Mueller Maneuver

Response in Normal Subjects

The Mueller maneuver involves inspiratory effort against a closed glottis; hence, it is often considered the opposite of the Valsalva maneuver. It is usually performed by having the subject inhale with maximal effort against a closed one-way valve attached to a transducer, so that the subject begins at his resting lung volume and generates -30 to -60 mm Hg for 20 to 30 sec. Since the inspiratory pressure that is generated (161, 162), the time period (163), and the initial lung volume (162) influence the direction and magnitude of hemodynamic alterations, these variables must be standardized if one is to interpret the results meaningfully.

During the Mueller maneuver, several hemodynamic alterations occur. Right ventricular filling increases for 2 to 3 sec (because of the negative intrathoracic pressure); this is followed by a prolonged period of diminished filling due to collapse of the superior and inferior vena cavae at the thoracic inlets (164-166). Left ventricular afterload rises, causing an increase in left ventricular end-diastolic and end-systolic volumes, a diminished stroke volume, and a reduced ejection fraction (162, 163, 165, 167, 168).

Responses in Subjects with Cardiac Disease

The hemodynamic alterations induced by the Mueller maneuver may be useful in distinguishing left- and right-sided heart murmurs (169). The transient increase in right-sided filling may briefly increase the intensity of right-sided murmurs, such as tricuspid regurgitation or stenosis (68). Despite its wide clinical use, there are no studies documenting the usefulness of the Mueller maneuver in differentiating left- and right-sided heart murmurs (154).

In patients with obstructive hypertrophic cardiomyopathy, the Mueller maneuver causes a striking reduction in the left ventricular outflow gradient, the intensity of the systolic murmur, and the echocardiographically-demonstrated systolic anterior movement of the anterior mitral valve leaflet (167, 170). These alterations are believed to be due to the increase in left ventricular afterload caused by this maneuver.

Cold Pressor Testing

Responses in Normal Subjects

The cold pressor test is performed by placing the patient's hand in ice for 1 to 3 min. The exposure to cold stimulates α-adrenergic receptors (171), leading to a modest increase in heart rate (5 to 15 bpm), systolic and mean arterial pressures (15 to 30 mm Hg), and cardiac output. A maximal response occurs within 2 min. Left ventricular end-diastolic volume increases during exposure to cold, whereas the response of end-systolic volume, stroke volume, and ejection fraction is heterogeneous (172-180). In normal subjects, α-adrenergic activation increases coronary blood flow, and coronary vascular resistance is decreased or unchanged despite a small (6 to 8%) decrease in coronary artery diameter (181, 182). Cold-induced, neurally mediated coronary vasoconstriction is offset by metabolically mediated vasodilation.

Responses in Subjects with Cardiac Disease

In patients with **coronary artery disease,** exposure to cold elicits similar modest elevations in heart rate and systemic arterial pressure (172, 173, 183-185), so that the heart rate-blood pressure product rises modestly (178, 180, 186). The precipitation of angina is caused by a concomitant reduction in oxygen supply which, in turn, is caused by increased coronary vascular resistance and diminished

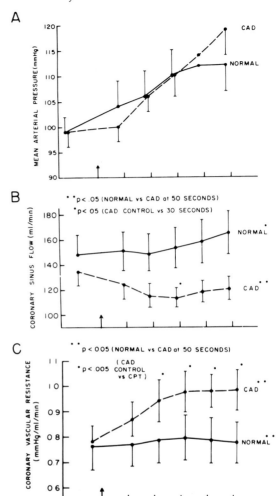

Figure 22.15. Changes in systemic and coronary vascular tone elicited by the cold pressor test (*CPT*) in normal subjects (*solid lines*) and in patients with *CAD* (*dashed lines*). Both groups demonstrate a systemic hypertensive response to cold (*A*). Unlike the normal subjects, however, patients with CAD have a cold-induced decrease in coronary blood flow (*B*) and an increase in coronary vascular resistance (*C*). (From Mudge GH Jr, Grossman W, Mills RM Jr, Lesch M, Braunwald E. Reflex increase in coronary vascular resistance in patients with ischemic heart disease. N Engl J Med 1976;295:1333–1337.)

coronary blood flow (Fig. 22.15) (172, 176, 181, 184). This cold-induced coronary vasoconstriction is mediated through stimulation of α-adrenergic receptors in diseased segments of coronary arteries (172, 174, 177); it is prevented with α-adrenergic blockade (181) and is potentiated by β-adrenergic blockade (184).

The usefulness of cold pressor testing in identifying patients with coronary artery disease is limited. Angina is precipitated uncommonly, even in the presence of documented ischemia; ECG changes are seldom observed (only in 25 to 30%) (177, 186). The cold pressor test is inferior to dynamic exercise testing in identifying patients with coronary artery disease: in direct comparisons of the two techniques, exercise offers a better sensitivity and specificity than exposure to cold (173, 187-189). Although stimulation of coronary α-adrenergic receptors has repeatedly been postulated as the etiology of vasospastic (Prinzmetal's) angina, recent studies have shown that exposure to cold usually does not induce focal coronary vasospasm (171, 180, 186), even though such spasm has occasionally been observed angiographically during cold provocation (182).

Hyperventilation

Responses in Normal Subjects

Besides ergonovine and cold pressor, hyperventilation has been used as a maneuver to induce coronary arterial spasm. It is usually performed by having the patient take 30 deep respirations/min for 5 min. If ischemia is precipitated, it may occur during hyperventilation; however, it more commonly develops within several minutes after the termination of hyperventilation (186). In response to hyperventilation, heart rate, oxygen consumption, the arteriovenous oxygen difference, and arterial pH increase, whereas mean arterial pressure, pulmonary arterial pressure, and arterial pCO_2 decline. Peripheral vascular resistance, cardiac output, and stroke volume are unchanged (190). In normal subjects, left ventricular ejection fraction increases (188).

Responses in Subjects with Cardiac Disease

Numerous reports have described ischemia induced by hyperventilation in patients with **stable** and **variant angina.** From 5 to 30% of patients with coronary artery disease develop angina and ischemic electrocardiographic

alterations during vigorous hyperventilation (191-194). The ischemia is rapidly relieved by sublingual nitroglycerin and frequently responds chronically to calcium antagonists (195). In both normal subjects and those with coronary artery disease, coronary sinus blood flow falls during hyperventilation (190, 196), and in those with atherosclerotic narrowings, hyperventilation may cause a significant reduction in coronary arterial diameter (by 25 to 100%) (193). In fact, patients with coronary artery disease and hyperventilation-induced myocardial ischemia have an increased mortality in comparison with those with coronary disease but without hyperventilation-induced ischemia (193). The sensitivity with which hyperventilation identifies patients with coronary vasospasm ranges from 70 to 80% (186, 188, 191, 194). It is thought that the hypocapnic alkalosis induced by hyperventilation decreases the concentration of hydrogen ions in vascular smooth muscle, thus allowing unbound calcium to induce smooth muscle contraction (195, 197, 198). In support of this mechanism, hyperventilation that is performed with rebreathed air (so that arterial pH and pCO_2 do not change) does not induce coronary arterial spasm (194).

Mental Stress

In some patients with coronary artery disease, mental stress may precipitate ischemia (199). Recent reports have documented a circadian variation in the occurrence of ischemia and infarction, with both occurring frequently in the early morning hours (200-205). The mental arousal state associated with awakening may contribute to this circadian variability, since periods of psychological stress increase the frequency of episodes of silent ischemia (206). Although only a small percentage (14%) of asymptomatic ischemic episodes occur at a time when **patients** consider that their mental state is stressful (207), many more episodes may occur with routine mental activity that is not perceived by the patient as stressful. In support of this, regional perfusion abnormalities may be demonstrated by positron tomography in a large percentage of patients with chronic stable angina during mental arithmetic that is not intended to upset or frustrate them (Fig. 22.16) (208).

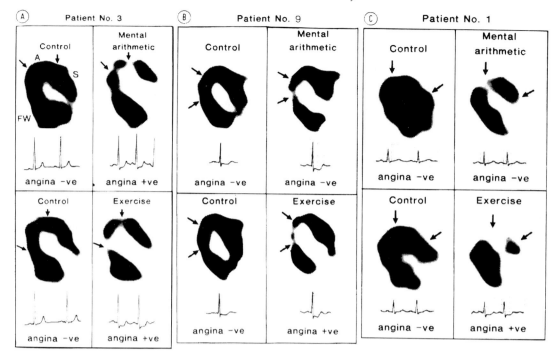

Figure 22.16. Changes in regional myocardial blood flow determined by rubidium-82 positron tomography before and after mental arithmetic in three patients with CAD. Resting (control) scans show homogenous uptake of cation. Mental arithmetic precipitates ischemic ECG changes and regional defects in rubidium uptake with angina, and similar changes with angina occur during exercise. (From Deanfield JE, Shea M, Kensett M, et al. Silent myocardial ischemia due to mental stress. Lancet 1984;2:1001–1005.)

In patients with coronary artery disease, the performance of difficult mental arithmetic causes an increase in heart rate, systemic arterial pressure, and myocardial oxygen consumption. Although quantitative coronary angiography in these patients demonstrates a reduction in the cross-sectional area of all coronary arterial segments (diseased and normal), coronary sinus blood flow rises modestly (199, 208, 209). Thus, in patients with coronary artery disease, mental stress may induce ischemia because it increases oxygen demand.

PHARMACOLOGIC STRESS

Nitroglycerin

Response in Normal Subjects

Nitrates cause relaxation of smooth muscle in the venous capacitance vessels; as a result, venous pooling occurs, and venous return to the heart is diminished. Although nitrates act predominantly on veins rather than arteries (210, 211), they acutely cause arterial vasodilation and decreased systemic vascular resistance at high doses. Thus, the hemodynamic responses that occur with nitrates depend on the dose administered.

At routine therapeutic doses, nitrates cause a modest decrease in systolic and mean arterial pressures, as well as a slight fall in systemic vascular resistance. At the same time, they induce a more profound reduction in pulmonary arterial and left ventricular end-diastolic pressures (212, 213). Left ventricular volumes decline, due to reduced preload and diminished impedance to ejection, and stroke volume is reduced. Since there is usually little change in heart rate, cardiac output falls (214-216). Nitrates exert no demonstrable influence on left ventricular performance (217), unless a large dose causes a profound fall in systemic arterial pressure, with resultant reflex sympathetic stimulation.

Figure 22.17. Changes in minimum cross-sectional area of normal and diseased coronary arteries after sublingual (*S.L.*) nitroglycerin. Coronary arteries are grouped according to severity of stenosis at baseline. All groups demonstrate significant increase in minimum cross-sectional area after nitroglycerin, regardless of severity of baseline stenosis. x, $p < 0.05$; *, $p < 0.01$; +, $p < 0.005$. *MOD* = moderate. (From Brown BG, Bolson E, Petersen RB, Pierce CD, Dodge HT. The mechanisms of nitroglycerin action: stenosis vasodilatation as a major component of the drug response. Circulation 1981;64:1089–1097. By permission of the American Heart Association, Inc.)

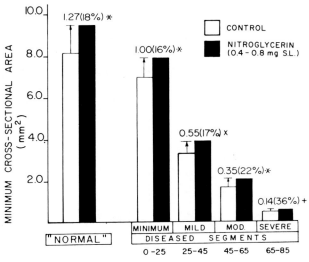

Nitroglycerin is a powerful coronary vasodilator (218, 219), which decreases coronary vascular resistance and increases coronary blood flow (220-222), even in the absence of systemic hemodynamic effects. With exposure to nitroglycerin, the luminal area of normal epicardial coronary arteries increases by about 20%, and smaller coronary arteries dilate even more impressively (219, 220). As shown in Figure 22.17, diseased coronary arteries also retain the ability to dilate in response to nitroglycerin. Nitroglycerin prevents sympathetic coronary vasoconstriction (218), relieves focal coronary arterial spasm, augments blood flow through collaterals to ischemic myocardium (221), and (in animal studies) improves subendocardial perfusion.

Responses in Subjects with Cardiac Disease

The beneficial effects of nitroglycerin in patients with **coronary artery disease** result from its vasodilatory influence on various vascular beds. Similar to the changes noted in normal subjects, nitroglycerin in patients with coronary artery disease induces a fall in left ventricular volumes and pressures, systemic vascular resistance, left ventricular wall tension, and myocardial oxygen demand. During dynamic exercise, patients with coronary artery disease who are pretreated with nitrates have an increased rate-pressure product at the onset of angina, a lower left ven-

tricular end-diastolic volume and pressure, a lower pulmonary-capillary wedge pressure, and a higher ejection fraction at peak exercise than when these same patients are studied during exercise without nitrate pretreatment (213, 214, 216, 223). In addition to their favorable effects on oxygen demand, oxygen supply is increased because of nitrate-induced coronary vasodilatation.

Since nitroglycerin may reverse the left ventricular asynergy associated with ischemia, it has been used to assess residual contractile function of ischemic myocardium. An improvement in global and regional left ventricular function has been noted in patients with coronary artery disease who are given nitroglycerin (224-226), and the regional ventricular response to nitroglycerin appears to be a reliable predictor of improvement in regional asynergy following successful coronary artery bypass surgery (227, 228). Asynergic areas that improve with nitroglycerin are thought to represent myocardium that is ischemic but not irreversibly injured.

When nitrates are given to subjects with **congestive heart failure,** they may induce a dramatic decrease in central venous and right atrial pressure, right ventricular end-systolic and end-diastolic pressures, and pulmonary arterial and left ventricular end-diastolic pressures. Heart rate is usually unchanged, whereas the response of stroke volume and cardiac output is variable. Those with a low cardiac output and a high left ventricular filling pressure before treatment are most likely to manifest an increase in stroke volume and cardiac output with nitrates (229, 230). In these individuals, cardiac output increases primarily because of a reduction in systemic vascular resistance (231).

Isoproterenol

Responses in Normal Subjects

Isoproterenol may be administered (as an intravenous infusion at 1 to 4 μg/min) as another means of provoking a stress response in the catheterization laboratory. Continuous hemodynamic and electrocardiographic monitoring is performed as the rate of infusion is increased until symptoms or electrocardiographic evidence of ischemia are observed. Its advantages are as follows: (*a*) it may be administered in situations where exercise is impossible; (*b*) as opposed to rapid atrial pacing, it may be given at the bedside without invasive monitoring; (*c*) the electrocardiogram is not obscured by motion or pacing artifact; and (*d*) it allows monitoring that may be technically difficult during active exercise. The hemodynamic changes that occur during an infusion of isoproterenol (232-239) are similar to those of dynamic exercise and are the consequence of β-adrenergic stimulation. Heart rate and cardiac output are increased. In young subjects, stroke volume increases substantially (236), whereas in older individuals the increased cardiac output is the result mainly of an increase in heart rate (237, 239, 240). The arterial pulse pressure widens as diastolic pressure falls and systolic pressure rises or is unchanged; mean arterial pressure declines. Systemic and pulmonary vascular resistances decline substantially, due to the vasodilating effects of β_2 stimulation. Pulmonary arterial pressure may decrease or be unchanged (233, 239).

During an isoproterenol infusion, left ventricular ejection fraction rises (241, 242). Increases in max dP/dt (234, 238), mean ejection rate (238, 240), and left ventricular work (in the setting of a decreased systemic vascular resistance) (233, 239, 243) provide evidence that ventricular contractility is enhanced. Left ventricular end-diastolic pressure is unchanged or falls (234, 238, 240). Myocardial oxygen consumption is increased, and coro-

nary blood flow rises markedly; in fact, the increase in flow is out of proportion to the increase in demand, so that myocardial oxygen extraction declines. Thus, isoproterenol causes direct coronary vasodilation (239, 244, 245).

Responses in Subjects with Cardiac Disease

The rate-pressure product that is achieved during an isoproterenol infusion is lower than that which occurs during dynamic exercise, primarily because isoproterenol does not cause a marked increase in systolic arterial pressure (236). Nevertheless, isoproterenol compares favorably with dynamic exercise in identifying patients with **coronary artery disease.** In these patients, an isoproterenol infusion has a sensitivity of 60 to 100% and a specificity of 70 to 80% in the identification of those with coronary artery disease (237, 246-248). Despite the similar hemodynamic responses to exercise and isoproterenol in subjects with coronary artery disease, global and segmental left ventricular performance is affected differently by the two interventions. As Figure 22.18 shows, left ventricular ejection fraction falls with exercise in patients with ischemic heart disease, whereas it increases in response to the infusion of a β-agonist in the same patients (242). Dynamic exercise causes a worsening of regional wall motion abnormalities, while isoproterenol improves regional wall dyskinesia.

The infusion of isoproterenol may be associated with several adverse effects, including sweating, apprehension, facial flushing, tremor, headache, and ventricular premature beats. If used carefully, however, it is safe, and its infusion rarely must be terminated because of intolerable side effects.

In patients with **congestive heart failure,** isoproterenol induces an increase in cardiac output, heart rate, stroke volume, and left and right ventricular stroke work, changes similar to those noted in normal subjects. Systemic and pulmonary vascular resistances fall. In those with heart failure, exercise causes pulmonary arterial pressure to rise, whereas isoproterenol is associated with a decrease in pulmonary arterial pressure (233, 243).

Ergonovine Maleate

Ergot alkaloids induce direct vasoconstriction by stimulating α-adrenergic and serotonin

Figure 22.18. Effects of exercise (*A*) and isoproterenol (isoprenaline)(*C*) on left ventricular ejection fraction in normal subjects (*open circles*) and patients with CAD (*closed circle*). Ejection fraction increases in normal subjects in response to both exercise and isoproterenol. In patients with CAD, left ventricular ejection fraction increases with isoproterenol but decreases with exercise. (From Sapru RP, Muir AL, Hannan WJ, Smith HJ, Brash HM, Wraith PK. Effect of exercise and isoprenaline on left ventricular ejection fraction in patients with angina pectoris as assessed by radionuclide angiography. Cardiology 1982;69:91–97. With permission from S. Karger AG, Basel.)

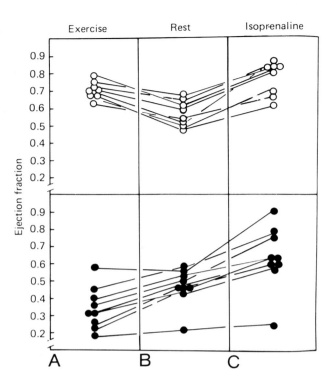

receptors in smooth muscle cells of veins and arteries. In 1949 Stein (249) introduced ergonovine as a provocative agent for coronary artery insufficiency, and in 1975 Heupler et al. (250) suggested that it was useful in provoking episodes of vasospastic angina. The reader is referred to the chapter on coronary arteriography for a description of its use in provoking coronary vasospasm.

Responses in Normal Subjects

The normal human subject responds to the administration of ergonovine with a small (10 to 15%) increase in systolic and mean arterial pressure and no change or a small increase (10%) in heart rate (251-256). Therefore, the rate-pressure product increases modestly (about 25%). Myocardial oxygen consumption usually increases (255, 256). Ergonovine causes an increase in left ventricular end-diastolic and end-systolic dimensions, due, in all probability, to increased venous return to the heart. Stroke volume and ejection fraction do not change significantly. Left ventricular end-diastolic pressure rises modestly (average, 3 mm Hg) with ergonovine (252). The epicardial coronary arteries demonstrate a 15 to 20%

decrease in luminal diameter with ergonovine (251, 255, 257), due to a direct vasoconstricting effect of the drug (257).

Responses in Subjects with Cardiac Disease

Patients with **coronary artery disease** may exhibit symptoms or electrocardiographic changes of ischemia with ergonovine, despite the absence of demonstrable coronary arterial spasm (258). In all probability, this occurs because of an ergonovine-induced increase in myocardial oxygen demand and a concomitant fall in oxygen supply (due to direct vasoconstriction). Subjects with ergonovine-induced ischemia may manifest an increase in left ventricular dimensions and left ventricular end-diastolic pressure, as well as a profound decrease in stroke volume (20 to 30%) and left ventricular ejection fraction (16 to 20%) (252-254).

Amyl Nitrite
Responses in Normal Subjects

Amyl nitrite is a rapidly acting, direct vasodilator that is administered by inhalation. Its

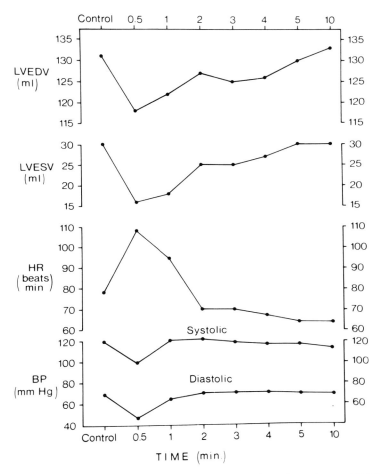

Figure 22.19. Time course of changes in left ventricular end-diastolic volume (*LVEDV*), end-systolic volume (*LVESV*), heart rate (*HR*), and blood pressure (*BP*) after the administration of amyl nitrite. Within 30 sec of amyl nitrite inhalation, there is a marked decline in left ventricular volumes and blood pressure, with a compensatory increase in heart rate. These variables return toward baseline 2 min after amyl nitrite administration. (From Burggraf GW, Parker JO. Left ventricular volume changes after amyl nitrite and nitroglycerin in man as measured by ultrasound. Circulation 1974;49:136–143. By permission of the American Heart Association, Inc.)

maximal hemodynamic effects are evident in 30 sec and resolve in 2 to 5 min (153, 259, 260). Because of its pronounced hypotensive effects, it should be administered to patients in the recumbent position. Its quick onset of action and rapid resolution make it an ideal agent for bedside use.

Within seconds of the inhalation of amyl nitrite, systolic, diastolic, and mean arterial pressures fall dramatically (by 25 to 35%) (153, 259-264), and a reflex tachycardia occurs, with the heart rate increasing 50 to 80%. Cardiac output increases proportionately to the increase in heart rate, since stroke volume does not change. Systemic and pulmonary vascular resistances decline. Left ventricular end-diastolic and end-systolic dimensions fall appreciably (18 and 57%, respectively) (260). Figure 22.19 demonstrates the time course of the changes in left ventricular volumes. Concomitant with a decline in left ventricular end-diastolic volume, end-diastolic pressure falls (259, 260). Myocardial contractility increases because of the sympathetic overdrive that is precipitated by a marked fall in arterial pressure.

Responses in Subjects with Cardiac Disease

In response to amyl nitrite, patients with **coronary artery disease** exhibit the same alterations in hemodynamic variables and ventricular volumes as normal subjects. Although it decreases myocardial oxygen demand and acts as a direct coronary vasodilator (265), it may reduce coronary blood flow because of its profound influence on systemic arterial pressure (266). In fact, some reports have noted that the administration of amyl nitrite may induce ischemic ST-T wave alterations (267, 268), and others have suggested that it may be used to identify subjects with coronary artery disease (262).

In summary, a complete understanding of cardiac hemodynamic function and its response to physiologic and pharmacologic maneuvers is essential for the cardiovascular specialist. In the cardiac catheterization laboratory these functional responses can be assessed directly and quantified in patients with a wide variety of disease states.

References

1. Mitchell JH, Blomqvist G. Maximal oxygen uptake. N Engl J Med 1971;284:1018–1022.
2. Douglas CG. Oliver–Sharpey lecture on the coordination of the respiration and circulation with variations in bodily activity. Lancet 1927;213:213–218.
3. Margaria R, Edwards HT, Dill DB. The possible mechanisms of contracting and paying the oxygen debt and the role of lactic acid in muscular contraction. Am J Physiol 1933;106:689–715.
4. Owles WH. Alterations in the lactic acid content of the blood as a result of light exercise, and associated changes in the CO_2 combining power of the blood and in the alveolar CO_2 pressure. J Physiol (Lond) 1930;69:214–237.
5. Wasserman K. Determinants and detection of anaerobic threshold and consequences of exercise above it. Circulation 1987;76:VI29–39.
6. Lorell BH, Grossman W. Dynamic and isometric exercise during cardiac catheterization. In Grossman W, ed. Cardiac catheterization and angiography, 3rd ed. Philadelphia: Lea & Febiger, 1986:251–266.
7. Mitchell JH. Cardiovascular control during exercise: central and reflex neural mechanisms. Am J Cardiol 1985;55:34D–41D.
8. Cohn JN. Quantitative testing for the cardiac patient: the value of monitoring gas exchange. Circulation 1987;76:VI1–2.
9. Robinson BF, Epstein SE, Beiser GD, Braunwald E. Control of heart rate by the autonomic nervous system. Studies in man on the interrelation between baroreceptor mechanisms and exercise. Circ Res 1966;19:400–411.
10. Thadani U, Parker JO. Hemodynamics at rest and during supine and sitting bicycle exercise in normal subjects. Am J Cardiol 1978;41:52–59.
11. Crawford MH, White DH, Amon KW. Echocardiographic evaluation of left ventricular size and performance during handgrip and supine and upright bicycle exercise. Circulation 1979;59:1188–1196.
12. Wilson M. Left ventricular diameter posture and exercise. Circ Res 1962;11:90–96.
13. Mitchell JH, Wildenthal K. Left ventricular function during exercise. In: Larsen OA, Malmborg RO, eds. Coronary heart disease and physical fitness. Copenhagen: Munksgaard, 1970:93–96.
14. Carroll JD, Hess OM, Studer NP, Hirzel HO, Krayenbuehl HP. Systolic function during exercise in patients with coronary artery disease. J Am Coll Cardiol 1983;2:206–216.
15. Dehmer GJ, Lewis SE, Hillis LD, Corbett J, Parkey RW, Willerson JT. Exercise–induced alterations in left ventricular volumes and the pressure–volume relationship: a sensitive indicator of left ventricular dysfunction in patients with coronary artery disease. Circulation 1981;63:1008–1018.
16. Shen WF, Roubin GS, Hirasawa K, et al. Left ventricular volume and ejection fraction response to exercise in chronic congestive heart failure: difference between dilated cardiomyopathy and previous myocardial infarction. Am J Cardiol 1985;55:1027–1031.
17. Francis GS, Goldsmith SR, Ziesche SM, Cohn JN. Response of plasma norepinephrine and epinephrine to dynamic exercise in patients with congestive heart failure. Am J Cardiol 1982;49:1152–1156.
18. Freeman MR, Berman DS, Staniloff H, et al. Comparison of upright and supine bicycle exercise in the detection and evaluation of extent of coronary artery disease by equilibrium radionuclide ventriculography. Am Heart J 1981;102:182–189.
19. Poliner LR, Dehmer GJ, Lewis SE, Parkey RW, Blomqvist CG, Willerson JT. Left ventricular performance in normal subjects: a comparison of the responses to exercise in the upright and supine positions. Circulation 1980;62:528–534.
20. Port S, McEwan P, Cobb FR, Jones RH. Influence of resting left ventricular function on the left ventricular response to exercise in patients with coronary artery disease. Circulation 1981;63:856–863.
21. Steingart RM, Wexler J, Slagle S, Scheuer J. Radionuclide ventriculographic responses to graded supine and upright exercise: critical role of the Frank–Starling mechanism at submaximal exercise. Am J Cardiol 1984;53:1671–1677.
22. Gorlin R, Cohen LS, Elliott WC, Klein MD, Lane FJ. Effect of supine exercise on left ventricular volume and oxygen consumption in man. Circulation 1965;32:361–371.
23. Sharma B, Goodwin JF, Raphael MJ, Steiner RE, Rainbow RG, Taylor SH. Left ventricular angiography on exercise. A new method of assessing left ventricular function in ischaemic heart disease. Br Heart J 1976;38:59–67.
24. Tebbe V, Hoffmeister N, Sauer G, Neuhaus K, Kreuzer H. Changes in left ventricular diastolic function in coronary artery disease with and with-

out angina pectoris assessed from exercise ventriculography. Clin Cardiol 1980;3:19–26.

25. Carroll JD, Hess OM, Hirzel HO, Krayenbuehl HP. Dynamics of left ventricular filling at rest and during exercise. Circulation 1983;68:59–67.

26. Bruce RA, Petersen JL, Kusumi F. Hemodynamic responses to exercise in the upright posture in patients with ischemic heart disease. In: Dhalla HS, ed. Myocardial metabolism. Baltimore: University Park Press, 1973:849–865.

27. Forrester JS, Diamond GA, Swan HJC. Correlative classification of clinical and hemodynamic function after acute myocardial infarction. Am J Cardiol 1977;39:137–145.

28. Bairey CN, Rozanski A, Levey M, Berman DS. Differences in the frequency of ST segment depression during upright and supine exercise: assessment in normals and in patients with coronary artery disease. Am Heart J 1987;114:1317–1323.

29. Reduto LA, Wickemeyer WJ, Young JB, et al. Left ventricular diastolic performance at rest and during exercise in patients with coronary artery disease. Assessment with first–pass radionuclide angiography. Circulation 1981;63:1228–1237.

30. Wiener L, Dwyer EM Jr, Cox JW. Left ventricular hemodynamics in exercise–induced angina pectoris. Circulation 1968;38:240–249.

31. Iskandrian AS, Heo J, Askenase A, Helfant RH, Segal BL. Factors affecting exercise left ventricular performance in patients free of obstructive coronary artery disease. Am J Cardiol 1987;60:1173–1176.

32. Sugishita Y, Koseki S. Dynamic exercise echocardiography. Circulation 1979;60:743–752.

33. Borer JS, Bacharach SL, Green MV, Kent KM, Epstein SE, Johnston GS. Real–time radionuclide cineangiography in the noninvasive evaluation of global and regional left ventricular function at rest and during exercise in patients with coronary artery disease. N Engl J Med 1977;296:839–844.

34. Caldwell JH, Hamilton GW, Sorensen SG, Ritchie JL, Williams DL, Kennedy JW. The detection of coronary artery disease with radionuclide techniques: a comparison of rest–exercise thallium imaging and ejection fraction response. Circulation 1980;61:610–619.

35. Kimchi A, Rozanski A, Fletcher C, Maddahi J, Swan HJC, Berman DS. The clinical significance of exercise–induced left ventricular wall motion abnormality occurring at a low heart rate. Am Heart J 1987;114:724–730.

36. Thadani U, West RO, Mathew TM, Parker JO. Hemodynamics at rest and during supine and sitting bicycle exercise in patients with coronary artery disease. Am J Cardiol 1977;39:776–783.

37. Clements IP, Gibbons RJ, Mankin HT, Zinsmeister AR, Brown ML. Guidelines for the interpretation of the exercise radionuclide ventriculogram for diagnosing coronary artery disease. Am J Cardiol 1987;60:1265–1268.

38. Rozanski A, Berman DS. The efficacy of cardiovascular nuclear medicine studies. Semin Nucl Med 1987;17:104–120.

39. Miller DD, Ruddy TD, Zusman RM, et al. Left ventricular ejection fraction response during exercise in asymptomatic systemic hypertension. Am J Cardiol 1987;59:409–413.

40. Ellestad MH. Stress testing: Principles and practice. Philadelphia: FA Davis, 1986:113–126.

41. Tristani FE, Hughes CV, Archibald DG, Sheldahl LM, Cohn JN, Fletcher R. Safety of graded symptom–limited exercise testing in patients with congestive heart failure. Circulation 1987;76:VI54–58.

42. Szlachcic J, Massie BM, Kramer BL, Topic N, Tubau J. Correlates and prognostic implication of exercise capacity in chronic congestive heart failure. Am J Cardiol 1985;55:1037–1042.

43. Weber KT, Kinasewitz GT, Janicki JS, Fishman AP. Oxygen utilization and ventilation during exercise in patients with chronic cardiac failure. Circulation 1982;65:1213–1223.

44. Franciosa JA, Baker BJ, Seth L. Pulmonary versus systemic hemodynamics in determining exercise capacity of patients with chronic left ventricular failure. Am Heart J 1985;110:807–813.

45. Franciosa JA, Leddy CL, Wilen M, Schwartz DE. Relation between hemodynamic and ventilatory responses in determining exercise capacity in severe congestive heart failure. Am J Cardiol 1984;53:127–134.

46. Francis GS, Goldsmith SR, Ziesche S, Nakajima H, Cohn JN. Relative attenuation of sympathetic drive during exercise in patients with congestive heart failure. J Am Coll Cardiol 1985;5:832–839.

47. Weber KT, Janicki JS. Lactate production during maximal and submaximal exercise in patients with chronic heart failure. J Am Coll Cardiol 1985;6:717–724.

48. Lipkin DP, Poole–Wilson PA. The mechanism of breathlessness in chronic heart failure (abstr). Circulation 1985;72:III–482.

49. Patterson JA, Naughton J, Pietras RJ, Gunnar RM. Treadmill exercise in assessment of the functional capacity of patients with cardiac disease. Am J Cardiol 1972;30:757–762.

50. Franciosa JA, Ziesche S, Wilen M. Functional capacity of patients with chronic left ventricular failure. Relationship of bicycle exercise performance to clinical and hemodynamic characterization. Am J Med 1979;67:460–465.

51. Benge W, Litchfield RL, Marcus ML. Exercise capacity in patients with severe left ventricular dysfunction. Circulation 1980;61:955–959.

52. Franciosa JA, Park M, Levine TB. Lack of correlation between exercise capacity and indexes of resting left ventricular performance in heart failure. Am J Cardiol 1981;47:33–39.

53. Francis GS, Goldsmith SR, Cohn JN. Relationship of exercise capacity to resting left ventricular performance and basal plasma norepinephrine levels in patients with congestive heart failure. Am Heart J 1982;104:725–731.

54. Hakki AH, Weinreich DJ, Depace L, Iskandrian AS. Correlation between exercise capacity and left ventricular function in patients with severely depressed left ventricular function. J Cardiac Rehabil 1984;4:38–43.

55. Higginbotham MB, Morris KG, Conn EH, Coleman RE, Cobb FR. Determinants of variable exercise performance among patients with severe left ventricular dysfunction. Am J Cardiol 1983;51:52–60.

56. DiBianco R, Shabetai R, Silverman BD, Leier CV, Benotti JR, and the Amrinone Multicenter Study Investigators. Oral amrinone for the treatment of chronic congestive heart failure: results of a multicenter randomized double–blind and placebo–controlled withdrawal study. J Am Coll Cardiol 1984;4:855–866.

57. Maskin CS, Forman R, Sonnenblick EH, Frishman WH, Lejemtel TH. Failure of dobutamine to increase exercise capacity despite hemodynamic improvement in severe chronic heart failure. Am J Cardiol 1983;51:177–182.

58. Franciosa JA, Wilen MM, Baker BJ. Functional capacity and long–term survival in chronic left ventricular failure (abstr). Circulation 1983;68:III–149.

59. Wilson JR, Schwartz JS, St John Sutton M, et al. Prognosis in severe heart failure: relation to hemodynamic measurements and ventricular ectopy. J Am Coll Cardiol 1983;2:403–410.

60. Clausen JP. Circulatory adjustments to dynamic exercise and effect of physical training in normal subjects and in patients with coronary artery disease. Prog Cardiovasc Dis 1976;18:459–495.

61. Franciosa JA, Cohn JN. Effect of isosorbide dinitrate on response to submaximal and maximal exercise in patients with congestive heart failure. Am J Cardiol 1979;43:1009–1014.

62. Franciosa JA, Cohn JN. Immediate effects of hydralazine–isosorbide dinitrate combination on exercise capacity and exercise hemodynamics in patients with left ventricular failure. Circulation 1979;59:1085–1091.

63. Franciosa JA, Goldsmith SR, Cohn JN. Contrasting immediate and long term effects of isosorbide dinitrate on exercise capacity in congestive heart failure. Am J Med 1980;69:559–566.

64. Rubin SA, Chatterjee KJ, Parmley WW. Metabolic assessment of exercise in chronic heart failure patients treated with short–term vasodilators. Circulation 1980;61:543–548.

65. Gorlin R, Sawyer CG, Haynes FW, Goodale WT, Dexter L. Effects of exercise on circulatory dynamics in mitral stenosis. Am Heart J 1951;41:192–203.

66. Ross J Jr, Gault JH, Mason DT, Linhart JW, Braunwald E. Left ventricular performance during muscular exercise in patients with and without cardiac dysfunction. Circulation 1966;34:597–608.

67. Arandi DT, Carleton RA. The deleterious role of tachycardia in mitral stenosis. Circulation 1967;36:511–516.

68. Braunwald E. Heart disease: a textbook of cardiovascular medicine, 2nd ed. Philadelphia: W.B. Saunders, 1984:1064–1135.

69. Flamm MD, Braniff BA, Kimball R, Hancock EW. Mechanism of effort syncope in aortic stenosis (abstr). Circulation 1967;35,36:II109.

70. Anderson FL, Tsagaris TJ, Tikoff G, Thorne JL, Schmidt AM, Kuida H. Hemodynamic effects of exercise in patients with aortic stenosis. Am J Med 1969;46:872–885.

71. Bache RJ, Wang Y, Jorgensen CR. Hemodynamic effects of exercise in isolated valvular aortic stenosis. Circulation 1971;44:1003–1013.

72. Richardson JW, Anderson FL, Tsagaris TJ. Rest and exercise hemodynamic studies in patients with isolated aortic stenosis. Cardiology 1979;64:1–11.

73. Henze E, Schelbert HR, Wisenberg G, Ratib O, Schon H. Assessment of regurgitant fraction and right and left ventricular function at rest and during exercise: a new technique for determination of right ventricular stroke counts from gated equilibrium blood pool studies. Am Heart J 1982;104:953–962.

74. Borer JS, Bacharach SL, Green MV, et al. Exercise–induced left ventricular dysfunction in symptomatic and asymptomatic patients with aortic regurgitation: assessment with radionuclide cineangiography. Am J Cardiol 1978;42:351–357.

75. Huxley RL, Gaffney FA, Corbett JR, et al. Early detection of left ventricular dysfunction in chronic aortic regurgitation as assessed by contrast angiography, echocardiography, and rest and exercise scintigraphy. Am J Cardiol 1983;51:1542–1550.

76. Johnson LL, Powers ER, Tzall WR, Feder J, Sciacca RR, Cannon PJ. Left ventricular volume and ejection fraction response to exercise in aortic regurgitation. Am J Cardiol 1983;51:1379–1385.

77. Massie B, Kramer B, Topic N, et al. Exercise hemodynamic responses in asymptomatic aortic regurgitation (abstr). J Am Coll Cardiol 1984;3:534.

78. Dehmer GJ, Firth BG, Hillis LD, et al. Alterations in left ventricular volumes and ejection fraction at rest and during exercise in patients with aortic regurgitation. Am J Cardiol 1981;48:17–27.

79. Bonow RO, Rosing DR, McIntosh CL, et al. The natural history of asymptomatic patients with aortic regurgitation and normal left ventricular function. Circulation 1983;68:509–517.

80. Gerstenblith G, Lakatta EG, Wesifeldt ML. Age changes in myocardial function and exercise response. Prog Cardiovasc Dis 1976;19:1–21.

81. Raven PB, Mitchell J. The effect of aging on the cardiovascular response to dynamic and static exercise. Aging 1980;12:269–296.

82. Rodeheffer RJ, Gerstenblith G, Becker LC, Fleg JL, Wesifeldt ML, Lakatta EG. Exercise cardiac output is maintained with advancing age in healthy human subjects: cardiac dilatation and increased stroke volume compensate for a diminished heart rate. Circulation 1984;69:203–213.

83. Donald KW, Lind AR, McNicol GW, Humphreys PW, Taylor SH, Staunton HP. Cardiovascular responses to sustained (static) contractions. Circ Res 1967;20,21:II5–30.

84. Matthews OA, Atkins JM, Houston JD, Blomqvist G, Mullins CB. Arrhythmias induced by isometric exercise (abstr). Clin Res 1971;19:23.

85. Amende I, Krayenbuehl HP, Rutishauser W, Wirz P. Left ventricular dynamics during handgrip. Br Heart J 1972;34:688–695.

86. Bodenheimer MM, Banka VS, Fooshee CM, Gillespie JA, Helfant RH. Detection of coronary heart disease using radionuclide determined regional ejection fraction at rest and during handgrip exercise: correlation with coronary arteriography. Circulation 1978;58:640–648.

87. Ewing DJ, Irving JB, Kerr F, Kirby BJ. Static exercise in untreated systemic hypertension. Br Heart J 1973;35:413–421.

88. Fisher ML, Nutter DO, Jacobs W, Schlant RC. Haemodynamic responses to isometric exercise

(handgrip) in patients with heart disease. Br Heart J 1973;35:422–432.

89. Flessas AP, Connelly GP, Handa S, et al. Effects of isometric exercise on the end–diastolic pressure, volumes, and function of the left ventricle in man. Circulation 1976;53:839–847.

90. Helfant RH, DeVilla MA, Banka VS. Evaluation of left ventricular performance in coronary heart disease: use of isometric handgrip stress test. Cathet Cardiovasc Diagn 1976;2:59–67.

91. Helfant RH, DeVilla MA, Meister SG. Effect of sustained isometric handgrip exercise on left ventricular performance. Circulation 1971;44:982–993.

92. Kivowitz C, Parmley WW, Donoso R, Marcus H, Ganz W, Swan HJC. Effects of isometric exercise on cardiac performance. The grip test. Circulation 1971;44:994–1002.

93. Krayenbuehl HP, Rutishauser W, Schoenbeck M, Amende I. Evaluation of left ventricular function from isovolumic pressure measurements during isometric exercise. Am J Cardiol 1972;29:323–330.

94. Krayenbuehl HP, Rutishauser W, Wirz P, Amende I, Mehmel H. High–fidelity left ventricular pressure measurements for the assessment of cardiac contractility in man. Am J Cardiol 1973;31:415–427.

95. Ludbrook P, Karliner JS, O'Rourke RA. Effects of submaximal isometric handgrip on left ventricular size and wall motion. Am J Cardiol 1974;33:30–36.

96. Payne RM, Horwitz LD, Mullins CB. Comparison of isometric exercise and angiotensin infusion as stress test for evaluation of left ventricular function. Am J Cardiol 1973;31:428–433.

97. Perez–Gonzales JF, Schiller NB, Parmley WW. Direct and noninvasive evaluation of the cardiovascular response to isometric exercise. Circ Res 1981;48:I138–148.

98. Savin WM, Alderman EL, Haskell WL, et al. Left ventricular response to isometric exercise in patients with denervated and innervated hearts. Circulation 1980;61:897–901.

99. Siegel W, Gilbert CA, Nutter DO, Schlant RC, Hurst JW. Use of isometric handgrip for the indirect assessment of left ventricular function in patients with coronary atherosclerotic heart disease. Am J Cardiol 1972;30:48–54.

100. Stefadouros MA, Grossman W, El Shahawy M, Stefadouros F, Witham AC. Noninvasive study of effect of isometric exercise on left ventricular performance in normal man. Br Heart J 1974;36:988–995.

101. Sagiv M, Hanson P, Besozzi M, Nagle F. Left ventricular responses to upright isometric handgrip and deadlift in men with coronary artery disease. Am J Cardiol 1985;55:1298–1302.

102. Broudy DR, Greenberg BH, Siemienczuk D, Reinhart S, Morris C, Demots H. Static exercise with congestive heart failure and the response to vasodilating drugs. Am J Cardiol 1987;59:100–104.

103. Elkayam U, Roth A, Weber L, et al. Isometric exercise in patients with chronic advanced heart failure: hemodynamic and neurohumoral evaluation. Circulation 1985;72:975–981.

104. Ricci DR, Orlick AE, Alderman EL, et al. Role of

tachycardia as an inotropic stimulus in man. J Clin Invest 1979;63:695–703.

105. Sonnenblick EH, Morrow AG, Williams JF Jr. Effects of heart rate on the dynamics of force development in the intact human ventricle. Circulation 1966;33:945–951.

106. Forrester JS, Helfant RH, Pasternac A, et al. Atrial pacing in coronary heart disease. Effect on hemodynamics, metabolism and coronary circulation. Am J Cardiol 1971;27:237–243.

107. Parker JO, Chiong MA, West RO, Case RB. Sequential alterations in myocardial lactate metabolism, S–T segments, and left ventricular function during angina induced by atrial pacing. Circulation 1969;40:113–131.

108. Dwyer EM Jr. Left ventricular pressure–volume alterations and regional disorders of contraction during myocardial ischemia induced by atrial pacing. Circulation 1970;42:1111–1122.

109. Khaja F, Parker JO, Ledwich RJ, West RO, Armstrong PW. Assessment of ventricular function in coronary artery disease by means of atrial pacing and exercise. Am J Cardiol 1970;26:107–116.

110. Krayenbuehl HP, Schoenbeck M, Rutishauser W, Wirz P. Abnormal segmental contraction velocity in coronary artery disease produced by isometric exercise and atrial pacing. Am J Cardiol 1975;35:785–794.

111. Linhart JW. Pacing–induced changes in stroke volume in the evaluation of myocardial function. Circulation 1971;43:253–261.

112. Linhart JW. Myocardial function in coronary artery disease determined by atrial pacing. Circulation 1971;44:203–212.

113. Mann T, Brodie BR, Grossman W, McLaurin LP. Effect of angina on the left ventricular diastolic pressure–volume relationship. Circulation 1977;55:761–766.

114. McLaurin LP, Rolett EL, Grossman W. Impaired left ventricular relaxation during pacing–induced ischemia. Am J Cardiol 1973;32:751–757.

115. Parker JO, Khaja F, Case RB. Analysis of left ventricular function by atrial pacing. Circulation 1971;43:241–252.

116. Parker JO, Ledwich JR, West RO, Case RB. Reversible cardiac failure during angina pectoris. Hemodynamic effects of atrial pacing in coronary artery disease. Circulation 1969;39:745–757.

117. Ross J Jr, Linhart JW, Braunwald E. Effects of changing heart rate in man by electrical stimulation of the right atrium. Studies at rest, during exercise, and with isoproterenol. Circulation 1965;32:549–558.

118. Dehmer GJ, Firth BG, Nicod P, Lewis SE, Hillis LD. Alterations in left ventricular volumes and ejection fraction during atrial pacing in patients with coronary artery disease: assessment with radionuclide ventriculography. Am Heart J 1983;106:114–124.

119. Markham RV Jr, Winniford MD, Firth BG, et al. Symptomatic, electrocardiographic, metabolic, and hemodynamic alterations during pacing–induced myocardial ischemia. Am J Cardiol 1983;51:1589–1594.

120. Leighton RF, Zaron SJ, Robinson JL, Weissler AM. Effects of atrial pacing on left ventricular perfor-

mance in patients with heart disease. Circulation 1969;40:615–622.

121. Aroesty JM, McKay RG, Heller GV, Royal HD, Als AV, Grossman W. Simultaneous assessment of left ventricular systolic and diastolic dysfunction during pacing–induced ischemia. Circulation 1985;71:889–900.

122. Mann T, Goldberg S, Mudge GH Jr, Grossman W. Factors contributing to altered left ventricular diastolic properties during angina pectoris. Circulation 1979;59:14–20.

123. DeMaria AN, Neumann A, Schubart PJ, Lee G, Mason DT. Systematic correlation of cardiac chamber size and ventricular performance determined with echocardiography and alterations in heart rate in normal persons. Am J Cardiol 1979;43:1–9.

124. Bahler RC, Macleod CA. Atrial pacing and exercise in the evaluation of patients with angina pectoris. Circulation 1971;43:407–419.

125. Kelemen MH, Gillilan RE, Bouchard RJ, Heppner RL, Warbasse JR. Diagnosis of obstructive coronary disease by maximal exercise and atrial pacing. Circulation 1973;48:1227–1233.

126. Boudoulas H, Cobb TC, Leighton RF, Wilt SM. Myocardial lactate production in patients with angina–like chest pain and angiographically normal coronary arteries and left ventricle. Am J Cardiol 1974;34:501–505.

127. Helfant RH, Forrester JS, Hampton JR, Haft JI, Kemp HG, Gorlin R. Coronary heart disease. Differential hemodynamic, metabolic, and electrocardiographic effects in subjects with and without angina pectoris during atrial pacing. Circulation 1970;42:601–610.

128. Linhart JW, Hildner FJ, Barold SS, Lister JW, Samet P. Left heart hemodynamics during angina pectoris induced by atrial pacing. Circulation 1969;40:483–492.

129. Mammohansingh P, Parker JO. Angina pectoris with normal coronary arteriograms: hemodynamic and metabolic response to atrial pacing. Am Heart J 1975;90:555–561.

130. Rios JC, Hurwitz LE. Electrocardiographic responses to atrial pacing and multistage treadmill exercise testing. Correlation with coronary arteriography. Am J Cardiol 1974;34:661–666.

131. Robson RH, Pridie R, Fluck DC. Evaluation of rapid atrial pacing in diagnosis of coronary artery disease. Evaluation of atrial pacing test. Br Heart J 1976;38:986–989.

132. O'Brien KP, Higgs LM, Glancy DL, Epstein SE. Hemodynamic accompaniments of angina. A comparison during angina induced by exercise and by atrial pacing. Circulation 1969;39:735–743.

133. Heller GV, Aroesty JM, McKay RG, et al. The pacing stress test: a reexamination of the relation between coronary artery disease and pacing–induced electrocardiographic changes. Am J Cardiol 1984;54:50–55.

134. Hecht HS, Chew CY, Burnam M, Schnugg SJ, Hopkins JM, Singh BN. Radionuclide ejection fraction and regional wall motion during atrial pacing in stable angina pectoris: comparison with metabolic and hemodynamic parameters. Am Heart J 1981;101:726–733.

135. Pasternac A, Gorlin R, Sonnenblick EH, Haft JI,

Kemp HG. Abnormalities of ventricular motion induced by atrial pacing in coronary artery disease. Circulation 1972;45:1195–1205.

136. Stone D, Dymond D, Elliott AT, Britton KE, Spurrell RAJ, Banim SO. Use of first–pass radionuclide ventriculography in assessment of wall motion abnormalities induced by incremental atrial pacing in patients with coronary artery disease. Br Heart J 1980;43:369–375.

137. Brooker JZ, Alderman EL, Harrison DC. Alterations in left ventricular volumes induced by Valsalva manoeuvre. Br Heart J 1974;36:713–718.

138. Gorlin R, Knowles JH, Storey CF. The Valsalva maneuver as a test of cardiac function. Pathologic physiology and clinical significance. Am J Med 1957;22:197–212.

139. Labovitz AJ, Dincer B, Mudd G, Aker UT, Kennedy HL. The effects of Valsalva maneuver on global and segmental left ventricular function in presence and absence of coronary artery disease. Am Heart J 1985;109:259–264.

140. Little WC, Barr WK, Crawford MH. Altered effect of the Valsalva maneuver on left ventricular volume in patients with cardiomyopathy. Circulation 1985;71:227–233.

141. Parisi AF, Harrington JJ, Askenazi J, Pratt RC, McIntyre KM. Echocardiographic evaluation of the Valsalva maneuver in healthy subjects and patients with and without heart failure. Circulation 1976;54:921–927.

142. Robertson D, Stevens RM, Friesinger GC, Oates JA. The effect of the Valsalva maneuver on echocardiographic dimensions in man. Circulation 1977;55:596–602.

143. Rubin SA, Brundage B, Mayer W, Chatterjee K. Usefulness of Valsalva manoeuvre and cold pressor test for evaluation of arrhythmias in long QT syndrome. Br Heart J 1979;42:490–492.

144. Zema MJ, Restivo B, Sos T, Sniderman KW, Kline S. Left ventricular dysfunction— bedside Valsalva manoeuvre. Br Heart J 1980;44:560–569.

145. Nishimura RA, Tajik AJ. The Valsalva maneuver and response revisited. Mayo Clin Proc 1986;61:211–217.

146. Palmero HA, Caeiro TF, Iosa DJ, Bas J. Baroreceptor reflex sensitivity index derived from phase 4 of the Valsalva maneuver. Hypertension 1981;3:II134–137.

147. Kalbfleisch JH, Reinke JA, Porth CJ, Ebert TJ, Smith JJ. Effect of age on circulating response to postural and Valsalva tests. Proc Soc Exp Biol Med 1977;156:100–103.

148. Ewing DJ, Campbell IW, Burt AA, Clark BF. Vascular reflexes in diabetic autonomic neuropathy. Lancet 1973;2:1354–1356.

149. Ibrahim MM, Tarazi RC, Dustan HP. Orthostatic hypotension: mechanisms and management. Am Heart J 1975;90:513–520.

150. Ruskin J, Harley A, Greenfield JC Jr. Pressure flow studies in patients having a pressor response to the Valsalva maneuver. Circulation 1968;38:277–281.

151. Pepine CJ, Wiener L. Effects of the Valsalva maneuver on myocardial ischemia in patients with coronary artery disease. Circulation 1979;59:1304–1311.

152. Levine HJ, McIntyre KM, Glovsky MM. Relief of angina pectoris by Valsalva maneuver. N Engl J Med 1966;275:487–489.

153. Benchimol A, Wang TF, Desser KB, Gartlan JL Jr. The Valsalva maneuver and coronary arterial blood flow velocity. Studies in man. Ann Intern Med 1972;77:357–360.

154. Rothman A, Goldberger AL. Aids to cardiac auscultation. Ann Intern Med 1983;99:346–353.

155. Moreyra E, Buteler B, Madoery R, Alday L. Drugs and maneuvers in the diagnosis of muscular subaortic stenosis. Am Heart J 1972;83:431–433.

156. Rosenblum R, Delman AJ. Valsalva's maneuver and the systolic murmur of hypertrophic subaortic stenosis: a bedside diagnostic test. Am J Cardiol 1965;15:868–870.

157. Barlow JB, Pocock WA, Marchand P, Denny M. The significance of late systolic murmurs. Am Heart J 1963;66:443–452.

158. Erfan A, Abdel–Salam R. The effect of the Valsalva maneuver on cardiac vibrations: a phonocardiographic study. J Egypt Med Assoc 1966;49:1–23.

159. Stefadouros MA, Mucha E, Frank MJ. Paradoxic response of the murmur of idiopathic hypertrophic subaortic stenosis to the Valsalva maneuver. Am J Cardiol 1976;37:89–92.

160. Polis 0, Cleempoel H, Hanson J, van Thiele E. Interet de l'epreuve de Valsalva en phonocardiographie. Acta Cardiol 1960;15:441–462.

161. Buda AJ, Pinsky MR, Ingels NB Jr, Daughters GT, Stinson EB, Alderman EL. Effect of intrathoracic pressure on left ventricular performance. N Engl J Med 1979;301:453–459.

162. Smucker ML, Cassidy SS, Nixon JV. Effect of the Mueller manoeuvre at different lung volumes on left ventricular performance in normal subjects. Clin Physiol 1983;3:411–421.

163. Scharf SM, Brown R, Tow DE, Parisi AF. Cardiac effects of increased lung volume and decreased pleural pressure in man. J Appl Physiol 1979;47:257–262.

164. Brinker JA, Weiss JL, Lappe DL, et al. Leftward septal displacement during right ventricular loading in man. Circulation 1980;61:626–633.

165. Condos WR Jr, Latham RD, Hoadley SD, Pasipoularides A. Hemodynamics of the Mueller maneuver in man: right and left heart micromanometry and Doppler echocardiography. Circulation 1987;76:1020–1028.

166. Sharpey–Schafer EP. Effect of respiratory acts on the circulation. In: Hamilton WF, Dow P, eds. Handbook of physiology, section 2. Washington, DC: Williams & Wilkins, 1965:1875–1886.

167. Buda AJ, MacKenzie GW, Wigle ED. Effect of negative intrathoracic pressure on left ventricular outflow tract obstruction in muscular subaortic stenosis. Circulation 1981;63:875–881.

168. Magder SA, Lichtenstein S, Adelman AG. Effects of negative pleural pressure on left ventricular hemodynamics. Am J Cardiol 1983;52:588–593.

169. Pennock RS, Kawai N, Segal BL. Physiologic and pharmacologic aids in cardiac auscultation. In: Fowler NO, ed. Diagnostic methods in cardiology. Philadelphia: FA Davis, 1975:29.

170. Bartall H, Amber S, Desser KB, Benchimol A. Normalization of the external carotid pulse tracing of hypertrophic subaortic stenosis during Muller's maneuver. Chest 1978;74:77–78.

171. Chierchia S, Davies G, Berkenboom G, Crea F, Crean P, Maseri A. α–adrenergic receptors and coronary spasm: an elusive link. Circulation 1984;69:8–14.

172. Feldman RL, Whittle JL, Marx JD, Pepine CJ, Conti CR. Regional coronary hemodynamic responses to cold stimulation in patients without variant angina. Am J Cardiol 1982;49:665–673.

173. Jordan LJ, Borer JS, Zullo M, et al. Exercise versus cold temperature stimulation during radionuclide cineangiography: diagnostic accuracy in coronary artery disease. Am J Cardiol 1983;51:1091–1097.

174. Malacoff RF, Mudge GH Jr, Holman BL, Idoine J, Bifolck L, Cohn PF. Effect of the cold pressor test on regional myocardial blood flow in patients with coronary artery disease. Am Heart J 1983;106:78–84.

175. Manyari DE, Nolewajka AJ, Purves P, Donner A, Kostuk WJ. Comparative value of the cold–pressor test and supine bicycle exercise to detect subjects with coronary artery disease using radionuclide ventriculography. Circulation 1982;65:571–579.

176. Mudge GH Jr, Goldberg S, Gunther S, Mann T, Grossman W. Comparison of metabolic and vasoconstrictor stimuli on coronary vascular resistance in man. Circulation 1979;59:544–550.

177. Shea MJ, Deanfield JE, deLandsheere CM, Wilson RA, Kensett M, Selwyn AP. Asymptomatic myocardial ischemia following cold provocation. Am Heart J 1987;114:469–476.

178. Stratton JR, Halter JB, Hallstrom AP, Caldwell JH, Ritchie JL. Comparative plasma catecholamine and hemodynamic responses to handgrip, cold pressor and supine bicycle exercise testing in normal subjects. J Am Coll Cardiol 1983;2:93–104.

179. Wainwright RJ, Brennand–Roper DA, Cueni TA, Sowton E, Hilson AJW, Maisey MN. Cold pressor test in detection of coronary heart disease and cardiomyopathy using technetium–99m gated blood–pool imaging. Lancet 1979;2:320–323.

180. Waters DD, Szlachcic J, Bonan R, Miller DD, Dauwe F, Theroux P. Comparative sensitivity of exercise, cold pressor and ergonovine testing in provoking attacks of variant angina in patients with active disease. Circulation 1983;67:310–315.

181. Mudge GH Jr, Grossman W, Mills RM Jr, Lesch M, Braunwald E. Reflex increase in coronary vascular resistance in patients with ischemic heart disease. N Engl J Med 1976;295:1333–1337.

182. Raizner AE, Chahine RA, Ishimori T, et al. Provocation of coronary artery spasm by the cold pressor test. Hemodynamic, arteriographic and quantitative angiographic observations. Circulation 1980;62:925–932.

183. Gondi B, Nanda NC. Cold pressor test during two–dimensional echocardiography: usefulness in detection of patients with coronary disease. Am Heart J 1984;107:278–285.

184. Kern MJ, Ganz P, Horowitz JD, et al. Potentiation of coronary vasoconstriction by beta–adrenergic blockade in patients with coronary artery disease. Circulation 1983;67:1178–1185.

185. Mueller HS, Rao PS, Rao PB, Gory DJ, Mudd JG, Ayres SM. Enhanced transcardiac 1-nore-

pinephrine response during cold pressor test in obstructive coronary artery disease. Am J Cardiol 1982;50:1223–1228.

186. Crea F, Davies G, Chierchia S, et al. Different susceptibility to myocardial ischemia provoked by hyperventilation and cold pressor test in exertional and variant angina pectoris. Am J Cardiol 1985;56:18–22.

187. Ahmad M, Dubiel JP, Haibach H. Cold pressor thallium–201 myocardial scintigraphy in the diagnosis of coronary artery disease. Am J Cardiol 1982;50:1253–1257.

188. Balino NAP, Liprandi AS, Masoli 0, et al. Usefulness of radionuclide ventriculography in assessment of coronary artery spasm. Am J Cardiol 1987;59:552–558.

189. Wynne J, Holman BL, Mudge GH Jr, Borow KM. Clinical utility of cold pressor ventriculography in coronary artery disease (abstr). Am J Cardiol 1981;47:444.

190. Rowe GG, Castillo CA, Crumpton CW. Effects of hyperventilation on systemic and coronary hemodynamics. Am Heart J 1962;63:67–77.

191. Girotti LA, Crosatto JR, Messuti H, et al. The hyperventilation test as a method for developing successful therapy in Prinzmetal's angina. Am J Cardiol 1982;49:834–841.

192. Rasmussen K, Bagger JP, Bottzauw J, Henningsen P. Prevalence of vasospastic ischemia induced by the cold pressor test or hyperventilation in patients with severe angina. Eur Heart J 1984;5:354–361.

193. Rasmussen K, Juul S, Bagger JP, Henningsen P. Usefulness of ST deviation induced by prolonged hyperventilation as a predictor of cardiac death in angina pectoris. Am J Cardiol 1987;59:763–768.

194. Ardissino D, De Servi S, Falcone C, et al. Role of hypocapnic alkalosis in hyperventilation–induced coronary artery spasm in variant angina. Am J Cardiol 1987;59:707–709.

195. Yasue H, Nagao M, Omote S, Takizawa A, Miwa K, Tanaka S. Coronary arterial spasm and Prinzmetal's variant form of angina induced by hyperventilation and tris–buffer infusion. Circulation 1978;58:56–62.

196. Neill WA, Hattenhauer M. Impairment of O_2 supply due to hyperventilation. Circulation 1975;52:854–858.

197. Fleckenstein A, Nakayama K, Fleckenstein–Grun B, Byron YK. Interaction of H ions, Ca antagonist drugs and cardiac glycosides with excitation contraction coupling of vascular smooth muscle. In: Betz E, ed. Ionic action on vascular smooth muscle. Berlin: Springer Verlag, 1976:117–125.

198. Mrwa U, Achtig I, Reugg JC. Influences of calcium concentration and pH on the tension development and ATPase activity of the arterial actomyosin contractile system. Blood Vessels 1974;11:277–286.

199. Specchia G, de Servi S, Falcone C, et al. Mental arithmetic stress testing in patients with coronary artery disease. Am Heart J 1984;108:56–63.

200. Deanfield JE, Selwyn AP, Chierchia S, Maseri A, Ribiero P, Krikler S. Myocardial ischemia during daily life in patients with stable angina: its relation to symptoms and heart rate change. Lancet 1983;2:753–758.

201. Johansson BW. Myocardial infarction in Malmo, 1960–1968. Acta Med Scand 1972;191:505–515.

202. Muller JE, Stone PH, Turi ZG, et al. Circadian variation in the frequency of onset of acute myocardial infarction. N Engl J Med 1985;313:1315–1322.

203. Pedoe HT, Clayton D, Morris JN, Brigden W, McDonald L. Coronary heart attacks in East London. Lancet 1975;2:833–838.

204. Pell S, D'Alonzo CA. Acute myocardial infarction in a large industrial population. Report of a 6 year study of 1356. JAMA 1963;185:831–838.

205. Rocco MB, Barry J, Campbell S, et al. Circadian variation of transient myocardial ischemia in patients with coronary artery disease. Circulation 1987;75:395–400.

206. Freeman LJ, Nixon PGF, Sallabank P, Reaveley D. Psychological stress and silent myocardial ischemia. Am Heart J 1987;114:477–482.

207. Campbell S, Barry J, Rebecca GS, et al. Active transient myocardial ischemia during daily life in asymptomatic patients with positive exercise tests and coronary artery disease. Am J Cardiol 1986;57:1010–1016.

208. Deanfield JE, Shea M, Kensett M, et al. Silent myocardial ischemia due to mental stress. Lancet 1984;2:1001–1005.

209. Bassan MM, Marcus HS, Ganz W. The effect of mild–to–moderate mental stress on coronary hemodynamics in patients with coronary artery disease. Circulation 1980;62:933–935.

210. Miller RR, Vismara LA, Williams DO, Amsterdam EA, Mason DT. Pharmacologic mechanisms for left ventricular unloading in clinical congestive heart failure. Differential effects of nitroprusside, phentolamine and nitroglycerin on cardiac function and peripheral circulation. Circ Res 1976;39:127–133.

211. Opie LH. Nitrates. Lancet 1980;1:750–753.

212. Mookherjee S, Fuleihan D, Warner RA, Vardan S, Obeid AI. Effects of sublingual nitroglycerin on resting pulmonary gas exchange and hemodynamics in man. Circulation 1978;57:106–110.

213. Parker JO, di Giorgi S, West RO. A hemodynamic study of acute coronary insufficiency precipitated by exercise. With observations on the effects of nitroglycerin. Am J Cardiol 1966;17:470–483.

214. Choong CYP, Roubin GS, Bautovich GJ, Harris PJ, Kelly DT. Antianginal effects of nitroglycerin during exercise–induced angina: hemodynamic and left ventricular function changes related to indexes of myocardial oxygen consumption. Am J Cardiol 1987;60:1OH–14H.

215. Mason DT, Braunwald E. The effects of amyl nitrite and nitroglycerin on the arterial and venous beds in man (abstr). Am J Cardiol 1965;15:139.

216. Udhoji VN, Heng MK. Hemodynamic effects of high–dose sustained–action oral isosorbide dinitrate in stable angina. Am J Med 1984;76:234–240.

217. Kingma I, Smiseth OA, Belenkie I, et al. A mechanism for the nitroglycerin–induced down–ward shift of the left ventricular diastolic pressure–diameter relation. Am J Cardiol 1986;57:673–677.

218. Brown BG. Response of normal and diseased epicardial coronary arteries to vasoactive drugs:

quantitative arteriographic studies. Am J Cardiol 1985;56:23E–29E.

219. Brown BG, Bolson E, Petersen RB, Pierce CD, Dodge HT. The mechanisms of nitroglycerin action: stenosis vasodilatation as a major component of the drug response. Circulation 1981;64:1089–1097.

220. Feldman RL, Marx JD, Pepine CJ, Conti CR. Analysis of coronary responses to various doses of intracoronary nitroglycerin. Circulation 1982;66:321–327.

221. Kern MJ, Miller JT, Henry RL. Attenuation of nitroglycerin–induced coronary hyperemic blood flow in patients with left anterior descending coronary collaterals. Clin Cardiol 1987;10:506–511.

222. May DC, Popma JJ, Black WH, et al. In vivo induction and reversal of nitroglycerin tolerance in human coronary arteries. N Engl J Med 1987;317:805–809.

223. Pepine CJ, Joyal M, Cremer KF, Hill JA, Feldman RL, Gelman JS. Hemodynamic effects of nitroglycerin combined with diltiazem in patients with coronary artery disease. Am J Med 1984;76:47–51.

224. Dumesnil JG, Ritman EL, Davis GD, Gau GT, Rutherford BD, Frye RL. Regional left ventricular wall dynamics before and after sublingual administration of nitroglycerin. Am J Cardiol 1975;36:419–425.

225. McAnulty JH, Hattenhauer MT, Rosch J, Kloster FE, Rahimtoola SH. Improvement in left ventricular wall motion following nitroglycerin. Circulation 1975;51:140–145.

226. Pepine CJ, Feldman RL, Ludbrook P, et al. Left ventricular dyskinesia reversed by intravenous nitroglycerin: a manifestation of silent myocardial ischemia. Am J Cardiol 1986;58:38B–42B.

227. Chesebro JH, Ritman EL, Frye RL, et al. Regional myocardial wall thickening response to nitroglycerin–a predictor of myocardial response to aortocoronary bypass surgery. Circulation 1978;57:952–957.

228. Helfant RH, Pine R, Meister SG, Feldman MS, Trout RG, Banka VS. Nitroglycerin to unmask reversible asynergy. Correlation with post coronary bypass ventriculography. Circulation 1974;50:108–113.

229. Franciosa JA, Blank RC, Cohn JN. Nitrate effects on cardiac output and left ventricular outflow resistance in chronic congestive heart failure. Am J Med 1978;64:207–213.

230. Gold HK, Leinbach RC, Sanders CA. Use of sublingual nitroglycerin in congestive heart failure following acute myocardial infarction. Circulation 1972;46:839–845.

231. Cohn JN. Role of nitrates in congestive heart failure. Am J Cardiol 1987;60:39H–43H.

232. Cokkinos DV, Tsartsalis GD, Heimonas ET, Gardikas CD. Comparison of the inotropic action of digitalis and isoproterenol in younger and older individuals. Am Heart J 1980;100:802–806.

233. Dodge HT, Lord JD, Sandler H. Cardiovascular effects of isoproterenol in normal subjects and subjects with congestive heart failure. Am Heart J 1960;60:94–105.

234. Firth BG, Tan LB, Rajagopalan B, Schultz DL, Lee GJ. Assessment of myocardial performance in ischaemic heart disease: from changes in left ventricular power output produced by graded-dose isoprenaline infusion. Cardiovasc Res 1981;15:351–364.

235. Fitzgerald DE, O'Shaughnessy AM. Cardiac and peripheral arterial responses to isoprenaline challenge. Cardiovasc Res 1984;18:414–418.

236. Kuramoto K, Matsushita S, Kuwajima I, Iwasaki T, Murakami M. Comparison of hemodynamic effects of exercise and isoproterenol infusion in normal young and old men. Jpn Circ J 1979;43:71–76.

237. Kuramoto K, Matsushita S, Mifune J, Sakai M, Murakami M. Electrocardiographic and hemodynamic evaluations of isoproterenol test in elderly ischemic heart disease. Jpn Circ J 1978;42:955–960.

238. Nathan D, Ongley PA, Rahimtoola SH. The dynamics of left ventricular ejection in "normal" man with infusion of isoproterenol. Chest 1977;71:746–752.

239. Stephens J, Ead H, Spurrell R. Haemodynamic effects of dobutamine with special reference to myocardial blood flow. A comparison with dopamine and isoprenaline. Br Heart J 1979;42:43–50.

240. Gundel W, Cherry G, Rajagopalan B, Tan LB, Lee G, Schultz D. Aortic input impedance in man: acute response to vasodilator drugs. Circulation 1981;63:1305–1314.

241. Sapru RP, Hannan WJ, Muir AL, Brash HM, Harper K. Effect of isoprenaline and propranolol on left ventricular function as determined by nuclear angiography. Br Heart J 1980;44:75–81.

242. Sapru RP, Muir AL, Hannan WJ, Smith HJ, Brash HM, Wraith PK. Effect of exercise and isoprenaline on left ventricular ejection fraction in patients with angina pectoris as assessed by radionuclide angiography. Cardiology 1982;69:91–97.

243. Dodge HT, Murdaugh HV Jr. Cardiovascular–renal effects of isoproterenol in congestive heart failure (abstr). Circulation 1957;16:873.

244. Horwitz LD, Curry GC, Parkey RW, Bonte FJ. Differentiation of physiologically significant coronary artery lesions by coronary blood flow measurements during isoproterenol infusion. Circulation 1974;49:55–62.

245. Krasnow N, Rolett EL, Yurchak PM, Hood WB, Gorlin R. Isoproterenol and cardiovascular function. Am J Med 1964;37:514–525.

246. Combs DT, Martin CM. Evaluation of isoproterenol as a method of stress testing. Am Heart J 1974;87:711–715.

247. Kerber RE, Abboud FM, Marcus ML, Eckberg DL. Effect of inotropic agents on the localized dyskinesis of acutely ischemic myocardium. An experimental ultrasound study. Circulation 1974;49:1038–1046.

248. Wexler H, Kuaity J, Simonson E. Electrocardiographic effects of isoprenaline in normal subjects and patients with coronary atherosclerosis. Br Heart J 1971;33:759–764.

249. Stein I. Observations on the action of ergonovine on the coronary circulation and its use in the diag-

nosis of coronary artery insufficiency. Am Heart J 1949;37:36–45.

250. Heupler F, Proudfit W, Siegel W, et al. The ergonovine maleate test for the diagnosis of coronary artery spasm (abstr). Circulation 1975;51,52:II–11.

251. Curry RC Jr, Pepine CJ, Sabom MB, Feldman RL, Christie LG, Conti CR. Effects of ergonovine in patients with and without coronary artery disease. Circulation 1977;56:803–809.

252. Curry RC Jr, Pepine CJ, Sabom MB, et al. Hemodynamic and myocardial metabolic effects of ergonovine in patients with chest pain. Circulation 1978;58:648–654.

253. Feldman RL, Pepine CJ, Whittle JL, Curry RC, Conti CR. Coronary hemodynamic findings during spontaneous angina in patients with variant angina. Circulation 1981;64:76–83.

254. Fragasso G, Davies GJ, Chierchia S, Crea F, Bencivelli V, Maseri A. Relative roles of preload increase and coronary constriction in ergonovine–induced myocardial ischemia in stable angina pectoris. Am J Cardiol 1987;60:238–243.

255. Orlick AE, Ricci DR, Cipriano PR, Guthaner DF, Harrison DC. Coronary hemodynamic effects of ergonovine maleate in human subjects. Am J Cardiol 1980;45:48–52.

256. Schwartz AB, Donmichael TA, Botvinick EH, Ishimori T, Parmley WW, Chatterjee K. Variability in coronary hemodynamics in response to ergonovine in patients with normal coronary arteries and atypical chest pain. J Am Coll Cardiol 1983;1:797–803.

257. Cipriano PR, Guthaner DF, Orlick AE, Ricci DR, Wexler L, Silverman JF. The effects of ergonovine maleate on coronary arterial size. Circulation 1979;59:82–89.

258. Crea F, Davies G, Romeo F, et al. Myocardial ischemia during ergonovine testing: different sus-

ceptibility to coronary vasoconstriction in patients with exertional and variant angina. Circulation 1984;69:690–695.

259. Burggraf GW, Parker JO. Hemodynamic effects of amyl nitrite in coronary artery disease. Am J Cardiol 1973;32:772–778.

260. Burggraf GW, Parker JO. Left ventricular volume changes after amyl nitrite and nitroglycerin in man as measured by ultrasound. Circulation 1974;49:136–143.

261. de Leon AC, Perloff JK. The pulmonary hemodynamic effects of amyl nitrite in normal man. Am Heart J 1966;72:337–344.

262. Mitake H, Sawayama T, Nezuo S, et al. Significant coronary artery disease detected by amyl nitrite and systolic time intervals. Am J Cardiol 1984;54:79–83.

263. Niarchos AP, Tahmooressi P, Tarazi RC. Comparison of heart rate and blood pressure response to amyl nitrite, isoproterenol, and standing before and during acute beta–adrenergic blockade with intravenous propranolol. Am Heart J 1978;96:47–53.

264. Perloff JK, Calvin J, De Leon AC, Bowen P. Systemic hemodynamic effects of amyl nitrite in normal man. Am Heart J 1963;66:460–469.

265. Miller H, Ostrzega E, Geva B, Laniado S. Effect of amyl nitrite on coronary blood flow (abstr). J Am Coll Cardiol 1983;1:695A.

266. Benchimol A, Desser KB, Raizada V. Effects of amyl nitrite on phasic aortocoronary bypass graft blood velocity in man. Am Heart J 1977;93:592–595.

267. Contro S, Haring DM, Goldstein W. Paradoxic action of amyl nitrite in coronary patients. Circulation 1952;6:250–256.

268. Kerber RE, Harrison DC. Paradoxical electrocardiographic effects of amyl nitrite in coronary artery disease. Br Heart J 1972;34:851–857.

23

Quantification of Vascular Stenoses

Charles R. Lambert, M.D., Ph.D.
James A. Hill, M.D.
Carl J. Pepine, M.D.

INTRODUCTION

Although the development and widespread application of coronary arteriography has revolutionized the evaluation and treatment of patients with coronary artery disease, the visual interpretation of angiograms in routine clinical practice has probably remained more art than science. In order to improve this situation, investigators have developed a number of methods designed to better estimate the pathophysiologic significance of a given lesion. These methods can be divided into two main categories. The first of these is quantitative angiography, which involves direct, usually computer-assisted measurement and analysis of stenosis dimensions. The second category includes techniques to assess the importance of a given lesion by measuring flow related variables either radiographically or directly, using invasive methods. Techniques in this latter category usually involve determination of baseline and vasodilator augmented coronary flow indices and attempt to quantitate coronary flow reserve, as defined below. In this chapter, an overview of these two methodologic categories will be given, and an assessment of current clinical utility will be made. Related material is discussed in Chapter 19 with regard to measurement of coronary blood flow.

QUANTITATIVE ANGIOGRAPHY

Before describing the methodology that has been developed for quantitative coronary angiography, it is pertinent to consider the reasons for development of such techniques in the first place. The first, and perhaps foremost, of these reasons has to do with the large and well-documented intraobserver and interobserver variability in coronary angiogram interpretation. Quantitative coronary angiography is one way to approach minimization of this variability and this may be considered a primary objective of the technique. A second objective of quantitative coronary angiography is to apply hydrodynamic and hemodynamic principles to analysis of stenosis geometry and, thus, to derive important information pertaining to the actual pathophysiologic significance of a given coronary lesion. Such information may not be evident from visual inspection of the angiogram alone. The principles applied to such analyses have been derived from the work of Young et al. (1), Mates et al. (2), and Logan (3), among others, and were originally applied to coronary angiography by Brown and co-workers (4). The basic premise used in such an analysis is that the hydraulic resistance (R) of a stenosis can be calculated by knowing the cross-sectional dimensions of the segment involved.

Although some methodologic differences exist between investigators, a typical basic quantitative angiographic analysis (5) separates resistance into viscous (R_v) and turbulent (R_t) components. For a series of i vessel cross sections reconstructed by the computer, viscous resistance is derived as $R_v = 30\mu \ \Sigma \ S_i/D_i^4$ where μ is blood viscosity, S_i is incremental section length, and D_i is diameter of the incremental section. Turbulent resistance is calculated as $R_t = (\rho_{0.266})(1/A_m - 1/A_d)^2$, where ρ is blood density, A_m is minimal stenotic area, and A_d is normal vessel diameter distal to the stenosis. For a given flow (Q), the pressure gradient (ΔP) across the stenosis is estimated as $\Delta P = Q^2 R_t + Q R_v$.

Thus, meaningful physiologic data can be derived from analysis of angiographic anatomy in this manner. Before examining the degree of success that has been achieved toward these objectives and their clinical applicability, it is of interest to consider briefly the methodology involved in quantitative coronary angiography. The reader is referred to a recent review by Brown and co-workers for a detailed discussion of this subject (6).

Manual Edge Detection

The simplest form of quantitative coronary angiography is the manual application of a ruler or set of calipers to visually measure the diameter of a narrowed coronary segment, and estimate percent diameter reduction with respect to the "normal adjacent vessel." Gensini and co-workers (7) described a mechanized system for this simple type of quantitative angiography in 1971. Their technique allowed movement of cursors on an angiographic viewing screen that were placed, by visual inspection, to define arterial diameters in normal and diseased vessel segments. By scaling measurements with reference to the size of the catheter tip, computation of absolute vessel dimensions could be done with a reported variability of ± 80 μm. A similar device using handheld electronic calipers was described by Scoblionko and co-workers (8), yielding a variability of ± 180 μm. This method was felt to be superior to visual estimation (± 260 μm) of stenosis dimensions. In our laboratories, Feldman and co-workers (9) described a similar method using 105-mm photospot angiography and a handheld magnifying comparator. These investigators reported 95% confidence limits for calculated measurements as $\leqslant 200$ μm.

The "next generation" techniques for quantitative coronary angiography attempt a more complete three-dimensional reconstruction of stenosis and arterial geometry. These techniques allow application of the principles outlined above to import hemodynamic significance to angiographic anatomy. Perhaps the most widely emulated of these methods is that of Brown and co-workers (4), who utilize a system in which angiographic images recorded on 35-mm cinefilm are projected at 5X magnification and traced on a digitizing tablet. Two views, at 90° from each other, are corrected for distortions introduced by the imaging train and then reconstructed and displayed in a three-dimensional format. Calculated geometric values include vessel diameters and cross-sectional areas along the length of the digitized vessel segment. If the "normal" ends of the vessel are defined, atheroma mass can be calculated. Based on hemodynamic principles and using hypothetical blood flow values, estimates of pressure drop and stenosis resistance are made as described above. An example of such an analysis is given in Figure 23.1. With high-quality angiograms this method yields an absolute accuracy of 0.08 mm, variability of 3% for percent stenosis, and 0.1 mm for minimum stenosis diameter. This method uses the human eye for edge detection, like the caliper methods described earlier. It is further limited in that in the series reported by Brown et al. a substantial number of determinations are based on only a single view because of difficulties associated with obtaining a comparable orthogonal view of each stenosis to be analyzed. The computer is used to perform geometric calculations that would be otherwise prohibitively tedious. Even with computer assistance, this method requires skill and attention to numerous methodological details and takes a finite period of time to utilize correctly (6).

Automated Edge Detection

The techniques reported above all yield specific quantitative parameters that may be used to characterize stenosis geometry. They do not, however, approach the problem of

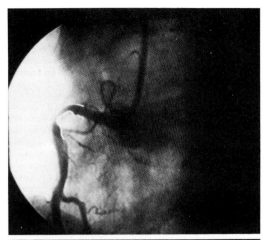

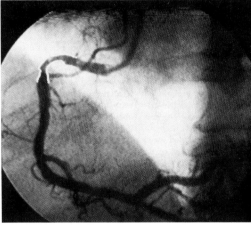

Figure 23.1. Video frames of a right coronary artery angiogram before (*upper*) and after (*lower*) balloon angioplasty. The stenosis is outlined with a computer-generated edge. (From Bove AA, Holmes DR, Owen RM, et al. Estimation of the effects of angioplasty on coronary stenosis using quantitative video angiography. Cathet Cardiovasc Diagn 1985;11:5–16.)

edge definition, which is a primary limiting issue in examining small vessels or severe stenoses. All of the methods mentioned above utilize the human eye to determine the border of the vessel lumen. Most, although not all, quantitative angiographic techniques developed subsequently to those mentioned above utilize some technique of computerized edge detection to eliminate this critical subjective element in defining the geometry of a stenosis. Principles important to application of com-

puterized methods in this regard have been examined in detail by Spears and co-workers (10, 11).

The methodology described by Sanders et al. (12) involves projection of cineframes into a television camera based video system with optical magnification. The selected image is then digitized into an 8-bit 480 × 512 pixel matrix. Approximate borders for the vessel segment of interest are drawn by the operator. The computer edge detection algorithm defines the lumen borders by doing densitometric scans perpendicular to the manually traced borders and computing the first derivative of pixel density along the scan lines. The lumen edge is defined at that point where the derivative is maximal. Magnification correction is performed and allows calculation of absolute lumen diameter, as well as segment area and volume. Reiber and co-workers (13) also utilize automated edge detection of projected cineframes with optical magnification. The operator defines the vessel centerline, and an edge detection algorithm, a weighted first-second derivative function, defines lumen dimensions within specified limits and using numeric interpolation for smoothing. Dimensional scaling is done using the cardiac catheter as a reference point, and orthogonal views can be utilized to form a three-dimensional representation of stenosis geometry. Barth and coinvestigators (14) utilized a system that digitizes cineframes using a Zeiss microscopic scanner. A cross-correlation operator defines the vessel centerline, and another correlative algorithm is used to define lumen borders. Vessel diameter measurements are then computed from these borders while lumen area is estimated by means of photodensitometry. The utility of this method is apparently limited to lumen diameters of ≥0.8 mm. Bove and co-workers utilize a similar algorithm (Fig. 23.1) for on-line quantitative angiographic analysis of video images (5).

Photodensitometry

As alluded to above, an alternative approach to edge detection for lesion analysis is photodensitometry. In theory, application of the Beer-Lambert principle to cineangiographic images should obviate need for edge detection and its inherent assumptions. The Beer-Lambert principle provides that the background-subtracted attenuation profile of a coronary angiogram gives a value directly proportional to the cross-sectional area of the vessel if viewed perpendicular to its central axis. This principle is applicable to photographic images, as well as to log-transformed digital images. A major possible advantage of this technique over other forms of quantitative analysis lies in evaluation of high-grade eccentric or irregular lesions, which may be particularly difficult to evaluate with other methodologies. According to the Beer-Lambert principle, and since photodensitometry does not rely on edge detection, orthogonal projections of lesions should give identical results for lesion severity. Possible sources of error in such applications include inadequate or improper background subtraction, as well as any degree of obliquity in viewing angle or misregistration from the perpendicular circumstance noted above. With these requirements, strict application of photodensitometry to the coronary arteries is difficult, and the technique has been used most often in peripheral arterial studies (15). Nevertheless, with careful attention to methodologic detail, photodensitometry can be a very useful tool.

For example, Sandor and co-workers (16) have adapted photodensitometric techniques to the coronary circulation by digitizing cineframes into a computer system and selecting an area for analysis. Density profiles are constructed for this window, and a smoothing algorithm is applied, after which the operator selects the boundaries of the density profiles for calculation of lumen area functions. This method may have a relatively large (30%) variability for area estimates in tubes of ≤ 1 mm^2, which may limit utility in the clinical situation. Nichols and co-workers (17) digitized cineframes into a 512×512 matrix from which regions of interest were selected and scanned, using an interpolated background subtraction algorithm. Percent area reduction (not absolute area) was then calculated by application of the principles referred to above. This method was found to give good results when premortem and postmortem studies were compared; however, few data were provided on small vessels (<1.0 mm) or critical stenoses.

A technique similar to those mentioned above, using photodensitometric analysis of digitized coronary angiograms, has been described by Collins and co-workers (18).

Johnson and co-workers (19) recently compared photodensitometry with intraoperative, high-frequency, epicardial echocardiographic measurement of stenosis dimensions. Although a correlation was present between these estimates ($r = 0.86$), significant scatter was observed. Excellent agreement was seen for photodensitometric measurements of eccentric stenosis severity in orthogonal projections. Silver and co-workers (20) recently validated a commercially available photodensitometry system, using standard cinefilm for input. This system performed well with regard to accuracy and reproducibility. In addition, as in the study by Johnson et al. (19), evaluation of orthogonal projections offered excellent agreement in terms of percentage relative stenosis estimates for eccentric lesions.

QUANTITATIVE CORONARY ANGIOGRAPHY: UTILITY

As noted previously, one objective of quantitative coronary angiography is to minimize the variability present in angiogram interpretation. This variability has been the subject of a number of studies, beginning with the report in 1966 of Robbins and co-workers (21), who used various media for postmortem analysis of coronary stenoses. Although observers were asked to give only rough estimates of stenosis severity by means of angiogram review, significant variance was noted in the moderate severity range. Detre and co-workers (22) evaluated the reliability of angiogram interpretation for 22 physicians and 13 angiograms. Again, significant interobserver and intraobserver variability was demonstrated, as was a probable effect of experience. In 1977 DeRouen and co-workers (23) reported results of having 10 coronary angiograms evaluated by 11 angiographers. The average standard deviation for estimation of any stenosis by any reader was 18% while agreement on the number of major vessels with a 70% stenosis occurred only 69% of the time. Variability in interpretation was manifested by both different estimation of lesion severity and also of lesion location. Again, experienced angiographers tended to be more accurate. Zir and co-workers (24) asked four angiographers to assess the location and severity of coronary artery stenoses in 20 angiograms. All observers agreed on the severity of a stenosis (defined as a ≥50% diameter reduction) only 65% of the time. Thus, all of these studies indicated significant variability in angiographic interpretation with respect to coronary artery stenoses.

From the figures quoted in the discussion of methodology, it is clear that most quantitative coronary angiographic techniques significantly decrease variability of angiographic interpretation with respect to stenosis severity. Although such an effect would be expected with machine-implemented, algorithm-dependent processing methods, it appears to hold, even for caliper-assisted or similar simple techniques that rely upon the human eye for edge detection. The marked decrease in variability that can be achieved with quantitative coronary angiography is illustrated by the work of Brown and co-workers (4). Their technique, which does not utilize automated edge detection, yields an accuracy of around 0.08 mm and repeatability of ±0.10 mm for estimates of minimum lesion diameter. The variability of this method vs. visual estimation of lesion severity is illustrated in Figure 23.2 (as adapted from Brown and co-workers (25)). Clearly, the quantitative method offers substantial improvement in minimization of variability for estimation of percent stenosis over a wide range of lesion severity. In contrast, techniques using photodensitometry have shown variability for percent stenosis estimates to be a function of lesion severity. Thus, variability may be 5% or so with high-grade (90%) lesions but up to 10% with moderate (50%) stenoses. This is compounded, as noted previously, by limitations in precision sometimes seen with these techniques for lumen diameters in the 1-mm range, which are of important clinical interest.

Another area in which the quantitative coronary angiographic technique developed by Brown and co-workers has been shown to be of use is in documentation of disease progression (26). In studying 290 coronary lesions in 26 patients at an interval of 18 months, disease progression was documented and stratified by lesion severity. The changes observed in magnitude of stenosis were well within the limitations in measurement imposed by the methodology. Reiber and co-workers (13) have assessed short-, medium-, and long-term variations in arterial dimensions using quantitative coronary angiography. Variability of

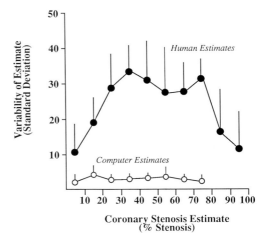

Figure 23.2. Variability of the estimate for lesions of varying severity by simple visual estimation vs. a computer-aided manual edge detection technique. (From Brown BG, Bolson EL, Dodge HT. Coronary arteriography and the objective assessment of coronary artery pathology. In: Kalsner S, ed. The coronary artery. New York: Oxford University Press, 1982:523–548.)

the analysis procedure itself was less than 0.12 mm while variability of obstruction diameter ranged from 0.22 to 0.36 mm. Variability in estimating a reference diameter of a "normal" vessel for a given stenotic segment ranged from 0.15 to 0.66 mm. Thus, biologic variability must be kept in mind when considering results of quantitative coronary angiographic studies.

Quantitative coronary angiography has proven useful in studying the effects of pharmacologic agents on the size of the coronary arteries and stenoses therein. In 1971 Gensini (7) described the effects of nitrates on coronary size, using a simple quantitative technique, and subsequently other investigators have confirmed his findings (27–29). Other compounds and maneuvers that have been studied with quantitative coronary angiography include the cold pressor test (25), verapamil (30), dipyridamole (31), isometric hand grip (32), combined epinephrine and propranolol (25), and ergonovine (33), among others.

MacMahon and co-workers (34) utilized quantitative coronary angiography to study the geometry of stenoses in patients with single-vessel coronary artery disease, unstable angina, and either no infarction or a non Q-wave infarction. Percent diameter reductions and percent area reductions were significantly higher in the patients with infarction. The predicted hemodynamic consequences of the differences in lesion geometry between the two groups were large, suggesting that such analysis might be necessary to accurately define a "critical stenosis," at least in this patient population. Thus, the application of quantitative coronary angiography in this study appears to offer information pertinent to both pathophysiology and the resultant clinical syndrome not necessarily evident by visual angiographic interpretation.

Quantitative coronary angiographic techniques have proven useful for following reperfusion during thrombolytic therapy (35) and in assessment of geometric changes after percutaneous transluminal coronary angioplasty (PTCA) (5,36,37). Serruys and co-workers (36) studied angiograms of 138 patients before and after PTCA using densitometric determination of percent area reduction, as compared with circular percent area reductions calculated from diameter measurements. Before PTCA the two methods showed a good correlation while after PTCA important deviations from linearity between the two methods were evident. It was concluded that these discrepancies were due to asymmetric changes in lumen morphology that were probably better assessed by densitometric methods of area change estimation, rather than by diameter-based measurements. Bove and co-workers (5) compared visual and computer estimation of the effects of PTCA in 14 patients. Results showed a tendency for visual overestimation of percent diameter reduction for severe lesions when compared with computer analysis and suggested that rapid estimation of stenosis geometry by quantitative angiographic techniques might be clinically useful during PTCA. Zijlstra and co-workers (37) recently utilized quantitative coronary angiography to document delayed increases in coronary dimensions that may occur after PTCA.

Perhaps the most interesting application of quantitative coronary angiography is in prediction of the physiologic importance of a given stenosis based on analysis of an angiographic image. White and co-workers (38) studied the relationship between percent diameter stenosis, as measured with calipers, to the reactive hyperemic response of the involved vessel, as determined at surgery by means of a Doppler technique after 20 sec of coronary occlusion. The basic premise of this investigation and others to be discussed below relies upon the concept of coronary flow reserve. The proponents of coronary flow reserve attest that the reactive hyperemic response after coronary occlusion (as used by White et al.) or the peak hyperemia induced by a potent coronary vasodilator can be used to assess the pathophysiological importance of a stenosis. This is based on the observation that the magnitude of inducible hyperemia possible decreases as a progressively more severe stenosis is imposed on the involved vessel. If severe enough, no inducible hyperemia will be observed. Coronary flow reserve is the ratio of peak to basal flow, as illustrated in Figure 23.3. Although this concept is attractive as a reference standard for assessment of stenosis significance, there are definite limitations to its application. These will be addressed below in more detail. White and co-workers (38) studied a total of 44 vessels in 39 patients with stenoses ranging in severity from 10 to 95%. No significant correlation between the percent diameter stenosis, as determined from the coronary angiogram, and the reactive hyperemic response was found ($r = -0.25$). These investigators concluded that their observations, combined with the large interobserver and intraobserver variability inherent in coronary angiographic interpretation, suggest that conventional methods of angiographic evaluation cannot give accurate results with respect to assessment of the physiologic importance of a stenosis.

Later studies by Harrison and co-workers (39) compared reactive hyperemic responses after coronary occlusion during surgery with more extensive quantitative angiographic parameters in a group of 23 patients with left anterior descending coronary artery stenoses. Computer-assisted quantitative coronary angiography was used to measure percent area stenosis, percent diameter stenosis, and minimal cross sectional area. There was a large overlap in both percent area and percent diameter stenosis measurements in vessels with and without an abnormal (diminished) reactive hyperemic response. In contrast, minimal cross-sectional area measurements appeared to separate those vessels with abnor-

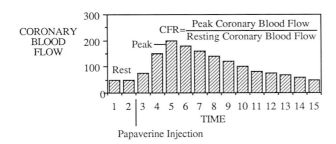

Figure 23.3. Schematic representation of data obtained during determination of papaverine-induced coronary flow reserve (*CFR*), as described in the text.

mal reactive hyperemia in almost every case, as illustrated in Figure 23.4. The minimum cross sectional area associated with a normal reactive hyperemia response seemed to be ⩾3.5 mm². The conclusion from this study was that while usual angiographic measurements, as well as quantitative determinations of percent area and diameter stenosis, cannot predict the hemodynamic severity of a stenosis, measurement of the minimal cross-sectional area of a lesion does this reliably.

Wilson and co-workers (40) reported similar studies in patients with single-vessel coronary artery disease, using Doppler measurements of hyperemia in response to intracoronary papaverine administration for determination of coronary flow reserve. Normality of coronary flow reserve was significantly related to percent area stenosis and less so with minimum cross-sectional area; however, an equally good correlation was found for maximal percent diameter narrowing, as shown in Figure 23.5. Reasons for the lack of correlation between percent diameter stenosis and flow reserve in the study by White et al. (38) cited previously and the presence of correlation in the study by Wilson and co-workers (40) are not clear. These differences may reside partially in methodologic differences, in the extent of coronary disease in the different patient groups, and in other factors addressed by the authors. Clear delineation of the reasons for such observed differences appears to be needed prior to clinical application of such techniques.

Wijns and co-workers (41) examined quantitative coronary angiographic variables in patients with left anterior descending lesions and compared percent area stenosis and translesional pressure gradients measured at catheterization with the presence of exercise-induced thallium perfusion defects. The translesional pressure gradient was found to show a sharp increase in the region of 2 to 4 mm² lumen area, supporting the findings of Harrison et al. (39) mentioned above. Normalized translesional pressure gradients and percent area stenosis predicted the occurrence of thallium perfusion defects induced by exercise in 83% of patients. Johnson and co-workers (42) studied videodensitometric (integrated optical density), as well as quantitative angiographic, parameters of coronary artery stenoses with either reactive or papaverine-induced hyperemic responses. Significant correlations were found between integrated optical density and both minimal lumen area determined by quantitative angiography and coronary flow reserve resulting from both forms of hyperemic stimuli.

CORONARY FLOW RESERVE TECHNIQUES

The concept of coronary flow reserve was introduced in the section on quantitative coronary angiography out of necessity since the former is being used by some investigators as a reference standard with which to gage the latter. It is important to realize, in this regard, that the acceptance of coronary flow reserve as a reference standard may not be justified in all circumstances and that application of this measurement has definite limitations, as recently reviewed by Klocke (43). Assuming perfect measurement technique, coronary flow reserve can be affected by alterations in aortic pressure, passive changes in stenosis geometry, preload, heart rate, and hypertrophy. The level of baseline flow, before vasodilation, varies widely with metabolic demand and antecedent ischemia. Other considerations include collateral blood flow and changes in the aortic pressure-flow relationship during maximal vasodilation on a

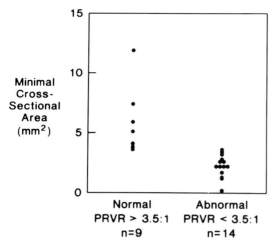

Figure 23.4. Separation of patients with "normal" vs. "abnormal" estimates of coronary flow reserve (*PRVR*) by minimal cross-sectional area determined by quantitative angiography. (From Harrison DG, White CW, Hiratzka LF, et al. The value of lesion cross-sectional area determined by quantitative coronary angiography in assessing the physiologic significance of proximal left anterior descending coronary arterial stenoses. Circulation 1984;69:1111–1119.)

chronic basis, if repeated evaluations are to be compared.

Doppler Catheter

Reference to use of the coronary Doppler velocity catheter to measure coronary flow reserve has already been made in the section on quantitative coronary angiography above and in Chapter 16. The Doppler catheter technique has the advantage of arterial selectivity. A disadvantage is inability to easily and accurately determine differences in baseline prevasodilation flow before and after a given intervention since velocity, not volumetric flow, is being measured. This limitation may be addressed by independent measurement of arterial cross-sectional area or infusion of an agent such as nitroglycerin continuously to minimize changes in epicardial coronary dimensions. Studies from expert investigators using this technique (38–40) have shown that, in general, coronary stenoses of 50% or less, as determined by diameter, are associated with coronary flow reserve of ≥3.5. Lesions of >60% diameter reduction are associated with

coronary flow reserve values <3.5. These data support selection of the flow reserve normal cutoff of 3.5. It is important to note that, even in these very select patients, substantial scatter of flow reserve exists at any particular level of stenosis (Fig. 23.5). Further discussion of the Doppler catheter and its use appears in Chapter 16.

Angiographic Techniques

Application of the coronary flow reserve concept to radiography depends primarily on the ability of radiography to measure coronary blood flow, as recently reviewed by Vogel (44). Providing that this can be done, the principles and limitations described above for coronary flow reserve determinations in general must be critically applied, just as for the Doppler catheter technique.

Use of angiographic techniques to measure or estimate coronary blood flow is based primarily on the use of contrast medium as an indicator and the application of the Stewart-Hamilton, Kety-Schmidt, or Sapirstein principles in some form (44). Since contrast media are not inert and have substantial vascular and hemodynamic effects, strict application of these methodologies is not possible, and a variety of alternative radiographic methods have been designed. Rutishauser and co-workers (45) developed the first such method, which involved determination of the transit time of contrast material at two points along an arterial segment with a measurable diameter and length. Volumetric flow can be calculated in such a segment as the ratio of vascular volume to transit time. Although such an approach may be ideal for study of bypass grafts, it cannot easily be applied to branching, distal, or tortuous arterial segments and requires attention to detail concerning image acquisition. Application of indicator dilution and videodensitometric methodologies to measure relative coronary flow ratios, as might be useful in flow reserve determinations, was described by Foerster and co-workers (46). Streaming and reflux of contrast material may present problems with this and related methods.

Digital subtraction coronary angiography has proven useful as a tool to indirectly assess coronary blood flow, again by application of indicator dilution principles and determina-

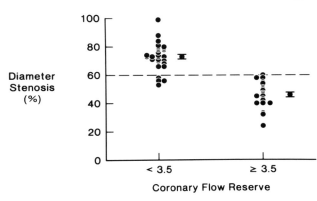

Figure 23.5. Separation of patients by "normal" (≥3.5) vs. "abnormal" (<3.5) coronary flow reserve values by means of percentage diameter stenosis. (From Wilson RF, Marcus ML, White CW. Prediction of the physiologic significance of coronary arterial lesions by quantitative lesion geometry in patients with limited coronary artery disease. Circulation 1987;75:723–732.)

tion of regional transit times for contrast medium (47, 48). This technique yields coronary flow reserve values for regions of interest and is commercially available in a package offering colored digital displays of flow patterns. Although these techniques may be useful in certain circumstances, validation studies (47, 48) have shown relatively large confidence limits for coronary flow reserve values when compared with electromagnetic flowmeter determinations in the animal laboratory. Until further validation studies provide guidelines to limit this variability in the clinical setting, this method will probably have limited practical applicability and will remain a research tool.

CONCLUSIONS

Quantitative coronary angiographic techniques minimize the variability inherent in visual angiogram interpretation and impart pathophysiologic significance to specific lesion geometry. Quantitative coronary angiography is useful in studying the mechanism of action of pharmacologic agents on the coronary circulation and in documenting the effects of maneuvers designed to alter coronary morphology (i.e., PTCA or thrombolysis). It should be emphasized, however, that useful application of quantitative angiography in these circumstances requires high quality angiographic studies and meticulous attention to technical detail.

The concept of coronary flow reserve is extremely useful in understanding the pathophysiology of coronary artery disease. Techniques such as the subselective Doppler catheter and digital subtraction angiography apply this concept in order to better assess the significance of coronary angiographic findings. Although useful data have been generated with these techniques, significant questions remain pertaining to the sensitivity and specificity of findings. Even in the hands of experienced investigators, data derived from measurements or estimates of coronary flow reserve, particularly in unselected patients with extensive coronary artery disease, may be ambiguous. In addition, it has not been shown that the application of quantitative coronary angiographic or coronary flow reserve techniques, no matter how sophisticated, will favorably alter the course of patient evaluation, treatment, and outcome when compared with routine methods of clinical and angiographic analysis. At this point in time, these techniques are not likely to alter the practice methods of experienced cardiologists since the proven benefits in terms of better patient evaluation do not outweigh the costs in time and other resources needed to set up and operate such systems. Further research is needed to determine whether quantitative coronary angiography and/or coronary flow reserve determination will have a substantial and definitive impact on the routine clinical practice of cardiology.

References

1. Young DF, Cholvin NR, Kirkeeide RL, Roth AC. Hemodynamics of arterial stenoses at elevated flow rates. Circ Res 1977;41:99–107.
2. Mates RE, Gupta RL, Bell AC, Klocke FJ. Fluid dynamics of coronary artery stenoses. Circ Res 1978;42:152–162.
3. Logan SE. On the fluid dynamics of human coronary stenosis. IEEE Trans Biomed Eng 1975;22:327–334.
4. Brown BG, Bolson E, Frimer M, Dodge HT. Quantitative coronary arteriography—estimation of

dimensions, hemodynamic resistance, and atheroma mass of coronary artery lesions using the arteriogram and digital computation. Circulation 1977;55:329–337.

5. Bove AA, Holmes DR, Owen RM, et al. Estimation of the effects of angioplasty on coronary stenosis using quantitative video angiography. Cathet Cardiovasc Diagn 1985;11:5–16.

6. Brown BG, Bolson EL, Dodge HT. Quantitative computer techniques for analyzing coronary arteriograms. Prog Cardiovasc Dis 1986;28:403–418.

7. Gensini GG, Kelly AE, Dacosta BCB, Huntington PP. Quantitative angiography: the measurement of coronary vasomobility in the intact animal and man. Chest 1971;60:522–530.

8. Scoblionko DP, Brown BG, Mitten S, et al. A new digital electronic caliper for measurement of coronary arterial stenosis: comparison with visual estimates and computer assisted measurements. Am J Cardiol 1984;53:689–693.

9. Feldman RL, Pepine CJ, Curry RC, Conti CR. Quantitative coronary arteriography using 105 mm photospot angiography and an optical magnifying device. Cathet Cardiovasc Diagn 1979;5:195–201.

10. Spears JR, Sandor T, Baim DS, Paulin S. The minimum error in estimating coronary luminal cross-sectional area from cineangiographic diameter measurements. Cathet Cardiovas Diagn 1983;9:119–128.

11. Spears JR, Sandor T, Als AV, et al. Computerized image analysis for quantitative measurement of vessel diameter from cineangiograms. Circulation 1983;68:453–461.

12. Sanders WJ, Alderman EL, Harrison DC. Coronary artery quantitation using digital image processing techniques. IEEE Comput Cardiol 1979;7:15–19.

13. Reiber JHC, Serruys PW, Kooijman CJ, et al. Assessment of short-, medium-, and long-term variations in arterial dimensions from computer-assisted quantitation of coronary cineangiograms. Circulation 1985;71:280–288.

14. Barth K, Faust U, Epple E. The objective measurement of coronary obstructions by digital image processing. IEEE Conference on physics and engineering in medical imaging. Asilomar, CA: IEEE, 1982:10–12.

15. Blankenhorn DH, Brooks SH, Selzer RH, Crawford DW, Chin HP. Assessment of atherosclerosis from angiographic images. Proc Soc Exp Biol Med 1974;145:1298–1300.

16. Sandor T, Als AV, Paulin S. Cine-densitometric measurement of coronary arterial stenoses. Cathet Cardiovasc Diagn 1979;5:229–245.

17. Nichols AB, Gabrieli CFO, Fenoglio JJ, Esser PD. Quantification of relative coronary arterial stenosis by cinevideodensitometric analysis of coronary arteriograms. Circulation 1984;69:512–522.

18. Collins SM, Skorton DJ, Harrison DG. Quantitative computer based videodensitometry and the physiological significance of coronary stenosis. Comput Cardiol 1982;10:219–222.

19. Johnson MR, McPherson DD, Fleagle SR, et al. Videodensitometric analysis of human coronary

stenoses: validation in vivo by intraoperative high-frequency epicardial echocardiography. Circulation 1988;77:328–336.

20. Silver KH, Buczek JA, Esser PD, Nichols AB. Quantitative analysis of coronary arteriograms by microprocessor cinevideodensitometry. Cathet Cardiovasc Diagn 1987;13:291–300.

21. Robbins SL, Rodrigues FL, Wragg AL, Fish SJ. Problems in the quantitation of coronary atherosclerosis. Am J Cardiol 1966;18:153–159.

22. Detre KM, Wright E, Murphey ML, Takaro T. Observer agreement in evaluating coronary angiograms. Circulation 1975;52:979–983.

23. DeRouen TA, Murray JA, Owen W. Variability in the analysis of coronary arteriograms. Circulation 1977;55:324–328.

24. Zir LM, Miller SW, Dinsmore RE, Gilbert JP, Harthorne JW. Interobserver variability in coronary angiography. Circulation 1976;53:627–632.

25. Brown BG, Bolson EL, Dodge HT. Coronary arteriography and the objective assessment of coronary artery pathology. In: Kalsner S, ed. The coronary artery. New York: Oxford University Press, 1982:523–548.

26. Brown BG, Pierce CD, Petersen RB, Bolson EL, Dodge HT. A new approach to clinical investigation of progressive coronary atherosclerosis (abstr). Circulation 1979;60:II–66.

27. Brown BG, Ross CR, Bolson E, Frimer M, Dodge HT. Quantitative effects of nitroglycerin in diseased human coronary arteries (abstr). Circulation 1977;56:II–866.

28. Feldman RL, Pepine CJ, Conti CR. Magnitude of dilation of large and small coronary arteries by nitroglycerin. Circulation 1981;64:324–333.

29. Feldman RL, Marx JD, Pepine CJ, Conti CR. Analysis of coronary responses to various doses of intracoronary nitroglycerin. Circulation 1982;66:321–327.

30. Chew CYC, Brown BG, Wong M, et al. The effects of verapamil on coronary hemodynamics and vasomobility in patients with coronary artery disease (abstr). Am J Cardiol 1980;45:389.

31. Brown BG, Petersen RB, Pierce CD, et al. Intravenous dipyridamole combined with isometric handgrip for maximal increase in coronary flow in patients with coronary disease (abstr). Circulation 1980;62:III–325.

32. Brown BG, Petersen RB, Pierce CD, Wong M, Bolson E, Dodge HT. Coronary artery constriction and hemodynamic responses during isometric handgrip in patients with coronary artery disease (abstr). Am J Cardiol 1980;45:431.

33. Curry RC, Pepine CJ, Sabom MB, Feldman RL, Christe LG, Conti CR. Effects of ergonovine in patients with and without coronary disease. Circulation 1977;56:803–809.

34. MacMahon MM, Brown BG, Cukingnan R, et al. Quantitative coronary angiography: measurement of the critical stenosis in patients with unstable angina and single vessel disease without collaterals. Circulation 1979;60:106–113.

35. Feldman RL, Crick WF, Conti CR, Pepine CJ. Quantitative coronary angiography during intracoronary streptokinase in acute myocardial infarction: how long to continue thrombo-

lytic therapy? Cathet Cardiovasc Diagn 1983; 9:9–18.

36. Serruys PW, Reiber JHC, Wijns W, et al. Assessment of percutaneous transluminal coronary angioplasty by quantitative coronary angiography: diameter versus densitometric area measurements. Am J Cardiol 1984;54:482–488.

37. Zijlstra F, Reiber JC, Juilliere Y, Serruys PW. Normalization of coronary flow reserve by percutaneous transluminal coronary angioplasty. Am J Cardiol 1988;61:55–60.

38. White CW, Wright CB, Doty DB, et al. Does visual interpretation of the coronary arteriogram predict the physiologic importance of a coronary stenosis? N Engl J Med 1984;310:819–824.

39. Harrison DG, White CW, Hiratzka LF, et al. The value of lesion cross–sectional area determined by quantitative coronary angiography in assessing the physiologic significance of proximal left anterior descending coronary arterial stenoses. Circulation 1984;69:1111–1119.

40. Wilson RF, Marcus ML, White CW. Prediction of the physiologic significance of coronary arterial lesions by quantitative lesion geometry in patients with limited coronary artery disease. Circulation 1987;75:723–732.

41. Wijns W, Serruys PW, Reiber JHC, et al. Quantitative angiography of the left anterior descending coronary artery: correlations with pressure gradient and results of exercise thallium scintigraphy. Circulation 1985;71:273–279.

42. Johnson MR, Fleagle SR, Aylward PE, et al. Analysis of right coronary artery stenoses using videodensitometry (abstr). Circulation 1985;72:III–262.

43. Klocke FJ. Measurements of coronary flow reserve: defining pathophysiology versus making decisions about patient care. Circulation 1987;76:1183–1189.

44. Vogel RA. The radiographic assessment of coronary blood flow parameters. Circulation 1985;72:460–465.

45. Rutishauser W, Bussman WD, Noseda G, Meier W, Wellauer J. Blood flow measurement through single coronary arteries by roentgen densitometry. Part I. A comparison of flow measured by a radiologic technique applicable in the intact organism and by electromagnetic flowmeter. AJR 1970;109:12–20.

46. Foerster J, Link DP, Lantz BMT, Lee G, Holcroft JW, Mason DT. Measurement of coronary reactive hyperemia during clinical angiography by video dilution technique. Acta Radiol 1981;22:209–216.

47. Hodgson JM, LeGrand V, Bates ER, et al. Validation in dogs of a rapid digital angiographic technique to measure coronary blood flow during routine cardiac catheterization. Am J Cardiol 1985;55:188–193.

48. Cusma JT, Toggart EJ, Folts JD, et al. Digital subtraction angiographic imaging of coronary flow reserve. Circulation 1987;75:461–472.

24

Valve Function: Stenosis and Insufficiency

John W. Hirshfeld, M.D.

GENERAL PRINCIPLES

Normal Valve Function

The heart is a pressure pump that propels blood through the circulatory system by raising chamber cavity pressure. When the pressure exceeds the pressure in the next chamber downstream, blood flows to the downstream chamber. The proper operation of this system depends on the cardiac valves whose purpose is to allow unidirectional blood flow. A normal valve performs this function without obstructing forward flow or allowing any reverse flow. Any of the four cardiac valves can become either stenotic (obstructing the normal forward flow of blood), regurgitant (allowing backward flow of blood), or both stenotic and regurgitant.

Objectives of the Catheterization Assessment

Most valvular dysfunction can be recognized by physical examination and noninvasive diagnostic techniques. Accordingly, it should be unusual to discover previously unrecognized valve disease during a cardiac catheterization procedure. Instead, the assessment of abnormal valve function by cardiac catheterization has two general purposes: to characterize and quantify the valvular dysfunction and to characterize and quantify the response of the affected chamber(s) to the excessive hemodynamic burden caused by the valvular dysfunction.

VALVULAR STENOSIS

Functional Problems Caused by a Stenosed Cardiac Valve

A stenotic cardiac valve predominantly affects the chamber immediately upstream from it. Although other cardiac chambers farther upstream may also be burdened, these effects are indirect, resulting from the altered conditions in the chamber immediately upstream from the stenotic valve.

The reduced orifice area of a stenotic valve presents an obstruction to normal forward blood flow requiring the generation of an abnormally increased pressure gradient across the valve. This, in turn, requires an increased cavity pressure in the chamber upstream from the stenosed valve. Thus, the stenotic valve places a pressure load on the upstream chamber, and the upstream chamber must adapt to the requirement to generate increased pressure.

Valvular stenosis, which can be either congenital or acquired, does not develop acutely. It is either present from birth or develops slowly over many years. Therefore, the affected cardiac chambers can adapt to the hemodynamic burden.

Determinants of Flow Velocity across a Cardiac Valve

When considering flow across a cardiac valve, it is important to distinguish between **flow rate** (which is measured in volume/unit time such as milliliters/second) and **flow velocity** (which is measured in length/unit time such as centimeters/second). Each unit of measurement has its own physiologic significance. **Flow rate** is related to the cardiac output and measures the total volume of flow across the valve. **Flow velocity,** on the other hand, measures the speed with which blood moves and (as will be explained below) is related to the pressure gradient across a valve orifice.

The flow velocity across any cardiac valve, stenotic or not, is determined by the interaction of two variables:

1. The **total flow rate** across the valve (generally the cardiac output divided by the **fraction of time** that flow actually occurs across the valve);
2. The **area of the valve orifice** through which flow must pass.

These variables are interrelated by the following mathematical expression:

$$\text{Flow} = \text{Area} \times \text{Velocity} \qquad (1)$$

This relationship, which is merely an expression of conservation of volume, has two pragmatic consequences:

1. At a given valve orifice area, an increase in flow rate requires a **direct** increase in flow velocity.
2. At a constant flow rate, a change in orifice area requires an **inverse** change in flow velocity.

Thus, either a decrease in orifice area or an increase in flow rate requires an increase in the flow velocity.

"Orifice Action": The Biophysics of Flow from One Cardiac Chamber to Another

The transfer of blood from a relatively stationary state within a cardiac chamber across an orifice to a downstream chamber or great vessel requires the addition of the kinetic energy associated with increase in velocity of the blood as it moves across the orifice. In the heart, this **kinetic** energy is derived from the **potential** energy associated with the cavity pressure in the chamber immediately upstream from the orifice. As the velocity of the stationary blood within the chamber cavity is accelerated, some of its potential (or pressure) energy is transformed to kinetic (or velocity) energy. The Bernoulli principle

(which is an expression of the conservation of energy) requires a decrease in pressure (pressure gradient) as the blood traverses the orifice (Fig. 24.1).

The following is a derivation of the relationship between orifice area, flow rate, and pressure gradient.

The hydraulic **potential** energy of a fluid is related to the volume of the fluid and its pressure:

$$E_p = PgV \qquad (2)$$

where E_p = potential energy (ergs), P = pressure (cm H_2O), g = gravitational acceleration (cm/sec), and V = volume (cm^3).

Hydraulic **kinetic** energy of a fluid is related to the volume of the fluid and its velocity.

$$E_k = \tfrac{1}{2}Vv^2 \qquad (3)$$

where E_k = kinetic energy (ergs), V = volume (cm^3), and v = velocity (cm/sec).

The V term is actually mass. ($E_k = \tfrac{1}{2}mv^2$). However, for simplicity of derivation, we are treating mass and volume as being interchangeable. This assumption would be correct if the specific gravity of blood (which is 1.06) were 1.00.

If energy is conserved in the passage of blood across the orifice, there is no change in total energy content, and the decrease in potential energy is equal to the increase in kinetic energy.

$$E_{p_1} + E_{k_1} = E_{p_2} + E_{k_2} \qquad (4)$$

Assuming that the blood contained in the chamber upstream from the orifice has zero kinetic energy, and also assuming that no potential energy is transformed in other processes (not exactly correct, but an adequate approximation for the purpose of this derivation), equations 1 and 2 can be combined.

$$P_1gV = P_2gV + (Vv_2^2/2)$$
$$(P_1 - P_2)g = v_2^2/2$$
$$(P_1 - P_2) = v_2^2/2g \qquad (5)$$

where $P_1 - P_2$ = the pressure gradient across the orifice (cm H_2O).

Since the potential energy content of blood is related linearly to pressure and the kinetic energy content of blood is related to the square of velocity, the decrement in

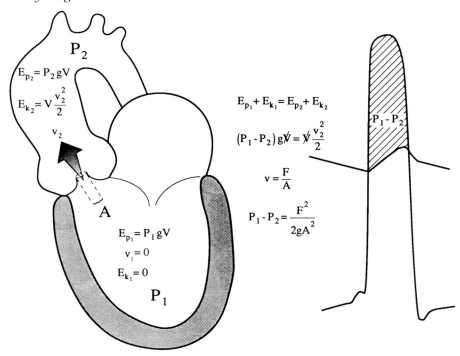

Figure 24.1. Diagram depicting biophysical events of energy transformation associated with blood flow across an orifice. In this example a stenotic aortic valve with an orifice area A is depicted. Blood in the chamber upstream from the orifice (in this case the left ventricle) has potential energy Ep_1 (ergs) determined by its pressure (P) and volume (V). Since the blood is relatively stationary, its kinetic energy E_{k_1} is considered to be zero. Blood in the chamber downstream from the orifice (in this case the aorta) has less potential energy E_{p_2} and has acquired kinetic energy E_{k_2}, which is determined by its velocity (v) and volume. Velocity (centimeters/second) of blood flow across the orifice is determined by the volume flow rate F (milliliters/ second) and orifice area A (square centimeters). As it passes through the orifice, the blood's loss of potential energy is equal to its gain of potential energy. Thus, the decrease in pressure ($P_1 - P_2$) as blood passes across the orifice is directly related to the square of the flow rate and inversely to the square of the orifice area. (See text for further details.)

pressure necessary to achieve a particular flow velocity is related directly to the square of the velocity.

The flow velocity in equation 4 may be derived by substituting measurements of flow rate into equation 1.

$$P_1 - P_2 = F^2/2gA^2 \qquad (6)$$

where F = flow rate (cm^3/sec), and A = orifice area (cm$^{2)}$.

Two consequences follow from equation 6: (*a*) At a particular flow rate, the pressure gradient across the orifice is related inversely to the square of the orifice area. (*b*) At a particular orifice area, the pressure gradient is related directly to the square of the flow rate.

Thus, curves describing the relationship between pressure gradient and flow rate across an orifice are parabolic (see Fig. 24.2).

The biophysical relationship derived above indicates that a pressure gradient should exist across a normal cardiac valve. This is, in fact, the case. Such a naturally occurring pressure gradient is termed "impulse gradient" to distinguish it from a gradient across a stenosed valve (1, 2). It is caused by the energy loss needed to (*a*) overcome resistive forces, (*b*) achieve the velocity needed to cross the orifice, and (*c*) accomplish the acceleration to that velocity. The magnitude of a typical impulse gradient is too small to be detected with a conventional fluid-filled catheter system because the obligatory artifacts in recordings made with such systems (see Chapter 18) are large

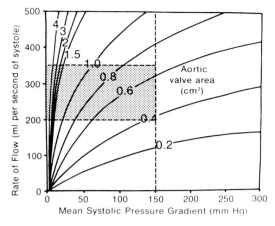

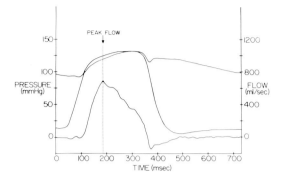

Figure 24.2. Hemodynamic characteristics of aortic stenosis. Graph of a family of curves illustrating the quadratic relationship between the aortic valve pressure gradient (mm Hg) and the transvalvular flow rate (milliliters/second) for different aortic valve orifice areas. The two *horizontal dashed lines* represent the normal aortic valve flow rate at rest and the flow rate achieved during moderately intense exercise, respectively. The *vertical dashed line* represents the maximum aortic valve pressure gradient. The *stippled area* enclosed by these lines illustrates the boundaries within which the heart must operate. Note the parabolic shape of the curves and that the curves become increasingly horizontal as valve area decreases. This relationship demonstrates why an aortic valve area of 0.5 cm^2, which only enters the lower right corner of the operating range, represents critical aortic stenosis. (Modified from Wallace AG. Pathophysiology of cardiovascular disease. In: Smith LH, Thier SO, eds. Pathophysiology. The Biological Principles of Disease. Philadelphia: WB Saunders, 1981:1200.)

Figure 24.3. Simultaneous recordings of left ventricular (*LV*) pressure, ascending aortic (*Ao*) pressure and ascending aortic flow velocity (*AoV*). Pressure recordings were made with catheter-mounted micromanometers and, accordingly, are free of the usual artifacts which distort recordings made with fluid-filled catheter systems. The velocity recording was made with a catheter-mounted velocity transducer. Flow velocity (centimeters/second) has been multiplied by the cross-sectional area of the ascending aorta to yield the flow rate (milliliters/second). Note the small systolic gradient between the left ventricle and aorta. As predicted by the Bernoulli theorem, peak magnitude of the pressure gradient coincides with peak magnitude of ascending aortic velocity.

Implications of Valve Orifice Area as a Quantification of the Severity of Valvular Stenosis

Ultimately, the most important determinant of the severity of a valvular stenosis is the actual size of the valve orifice. It should be clear from the biophysics presented above that, in the setting of a stenosed cardiac valve, the absolute magnitude of the affected cardiac chamber's pressure and the pressure gradient across the valve change as hemodynamic conditions change. Thus, a particular valve orifice area is associated with a range of intracardiac pressures and pressure gradients. **Consequently, measurement of the valve pressure gradient alone is not adequate to define the stenosis severity.**

Since the relationship between the flow across a valve orifice and the pressure gradient required to generate the flow is quadratic, small changes in certain hemodynamic parameters, such as heart rate and cardiac output, can cause large changes in the pressure

compared with the magnitude of the impulse gradient. Such gradients are recognizable, however, when pressure is recorded with precisely calibrated catheter-tip micromanometers (Fig. 24.3).

At rest, and probably during exercise, the "normal" pressure gradient that occurs across a normal cardiac valve does not contribute significantly to the hydraulic load faced by the cardiac chamber which generated it. This is because the orifice area of a normal cardiac valve is large enough to permit flow to occur at a relatively high velocity (3).

gradient. For example, a small pressure gradient may exist across a severely stenotic valve if the cardiac output is low. Also, a change in heart rate may, because of its effect on the flow time, cause a substantial change in the pressure gradient across a valve even if the cardiac output does not change.

Application of the Bernoulli Principle to the Calculation of Valve Orifice Area

Theory of the Calculation of the Valve Orifice Area by the Gorlin Equation

The concept of calculation of valve orifice area from hemodynamic measurements was originally conceived by Gorlin and Gorlin as a means of explaining the wide range of variability of hemodynamic findings in valvular stenosis (4). Despite the fact that it was published over 35 years ago, the validity of this concept has stood the test of time. The Gorlin equation applies the Bernoulli principle, as expressed in equation 5, to the hemodynamic behavior of a stenotic cardiac valve.

Equation 5 may be rearranged:

$$A^2 = F^2/2g(P_1 - P_2)$$
$$A = F/\sqrt{2g(P_1 - P_2)}$$

since $\sqrt{2g} = 44.3$

$$A = F/C\,(44.3)\,\sqrt{P_1 - P_2} \qquad (7)$$

where A = valve orifice area (cm^2), F = flow across the valve (cm^3/sec), $P_1 - P_2$ = pressure gradient (mm Hg), and C = an empiric constant to correct for viscous properties of blood and complexities of the geometry of the orifice and to convert the pressure units from cm H_2O to the clinically used mm Hg.

Equation for the Aortic Valve

In calculating the aortic valve orifice area, the average systolic pressure gradient between the left ventricle and the aorta is measured and substituted into the equation. Since aortic valve flow occurs during systole, the flow term (in milliliters/second) is the cardiac output divided by the systolic ejection period in seconds of systole/minute. The value of the constant was empirically determined by Gor-

lin and Gorlin to be 1.0 (4). Thus, for the aortic valve:

$$A = (CO/sep)/44.3\,\sqrt{P_1 - P_2} \qquad (8)$$

where CO = cardiac output (milliliters per minute), sep = systolic ejection period (seconds per minute), and $(P_1 - P_2)$ = mean (time averaged) systolic gradient, between the left ventricle and the aorta in mm Hg.

Equation for the Mitral Valve

In calculating the mitral valve orifice area, the average diastolic pressure gradient between the left atrium and the left ventricle is measured and substituted into the equation. The flow term (milliliters/second) in the equation is the cardiac output in milliliters/minute divided by the diastolic filling period in seconds of diastole/minute. The value of the constant (C) was originally determined by Gorlin and Gorlin to be 0.7. However, in the original determinations, left heart catheterization was not done. Left atrial pressure was estimated from the pulmonary-capillary wedge pressure; left ventricular diastolic pressure was assumed to be 5 mm Hg; and the pressure gradient was calculated by subtracting 5 from the pulmonary-capillary wedge pressure. The diastolic filling period was estimated by subtracting the systolic ejection period (determined from a peripheral arterial recording) from 1 min. However, these approximations tend to overestimate the actual pressure gradient and diastolic flow period. Subsequent validation studies using direct measurement of left atrial and left ventricular pressure have recalculated the value of the constant to be 0.85 (5) or 0.90 (6). The value of 0.85 was determined using pulmonary-capillary wedge pressure recordings; the value of 0.90 was determined using direct left atrial pressure measurements. Thus, for the mitral valve when a direct left atrial pressure measurement is used:

$$A = (CO/dfp)/40.0\,\sqrt{P_1 - P_2} \qquad (9)$$

where CO = cardiac output (milliliters per minute), dfp = diastolic filling period (seconds per minute), $40.0 = (44.3)(0.902)$, and $(P_1 - P_2)$ = mean (time averaged) diastolic pressure gradient between the left atrium and the left ventricle in mm Hg. If the pulmonary-capillary wedge pressure is used, the constant 40.0 should be replaced by 37.6.

It is noteworthy to point out that the same principle (Bernoulli) on which the Gorlin equation is based is used to determine transvalvular pressure gradients from Doppler ultrasound measurements of flow velocity (7, 8). In this procedure, the principle is applied somewhat differently. The flow velocity is measured, and the estimated pressure gradient is calculated from it.

Simplifications Inherent in the Gorlin Equation

The Gorlin equation is a simplified application of a physical principle to the circulation. There are two approximations, which are not exactly correct, that are involved in the actual calculation:

1. The equation uses the average pressure gradient and average flow across the valve orifice. These variables change from one cardiac cycle to the next and, over time, within each cardiac cycle.
2. The equation assumes that valve orifice is a so-called "ideal" orifice. This is known not to be the case.

In fact, the geometry of the orifices of stenotic cardiac valves is so complex as to defy precise measurement of orifice area. The equation attempts to deal with this problem by the insertion of a correction factor that was derived by comparing orifice areas calculated from the uncorrected equation with estimations of actual orifice area at the time of surgical exposure of the valve.

Despite these approximations, the valve orifice area calculated from the Gorlin equation is a measure of the hemodynamic behavior of a stenosed orifice even if it does not exactly measure the actual anatomic orifice area.

Requirements for Accurate Determination of Valve Area

Accurate determination of valve area requires a thorough understanding of the biophysical principles that underlie the Gorlin equation and acquisition of accurate valid hemodynamic data. Several basic principles apply:

1. Since cardiac output, pressure gradient, and flow time all appear in the equation, they must be measured **simultaneously.** It is not correct to measure cardiac output at one point in the study, pressure gradient at another, and then

to substitute the two values into the same equation. If the hemodynamic situation changes between the two determinations, the calculated valve area is not valid.
2. Since transvalvular flow enters the equation linearly and the pressure gradient enters the equation as a square root function, the valve area calculation is more strongly influenced by the cardiac output and the flow time measurements. Thus, it is particularly important that these measurements be precise. **In a low cardiac output state, a deceptively small valve pressure gradient can exist across a valve with a very small orifice area.**
3. Accurate determination of the transvalvular pressure gradient requires simultaneous, high-fidelity, properly damped pressure recordings from the chambers upstream and downstream from the valve in question. Pullback gradients are not accurate enough and should not be used. If the pulmonary-capillary wedge pressure is used to represent left atrial pressure, great care must be taken to obtain a recording with as high a frequency response as possible. Recordings from balloon-tipped catheters are not acceptable because attenuation of the rate of descent of pressure from the peak of the V wave will cause a systematic overestimation of the pressure gradient. Recordings should be made at a paper speed of 100 mm/sec at a gain which produces a recorded image of the gradient which is large enough to measure accurately. Average gradients should be determined by planimetric methods. If the patient is in sinus rhythm, five **consecutive** cardiac cycles should be measured and averaged. If the patient is in atrial fibrillation, no less than 10 **consecutive** cardiac cycles should be measured and averaged. Failure to use consecutive cardiac cycles risks the selection of nonrepresentative beats.

VALVULAR INSUFFICIENCY

Functional Problems Caused by a Regurgitant Cardiac Valve

In contrast to a stenotic cardiac valve, which directly affects only the chamber immediately upstream from it, a regurgitant valve always affects at least two chambers. One of the affected chambers is always a ventricle.

The fundamental physiologic consequence of a regurgitant cardiac valve is that the **regurgitant volume** (the blood that the valve allows to regurgitate) moves uselessly back and forth between the cardiac chambers upstream and downstream from the regurgitant valve. Thus, both chambers are subjected to an increased volume load. This requires both affected chambers to be distended to larger than normal volumes during their respective filling periods. This also requires that the ventricle affected by the regurgitant valve generate a stroke volume, which is the sum of the net forward and regurgitant stroke volumes.

Valvular insufficiency also differs from stenosis in that insufficiency can develop **acutely.** Disorders such as infective endocarditis, rupture of chordae tendineae, and aortic dissection can cause severe, acute valvular insufficiency. The hemodynamic consequences of abruptly developing insufficiency are different from those of gradually developing insufficiency because the heart does not have time to develop an appropriate hypertrophic response to deal with the abnormal loading condition (9–12).

Determinants of the Severity of Valvular Insufficiency

The biophysics of antegrade flow across stenotic orifices should also apply to regurgitant flow across incompetent valves. Thus, the quantitative severity of insufficiency through a cardiac valve should be determined by the pressure gradient between the two chambers during the period of insufficiency and the size of the regurgitant orifice. Accordingly, attempts have been made to extend the principle of the Gorlin equation to calculate an effective regurgitant orifice area in order to explain the behavior of regurgitant cardiac valves (13, 14). Ideally, the size of the regurgitant orifice area should predict the performance of the heart under all conceivable hemodynamic conditions. Unfortunately, this concept has not worked well in clinical practice because the nature of the pathology of many regurgitant valves causes regurgitant orifices that vary in size with changes in hemodynamic conditions (15).

Implications of Regurgitant Volume as a Quantification of the Severity of Valvular Insufficiency

The **total stroke volume** of the ventricle, which is directly affected by a regurgitant valve, is the sum of the **effective stroke volume** (the net forward stroke volume) and the

regurgitant stroke volume (the volume of blood which travels retrogradely across the regurgitant valve). Thus, if systemic cardiac output (and, consequently, effective stroke volume) is to remain in the normal range, the total stroke volume must be increased by the regurgitant volume. Two other consequences are derived from this principle.

1. The peak volume of both of the affected chambers must equal the sum of the total stroke volume and the volume at the point of maximum emptying. Thus, the increase in ventricular volume required by valvular insufficiency is determined by the magnitude of the regurgitant volume and by the quality of ventricular ejection performance.
2. The magnitude of chamber cavity pressure at the point of maximal filling is one of the determinants of the impact of the insufficiency on the overall performance of the heart. This pressure is determined by the chamber's pressure-volume relationship and the volume to which it must be distended.

Thus, the effect of valvular insufficiency on the circulation is determined by regurgitant volume, ventricular ejection performance, and the pressure-volume relationships of the affected cardiac chambers.

Regurgitant volume is not constant. Many changes in the operating parameters of the circulatory system can change the magnitude of the regurgitant volume (16–18). Changes in heart rate alter the amount of time available for insufficiency. Changes in arterial pressure can change the driving pressure responsible for the insufficiency. Changes in ventricular volume and contractile state can change the actual geometry of the regurgitant mitral orifice (14).

Measurement of the Severity of Valvular Insufficiency

Regurgitant Volume and Regurgitant Fraction

The most rigorous way to quantify the severity of valvular insufficiency is technically the most difficult (i.e., to measure the regurgitant volume). No practical technique exists to measure regurgitant volume directly in intact humans. Therefore, indirect measures are employed. Aortic regurgitant volume has been measured in humans by using catheter-mounted flow velocity transducers and scaling the velocity signal by measuring the aortic cross-sectional area (19). However, this technique is difficult to perform with precision and is not practical for routine clinical catheterization. The most practical technique is to measure the total stroke volume of the affected ventricle by quantitative angiography (see Chapter 12), and the net forward stroke volume by measuring cardiac output either by the Fick or indicator dilution technique (see Chapter 9). The regurgitant volume is then given by the difference between the total stroke volume and the regurgitant stroke volume (20).

$$RV = SV_{ANGIO} - SV_{CO} \qquad (10)$$

where RV = regurgitant volume (ml), SV_{ANGIO} = ventricular stroke volume (ml) measured from ventriculography, and SV_{CO} = net forward stroke volume (ml) measured from a cardiac output determination.

The regurgitant volume index may be calculated by normalizing the regurgitant volume-to-body surface area in the same manner as cardiac output is normalized to body surface area to calculate the cardiac index.

$$RVI = RV/BSA \qquad (11)$$

where RVI = regurgitant volume index (ml/min/m²), and BSA = body surface area (m²).

In general, a regurgitant volume index of <700 ml/min/m² represents mild insufficiency, 700 to 1700 ml/min/m² represents moderate insufficiency, 1700 to 3000 ml/min/m² represents moderately severe insufficiency, and >3000 ml/min/m² represents severe insufficiency (21, 22).

The regurgitant volume may be normalized to total stroke volume by dividing the former by the latter, yielding the **regurgitant fraction.**

$$RF = RV/SV_{ANGIO} \qquad (11)$$

where RF = regurgitant fraction (%).

The regurgitant fraction, like the ejection fraction, is a dimensionless variable which is the percent of the total stroke volume that regurgitates through the incompetent valve. In general, a regurgitant fraction of 0 to 20% represents mild insufficiency, 20 to 40% represents moderate insufficiency, 40 to 60% represents moderately severe insufficiency, and >60% represents severe insufficiency (22).

Measurements of regurgitant volume and regurgitant fraction are not widely used in routine clinical cardiac catheterization because of the complexity of making accurate measurements. There are several potential sources of error that must be carefully controlled. The independent determinations of cardiac output and stroke volume cannot be made simultaneously but must be made as close together in time as possible. The accuracy of determination of left ventricular volume is dependent on having optimal radiographic image quality, optimal chamber opacification, precise identification of chamber borders, normal chamber geometry, a representative cardiac cycle for analysis, and accurate magnification correction.

Since many of the conditions necessary for optimal ventricular volume measurement are compromised by the enlargement and distortion of the left ventricle, which occurs in chronic aortic and mitral insufficiency, precise determination of regurgitant volume and regurgitant fraction is difficult.

Qualitative Angiographic Assessment

The severity of insufficiency may also be judged by a qualitative assessment of a properly performed angiogram. This method is less rigorous but is convenient, pragmatically useful, and hence, most commonly used clinically. A qualitative system for assessing insufficiency has been been in place essentially unmodified since 1964 (23). The system is as follows:

1+ (*mild*) A trace of contrast agent insufficiency is visible in the receiving chamber but clears out during the emptying phase of the cardiac cycle.

2+ (*moderate*) Regurgitant contrast agent is visible within the entire receiving chamber and does not clear during the emptying phase of the cardiac cycle.

3+ (*moderately severe*) Regurgitant contrast agent opacifies the receiving chamber, and the opacification becomes more dense with each cardiac cycle.

4+ (*severe*) Regurgitant contrast agent completely opacifies the receiving chamber during the first cardiac cycle after full opacification of the injected chamber.

In general, these qualitative grades correspond roughly to the quantitative ranges of insufficiency severity outlined above. However,

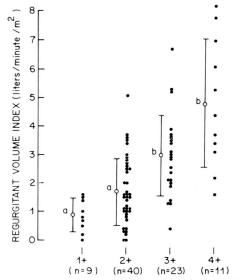

ANGIOGRAPHIC SEVERITY OF AORTIC REGURGITATION

Figure 24.4. Aortic insufficiency. Relationship between qualitative angiographic grade and quantitative measured regurgitant volume index. Each *dot* represents data from an individual patient (*n*), and the mean + 1 SD is shown to the *left* of each set of dots. Mean values of groups marked with the same letter are statistically indistinguishable. Mean values of groups marked with different letters are statistically different (*p* < 0.05). Note that although there is a statistical relationship between increasing grade of insufficiency and increasing regurgitant volume index, there is considerable scatter of the data. (From Croft CH, Lipscomb K, Mathis K, et al. Limitations of qualitative grading in aortic or mitral regurgitation. Am J Cardiol 1984; 53: 1593–1598. Reproduced with permission of the American Journal of Cardiology.)

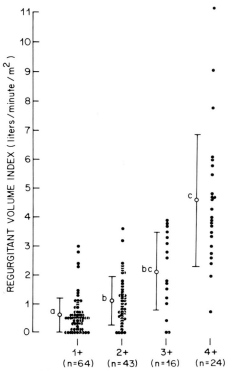

ANGIOGRAPHIC SEVERITY OF MITRAL REGURGITATION

Figure 24.5 Mitral insufficiency. Relationship between qualitative angiographic grade and quantitative measured regurgitant volume index. Format of the graph is identical to that of Figure 24.4. Note that the same semiquantitative relationship exists as for aortic insufficiency. For mitral insufficiency the quantitative magnitude of insufficiency in the lower angiographic grades is slightly less than for aortic insufficiency. (From Croft CH, Lipscomb K, Mathis K, et al. Limitations of qualitative grading in aortic or mitral regurgitation. Am J Cardiol 1984;53:1593–1598. Reproduced with permission of the American Journal of Cardiology.)

it is important to bear in mind that this system is qualitative and that the grading of a particular angiogram is influenced by a variety of other factors not directly related to the quantitative severity of the insufficiency. These include (*a*) the volume of the chamber into which the contrast agent is injected, (*b*) the volume of the chamber that receives the regurgitant volume, (*c*) the heart rate and the systemic cardiac output, and (*d*) observer bias.

Each of these factors affects the degree of dilution of the regurgitant contrast agent and, as a result, the extent of opacification of the chamber that receives it. These factors must be taken into account when assessing angiograms for insufficiency.

Studies that have examined the validity of this system have shown a reasonable semiquantitative relationship between the angiographic grade of insufficiency and a quantitative measure of insufficiency (21, 22). However, within any particular angiographic grade of insufficiency severity, there is substantial scatter of the measured regurgitant volume index (Figs. 24.4 and 24.5).

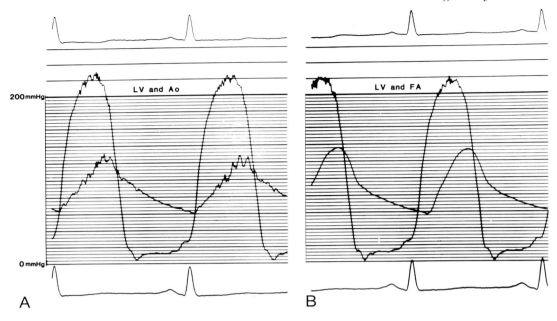

Figure 24.6. Aortic stenosis. Simultaneous recordings of left ventricular (*LV*) pressure and central aortic (*Ao*) pressure (*A*), and left ventricular and femoral arterial (*FA*) pressure (*B*) from the same patient. Note that the femoral arterial pressure has a phase lag and that the systolic peak is artifactually elevated by summation of the antegrade pulse wave with reflected waves. In order to determine a valid aortic valve gradient using a peripheral arterial pressure recording, the recording must first be corrected for phase lag and downstream distortion. (See text for details.)

AORTIC VALVE

Aortic Stenosis

Hemodynamic Assessment

Aortic stenosis is usually valvular, but occasionally is subvalvular, and rarely supravalvular. The hemodynamic alterations of aortic stenosis include the aortic valve pressure gradient, an elevated left ventricular systolic pressure, a variable elevation of left ventricular filling pressure, and a slowing of the rate of the upstroke of the aortic pressure during systole.

The quantitative severity of aortic stenosis is assessed by calculation of the aortic valve area. This requires simultaneous measurement of left ventricular pressure, aortic pressure, and cardiac output. Optimally, the aortic pressure recording should be obtained from the ascending aorta rather than from a peripheral arterial site. This is because the peripheral arterial pulse waveform is delayed by the time required for transmission of the pulse wave

from the central aorta and is distorted by reflected pulse waves (24) (Fig. 24.6). If a peripheral arterial pressure is used, it should also be recorded simultaneously with central aortic pressure in order to judge the magnitude of phase delay and pulse amplification. The peripheral arterial waveform can then be corrected to approximate the central aortic waveform.

Catheterization Technique

Two principal techniques are employed for obtaining left ventricular pressure recordings. The left ventricle may be entered either retrogradely across the aortic valve (25) or antegradely across the mitral valve via the transseptal route (26). A third, infrequently used technique for obtaining left ventricular pressure is direct left ventricular puncture. This technique is reserved for selected cases such as patients with prosthetic mechanical mitral valves and is discussed in Chapter 6.

The retrograde approach is most commonly used but occasionally can be difficult in a patient with extreme poststenotic dilation of the aorta or an eccentrically located valve orifice. Occasionally, retrograde crossing of a stenotic aortic valve dislodges calcific fragments which embolize. In patients with extremely tight aortic stenosis, the cross-sectional area of the catheter shaft occasionally can constitute a significant fraction of the aortic valve orifice area. In this circumstance the presence of the catheter shaft in the aortic valve orifice reduces the effective cross-sectional area of the valve orifice. In such circumstances the aortic pressure has been observed to rise after withdrawal of the catheter (27). The aortic pressure may be measured from a second retrograde catheter positioned in the ascending aorta or the peripheral arterial pressure may be measured from the side port of the sheath used to introduce the retrograde catheter into the arterial system. If a peripheral arterial pressure is used, it should be corrected as described above. If the side port of the arterial introducing sheath is used as a source of the pressure signal, the inside diameter of the sheath should be a full French size larger than the outside diameter of the catheter within it.

The transseptal approach has the advantage of not having to cross the aortic valve and of using the retrograde aortic catheter, inserted for aortography and coronary arteriography, to obtain a high quality central aortic pressure. On the other hand, the transseptal approach is dangerous in inexperienced hands and should be employed only by those who have mastered the technique.

When measuring left ventricular pressure with a multiple-hole catheter (e.g., a pigtail), one should be careful to be certain that all of the holes are fully in the left ventricle. Otherwise, depending on the route of access, a hybrid left ventricular-left atrial pressure or a hybrid left ventricular-aortic pressure will be obtained which superficially appears to be a valid left ventricular pressure but gives an inappropriately low value for pressure during systole. This would cause an underestimation of the aortic valve pressure gradient (see Figs. 24.7 and 24.8).

Determination of Severity

Aortic stenosis becomes hydraulically significant when the aortic valve area approaches 1 cm^2. Normal resting aortic valve flow rates are approximately 200 ml/sec. During moderately intense exercise, aortic valve flow rates increase to 300 ml/sec. A valve area of 1.0 cm^2 can transmit a 200 ml/sec flow at a pressure gradient of 21 mm Hg and a flow of 300 ml/sec at a pressure gradient of 47 mm Hg. As valve area is progressively reduced below 1.0 cm^2, the parabolic relationship between valve pressure gradient and flow rate requires a large increase in the pressure gradient (see Fig. 24.2). A valve area of 0.5 cm^2 requires a pressure gradient of 84 mm Hg to transmit 200 ml/sec and 188 mm Hg to transmit 300 ml/sec. An aortic valve pressure gradient >150 mm Hg is probably unattainable since the left ventricle generally cannot generate a systolic pressure >300 mm Hg. Thus, an aortic valve area of 0.5 mm Hg constitutes "critical" aortic stenosis. At this valve area a large resting pressure gradient is required to maintain a normal resting cardiac output, and the ability to increase cardiac output is severely limited or absent.

One should be cautious not to be misled by an apparently small systolic pressure gradient in patients with congestive heart failure and low cardiac output. A patient with an aortic valve pressure gradient of 25 mm Hg and a cardiac output of 3.0 liters/min may have an aortic valve area of 0.5 cm^2. An accurate valve area determination should be performed in all patients who have an aortic valve pressure gradient >10 mm Hg.

Aortic Insufficiency

Hemodynamic Assessment

Hemodynamic assessment of aortic insufficency requires measurement of central aortic pressure, left ventricular pressure, right heart pressures, and cardiac output. The severity of the insufficency is assessed by aortic root angiography. Since the aortic valve is not obstructive, no particular obstacle is presented to gaining access to the left ventricle by the retrograde route. In pure aortic insufficency, the left ventricular systolic pressure should be nearly equal to aortic systolic pressure.

Chronic Aortic Insufficiency

The hemodynamic alterations of **chronic** severe aortic insufficency include a large

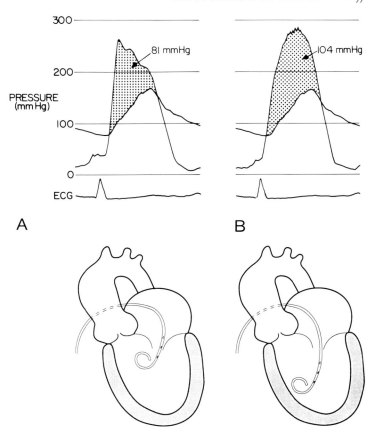

Figure 24.7. Aortic stenosis. Artifact caused by incorrect placement of a transseptal catheter in the left ventricle. *A* shows a central aortic pressure recording and an inaccurate left ventricular pressure recording obtained from an improperly positioned pigtail catheter. The left ventricular catheter is positioned such that some of its proximal holes are on the atrial side of the mitral valve. (See corresponding diagram immediately below pressure recording). This produces a recording that superficially appears to be a valid left ventricular pressure but actually underestimates the peak value of left ventricular systolic pressure. Consequently, it underestimates the aortic valve pressure gradient. *B* shows a central aortic pressure recording and an accurate left ventricular pressure recording in the same patient, obtained by advancing the transseptal catheter until all of its holes are on the left ventricular side of the mitral valve. (See text for details.)

aortic pulse pressure, a low aortic diastolic pressure (16) (Fig. 24.9*A*), and depending upon the severity of insufficiency and the quality of left ventricular function, a variable elevation of left ventricular filling pressure.

Acute Aortic Insufficiency

The hemodynamics of **acute** severe aortic insufficiency differ substantially from those of long-standing aortic insufficiency (9) (Fig. 24.9*B*). When severe aortic insufficiency develops acutely, the left ventricle cannot accept a large regurgitant volume at a normal or even moderately elevated filling pressure. Patients with acute severe aortic insufficiency are generally acutely ill with tachycardia, narrow aortic pulse pressure, and a normal aortic diastolic pressure. The aortic diastolic pressure is not low because it is supported by equilibration with a greatly elevated left ventricular end-diastolic pressure. Left ventricular end-diastolic pressure frequently exceeds left atrial pressure, causing premature closure of the mitral valve.

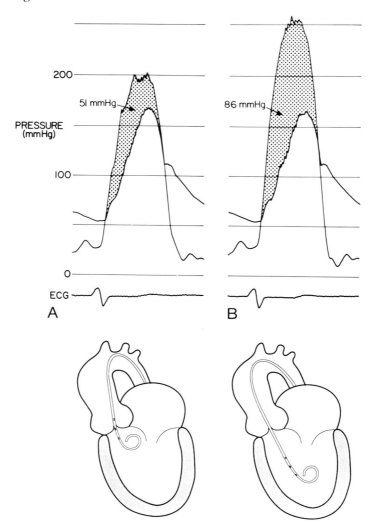

Figure 24.8. Aortic stenosis. Artifact caused by incorrect placement of a retrograde catheter in the left ventricle. The format of this figure is identical to that of Figure 24.7. *A* shows a central aortic pressure recording and an inaccurate left ventricular pressure recording obtained from an improperly positioned pigtail catheter. The left ventricular catheter is positioned such that some of its proximal holes are on the aortic side of the aortic valve. (See corresponding diagram immediately below the pressure recording.) As in Figure 24.7, this produces a recording which underestimates the peak left ventricular systolic pressure and, accordingly, the aortic valve pressure gradient. *B* shows a central aortic pressure recording and an accurate left ventricular pressure recording in the same patient, obtained by advancing the retrograde catheter until all of its holes are on the left ventricular side of the aortic valve. (See text for details.)

Catheterization Technique

Contrast aortography is performed by injecting 40 to 50 ml of contrast agent into the aortic root at 20 to 30 ml/sec. Cinefilming should be carried out with the patient positioned so that the ascending aorta, the **entire left ventricle,** and the left atrium are included in the image.

If the procedure is being performed with single-plane radiographic equipment, the left anterior oblique projection is preferable to the right anterior oblique because it is the optimal projection to demonstrate the anatomy of the aortic root. An interpretable study must provide rapid dense opacification of the aortic root without the catheter touching the aortic

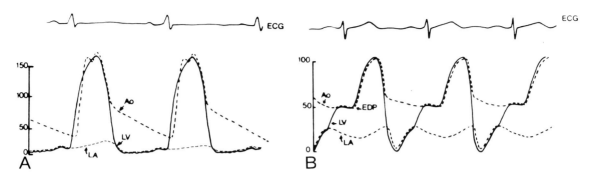

Figure 24.9. Aortic insufficiency. Representative recordings of aortic (*Ao*) and left ventricular (*LV*) pressure in chronic severe aortic insufficiency (*A*), and acute severe aortic insufficiency (*B*). A representation of left atrial (*LA*) pressure has been drawn into the figures to illustrate the behavior of the mitral valve in the two conditions. In the example of chronic aortic insufficiency, note the large aortic pulse pressure, low aortic diastolic pressure, and relatively normal left ventricular filling pressure and left atrial pressure. In the example of acute aortic insufficiency, note the normal aortic pulse pressure, normal aortic diastolic pressure, and strikingly elevated left ventricular filling pressure that equilibrates with aortic pressure and, during the latter portion of diastole (*EDP*), exceeds left atrial pressure, passively closing the mitral valve. *ECG*, electrocardiograph. (Modified from Morganroth J, Perloff JK, Zeldis SM, Dunkman WB. Acute severe aortic regurgitation: pathophysiology, clinical recognition, and management. Ann Intern Med 1977;87:223–232.)

valve. Accordingly, the catheter should be positioned with its tip just above the aortic valve. During the injection, the catheter should be allowed neither to recoil into the upper ascending aorta nor to advance into contact with the aortic valve. In patients with severe aortic insufficiency who are hemodynamically precarious and can only tolerate a single contrast agent injection, this study, if properly executed, will both define the severity of the aortic insufficiency and opacify the left ventricle sufficiently to assess its function and mitral valve competence.

MITRAL VALVE

Mitral Stenosis

Hemodynamic Assessment

The hemodynamics of mitral stenosis are characterized by the mitral valve pressure gradient and elevated left atrial pressure. Chronic left atrial hypertension causes reactive pulmonary arteriolar vasoconstriction, which may lead to a chronic obliterative destruction of the pulmonary arterioles. Consequently, patients with mitral stenosis can have both a reactive and a fixed elevation of pulmonary vascular resistance. The left ventricle is underfilled because of the valvular obstruction to

filling, and its function is affected only by whatever distortion of its geometry is caused by enlargement and hypertrophy of the right ventricle (28). Pulmonary artery pressure and left atrial pressure are variably elevated, and cardiac output is normal or variably reduced (29).

This wide variation in hemodynamic profile, in which some patients have normal cardiac output and substantially elevated left atrial and right heart pressures while others have reduced cardiac output and normal or only slightly elevated left atrial and right heart pressures, provided the original stimulation for the research which led to the Gorlin valve orifice area formula.

Like aortic stenosis, the severity of mitral stenosis is quantified by the calculation of the mitral valve area. This requires simultaneous measurement of left atrial pressure, left ventricular pressure, and cardiac output. Optimally, the left atrial pressure should be obtained directly from the left atrium rather than indirectly from a pulmonary-capillary wedge recording. However, in practice, the pulmonary-capillary wedge pressure is frequently substituted for the direct left atrial pressure because many operators are not experienced in the transseptal technique.

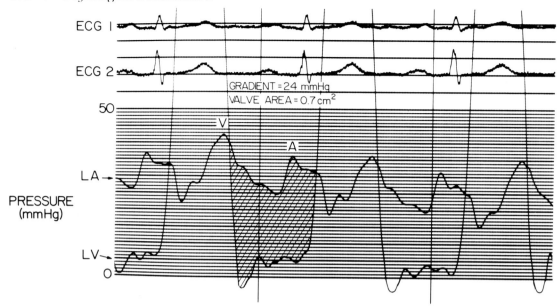

Figure 24.10. Severe mitral stenosis. Simultaneous recording of left atrial (*LA*) and left ventricular (*LV*) pressure illustrating the mitral valve pressure gradient. Note that the descent of the V wave begins promptly at the time of the early diastolic pressure crossover. Note also that the stenotic mitral valve impedes transmission of the A wave of left atrial systole to the left ventricle. Thus, during atrial systole the pressure gradient increases.

Catheterization Technique

The mitral valve pressure gradient is determined by simultaneously recording left atrial and left ventricular pressure (Fig. 24.10). If a pulmonary-capillary wedge recording is to be used, great care must be taken to maximize the fidelity of the recording. This may be difficult in patients with mitral stenosis because right heart enlargement frequently complicates catheter manipulation. The pulmonary-capillary wedge pressure is damped and has a phase lag compared with the directly recorded left atrial pressure. The damping attenuates the *y* descent of left atrial pressure and the phase lag delays it. Both of these phenomena can cause an incorrect overestimation of the mitral valve pressure gradient (see Fig. 24.11). The recording should only be made with a standard end-hole catheter such as a Cournand or a Goodale-Lubin. A pulmonary-capillary wedge pressure estimated from the pulmonary artery balloon occlusion pressure recorded from a balloon-tipped catheter is unacceptably damped and has an even greater phase lag.

Patients with mitral stenosis are frequently in atrial fibrillation, and accordingly, at least 10 consecutive cardiac cycles should be averaged to determine the mean diastolic gradient.

Left ventricular pressure is generally obtained by retrograde catheterization using standard techniques. A technique for antegrade crossing of the mitral valve, using a balloon-tipped catheter introduced through a transseptally placed sheath, has been developed (30). Since left atrial pressure can then be measured using the side port of the sheath, this provides a simultaneous measurement of left ventricular pressure and left atrial pressure from a single venous entry. However, since most assessments of mitral stenosis require a separate arterial entry, left ventricular pressure is most commonly recorded from a retrograde entry into the left ventricle.

Determination of Severity

Mitral stenosis becomes hydraulically significant when mitral valve area approaches 1.5 cm² and critical at a valve area of 1.0 cm². This is a larger area than the corresponding range for the aortic valve because the maximum mitral valve pressure gradient that can be

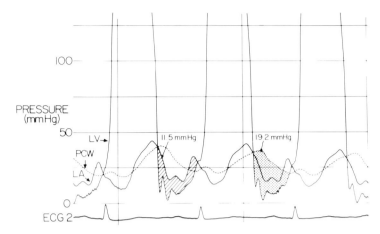

Figure 24.11. Moderate mitral stenosis. Simultaneous recording of pulmonary-capillary wedge pressure (*PCW*), left atrial (*LA*) pressure, and left ventricular (*LV*) pressure to illustrate the relationship between pulmonary-capillary wedge pressure and the directly recorded left atrial pressure. The pulmonary-capillary wedge pressure recording is shown by a *dashed line* in order to distinguish it from the left atrial recording. Mitral valve pressure gradients determined from the two recordings are *shaded* in different beats, and their planimetered values are indicated. Note that, compared to the left atrial recording, the pulmonary-capillary wedge pressure has a phase lag and that oscillations are damped. Damping attenuates the rate of the *y* descent from the peak of the V wave causing overestimation of the mitral valve pressure gradient. The degree of overestimation could be even greater if a poor quality pulmonary-capillary wedge recording were used. Note also that, in this case of moderate mitral stenosis, the left atrial A wave is partially transmitted to the left ventricle. *ECG,* electrocardiograph.

tolerated is substantially lower than the corresponding gradient for the aortic valve. Since the lungs generally do not tolerate a pulmonary-capillary wedge pressure >30 mm Hg, the maximum tolerable mean mitral valve pressure gradient is approximately 20 mm Hg.

Normal resting mitral valve flow rates are approximately 150 ml/sec. Because the duration of diastole is abbreviated as heart rate increases, mitral valve flow rate must increase markedly when heart rate and cardiac output increase. A mitral valve area of 1.5 cm^2 requires a pressure gradient of 7 mm Hg to transmit a flow rate of 150 ml/sec. If left ventricular filling pressure is normal, this would require a mean left atrial pressure of 15 mm Hg. At the maximum allowable pressure gradient of 20 mm Hg, a mitral valve area of 1.5 cm^2 can transmit a flow rate of 250 ml/sec. However, if mitral valve area is reduced to 1.0 cm^2, a 16 mm Hg pressure gradient is required to transmit the normal resting flow rate of 150 ml/sec. This requires a resting left atrial pressure of 20 to 25 mm Hg. The parabolic relationship between valve pressure gradient and transvalvular flow (Fig. 24.12) dictates that, at a valve area of 1.0 cm^2, the

transvalvular flow rate is essentially fixed. Thus, a mitral valve area of 1.0 cm^2 represents critical mitral stenosis.

Mitral Insufficiency

Hemodynamic Assessment

The hemodynamic assessment of mitral insufficiency requires measurement of left ventricular pressure, left atrial or pulmonary-capillary wedge pressure, aortic pressure, right heart pressures, and cardiac output. The severity of mitral insufficiency is assessed by left ventriculography.

Chronic Mitral Insufficiency

The hemodynamics of **chronic** severe mitral insufficiency are characterized by a brisk systolic upstroke of aortic pressure (31, 32) and highly variable elevations of left atrial pressure and left ventricular filling pressure (33). The striking variation in left atrial pressure and left ventricular filling pressure is attributable to variations in intravascular volume, left atrial compliance, left ventricular function, and systemic vascular resistance. Similarly,

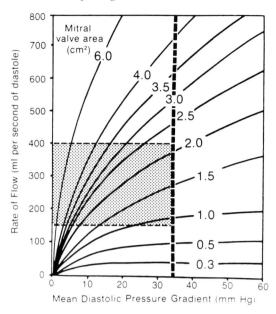

Figure 24.12. Hemodynamic characteristics of mitral stenosis. Graph of a family of curves illustrating quadratic relationship between mitral valve pressure gradient (mm Hg) and the transvalvular flow rate (milliliters/second of diastole) for different mitral valve orifice areas. The two *horizontal lines* represent the normal mitral valve flow rate at rest and the flow rate achieved during moderately intense exercise, respectively. The *vertical line* represents the upper limit of allowable left atrial pressure. The *stippled area* enclosed by the lines illustrates boundaries within which the heart must operate. Note the parabolic shape of the curves and that the curves become increasingly horizontal as valve area decreases. This relationship demonstrates why a mitral valve area of $1.0 \, cm^2$, which only enters the lower right corner of the operating range, represents critical mitral stenosis. (Modified from Wallace AG. Pathophysiology of cardiovascular disease. In: Smith LH, Thier SO, eds. Pathophysiology. The Biological Principles of Disease. Philadelphia: WB Saunders, 1981:1192.)

the prominence of the left atrial V wave is variable. It is important to emphasize that the V wave of left atrial pressure is neither a sensitive nor a specific criterion for including or excluding the presence of chronic mitral insufficiency of any severity (34).

Acute Mitral Insufficiency

The hemodynamics of **acute** severe mitral insufficiency differ from those of the chronic severe form of the disease. The aortic pressure is generally low, left atrial pressure is generally elevated and has a prominent V wave, and left ventricular filling pressure is variably elevated (Fig. 24.13). Patients with acute severe mitral insufficiency are generally acutely ill with tachycardia, pulmonary vascular congestion, and reduced forward cardiac output. In this circumstance, the reflex elevation of systemic vascular resistance is detrimental to the generation of systemic cardiac output. Such patients often exhibit dramatic acute hemodynamic improvement when treated with vasodilators (35).

Catheterization Technique

Contrast ventriculography is performed by injecting 40 to 50 ml of contrast agent into the left ventricle at 10 to 14 ml/sec. Care should be taken to position the catheter within the left ventricle not too close to the mitral valve and to select an injection rate that provides satisfactory opacification but does not cause ventricular ectopy. If the study is performed with single-plane radiographic equipment, the right anterior oblique projection should be used. The degree of obliquity should be slightly greater than usual in order to separate the left atrium from the thoracic spine. If biplane radiographic equipment is used, the left anterior oblique projection should be steep enough to separate the left atrium from the thoracic spine and should be cranially angulated in order to separate the left atrium from the left ventricle. The angiographic study should, if properly executed, quantify left ventricular size and function and the severity of the mitral insufficiency.

PULMONIC VALVE

Pulmonic Stenosis

Hemodynamic Assessment

Pulmonic stenosis is almost invariably congenital. The stenosis can be either at the level of the pulmonic valve itself, above or below the valve, or at multiple locations. The most common form of pulmonic stenosis is the combination of valvular and subvalvular (or infundibular) stenosis. The hemodynamics of pulmonic stenosis are characterized by the pulmonic valve pressure gradient and the

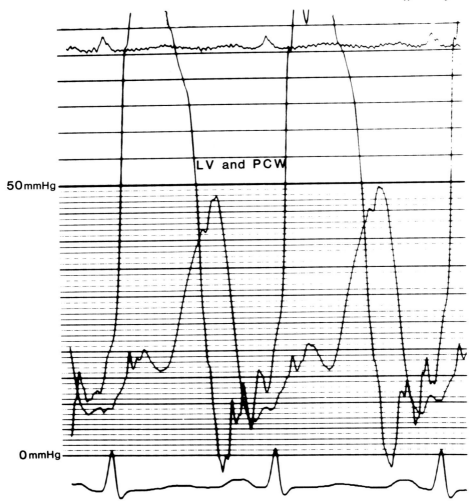

Figure 24.13. Acute severe mitral insufficiency. Simultaneous recording of pulmonary-capillary wedge (*PCW*) and left ventricular (*LV*) pressures. Note the large V wave, which frequently occurs in acute severe mitral insufficiency. The apparent early diastolic mitral valve pressure gradient is attributable to a somewhat damped pulmonary-capillary wedge tracing and rapid diastolic transmitral flow velocity, which is required by the insufficiency.

right ventricular response to the pressure load. The pulmonary artery pressure is invariably normal or low. Therefore, the right ventricular pressure is an accurate reflection of the severity of the obstruction.

Catheterization Technique

The three purposes of the catheterization study in pulmonic stenosis are to localize the obstruction, to quantify its severity, and to identify any other congenital abnormalities. Accordingly, the pressure gradient across the

pulmonic valve is measured by simultaneous recording of right ventricular and pulmonary artery pressure, and cardiac output is determined.

Particular care must be taken to localize the obstruction by pressure recording during a careful pullback across the pulmonary outflow tract. Subvalvular obstruction may be identified by finding a zone in the right ventricular outflow tract in which the pressure contour is clearly ventricular but has a lower systolic peak than does the body of the ventricle (Fig. 24.14). Right ventricular angiography

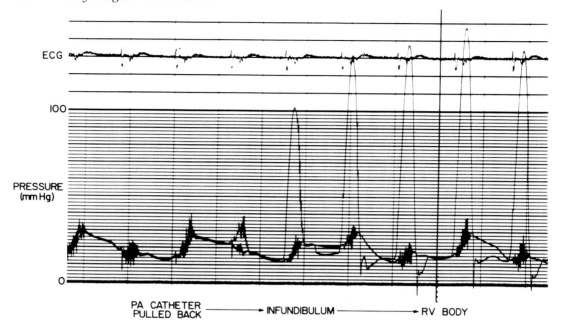

Figure 24.14. Severe valvular and subvalvular pulmonic stenosis. Recording of pulmonary artery (*PA*) pressure with two catheter-mounted micromanometers. During the recording, one of the two micro-manometers was gradually pulled back across the pulmonic valve into the right ventricle (*RV*). During one cardiac cycle, it was located in the subvalvular infundibular chamber where it recorded a right ventricular pressure with a peak systolic pressure 30 mm Hg below the systolic pressure recorded in the body of the ventricle. This demonstrates the two zones of obstruction to right ventricular outflow.

delineates the anatomy of the right ventricular outflow tract. This also helps to localize the obstruction.

Determination of Severity

Although the valve area concept should apply to the pulmonic valve, it is rarely used in specifying the severity of pulmonic stenosis. In general, a right ventricular outflow gradient of <50 mm Hg constitutes mild, and a gradient >75 mm Hg a severe, pulmonic stenosis (36).

TRICUSPID VALVE

Tricuspid Stenosis

Hemodynamic Assessment

The hemodynamics of tricuspid stenosis are characterized by the tricuspid valve pressure gradient and consequent elevation of right atrial pressure and relative underfilling of the right ventricle. Tricuspid stenosis, which is almost invariably a sequella of rheumatic

fever, almost always coexists with disease of other cardiac valves. Consequently, the other right heart pressures will be influenced by the severity and type of other valve disease.

Catheterization Technique

The tricuspid valve must be crossed in order to measure the gradient. This may be technically difficult because patients with tricuspid stenosis frequently have very large right atria, which makes catheter manipulation difficult. The difficulty of crossing the tricuspid valve generally discloses the presence of previously unrecognized tricuspid stenosis.

Because the degree of pressure elevation tolerable is less for the right atrium than for the left atrium, the magnitude of the pressure gradient found across a stenotic tricuspid valve is less than that commonly found across a stenotic mitral valve. Patients with tricuspid stenosis frequently have atrial fibrillation. The combination of atrial fibrillation and the small pressure gradient makes simultaneous right atrial and right ventricular pressure recording essential to the detection and accurate assessment of tricuspid stenosis.

The tricuspid valve area may be calculated using the same equation as for the mitral valve.

Determination of Severity

As mentioned above, tricuspid stenosis is clinically significant at a larger valve area than is mitral stenosis. Thus, a tricuspid valve area as large as 1.5 cm^2 constitutes severe tricuspid stenosis.

ACKNOWLEDGMENTS

The author would like to thank Howard C. Herrmann M.D., William G. Kussmaul M.D., and Warren K. Laskey M.D. and his colleagues on the faculty of the Cardiac Catheterization Laboratory at the Hospital of the University of Pennsylvania for contributing some of the pressure recordings used in this chapter; John H. Miller M.D., faculty of the Clinical Electrophysiology Laboratory at the Hospital of the University of Pennsylvania, for assistance in preparing illustrations; and Nancy S. Ripley for expert secretarial assistance.

References

1. Murgo JP, Altobelli SA, Dorethy JF, Logsdon JR, McGranahan GM. Normal ventricular ejection dynamics in man during rest and exercise. Am Heart Assoc Monogr 1975;46:92–101.
2. Nichols WW, Pepine CJ, Geiser EA, Conti CR. Vascular load defined by the aortic input impedance spectrum. Fed Proc 1980;39:196–201.
3. Murgo JP, Westerhof N, Giolma JP, Altobelli SA. Effects of exercise on aortic input impedance and pressure wave forms in normal humans. Circ Res 1981;48:334–343.
4. Gorlin R, Gorlin SG. Hydraulic formula for calculation of stenotic mitral valve, other cardiac valves, and central circulatory shunts. Am Heart J 1951;41:1–29.
5. Hammermeister KE, Murray JA, Blackmon JR. Revision of Gorlin constant for calculation of mitral valve area from left heart pressures. Br Heart J 1972;35:392–396.
6. Cohen MV, Gorlin, R. Modified orifice equation for the calculation of mitral valve area. Am Heart J 1972;84:839–840.
7. Young JB, Quinones MA, Waggoner AD, Miller RR. Diagnosis and quantification of aortic stenosis with pulsed Doppler echocardiography. Am J Cardiol 1980;45:487–494.
8. Holen J, Aaslid R, Landmark K, Simonsen S. Determination of pressure gradient in mitral stenosis with noninvasive ultrasound Doppler technique. Acta Med Scand 1976;199:455–460.
9. Morganroth J, Perloff JK, Zeldis SM, Dunkman WB. Acute severe aortic regurgitation: pathophysiology, clinical recognition, and management. Ann Intern Med 1977;87:223–232.
10. Auger P, Wigle ED. Sudden severe mitral insufficiency. Can Med Assoc J 1967;96:1493–1503.
11. Braunwald E. Mitral regurgitation: physiological, clinical and surgical considerations. N Engl J Med 1969;281:425–433.
12. Sasayama S, Takahashi M, Osakada G, et al. Dynamic geometry of the left atrium and left ventricle in acute mitral regurgitation. Circulation 1979;60:177–186.
13. Gorlin R, Dexter L. Hydraulic formula for the calculation of the cross sectional area of the mitral valve during regurgitation. Am Heart J 1952;43:188–205.
14. Yellin EL, Yoran EL, Sonnenblick EH, Gabbay S, Frater RWM. Dynamic changes in the canine mitral regurgitant orifice area during ventricular ejection. Circ Res 1979;45:677–683.
15. Yoran C, Yellin EL, Becker RM, Gabbay S, Frater RWM, Sonnenblick EH. Dynamic aspects of acute mitral regurgitation: effects of ventricular volume, pressure and contractility on the effective regurgitant orifice area. Circulation 1979;60:170–176.
16. Judge TP, Kennedy JW, Bennett LJ, Willis RE, Murray JA, Blackman JR. Quantitative hemodynamic effects of heart rate on aortic regurgitation. Circulation 1971;44:355–367.
17. Dehmer GJ, Firth EG, Hillis LD, et al. Alterations in left ventricular volumes and ejection fraction at rest and during exercise in patients with aortic regurgitation. Am J Cardiol 1981;48:17–27.
18. Yoran C, Yellin EH, Becker RM, Gabbay S, Frater RW, Sonnenblick EH. Mechanism of reduction of mitral regurgitation with vasodilator therapy. Am J Cardiol 1979;43:773–777.
19. Nichols WW, Pepine CJ, Conti CR, Christie LG, Feldman RL. Quantitation of aortic insufficiency using a catheter-tip velocity transducer. Circulation 1981;64:375–380.
20. Sandler H, Dodge HT, Hay RE, Rackley CE. Quantitation of valvular insufficiency in man by angiocardiography. Am Heart J 1963;65:501–513.
21. Hunt D, Baxley WA, Kennedy JW, Judge TP, Williams JE, Dodge HT. Quantitative evaluation of cineaortography in the assessment of aortic regurgitation. Am J Cardiol 1973;31:696–700.
22. Croft CH, Lipscomb K, Mathis K, et al. Limitations of qualitative grading in aortic or mitral regurgitation. Am J Cardiol 1984;53:1593–1598.
23. Sellers RD, Levy MJ, Amplatz KW, Lillehei CW. Left retrograde cardioangiography in acquired cardiac disease. Am J Cardiol 1964;14:437–447.
24. Murgo JP, Westerhof N, Giolma JP, Altobelli SA. Aortic input impedance in normal man: relationship to pressure wave forms. Circulation 1980;62:105–116.
25. Laskey WK, Hirshfeld JW, Untereker WJ, Kusiak V, Martin JL, Groh WC. A safe and rapid technique for retrograde catheterization of the left ventricle in aortic stenosis. Cathet Cardiovasc Diagn 1982;8:429–435.
26. Laskey WK, Kusiak V, Untereker WJ, Hirshfeld JW.

Transseptal left heart catheterization: utility of a sheath technique. Cathet Cardiovasc Diagn 1982;8:535–542.

27. Carabello BA, Barry WH, Grossman W. Changes in arterial pressure during left heart pullback in aortic stenosis; a sign of severe aortic stenosis. Am J Cardiol 1979;44:424–427.

28. Ahmed SS, Regan TJ, Fiore JJ, Levinson GE. The state of the left ventricular myocardium in mitral stenosis. Am Heart J 1977;94:28–36.

29. Hugenholtz PG, Ryan TJ, Stein SW, Abelmann WH. The spectrum of pure mitral stenosis. Hemodynamic studies in relation to clinical disability. Am J Cardiol 1962;10:773–784.

30. Lam W, Jones J, Pietras R. Transseptal balloon catheterization of the left ventricle in adult valvular heart disease. Am Heart J 1984;107:147–152.

31. Braunwald E, Welch GH, Sarnoff SJ. Hemodynamic effects of quantitatively varied experimental mitral regurgitation. Circ Res 1957;5:539–545.

32. Ross J, Braunwald E, Morrow AG. Clinical and hemodynamic observations in pure mitral insufficiency. Am J Cardiol 1958;2:11–23.

33. Braunwald E, Awe WC. The syndrome of severe mitral regurgitation with normal left atrial pressure. Circulation 1963;27:29–35.

34. Fuchs RM, Heuser HR, Yin FCP, Brinker JA. Limitations of pulmonary wedge V waves in diagnosing mitral regurgitation. Am J Cardiol 1982;49:849-854.

35. Harshaw CW, Grossman W, Munro AB, McLaurin LP. Reduced systemic vascular resistance as therapy for severe mitral regurgitation of valvular origin. Ann Intern Med 1975;82:312–316.

36. Johnson LW, Grossman W, Dalen JE, Dexter L. Pulmonic stenosis in the adult: long term followup results. N Engl J Med 1972;287:1159–1163.

25

The Cardiac Catheterization Report, Records, and Data Base

James A. Hill, M.D.
Charles R. Lambert, M.D., Ph.D.
Carl J. Pepine, M.D.

INTRODUCTION

The ability to communicate, store, and retrieve data is an essential function of the cardiac catheterization laboratory. The record generated to communicate the results of a catheterization procedure is an important source of information about a patient. In most cases, it is essential for medical care and, as such, is an important legal document. It also provides information to discover trends in catheterization practice, information for quality assurance monitoring, and a data base to conduct and guide clinical investigation. A variety of commercial computer-based systems have been developed to provide the catheterization laboratory with reporting systems to meet many of these needs. However, as with any system that is generically developed, often the specific needs of any given laboratory or group of operators are poorly addressed. It is not our purpose to discuss in detail the various commercial report generating systems currently available. Instead, in this chapter we will define the essential elements of a catheterization report to help in the assessment of current systems or development of custom systems by the user.

ELEMENTS OF REPORT

General

The most fundamental general feature of any successful automated catheterization record system, particularly when it is computer-based, is that it must be a by-product of the physician's routine. When the record-keeping system hinders daily catheterization laboratory practice, it is destined to failure.

Patient Identification

The obvious beginning of any record is the patient demographic data that should include name, sex, date of the procedure, date of birth, Social Security number, height, weight, body surface area, and medical record number for local identification. Many physicians also add data from the history and physical examination. This may be extensive, including the electrocardiogram, chest x-ray, exercise test, and other ancillary laboratory data, or only a brief summary. This is particularly helpful if the catheterizing physician also provides the major cardiac consultation. Often the catheterization report is the easiest portion of the medical record to obtain and, to the person who reads the report at some later date, it can provide a major amount of useful historical information. How much information any particular laboratory and physician chooses to include in the patient demographic section will vary according to local need and practice patterns.

Indications for the Procedure

Indications for the procedure should be included in the report. This gives anyone reading it some idea as to why the procedure was performed and is good medical practice.

Moreover, it provides information for quality assurance monitoring. Certification organizations including the Joint Commission for the Accreditation of Health Organizations (JCAHO), various third party insurance providers, and Medicare all stipulate that the indications for any procedure should be made clear in the medical record. Documenting indications in the catheterization report assures that this information is available in a legible form should it be needed at a later date.

As noted in other chapters of this book, the American College of Cardiology, the American Heart Association, and other professional organizations have formed task forces to provide guidelines for indications of the various cardiac catheterization procedures. These include cardiac catheterization laboratories, coronary angiography, coronary angioplasty, permanent pacemaker implantation, and invasive electrophysiologic testing. It is prudent to have these reports filed in the catheterization laboratory and to utilize them for quality assurance. It is the authors' practice to include the indications for any procedure in the same terminology used in these published reports and to provide a reference to these indications in the catheterization report. This practice permits accurate communication in a common language among various groups.

Complications

Complications occurring either during or as a result of a catheterization procedure must be included in the report. Again, these should be reported in a uniform fashion among the various operators with an explanation of the occurrence and outcome. It is the authors' practice to have a complication list filled out and signed by the attending physician immediately prior to the patient's leaving the laboratory. An example is illustrated in Table 25.1. Note that this practice requires the physician to certify that either no complication occurred or a specific problem developed. If a major problem occurs, it is also useful to provide a detailed narrative summary of events surrounding the occurrence immediately on leaving the laboratory. In all patients, at the time of discharge or no later than 24 hr postcatheterization, either a nurse or physician from the laboratory should record results of a postcatheterization visit for inclusion into the final report. This report should include any adverse events that may have occurred since the patient left the laboratory and a follow-up about any adverse event that may have occurred in the laboratory. If the patient experienced an adverse reaction during the procedure, it is a good practice for the catheterizing physician to perform the follow-up visit.

Technical Aspects of the Procedure

All events that occur in the catheterization laboratory should be recorded. The record should be sufficiently detailed to permit a reconstruction of the procedure days or even months later. This will frequently be done by maintaining a chronological log of any actions or events that occur. This log should also include the time that any actions or events occurred. Pertinent times that should be listed include starting and finishing, medication administration, catheter exchanges, performance of angiography, blood sampling, and other items relevant to the performance and interpretation of the procedure. In addition, views used for cineangiography, duration of fluoroscopy, fluid volume administered, contrast volume and type given, patient condition, estimated blood loss, and the number of angiograms should be recorded. The log should also include sites used for pressure recording and blood sampling. This log should also include nurses' notes and be maintained as part of the patient file. All of this information does not necessarily need to be incorporated into the report but is maintained in the catheterization laboratory files as part of the permanent record. A sample of such a log is included in Figure 25.1.

Many technical aspects of the procedure are important enough to include in the final report because they may be relevant to complications and important to those who may need to perform catheterization at some future time in the same patient. These include: approach utilized; any peculiar problems of technique such as difficulty in manipulating catheters beyond vascular obstructions; catheters utilized; and condition of the pulses before and after the procedure. Too often many extraneous, irrelevant details are included such as "the patient was placed on the table, prepped, and draped." This tendency should be avoided.

Hemodynamic Data

Hemodynamic measurements are an essential part of any cardiac catheterization

Table 25.1.
Report Form of Complications of Cardiac Catheterization

Major	Minor
Circle appropriate responses in each column:	
Death in catheterization laboratory	Allergic reaction
Death within 48 hr	Vasovagal reaction
Myocardial infarction	Transient ECG changes
Cerebrovascular complications	Hypotension
Local femoral artery complications	Infection
Local brachial artery complications	Phlebitis
Cardiac perforation	Other (describe)_____
Great vessel perforation	
Coronary artery dissection	
Ventricular fibrillation	
Ventricular tachycardia	
Asystole	
Complete heart block	
Atrial fibrillation	
Atrial flutter	
Supraventricular tachycardia	
Allergic reaction	
Vasovagal reaction	
Hypotension requiring transfusion	
Bleeding requiring transfusion	
Renal dysfunction	
Incomplete study	
Other (describe)_____	
Explanation:	
Resolution:	
None	
Attending:_____Assistant/Fellow:_____	

procedure and thus the report should document these data and contain an accurate interpretation of these results. These descriptions can be of varying degree of complexity depending on the techniques utilized. Many currently available computer systems for catheterization laboratories have the ability to automatically record the hemodynamic data by converting from analog to digital format. They also often provide an example of the specific pressure recording for the report. A major problem with these systems is that often the measurements are taken at slightly different phases of respiration and at different parts of the procedure or do not account for beat-to-beat variability of cardiac function, particularly in patients with an irregular rhythm. This is particularly true with "pullback" measurements, and often physiologically impossible data are reported such as systolic aortic pressure higher than systolic left

ventricular pressure. If such a system is used, it must be "over read" before it becomes a final report.

A more significant problem may be the reporting of pressure gradients where none exist. Because such systems have the ability to calculate a number of indices using the numbers generated, the computer-generated report that automatically reads the analog pressure data often is cluttered with meaningless information. The recording fidelity of standard fluid-filled catheters used for cardiac angiography and the care with which they are calibrated and flushed do not yield measurements that are accurate enough to derive some of the indices (e.g., dp/dt) that are available with many currently available computer-generated catheterization reports. Moreover, many of these parameters are poorly understood by most of those who will read and use the report. Thus, such findings

DATE		PHYSICIAN		

☐ Patient Consent   ☐ History & Physical   DATE OF BIRTH
☐ 12 Lead Electrocardiogram

HEIGHT	WEIGHT	B.S.A.	ARRIVAL TIME ☐ AM ☐ PM	FROM (Ward)

PATIENT INFORMATION

VITALS:BP	HR.	TEMP	PULSES ☐ Doppler	LOCATION(S)
/			☐ 1+ ☐ 2+ ☐ 3+	

LABS   Hct _____ BUN _____ PT _____ Glucose _____
       Hgb _____ Creat _____ K+ _____ PTT _____ ☐ T&S ☐ T&CM

HISTORY _____

PRE-OP MEDICATIONS _____

ALLERGIES _____

ANCILLARY EQUIPMENT _____

PROCEDURE(S):

☐ Left Heart Only	☐ Temp. Pacer Insertion
☐ Right Heart Only	☐ Permanent Pacemaker
☐ Combined Heart	☐ Biopsy
☐ P.T.C.A.	☐ Electrophysiology Study
☐ P.T.A.	☐ Transseptal
☐ Pacing	☐ IAB Insertion
☐ Ergonovine Provocation	☐ Cardioversion
☐ Exercise Testing	☐ Thrombolytic Therapy
☐ Valvuloplasty	☐ Investigational Protocol
☐ Pericardiocentesis	☐ Other _____

IV SITE	DRUG	RATE

ROUTE:

☐ Right Femoral Percutaneous	☐ Right Brachial Cutdown
☐ Left Femoral Percutaneous	☐ Left Brachial Cutdown
☐ Right Brachial Percutaneous	☐ Internal Jugular
☐ Left Brachial Percutaneous	☐ Other _____

PROCEDURE

LOCAL: ☐ AM   ☐ PM
Time(s) _____
Site(s) _____
☐ 1% Lidocaine
☐ 2% Lidocaine

TIME	CATHETER	SITE	TIME	CATHETER	SITE
1			8		
2			9		
3			10		
4			11		
5			12		
6			13		
7			14		

CARDIAC OUTPUT:
☐ Thermodilution
☐ Green Dye
Sites _____
C.O. _____ L/min
_____ L/min
_____ L/min
_____ L/min

TIME	SITE	SENSITIVITY	COMMENTS	TIME	SITE	SENSITIVITY	COMMENTS
	1				5		
	2				6		
	3				7		
	4				8		

TIME	MEDICATION	DOSAGE	ROUTE	TIME	MEDICATION	DOSAGE	ROUTE

ANGIOGRAPHY: Midchest _____ cm

SITE	GRID	ANGLE	PROGRAM	SITE	PROJECTION	SITE	PROJECTION
				1		6	
				2		7	
				3		8	
				4		9	
				5			

FLOUROSCOPY TIME _____ min.

CATH. REMOVAL TIME ☐ AM ☐ PM	DEPARTURE TIME ☐ AM ☐ PM	TO (Ward)	VITALS: BP	HR.	TEMP.	PULSES ☐ Doppler	LOCATION(S)
			/			☐ 1+ ☐ 2+ ☐ 3+	

INTAKE AND OUTPUT   ☐ IN   ☐ OUT
_____ ml. contrast _____ ml. fluids _____ ml _____ ml. total _____ ml. voided _____ ml. blood

COMPLICATIONS: ☐ None ☐ Yes, Letter(s) _____ Explanation _____

RECORDER	PHYSICIAN

CARDIAC CATHERIZATION PROCEDURE SHEET   WHITE COPY—CHART   CANARY COPY—DEPARTMENT   PINK COPY—OUTPATIENT/INPATIENT SUMMARY

Figure 25.1. An example of a flow sheet log used during the cardiac catheterization procedure.

have very little clinical importance. It is important to remember that the burden of accuracy and the clarification and interpretation of data remain with the operator, not with the computer.

Hemodynamic measurements should be recorded and reported as either simultaneously obtained or direct pullback. They can be listed in any order, but it is the authors' practice to list hemodynamic measurements in the order in which blood passes into the heart from the venous circulation. Calculated indices are listed only when the accuracy of the measurements can be reasonably assured, as with systemic and pulmonary resistance in a standard catheterization. When high-fidelity micromanometers are used, additional data may be added if there is clinical relevance. If this is done appropriately, there is little to be gained by having analog or digital pressure displays reproduced in the report. There is also no point to including valve areas when patients don't have valvular stenosis. Finally, the essential data should include heart rate, rhythm, and systolic, end-diastolic, and mean pressures, where appropriate, cardiac output, and arteriovenous oxygen saturation data, when measured.

Angiographic Data

Every angiogram or series of angiograms performed should be described in detail. This should include the views utilized, whether medications such as nitroglycerin or ergonovine were administered prior to the angiogram, and specific details as to the anatomic findings. It is not important to report angiographic findings in the order in which the angiography is performed but this is a convenient method.

Coronary angiography should be reported in enough detail to give the reader an accurate picture of the coronary anatomy. The various branches should be described in terms of size, location of their course, calcification, and any stenoses present. It is not important, however, to include a "lesson in normal anatomy" in each report, but one should point out pertinent variations. Each stenosis should be characterized as to its length, eccentricity, and degree of diameter narrowing in addition to the presence of thrombus or filling defects, spasm, and collaterals. Further details relating

to coronary angiography are discussed in Chapter 13.

Ventricular angiography should be described in terms of the views used, the wall motion in general (as ejection fraction) and specific regions, any filling defects suggesting ventricular thrombus, wall thickness, and the presence of mitral valve prolapse or regurgitation. Details of technique and wall motion analysis are discussed in Chapter 12.

Any other angiography that was performed, such as pulmonary artery or ascending aorta, should be described in a similarly detailed fashion and are discussed in Chapter 14.

Many currently available computer systems that generate reports will provide graphics of the coronary anatomy and ventricular wall motion with different degrees of detail. These diagrams are variably schematic in type and are thus of value only for modification of the text. They will not substitute for review of the cineangiogram or video playback when a clinical decision needs to be made regarding revascularization. In our opinion, a narrative summary of the angiographic findings is usually appropriate. We also use a diagram, filled out by hand, as part of the immediate report. Many operators prefer to include either a photograph of certain frames of the angiogram or an x-ray film generated from digital images for inclusion in the final report. The possibility also exists that videotape copies can be sent to referring physicians for local reviewing and record keeping. Whatever is appropriate for local circumstances of a particular laboratory should be determined beforehand. Then this form of reporting should be consistently used.

Conclusions

Often the only parts of a report that may be transmitted, particularly over the phone, are the conclusions. This portion should reflect in a few words the salient features of the procedure. This should include summary sentences about the hemodynamics and all the angiography performed. It is the authors' practice to do this in a list format rather than narrative listing the findings in order of importance.

Recommendations

As with the patient historical data, recommendations may or may not be appropriate to include in the report, depending on local practice. This may include management suggestions and treatment options, the suitability of the vessels for PTCA or coronary artery bypass, or details regarding prognosis. It is the authors' practice to confine the report to the objective information obtained. We either discuss the recommendations with the referring physician directly or in a letter or provide this opinion in an area of the hospital record other than the catheterization report.

DATA BASE

In this era of powerful microcomputers and inexpensive digital storage systems, data base systems and software abound. In addition, many custom commercial systems have been designed to handle cardiac catheterization laboratory data from acquisition to storage and retrieval. Some of these systems are designed to handle catheterization data alone, while others integrate data from other stations including echocardiography, electrocardiography, ambulatory electrocardiographic monitoring, exercise stress testing, radiology, and others. These latter systems are necessarily large, sometimes require extensive networking, and may be quite expensive both for initial installation and, more importantly, to maintain. The larger and more comprehensive a data base system is, the more people are required to input data on a daily basis. The cost/benefit ratio of a given data base system must be carefully weighed for a given installation.

A data base system for basic cardiac catheterization data, as reported in the medical record, is relatively simple to set up using almost any commercially available data base software. One must simply index items, which will be cataloged along with appropriate descriptors and demographic data, and set up an output format. Hemodynamic data are straightforward, as are patient demographics. Angiographic data can be data based in as simple or complex a format as desired. A convenient method to catalog segments of the coronary arterial tree can be custom-made or borrowed from formats such as that used for the Coronary Artery Surgery Study (CASS). Descriptors of coronary artery morphology to describe calcification, eccentricity, ectasia, spasm, etc. can be added, as can be quantita-

tive angiographic data if locally available. Similar descriptive systems can be used to describe ventriculographic findings and data obtained from great vessel angiography or during coronary angioplasty.

Primary requirements of a data base system include speed, substantial capacity with regard to record, field, and file size, and good report generation capabilities. Graphic capabilities may be especially useful if digital representations of angiographic data are available for importation. Storage today will be based primarily on hard disk technology although write-only optical disks (WORM) may be used. If magnetic media are used for data base storage, high quality back-up devices and uninterruptable power supplies are required. Digital storage technology is rapidly advancing, and newer devices will likely become available in the future.

The perfect data base system for the cardiac catheterization laboratory has not yet been implemented. Such a system would track the patient from initial referral to the catheterization laboratory and to ultimate disposition. This system would be all electronic with entry of data from the on-line laboratory flow sheet, to complications, catheter inventory, hemodynamics, angiographic findings, and report generation, all via the same system. The data base would allow storage of 8 bit digital images for recall and review, and reports would be generated on a laser or other printer having a resolution of 600 dpi or greater for reproduction of angiograms. The data base could be accessed from the physician's desktop terminal or in the emergency room. Such a system should not be too far into the future and will be an integral part of the filmless digital cardiac catheterization laboratory.

SUMMARY

The catheterization report provides an important medical and legal record and delineates elements of the catheterization laboratory data base. The details of the procedure performed and interpretation of the results should be accurately described and recorded. When properly designed, this report can provide a great deal of information that can be utilized in virtually any type of catheterization practice to improve patient care.

SPECIFIC CLINICAL STATES: THEIR ASSESSMENT AND INTERVENTION BY CATHETER TECHNIQUES

26

The Patient with Known or Suspect Coronary Heart Disease: Stable Ischemic Syndromes

Carl J. Pepine, M.D.
Barry Rose, M.D.
James A. Hill, M.D.
Charles R. Lambert, M.D., Ph.D.

INTRODUCTION

Patients with apparent clinically stable ischemic heart disease comprise a significant proportion of those undergoing cardiac catheterization studies. There is a consensus that the stable ischemic syndromes are due to transient myocardial ischemia. Transient ischemia is a result of variable contributions by processes acting to limit or reduce myocardial blood supply and/or increase myocardial oxygen demand. Atherosclerosis, dynamic coronary artery narrowing, and perhaps, thrombus may act alone or in combination to transiently reduce coronary blood flow. Increases in heart rate, blood pressure, contractility, and ventricular size act alone or in combination to increase myocardial oxygen demands. What is needed from cardiac catheterization studies in order to adequately assess these patients with known or suspect coronary artery disease (CAD) who are clinically stable?

Numerous studies have shown that the **extent and severity of CAD** are among the most important predictors of outcome in these patients. The status of **left ventricular function** clearly interacts with CAD severity to determine outcome. Coronary angiography with left ventriculography will permit identification and quantification of these processes. Noninvasive assessment of the magnitude of ischemia and/or magnitude of myocardium at risk for ischemia is important within coronary anatomic subsets (1). Other conditions can also be identified and quantified at cardiac catheterization (e.g., mitral insufficiency, pulmonary hypertension, ventricular aneurysm). Once this information is obtained, the role of catheterization-based therapy such as percutaneous transluminal coronary angioplasty (PTCA) and/or bypass surgery also needs to be addressed.

The aim of this chapter is to provide a synthesis of these topics relative to specific clinical states associated with stable myocardial ischemic syndromes. To do this we will integrate selected data from clinical trials. From this information the practitioner should be better equipped to recommend and use cardiac catheterization in the management of these patients. Patients with stable ischemic heart disease will be considered according to the following groups: (*a*) those who have **stable symptoms suggesting CAD,** (*b*) those who have **survived myocardial infarction,** and (*c*) those who are and always have been **asymptomatic** but have findings which suggest that they may be at **high risk for CAD.**

CHRONIC STABLE ANGINA PECTORIS

General Considerations

Factors Predicting Prognosis

It is important to briefly review some of the factors that relate to prognosis in chronic stable angina patients. Years ago, Burggraf and Parker were among the first to recognize the importance of the extent and severity of CAD, defined by coronary angiography, on long-term survival in patients with angina (Fig. 26.1*A*) (2). Extent of CAD and severity of left ventricular dysfunction have been repeatedly documented to be two very important, if not the most important, predictors of mortality in patients with chronic stable angina pectoris (Figs. 26.1*B* and 26.2) (3). As currently performed, however, coronary angiography provides only anatomic data, but functional data are also important. It is well-established that there is an increased risk of cardiac events, including death, in angina patients who develop objective evidence for transient myocardial ischemia during stress testing (4). A number of exercise test findings may be used to identify those patients at "high risk" as outlined in Chapter 2. The exercise test also yields other important functional parameters that help predict prognosis among patients with comparable coronary anatomic disease (1). Therefore, exercise testing is very useful in patients with chronic stable angina. Exercise testing may even be done after coronary angiography has defined the anatomic pattern. Other demographic factors that interact with the severity of CAD, such as age, sex, and diabetes are also important determinants of morbidity among patients with various anatomic patterns of coronary artery disease. Thus, coronary angiography provides the most essential anatomic data that interacts with functional and demographic data to yield information important for management.

Patients with Disabling Symptoms and "Optimal" Therapy

There is general agreement that coronary angiography, to identify patients for revascularization, is of proven value in patients with **disabling** symptoms, due to transient myocardial ischemia, that recur with **optimal medical therapy** (5). Optimal medical therapy is expected to vary from patient to patient and is meant to be individualized. Optimal medical therapy should include modification of aggravating factors, for example, obesity, hypertension, anemia, and smoking, in addition to adjusting medications, such as nitrates, calcium antagonists, and β-adrenergic blockers. Failure of optimal therapy then implies that

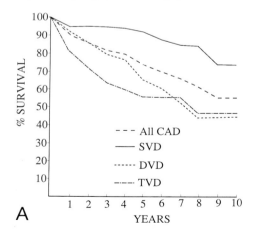

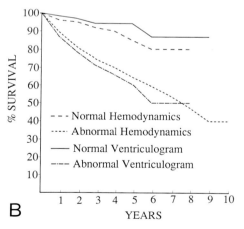

Figure 26.1. *A*, Survival of patients with chronic stable angina related to extent of coronary artery involvement. *DVD*, double-vessel disease; *SVD*, single-vessel disease; *TVD*, triple-vessel disease. *B*, Survival with coronary artery disease related to hemodynamics and ventriculography. It is apparent that the outcome of patients with stable ischemic syndromes is directly dependent upon the extent of coronary artery disease and abnormal ventricular function. (From Burggraf GW, Parker JO. Prognosis in coronary artery disease: angiographic, hemodynamic and clinical factors. *Circulation* 1975;51:146–156.)

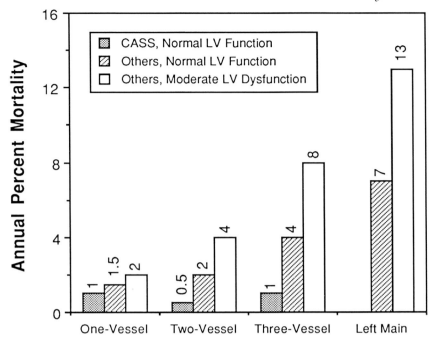

Figure 26.2. Expected annual mortality among medically treated patients with coronary-artery disease and chronic angina pectoris. Percentages (rounded off) are from the CASS trial or are estimates based on a number of other studies and are presented according to the number of diseased vessels and the extent of left ventricular (*LV*) dysfunction. Patients with left main coronary disease were excluded from the CASS trial. (Modified with permission of the New England Journal of Medicine from Silverman KJ, Grossman W. Current concepts. Angina pectoris: natural history and strategies for evaluation and management. N Engl J Med 1984;310:1712–1717.)

symptoms due to either myocardial ischemia or side effects of medications result in an **unacceptable life-style.** In patients meeting this definition the decision for catheterization and possible revascularization is usually not difficult. The majority of these patients with chronic stable symptoms will have multivessel CAD and relatively well-preserved left ventricular function. Only about 3 to 5% will have left main CAD. In 85 to 90% of patients with CAD, symptoms will be markedly improved with a revascularization procedure. Approximately 10% will have normal coronary arteries and no evidence for coronary spasm, excluding coronary artery disease and transient ischemia as the basis for their symptoms. In these latter patients the burden and side effects of costly antiischemic medication can be removed and they can be reassured that their long-term outcome is excellent (6).

The more difficult decision is when to recommend these measures in patients who are **less symptomatic.** In such patients the justification for catheterization is to confirm the diagnosis and **attempt to improve long-term prognosis** as opposed to assuming that the diagnosis is accurate and using medical therapy alone. In order to use catheterization optimally in these patients, it is appropriate to review results that can be obtained with revascularization procedures that are based upon management directed by specific catheterization findings.

Results in Specific Practice Environments

Before addressing results of revascularization procedures, it is important to note that results of highly technical procedures like coronary artery bypass graft (CABG) surgery and PTCA vary widely from one practice setting to another even in similar patients. For example, while the overall average surgical mortality in the Coronary Artery Surgery Study (CASS) report was approximately 3%, the actual mortality rate at individual sites, all of which were selected because of excellence in CABG surgery, ranged from <1% to >12% (7). A similarly wide range of surgical mortality rates was also noted in the Veterans Administration (VA) Cooperative Study (8). Some of this variability can be accounted for by the varied patient mix at different centers. For example, in the CASS, mortality for patients over 60 years of age was >6%, and women of all ages had approximately twice the mortality of men. A substantial proportion of the remaining variability, however, probably relates to technical factors that differ between the centers. There is no doubt that similar variability is present when examining results of PTCA. Thus, it is imperative for clinicians to interpret results discussed below in light of their own practice settings when attempting to make decisions relative to coronary angiography and revascularization in any given patient.

Coronary Bypass Graft Surgery in Coronary Angiographically Defined Subsets

Left Main and Single-Vessel Coronary Stenosis

Three major multicenter randomized trials addressed results of surgery in chronic effort angina. The VA Cooperative Study randomized patients to either surgical (286 patients) or medical (310 patients) treatment (8). Despite criticisms regarding high surgical mortality and graft occlusion rates, this study clearly demonstrated improved survival in the subgroup of patients with left main obstruction randomized to initial surgery. These results were confirmed by the European Coronary Surgery Study Group (ECSSG) (9, 10) (Fig. 26.3). As a result, the CASS excluded patients with left main obstruction from randomization (11). Data from several observational studies also support the beneficial effect of surgery on survival in patients with left main obstruction (12). Because it was evident from nonrandomized trials that, as a group,

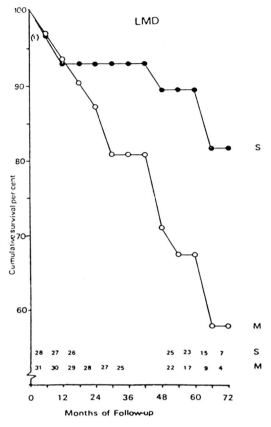

Figure 26.3. Cumulative survival curves for patients with left main disease (*LMD*). *M*, medical group; *S*, surgical group. (From European Coronary Surgery Study Group. Prospective randomized study of coronary artery bypass surgery in stable angina pectoris: a progress report on survival. Circulation 1982;65:II-67–71.)

patients with single-vessel disease had relatively low mortality over 5 to 10 years of follow-up (e.g., 2 to 3% per year), the ECSSG excluded patients with single-vessel obstruction. The other two randomized trials (VA and CASS) found similar 5- to 7-year survival rates in patients with single-vessel obstruction when comparing initial medical and surgical treatment.

Synthesis

When coronary angiography identifies left main coronary obstruction >50% diameter reduction, initial surgery is considered the treatment of choice, regardless of symptom status. There is no clear advantage with single-vessel obstruction, in terms of improved mortality over 5 to 7 years, employing initial surgery compared with medical treatment. Therefore, treatment choices for patients with single-vessel obstruction should be based on other considerations (i.e., symptoms, life-styles, and indicators of high risk). It should be emphasized that all of the randomized trials compare initially assigned treatment groups. Hence, those assigned initial medical therapy, who undergo CABG surgery for whatever reason several months later, continue to remain in the medically assigned group for the purposes of the study. Thus, these results refer only to initial treatment choice. Furthermore, these choices can only be made after coronary angiography has been done.

Multivessel Coronary Artery Obstruction

Despite general agreement in the above mentioned groups, disagreement results when comparing stable patients with those with multivessel coronary disease. In patients with multivessel disease and good ventricular function, both the CASS and VA studies demonstrated similar survival rates for those assigned initial medical and surgical treatment. However, the ECSSG found significantly increased survival in patients with triple-vessel disease when treated surgically compared with those assigned medical treatment (94 vs. 80.4%, 6-year survival rate). The reason for this difference is probably related to the severity of ischemia in patients in the ECSSG.

Evidence to support this suggestion is provided by the fact that 42% of ECSSG patients had either **class III or IV angina,** whereas, CASS excluded patients with severe angina from randomization (13). An observational study of patients with severe angina from the nonrandomized CASS registry did demonstrate improved survival in surgically treated patients who had multivessel CAD (14). It seems reasonable to conclude that patients with multivessel disease and signs or symptoms suggesting severe ischemia may have improved survival with CABG surgery compared with medical therapy. Since 5-year survival rates in surgically treated patients

are similar in both CASS and ECSSG, some of the disparity may be attributed to higher mortality in medically assigned patients. In a group of 117 patients with mild angina or who were asymptomatic and prospectively followed for 4 years after referral, it has been suggested that a subgroup of patients with triple-vessel CAD and preserved left ventricular function who are at high risk for death when treated medically may be identified by exercise testing (15). Forty-three patients with triple-vessel CAD had a 4-year survival of 88%. No deaths occurred in the 12 patients without exercise-induced ST shifts, whereas 31 patients with an ischemic ST segment response during exercise had a 4-year survival of 82% (annual mortality 4.5%). Data from the CASS Registry on 5303 patients who underwent treadmill testing at the time of catheterization showed surgical treatment to be more beneficial in patients exhibiting ≥ 1 mm of ST segment depression and in those who could only exercise to stage I or less of the Bruce protocol (16). Seven-year survival of patients in this subgroup was 58% when treated medically compared with 81% when treated surgically.

The ECSSG patients with two-vessel CAD who had one stenosis involving the **proximal left anterior descending** artery also had improved survival after surgery (Fig. 26.4). Several nonrandomized, observational studies provide further support for the prognostic importance of proximal left anterior descending artery stenoses (17). A report from CASS Registry data suggested that patients with proximal stenosis in any vessel had a poorer prognosis than patients with the same number of diseased vessels but with distal stenosis (18). Review of data from 903 patients with combined proximal left anterior descending and left circumflex stenosis (the majority not meeting randomization criteria) demonstrated improved 5-year survival in those treated surgically vs. medically (85 vs. 55%) (19).

When comparing patients who had both **multivessel disease and poor left ventricular function,** defined as an ejection fraction <50%, long-term follow-up from both the VA and CASS studies suggests that surgery improves survival (20–23). Patients with an ejection fraction of <50% were excluded from the ECSSG.

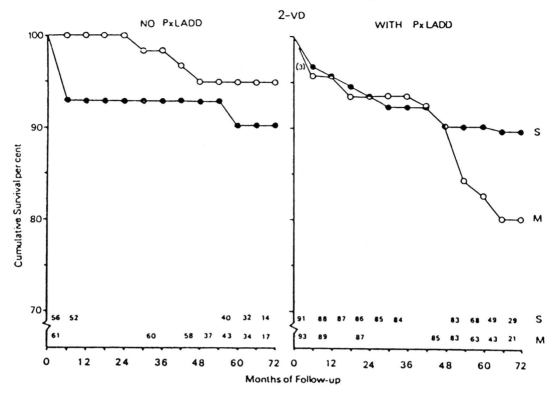

Figure 26.4. Cumulative survival curves for patients with two-vessel disease (*2-VD*) subdivided into two subsets according to absence (*NO*) and presence (*WITH*) of proximal left anterior descending disease (*PxLADD*). *M*, medical group; *S*, surgical group. (From European Coronary Surgery Study Group. Prospective randomized study of coronary artery bypass surgery in stable angina pectoris: a progress report on survival. Circulation 1982;65:II-67–71.)

Synthesis

Based on review of results of major trials in patients with chronic stable angina and our knowledge of predictors of high risk from noninvasive testing studies, it would appear that coronary angiography directed toward identifying sites for revascularization should be recommended in all patients with chronic stable angina who have "failed optimal medical therapy" as discussed above. In angina patients who have not failed medical therapy, a recommendation for coronary angiography is often useful, based upon results of stress testing. Important prerequisites in the patient with lesser symptoms seem to be documentation that reversible ischemia is present and the possibility from the characteristics of the ischemic response that suggest a large amount of myocardium may be at risk. The following coronary angiographically de-

fined subgroups should have improved survival with surgery: (*a*) left main stenosis; (*b*) triple-vessel disease with depressed left ventricular function; (*c*) triple-vessel disease with normal left ventricular function in patients with moderate to severe angina; (*d*) double-vessel disease with normal left ventricular function when one of the occluded vessels is the proximal left anterior descending artery; and (*e*) patients who appear to be at high risk based upon risk stratification by noninvasive tests, that is those with ischemia provokable at low workloads or of severe magnitude. When these findings are documented, a recommendation for revascularization seems warranted.

Percutaneous Transluminal Coronary Angioplasty

Initially, PTCA was introduced for use only in the highly select group of patients described in Chapter 15. Since such patients (recent onset angina and single-vessel disease) usually do well with medical therapy in terms of 5-year survival, and surgery has not been shown to reduce mortality or myocardial infarction rates in such patients, PTCA was reserved for those with unsatisfactory symptom responses to medical therapy. As the primary success rates with PTCA improved (≥90%) and the need for emergency CABG declined (≤3%), PTCA emerged as an alternative treatment to chronic drug therapy. The question remains as to whether PTCA, as an alternative form of revascularization, will offer results different from CABG surgery or even medical therapy. These issues are currently being addressed in the United States by National Heart, Lung and Blood Institute (NHLBI)- and VA-sponsored clinical trials, as well as several European trials. More recently, PTCA has also been applied to increasing numbers of patients with multivessel disease. This issue is also being addressed by the controlled trials. It is likely, however, that no trial currently underway or planned will yield information on PTCA and mortality, as compared with surgery or drugs. At this time, PTCA has **some favorable cost and logistical advantages over CABG surgery.** However, until results of controlled trials are available, clinical judgment must be used to select candidates. Some arbitrary guidelines based on the coronary angiogram are in order (see Chapter 15).

Left Main and Single-Vessel Disease

Presently, in patients with single-vessel disease, PTCA appears more clearly indicated for those whose life-styles are limited by symptoms, drug therapy itself, or stress tests suggesting high-risk ischemia based upon recent guidelines (12). With respect to left main disease, it would appear that surgery is the currently preferred revascularization approach because of unacceptable long-term results in a few patients who were treated with PTCA when the procedure was introduced (1). However, patients with "protected" left main disease, where at least one patent graft supplies a left coronary branch, are usually acceptable PTCA candidates.

Multivessel Disease

Frequently, the question arises as to whether patients with multiple vessel disease, who would be expected to benefit from CABG revascularization, should be given the option for revascularization by PTCA. This question is important because of concerns about PTCA efficacy in multivessel disease related to primary success rate, completeness of revascularization, and possible increased rates of complication and restenosis.

Dorros et al. reported results of multivessel PTCA in a series of 309 patients (24). Initial angiographic success was achieved in 87% of lesions and in 285 (92%) patients. The complication rate was similar to that of PTCA performed in patients with single-vessel disease. Follow-up studies showed that only 20% had clinical evidence of lesion recurrence, including those who underwent repeat PTCA. On long-term follow-up, 85% of patients had sustained clinical improvement. Cowley et al. reported results of PTCA on 84 patients with two-vessel disease, 14 with triple-vessel disease, and two with four-vessel disease (25). Two hundred and seventy-three lesions were attempted in these 100 patients with an angiographic success rate of 90% and clinical improvement in 95%. These investigators reported the clinical success rate to be higher than in their total PTCA population (including patients with single-vessel disease) for the same time period. It should be noted that case selection may have affected results, as revascularization by PTCA was recommended when lesions were felt amenable to such therapy. Most importantly, in this report the incidence of complications was not appreciably different from that of PTCA done in patients with single-vessel disease. Sustained improvement was noted in many patients, as 64% were event-free and 50% were asymptomatic after a mean follow-up of approximately 2 years. There was no statistically significant difference in recurrence rate comparing patients with multi-vessel PTCA (34%) and patients with single vessel PTCA (28%) who had PTCA performed during the same time period at that institution.

The importance of **complete revascularization** for relief of angina with CABG surgery has been emphasized (26). One study followed consecutive patients undergoing

CABG surgery, with repeat angiography 1 year after operation (27). Complete revascularization was defined as all major vessels ≥1.5 mm in diameter with stenosis of ≥50% being bypassed. When correlating symptoms with both graft patency and completeness of revascularization, **asymptomatic** patients had 91% graft patency as compared with only 27% graft patency in **unimproved** patients. Likewise, 87% of patients completely revascularized with all grafts patent were asymptomatic. Only 42% of those patients incompletely revascularized were asymptomatic. From these findings after CABG surgery, one would expect that complete revascularization should be important after PTCA in patients with multivessel disease.

Mabin et al. addressed "completeness of revascularization" in an experience with 229 patients undergoing PTCA, 86 of whom had multivessel disease (28). Success rate was 67% (153 patients) for the series, 61% for patients with single-vessel disease, and 77% for those with multivessel disease. Of the 153 patients in whom PTCA was initially successful, revascularization was considered complete, that is there was no residual diameter stenosis >70%, in 87 of 143 patients with single-vessel disease and 31 of 86 patients with multivessel disease. The chance of event-free survival (e.g., no angina recurrence, myocardial infarction, death, repeat PTCA or CABG

surgery) was directly influenced by completeness of revascularization. All patients with multivessel disease, obtaining complete revascularization, had no angina on follow-up; whereas, only 57% of those patients with partial revascularization were asymptomatic. At 6 months, 79% of patients with complete revascularization had event-free survival compared with only 43% of those who had a residual stenosis (Fig. 26.5).

A subsequent study suggested that, despite high primary success rates, defined as dilatation of the critical lesion, complete revascularization was obtained in only 46% of patients with multivessel disease who had obtained primary success (29). As with the Mabin et al. study, cardiac events, need for second revascularization procedure, and evidence for residual myocardial ischemia by exercise testing were more frequent in the incompletely revascularized group despite initial clinical improvement.

Synthesis

It is apparent that with optimal case selection, based on coronary angiography, initial success rates with PTCA may be similar for patients with single- and multivessel CAD. On long-term follow-up, patients with single-vessel disease are more likely to sustain clinical and angiographic improvement than patients with

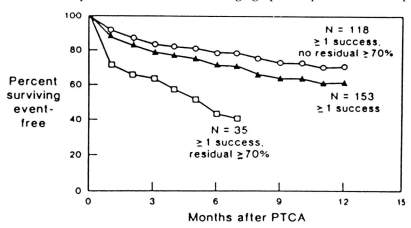

Figure 26.5. Event-free survival after successful dilatation of at least one vessel (triangles, *n* = 153) and in subgroups: with complete revascularization (no residual stenosis, circles, *n* = 118) and with incomplete revascularization (one or more residual stenoses ≥70%, squares, *n* = 35). The difference between results in the two subgroups is significant (p < 0.001). (From Mabin TA, Holmes DR, Smith HC, et al. Follow-up clinical results in patients undergoing percutaneous transluminal coronary angioplasty. Circulation 1985;71:754–760.)

multivessel CAD. Many patients with multivessel disease, however, also may have sustained long-term benefit after PTCA. In patients who have recurrence of signs or symptoms of ischemia and in those with angiographically documented restenosis, either repeat PTCA or CABG surgery may be readily performed with a very high success rate. It is our opinion that PTCA and CABG surgery are complimentary revascularization techniques that are best used at different stages in the course of a given patient's generally progressive coronary obstructive disease. Even when PTCA results in acute occlusion, surgical treatment may be performed with the same relatively low operative mortality/morbidity rates that are enjoyed without the attempted PTCA. For those in whom PTCA is unsuccessful and without complication, CABG surgery may be performed electively (6, 30, 31). Event-free survival in patients treated unsuccessfully by PTCA followed by prompt CABG surgery is as good as or better than that in patients who had successful PTCA of at least one vessel.

So currently available information suggests that it is possible to identify subgroups of patients with chronic stable angina, based on coronary angiographic findings, in whom CABG surgery improves prognosis. At this time similar information is not available for PTCA but may evolve in the future. Until then, use of PTCA is governed by clinical judgment based upon coronary angiographic findings, suggesting that PTCA appears to offer a reasonable alternative to CABG surgery.

Special Considerations

Repeat Revascularization

It must be recognized that any revascularization therapy directed towards CAD is often temporary because of the generally progressive course of atherosclerosis. With regard to CABG surgery, follow-up angiographic studies have shown that 15 to 20% of saphenous vein CABGs are occluded by 1 year and that only about 60% remain patent at 11 years (32). Grafts remaining patent often have evidence of important stenosis. There may also be increased progression of native CAD in vessels that have been bypassed. Thus, as a consequence of graft occlusion, stenosis, and/or progression of native CAD, disabling angina recurs at a rate of up to 5%/year following initially successful CABG surgery and silent ischemia may even recur at a higher rate. Thus, many patients will become candidates for reoperation with fewer options for conduits, increased risk of complications, and possibly increased mortality (33). Long-term relief of angina is not as effective with repeat surgery (27, 34). For example, in one series of 1000 patients undergoing reoperation from 1969 to 1982, angina was completely relieved in about 70% of patients 5 years after initial CABG surgery, while only 50% were angina-free 5 years after reoperation. Internal mammary arteries are increasingly used as conduits since patency rates in uncontrolled series appear higher than veins, averaging about 90% at 10 years (35-37). Nonrandomized studies suggest that this improved patency may be translated to improved survival compared with saphenous vein CABGs (38, 39).

Although reoperation can be performed successfully with only a small increase in mortality and complications, PTCA is an attractive alternative form of therapy for patients with signs or symptoms of recurrent ischemia due to bypass graft occlusion. PTCA can be performed on either grafted native vessels or bypass grafts (40–43). In reports which evaluate the occurrence of restenosis with respect to the site of PTCA, the distal graft-native artery anastomosis seems to behave similarly to a native coronary artery, whereas the aortosaphenous vein graft anastomosis and vein graft body are associated with high rates of restenosis. Also, the risk of infarction is higher with PTCA of lesions in the body of saphenous vein grafts presumably due to embolic debris.

It is important to recognize that graft occlusion after CABG surgery is not the same as restenosis after PTCA. Restenosis occurs in 20 to 45% of cases undergoing successful PTCA and usually occurs within 4 to 6 months of dilation. The etiology of restenosis remains unclear. This process probably is related to a form of accelerated atherosclerosis and includes platelet activation, thrombosis, noncellular components, and smooth muscle cell injury and proliferation. As opposed to reoperation following CABG surgery, repeat PTCA for restenosis can be done with a high success rate and few complications (44, 45).

Furthermore, a valuable "conduit" (e.g., vein or internal mammary artery) has not been used or damaged.

Other Special Risk Groups

Although some report that **elderly patients** undergoing CABG surgery have similar perioperative mortality when compared with younger individuals, the CASS demonstrated a significantly increased risk (46, 47). Part of the reason for this disparity may relate to chronologic vs. physiologic age. Reports on the role of PTCA in the elderly vary. One suggests similar initial success rates, complications, and long-term clinical improvement as compared with younger individuals (48). Another suggests a slightly lower primary success rate and higher complication rate (49). However, in this latter study the magnitude of difference, though statistically significant, was small and may not be clinically important. Thus, both PTCA and CABG surgery are feasible in the elderly. Others considered at high risk for CABG surgery include those with depressed left ventricular function and those with poor general medical condition. In select patients, PTCA may be considered palliative for those at high risk for CABG surgery (50).

CORONARY ARTERY SPASM

General Considerations

Among patients with transient myocardial ischemia, coronary spasm is responsible in two subgroups. One of these subgroups is termed **"variant angina"** and comprises about 3 to 4% of patients undergoing coronary angiography for chest pain. Variant angina refers specifically to individuals who have chest pain primarily at rest associated with ST segment elevation. In a larger subgroup of patients who also have coronary spasm during chest pain, there is a wide variety of ST segment and/or T wave changes. A small portion of both subgroups has little atherosclerotic obstruction. These patients respond well to nitrates and calcium antagonists, and their long-term outcome is excellent (50) (Fig. 26.6).

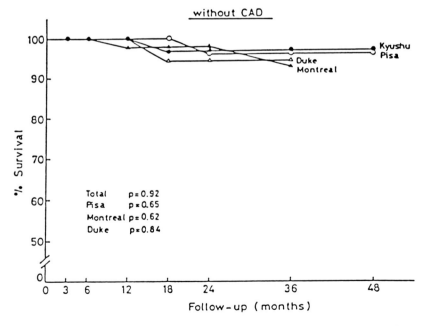

Figure 26.6. Comparison of long-term survival among four reports from different regions: Japan (Kynshu), North American (Montreal and Duke), and Europe (Pisa) for variant angina patients without significant coronary artery disease. Survival for this subpopulation is excellent, approximating 95% at 4 years, and there are no significant differences between reports. (From Shimokawa H, Nagasawa K, Irie T, et al. Clinical characteristics and long-term prognosis of patients with variant angina. A comparative study between western and Japanese populations. Int J Cardiol 1988;18:331-349.)

However, the majority of patients with coronary spasm seen in North America and Europe are much more likely to have dynamic obstruction superimposed on important atherosclerotic stenosis. Patients with spasm and CAD have an impaired prognosis related to the extent and severity of atherosclerotic CAD and their left ventricular function (Fig. 26.7). Thus, identification of spasm and CAD are very important in terms of patient management. The definitive diagnosis of coronary spasm can be made only during coronary angiography.

Coronary spasm is considered present when a reversible change in coronary artery size is observed to reduce the diameter ≥50% and is associated with transient ischemia. Objective evidence for myocardial ischemia may include any of the following: (*a*) transient ECG changes, such as ST segment shifts, normalization of previously depressed ST segments, and peaking of T waves; (*b*) exaggerated rise in left ventricular end-diastolic pressure (The rise in left ventricular end-diastolic pressure must be greater than expected from loading effects due to ergonovine-related increases in aortic pressure and venoconstriction.); (*c*) reversible decrease in regional thallium-201 uptake or wall motion; and (*d*) abnormal changes in myocardial metabolic indicators.

When spasm does not occur spontaneously during coronary angiography, a provocative test is used. In general, ergonovine testing is used for this purpose (see Chapter 13). The broad indication for ergonovine testing is the need to know if coronary spasm is contributing to a patient's chest pain syndrome in the absence of contraindications. Some specific clinical situations for testing in patients with coronary angiograms that do not show sufficient obstruction to explain an angina syndrome appear in Table 26.1. These suggestions may also apply to patients with more severe coronary atherosclerosis if suspicion of spasm is high (e.g., rest angina and relatively well-preserved or widely variable effort tolerance). Goals of testing are to: (*a*) confirm the presence of spasm; (*b*) define the location and degree of spasm, number of vessels involved, and relationship to atherosclerotic coronary narrowing (e.g., at the site, proximal, distal); and (*c*) provide baseline data for later evalua-

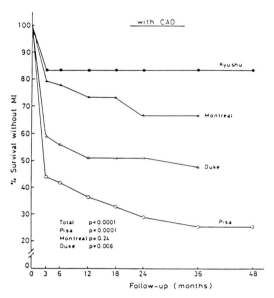

Figure 26.7. Outcome (survival without myocardial infarction (*MI*)) from the four reports shown in Figure 26.6 for variant angina patients with significant coronary artery disease. Prognosis is poor in all four studies and depends directly upon the severity of coronary disease in the population studied. For example, multivessel CAD was present in 56% of patients in the Pisa study where outcome was worst and only 4% of the Kyushu study where relative outcome is best. (From Shimokawa H, Nagasawa K, Irie T, et al. Clinical characteristics and long-term prognosis of patients with variant angina. A comparative study between western and Japanese populations. Int J Cardiol 1988;18:331–349.)

tion of therapy or course of disease (e.g., spontaneous remission). This information is important in terms of prognosis, drug selection, and potential for cardiac surgery (e.g., bypass, plexectomy). Contraindications to ergonovine testing appear in Table 26.2. The first three contraindications are relative because, even though risks may increase in some instances, it is necessary to know if spasm is present. The latter five are absolute.

Although tests for coronary spasm can be performed outside the catheterization laboratory, we believe that **the initial test** in any patient, and whenever possible **all tests,** should be done during catheterization (52). This practice allows hemodynamic, as well as ECG monitoring and ensures the safest approach to manage potentially serious effects of spasm-related ischemia, such as

Table 26.1.
Specific Clinical Situations Where Provocative Testing for Coronary Spasm May Be Helpful[a]

Rest pain associated with
  No preceding rise in heart rate and/or blood pressure
  Preserved effort tolerance
  Cyclic recurrence often in early AM
  Transient ST segment elevation or ventricular arrhythmias
  Nonspecific or no ECG change
  ECG pattern prohibiting interpretation of ST segment (e.g., pacer, left bundle branch block, Wolff-Parkinson-White)
Angina associated with
  Variable exercise threshold
  ST segment elevation during stress testing
  Syncope and/or ventricular dysrhythmias
  Patent coronary bypass grafts
Assess efficacy of therapy or spontaneous remission

[a] From Pepine CJ, Lambert CR. Coronary artery spasm: pathophysiology, natural history, recognition, and treatment. In: Hurst JW, ed. The Heart. 7th ed. New York: McGraw-Hill, 1989.

heart block, ventricular arrhythmias, and hypotension.

Currently, there are no published controlled studies comparing medical with revascularization therapy in coronary spasm patients. David et al. reported results of PTCA in 11 patients with variant angina who had coexisting coronary stenosis (53). Despite initial success, persistence of symptoms requiring calcium antagonists and a high restenosis rate were noted. Corcos and colleagues also demonstrated a high restenosis rate in a series of 21 patients (54). But after repeat angioplasty 75% of patients were asymptomatic requiring no medical therapy, suggesting that PTCA may play a role in management when spasm was superimposed on organic stenosis (54). More recently, Bertrand et al. suggested a high incidence of restenosis when PTCA was performed in patients with dynamic narrowing (55). Leisch et al. have suggested that, although PTCA may initially be effective in patients with variant angina, there is a higher restenosis rate (56).

Results of surgical treatment of patients with proven or suspected coronary spasm are very limited. It is apparent, however, that CABG surgery can be done on patients with spasm superimposed on atherosclerotic lesions, but results are not as favorable as those found when CABG surgery is done in patients without spasm (57). Perioperative death, myocardial infarction, and recurrent angina or myocardial infarction are frequent. Likewise, isolated case reports suggest that CABG surgery is not useful in patients with coronary spasm who do not have important atherosclerotic obstruction. Plexectomy combined with CABG surgery has been suggested, but these results are not very encouraging.

Synthesis

It would appear that patients with suspect coronary spasm should have coronary angiography and ergonovine testing, if necessary, in an attempt to identify spasm and associated CAD. Medical therapy (nitrates plus calcium antagonists) should be utilized in patients with documented coronary spasm. If symptoms or signs of ischemia recur and can be documented as due to spasm, PTCA may be an appropriate consideration for a very select few patients. Because of the reported high restenosis rate, the procedure may have to be done several times. CABG surgery may be a consideration in a very few patients with severe associated CAD. These few patients probably should have multivessel disease and evidence suggesting that spasm is not diffuse along the course of any vessel.

Because of the possibility of recurrent spasm, patients undergoing either PTCA or CABG surgery should continue to receive intravenous nitroglycerin and calcium antagonists during and following the procedure.

Table 26.2.
Contraindications to Provocative Testing for Coronary Spasm[a]

Relative
  Recent myocardial infarction (within 5 days)
  Uncontrolled angina
  Uncontrolled ventricular arrhythmias
Absolute
  Amenorrhea in a premenopausal female
  Severe hypertension
  Severe left ventricular dysfunction
  Severe aortic stenosis
  Significant left main coronary stenosis

[a] From Pepine CJ, Lambert CR. Coronary artery spasm: pathophysiology, natural history, recognition, and treatment. In: Hurst JW, ed. The Heart. 7th Ed. New York: McGraw-Hill, 1989.

These patients, as well as those treated without revascularization, should be maintained on oral nitrates and calcium antagonists for at least a year. Judicious withdrawal of antispasm therapy should be contemplated only after an appropriate asymptomatic interval and with proof (i.e., ambulatory monitoring) that recurrent ischemia does not occur in either a painful or silent form. In many of these patients remission will have occurred, and antispasm medication will no longer be required.

POSTMYOCARDIAL INFARCTION PATIENTS

General Considerations

The postmyocardial infarction period is known to be associated with substantial morbidity and mortality. Risks for reinfarction and death, however, decrease throughout the first year. Accordingly, identification of those at high risk is standard medical practice in the postinfarction period. In addition to the status of left ventricular function, other factors have been identified as important in predicting prognosis during this period (58, 59). Of these, the presence of postinfarction angina or ischemia detected by stress testing appear to significantly alter prognosis in patients with similar degrees of left ventricular function. Schuster and Bulkley followed 70 patients with early postinfarction angina with either "ischemia at a distance" or ischemia in the infarct zone and noted a 56% mortality at 6 months (60). Ischemia at a distance was associated with a particularly high mortality rate of 72%.

Ischemia interacts with left ventricular dysfunction to increase risks. For example, De Feyter et al. noted increased mortality in patients with either ejection fractions <30% or with triple-vessel CAD compared with patients with either ejection fractions >30% or single- or double-vessel CAD (61). Patients who were able to complete 10 min of exercise had a much lower reinfarction rate as compared with those who did not complete 10 min. Thus, among patients with postinfarction angina, those with left ventricular dysfunction and ischemia, as well as those with triple-vessel CAD, might be expected to have an improved prognosis if these findings were identified at catheterization and if revascularization were performed.

Coronary Artery Bypass Graft Surgery

One might expect that CABG surgery in the postinfarction period would be associated with improved survival. In an observational study, Akhras et al. followed 119 patients with relatively uncomplicated myocardial infarction and performed exercise testing 2 weeks postinfarction (62). Those patients who had positive treadmill tests underwent coronary angiography at 6 weeks. Patients with triple-vessel CAD, those with critical proximal left anterior descending stenosis as a component of double- or triple-vessel disease, and those with refractory angina despite optimal medical therapy underwent CABG surgery within 3 months of infarction. The majority of these patients had triple-vessel disease, and their exercise time averaged only 5.5 min. Thus, they would be considered high risk. Yet CABG surgery resulted in a 1-year mortality of only 2%. Singh et al., in a study of 108 consecutive patients with angina within 30 days of infarction, undergoing CABG surgery, found 5-year actuarial survival to be 87% (63). Although the limitations associated with this type of analysis are numerous, one might infer that CABG surgery may be associated with reduced mortality when done in patients with postinfarction angina.

In patients who were asymptomatic or mildly symptomatic postinfarction, three randomized controlled trials of CABG surgery vs. medical therapy have shown no distinct benefit in favor of surgery. Norris et al. addressed this issue in 100 consecutive patients believed to be at high risk because they had second or third infarctions (64). The majority had triple-vessel CAD, and most had depressed left ventricular function (ejection fraction <50%). Those with left main CAD and severe symptoms were not included. All were either asymptomatic or only minimally symptomatic and were randomized to received either CABG or medical therapy. No difference in mortality was found in follow-up to 4.5 years (mean). These same investigators also terminated a similar randomized trial done in patients following "first" infarction when no trends were observed in favor of surgery (65). Likewise, Group C of the CASS report (i.e., those asymptomatic for more than 3 weeks after documented infarction) included 160 postmyocardial infarction patients randomized to either CABG or medical therapy. Again, no significant improvement was seen after CABG surgery compared with medical therapy (18).

Synthesis

In the postmyocardial infarction period, coronary angiography and revascularization are clearly indicated in patients who have signs or symptoms of recurrent myocardial ischemia. Recurrence of ischemia in this setting is in itself indicative of high risk, and successful CABG surgery will prevent recurrent ischemia and has the potential to improve survival. The latter has not been proven in controlled trials and is unlikely to be tested on ethical grounds. For postinfarction patients who are not symptomatic, risk stratification is in order. Many, including ourselves, consider patients with non-Q-wave infarction to be at high risk. For those with either clinical or noninvasively detected indicators of high risk, coronary angiography is indicated. If high-risk anatomy is found, for example, left main or three-vessel disease, or high risk ventricular dysfunction (i.e., ejection fraction ≤40%), strong consideration should be given to a recommendation for CABG surgery. It should be emphasized that this recommendation relates to potential for modifying risk and has not been tested in controlled trials.

Percutaneous Transluminal Coronary Angioplasty

Recently, De Feyter et al. performed PTCA between 48 hr and 30 days after acute myocardial infarction in 53 patients with angina (66). PTCA was initially successful in 89% and four of the six patients with unsuccessful PTCA had reinfarctions. The procedure-related myocardial infarction rate was somewhat higher than that expected for elective PTCA done for chronic stable angina. The majority of patients in this study had single-vessel disease, as patients with multivessel disease were often offered CABG surgery. Angina recurred more frequently in patients with multivessel disease who had undergone PTCA of only the "ischemia-related vessel" (8 of 17, 47%) than in patients with single-vessel disease (6 of 30, 20%). This difference, however, apparently was not statistically signifi-

cant. During 6 months of follow-up, there were no late cardiac deaths, but recurrent myocardial infarction developed in two patients.

Synthesis

It would appear that postmyocardial infarction patients, with abnormal left ventricular function, recurrent signs or symptoms of ischemia, or multivessel disease, are at increased risk. Revascularization with PTCA may be offered in certain settings as an alternative to CABG surgery as discussed above. It would appear at present that patients with single-vessel CAD excluding the left main stenosis may be better PTCA candidates; whereas, the majority of those with multivessel CAD may be better CABG surgery candidates.

ASYMPTOMATIC PATIENTS AT RISK FOR CORONARY ARTERY DISEASE

General Considerations

Individuals who are totally asymptomatic but at high risk for CAD constitute a very large subgroup. Included are those who have evidence for **silent myocardial ischemia** documented by noninvasive testing, those who have ECG changes suggesting **silent or unrecognized myocardial infarction,** and those without noninvasive test findings suggesting CAD but who are at **extreme high risk** due to other factors. Although subjects in these three subsets are all totally asymptomatic, concern arises because the initial clinical manifestation of CAD may be sudden death or acute myocardial infarction. Rates for these events will determine the level of concern and ultimately play an important role in weighing the potential risks and benefits to be derived from a catheterization procedure directed towards diagnosis and finding candidates for revascularization. Although specific CAD event rates for these patients are not known with certainty, some data are available to help in their management.

Ellestad and Wan were among the first to suggest that treadmill tests demonstrating ischemic ST segment responses appear to have the same prognostic significance regardless of whether or not the ST segment changes are accompanied by symptoms (67). Recently, Falcone et al. examined the clinical significance of exercise-induced silent myocardial ischemia in patients with CAD documented by angiography (68). Patients with chest pain and ischemic ST segment changes were compared with patients who had exercise-induced ischemic ST segment changes but no chest pain. The two groups had similar left ventricular function and severity of coronary artery disease. CABG surgery was performed in approximately one-half of those with symptoms and one-quarter of those without symptoms. After 3 years' follow-up, survival rates of medically treated patients with exercise-induced symptoms and medically treated patients without exercise-induced symptoms were not statistically different even when patients were classified according to the number of diseased vessels.

Recently, Weiner et al. reported on a large group of patients from the CASS Registry who underwent coronary angiography and treadmill testing at approximately the same time and were then followed for 7 years (69). The patients were divided into four groups. Group one (Fig. 26.8) consisted of 424 patients who had exercise-induced ST segment depression without angina during exercise testing (i.e., silent ischemia). Thirty-five percent of these patients were asymptomatic (class I) and another 44% had only mild angina (class II) during other activities. Group two had 232 patients all of whom had angina during exercise testing without clearly ischemic ST segment changes. Group three was comprised of

456 patients who had both ischemic ST segment depression and angina during exercise. Group four patients had no ST segment depression or symptoms during exercise. All groups had similar frequencies of single- and multivessel CAD, left ventricular function, and exercise tolerance. The 7-year survival rates from the first three groups with signs and/or symptoms of ischemia were very similar (approximately 78%). Survival of these patients was significantly different compared with group four patients who had no signs or symptoms of ischemia during exercise testing.

These findings suggest that patients with silent myocardial ischemia detected by treadmill testing may have a long-term prognosis that is not different from patients who experience angina. Also, those without signs or symptoms of ischemia during exercise testing have a significantly better prognosis than those with ischemia despite similar degrees of CAD and left ventricular dysfunction. Further analysis of survival according to severity of CAD of those patients in group one, who had silent ischemia during exercise, were particularly impressive (Fig. 26.9). Those with two-vessel CAD had a 7-year survival of approximately 70%, and those with three-vessel CAD had a 7-year survival of only 50%.

Weiner et al. also compared survival rates of group one silent ischemia patients (e.g., exercise-induced ST segment depression and no angina) with a group of 282 patients with-

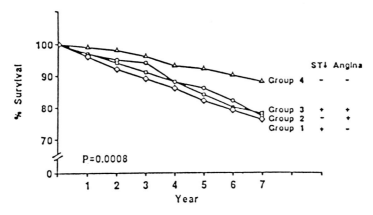

Figure 26.8. Cumulative survival for patients with and without exercise-induced silent ischemia. The 7-year survival was similar for patients in group one (silent ischemia) compared with groups two and three (painful ischemia). Group four patients had a substantially better 7-year survival. (From Weiner DA, Ryan TJ, McCabe C, et al. Significance of silent myocardial ischemia during exercise testing in patients with coronary artery disease. Am J Cardiol 1987;59:725–729.)

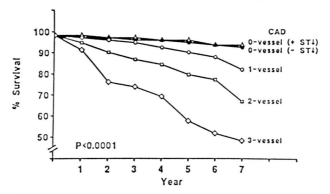

Figure 26.9. Seven-year survival rates for group one patients (silent ischemia) based on the severity of CAD; a separate group of 282 patients without CAD who had ischemic ST segment depression without angina during exercise testing, and a control group of 1117 patients without CAD and without either ischemic ST depression or angina during exercise testing. (From Weiner DA, Ryan TJ, McCabe C, et al. Significance of silent myocardial ischemia during exercise testing in patients with coronary artery disease. Am J Cardiol 1987;59:725-729.)

out CAD who had ischemic-type ST segment depression during exercise and also with 1117 patients with neither CAD nor ST segment depression. Both of these latter groups showed 7-year survival rates of 95% or better, illustrating the lack of prognostic importance of ST segment depression during exercise when CAD is not present. The frequency of such "false-positive" responses depends upon the prevalence of CAD in the group being tested.

Middle-aged, asymptomatic men with multiple risk factors and abnormal exercise ECGs suggesting silent ischemia have an approximately 4-fold increase in CAD mortality over 7 years compared with patients who have normal exercise ECG responses (70). Considering that some (perhaps 25% or more) of these patients with exercise-induced ECG changes suggesting ischemia probably have false-positive ECG responses (i.e., ST segment depression but no CAD), these mortality rates underestimate the true prognostic importance of silent ischemia associated with CAD in high-risk, asymptomatic middle-aged men.

Finally, Framingham study data documented that approximately 25% of the men and 30% of the women who had myocardial infarction documented by new Q waves on a biannual ECG had unrecognized, frequently silent, myocardial infarctions (71). Ten-year follow-up of these patients indicates that the frequencies of death,

recurrent myocardial infarction, and most other CAD endpoints were essentially the same as those of patients who had painful myocardial infarction. It has been well-known that postmortem studies often identify a substantial amount of severe coronary atherosclerosis and myocardial scarring in many patients who were thought to be completely asymptomatic.

Synthesis

Although the mechanism by which such patients have important CAD and episodes of myocardial ischemia and necrosis without warning is unclear, this is not a rare finding. While family history and other risk factors (e.g., smoking, hypercholesteremia) predispose patients to CAD, it is clear that many will not have CAD. The question of when and for which patients to recommend coronary angiography is asked with increasing frequency. Risk factors alone are not as useful when applied to the general asymptomatic population where the likelihood of CAD is low. Furthermore, when exercise testing is applied to a population where CAD probability is low, even ≥ 1.0 mm of ST segment depression is associated with a very low abnormal event rate of approximately 2 to 4%/year. Even when applied to middle-aged patients with chest pain (e.g., high pretest CAD probability), the sensitivity and specificity for CAD of ≥1.0 mm of ST segment depression on exercise testing range between approximately 60 and 80%. Thus, some decision-making schema relative to recommendations for coronary angiography is required in the evaluation of these asymptomatic patients.

We suggest the schema represented in Figure 26.10. It is similar to that recommended by others (72). Patients over 35 years of age who have more than one risk factor (e.g., are male, hypercholesteremic, hypertensive, smoke cigarettes, or have a family history) should undergo exercise stress testing. If high-risk ischemic responses are found, coronary angiography is indicated. If ST segment depression suggesting ischemia is present without evidence for high risk, radionuclide testing is suggested to further define the likelihood of CAD and risk of events. When the likelihood is high, coronary angiography is recommended. In the absence of these high-risk noninvasive findings, it is appropriate to examine the exercise workload achieved to provide more information relative to risk. If a high level was achieved, then the risk of CAD events is too low to recommend coronary angiography. If a high level workload was not reached during exercise testing, however, it is appropriate to also recommend a radionu-

clide test and possibly coronary angiography based upon the results of the radionuclide study.

Treatment Based upon Coronary Angiographic Findings

We believe that strong consideration should be given to treating asymptomatic patients with coronary angiographic findings suggesting high risk (e.g., left main and three-vessel CAD or ejection fraction ≤35%) with revascularization therapy so that asymptomatic ischemia is not inducible. Although not yet proven, we believe this approach is a rational attempt to prevent myocardial infarction and sudden death in such patients. At the current time there are no controlled studies of asymptomatic patients with definite ischemia comparing revascularization with medical therapy in order to determine the effect on future events or life expectancy. Patients who are asymptomatic postinfarction were discussed earlier in this chapter.

It seems reasonable to conclude that certain asymptomatic patients should be approached for cardiac catheterization in a manner similar to patients who have symptoms. Presently, no studies are available randomizing patients with mild or no symptoms to

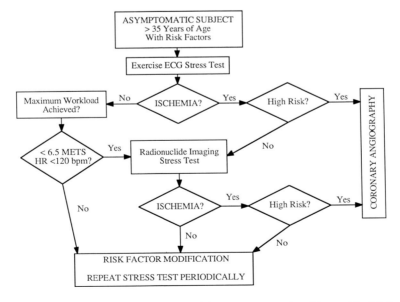

Figure 26.10. Proposed algorithm for evaluation of the asymptomatic subject with risk factors for coronary artery disease. *HR*, heart rate; *METS*, metabolic equivalents.

either PTCA vs. CABG surgery or PTCA vs. medical therapy. It is uncertain as to which asymptomatic patients with silent ischemia should be referred for revascularization. Based on results of exercise testing that demonstrate that patients have similar prognoses regardless of whether or not symptoms are present, patients with silent ischemia and stress tests suggesting high risk should undergo coronary angiography. If high-risk anatomy (left main stenosis or three-vessel disease with poor left ventricular function) is present, either CABG surgery (for left main) or PTCA (dependent on anatomy) should be considered. Asymptomatic CAD patients with high-risk radionuclide studies despite medical therapy may also be considered for revascularization.

SUMMARY AND CONCLUSION

Diagnostic and therapeutic cardiac catheterization procedures play a central role in the management of many patients with stable ischemic syndromes. In many subsets of patients with these syndromes, revascularization directed by integration of clinical and coronary angiographic findings will result in an improved outcome and even reduced mortality. As more and more patients undergo noninvasive testing and more catheter-based therapeutic techniques are developed this role will continue to expand.

References

1. McNeer JF, Margolis JR, Lee KL, et al. The role of the exercise test in the evaluation of patients for ischemic heart disease. Circulation 1978;57:64–70.
2. Burggraf, GW, Parker JO. Prognosis in coronary artery disease: angiographic, hemodynamic and clinical factors. Circulation 1975;51:146–156.
3. Silverman KJ, Grossman W. Current concepts. Angina pectoris: natural history and strategies for evaluation and management. N Engl J Med 1984;310:1712–1717.
4. Schlant RC, Blomqvist CG, Bradenburg RD, et al. A report of the American College of Cardiology/American Heart Association Task Force on Assessment of Cardiovascular Procedures (Subcommittee on Exercise Testing). Guidelines for exercise testing. J Am Coll Cardiol 1986;8:725–738.
5. Ross J, Brandenburg RO, Dinsmore RE, et al. A report of the American College of Cardiology/American Heart Association Task Force on Assessment of Diagnostic and Therapeutic Cardiovascular Procedures (Subcommittee on Coronary Angiography). Guidelines for coronary angiography. J Am Coll Cardiol 1987;10:935–950.
6. Bemiller CR, Pepine CJ, Rogers AK. Long-term observations in patients with angina and normal coronary arteriograms. Circulation 1973;47:36–43.
7. Kennedy JW, Kaiser GC, Fisher LD, et al. Multivariate discriminant analysis of clinical and angiographic predictors of operative mortality from the Collaborative Study in Coronary Artery Surgery (CASS). J Thorac Cardiovasc Surg 1980;80:876–887.
8. Murphy ML, Hultgren HN, Detre K, et al. Treatment of chronic stable angina: a preliminary report of survival data of the Randomized Veterans Administration Cooperative Study. N Engl J Med 1977;297:621–627.
9. Varnaukas E, European Coronary Surgery Study Group. Twelve-year follow-up of survival in the randomized European Coronary Surgery Study. N Engl J Med 1988;319:332–337.
10. European Coronary Surgery Study Group. Prospective randomized study of coronary artery bypass surgery in stable angina pectoris: a progress report on survival. Circulation 1982;65:II–67–71.
11. CASS Principal Investigators and their Associates. Coronary Artery Surgery Study (CASS): a randomized trial of coronary artery bypass surgery (survival data). Circulation 1983;68:939–950.
12. Conti CR, Selby JH, Christie LG, et al. Left main coronary artery stenosis: clinical spectrum, pathophysiology and management. Prog Cardiovasc Dis 1979;22:73–106.
13. Bonow RO, Epstein SE. Indications for coronary artery bypass surgery in patients with chronic angina pectoris: implications of the multicenter randomized trials. Circulation 1985;72:V–23–30.
14. Kaiser GC, Davis KB, Fisher LD, et al. Survival following coronary artery bypass grafting in patients with severe angina pectoris (CASS). An observational study. J Thorac Cardiovasc Surg 1985;89:513–524.
15. Bonow RO, Kent KM, Rosing DR, et al. Exercise-induced ischemia in mildly symptomatic patients with coronary-artery disease and preserved left ventricular function. N Engl J Med 1984;311:1339–1345.
16. Weiner DA, Ryan TJ, McCabe CH, et al. The role of exercise testing in identifying patients with improved survival after coronary artery bypass surgery. J Am Coll Cardiol 1986;8:741–748.
17. Klein LW, Weintraub WS, Agarwal JB, et al. Prognostic significance of severe narrowing of the proximal portion of the left anterior descending coronary artery. Am J Cardiol 1986;58:42–46.
18. Mock MB, Ringqvist I, Fisher L, et al. The survival of nonoperated patients with ischemic heart disease: the CASS experience (abstr). Am J Cardiol 1982;49:1007.
19. Chaitman BR, Davis KB, Kaiser GC, et al. Participating CASS Hospitals. The role of coronary bypass surgery for "left main equivalent" coronary disease: The Coronary Artery Surgery Study Registry. Circulation 1986;74:III–17–25.
20. Passamani E, Davis KB, Gillespie MJ, Killip T. A randomized trial of coronary artery bypass surgery: survival of patients with a low ejection fraction. N Engl J Med 1985;312:1665–1671.
21. Killip T, Passamani E, Davis K. Coronary artery surgery study (CASS): a randomized trial of

coronary bypass surgery. Eight years follow-up and survival in patients with reduced ejection fraction. Circulation 1985;72:V–102–109.

22. Detre KM, Takaro T, Hultgren H, Peduzzi P. Long-term mortality and morbidity results of the Veterans Administration randomized trial of coronary artery bypass surgery. Circulation 1985;72:V–84–89.

23. The Veterans Administration Coronary Artery Bypass Surgery Cooperative Study Group. Eleven-year survival in the Veterans Administration Randomized Trial of Coronary Bypass Surgery for Stable Angina. N Engl J Med 1984;311:1333–1339.

24. Dorros G, Stertzer SH, Cowley MJ, et al. Complex coronary angioplasty: multiple coronary dilatations. Am J Cardiol 1984;53:126C–130C.

25. Cowley MJ, Vetrovec GW, DiSciasco G, et al. Coronary angioplasty of multiple vessels: short-term outcome and long-term results. Circulation 1985;72:1314–1320.

26. Cukingnan RA, Carey JS, Wittig JH, Brown BG. Influence of complete coronary revascularization on relief of angina. J Thorac Cardiovasc Surg 1980;79:188–193.

27. Loop FD, Lytle BW, Gill CC, Golding LA, Cosgrove DM, Taylor PC. Trends in selection and results of coronary artery reoperations. Ann Thorac Surg 1983;36:380–388.

28. Mabin TA, Holmes DR, Smith HC, et al. Follow-up clinical results in patients undergoing percutaneous transluminal coronary angioplasty. Circulation 1985;71:754–760.

29. Vandormael MG, Chaitman BR, Ischinger T, et al. Immediate and short-term benefit of multilesion coronary angioplasty: influence of degree of revascularization. J Am Coll Cardiol 1985;6:983–991.

30. Pelletier LC, Pardini A, Renkin J, David PR, Hebert Y, Bourassa MG. Myocardial revascularization after failure of percutaneous transluminal coronary angioplasty. J Thorac Cardiovasc Surg 1985;90:265–271.

31. Akins CW, Block PC. Surgical intervention for failed percutaneous transluminal coronary angioplasty. Am J Cardiol 1984;53:108C–111C.

32. Bourassa MG, Fisher LD, Campeau L, Gillespie MJ, McConney M, Lesperance J. Long-term fate of bypass grafts: the Coronary Artery Surgery Study (CASS) and Montreal Heart Institute experiences. Circulation 1985;72:V–71–78.

33. Foster ED. Reoperation for coronary artery disease. Circulation 1985;72:V–59–64.

34. Schaff HV, Orszulak TA, Gersh BJ, et al. The morbidity and mortality of reoperation for coronary artery disease and analysis of late results with use of actuarial estimate of event-free interval. J Thorac Cardiovasc Surg 1983;85:508–515.

35. Barner HB, Standeven JW, Reese J. Twelve-year experience with internal mammary artery for coronary artery bypass. J Thorac Cardiovasc Surg 1985;90:668–675.

36. Lewis MR, Dehmer, GJ. Coronary bypass using the internal mammary artery. Am J Cardiol 1985;56:480–482.

37. Bashour TT, Hanna ES, Mason DT. Myocardial revascularization with internal mammary artery bypass: an emerging treatment of choice. Am Heart J 1986;111:143–151.

38. Loop FD, Lytle BW, Cosgrove DM, et al. Influence of the internal-mammary-artery graft on 10-year survival and other cardiac events. N Engl J Med 1986;314:1–6.

39. Cameron A, Kemp HG, Green GE. Bypass surgery with the internal mammary artery graft: 15 year follow-up. Circulation 1986;74:III–30–36.

40. Corbelli J, Franco I, Hollman J, Simpfendorfer C, Galan K. Percutaneous transluminal coronary angioplasty after previous coronary artery bypass surgery. Am J Cardiol 1985;56:398–403.

41. Block PC, Cowley MJ, Kaltenbach M, Kent KM, Simpson J. Percutaneous angioplasty of stenoses of bypass grafts or of bypass graft anastomotic sites. Am J Cardiol 1984;53:666–668.

42. Douglas JS, Gruentzig AR, King SB, et al. Percutaneous transluminal coronary angioplasty in patients with prior coronary bypass surgery. J Am Coll Cardiol 1983;2:745–754.

43. El Gamal M, Bonnier H, Michels R, et al. Percutaneous transluminal angioplasty of stenosed aorto-coronary bypass grafts. Br Heart J 1984;52:617–620.

44. Meier B, King SB, Gruentzig AR, et al. Repeat coronary angioplasty. J Am Coll Cardiol 1984;4:463–466.

45. Williams DO, Gruentzig AR, Kent KM, et al. Efficacy of repeat percutaneous transluminal coronary angioplasty for coronary restenosis. Am J Cardiol 1984;53:32C–35C.

46. Rahimtoola SH, Grunkemeier GL, Starr A. Ten year survival after coronary artery bypass surgery for angina in patients aged 65 years and older. Circulation 1986;74:509–517.

47. Gersh BJ, Kronmal RA, Frye RI, et al. Coronary arteriography and coronary artery bypass surgery: morbidity and mortality in patients ages 65 years or older. A report from the Coronary Artery Surgery Study. Circulation 1983;67:483–491.

48. Raizner AE, Hust RG, Lewis JM, et al. Transluminal coronary angioplasty in the elderly. Am J Cardiol 1986;57:29–32.

49. Mock MB, Homes DR, Vliestra RE, et al. Percutaneous transluminal coronary angioplasty (PTCA) in the elderly patient: experience in the National Heart, Lung, and Blood Institute PTCA Registry. Am J Cardiol 1984;53:89C–91C.

50. Taylor GJ, Rabinovich E, Mikell FL, et al. Percutaneous transluminal coronary angioplasty as palliation for patients considered poor surgical candidates. Am Heart J 1986;111:840–844.

51. Shimokawa H, Nagasawa K, Irie T, et al. Clinical characteristics and long-term prognosis of patients with variant angina. A comparative study between western and Japanese populations. Int J Cardiol 1988;18:331–349.

52. Pepine CJ, Feldman RL, Conti CR. Recommendations for use of ergonovine to provoke coronary artery spasm. Cathet Cardiovasc Diagn 1980;6:423–426.

53. David PR, Waters DD, Scholl JM, et al. Percutaneous transluminal coronary angioplasty in patients with variant angina. Circulation 1982;66:695–702.

54. Corcos T, David PR, Bourassa MG, et al. Percutaneous transluminal coronary angioplasty for the treatment of variant angina. J Am Coll Cardiol 1985;5:1046–1054.

55. Bertrand ME, LaBlanche JM, Thieureux F, Fourrier JL, Traisnel G, Asseman P. Comparative results of percutaneous transluminal coronary angioplasty in patients with dynamic versus fixed coronary stenosis. J Am Coll Cardiol 1986;8:504–508.

56. Leisch F, Schutzenberger W, Kerschner K, et al. Influence of variant angina of the results of percutaneous transluminal coronary angioplasty. Br Heart J 1986;56:341–345.

57. Conti CR. Large vessel coronary vasospasm: diagnosis, natural history and treatment. Am J Cardiol 1985;55:41B–49B.

58. Beller GA, Gibson RS. Risk stratification after myocardial infarction. Mod Concepts Cardiovasc Dis 1986;55:5–10.

59. DeBusk RF, Blomqvist CE, Kouchoukos NT, et al. Identification and treatment of low-risk patients after acute myocardial infarction and coronary-artery bypass graft surgery. N Engl J Med 1986;314:161–166.

60. Schuster EH, Bulkley BH. Early post-infarction angina: ischemia at a distance and ischemia in the infarct zone. N Engl J Med 1981;305:1101–1105.

61. De Feyter PJ, van Eenige MJ, Dighton DH, Visser FC, De Jong J, Roos JP. Prognostic value of exercise testing, coronary angiography and left ventriculography 6–8 weeks after myocardial infarction. Circulation 1982;66:527–536.

62. Akhras F, Upward J, Keates J, Jackson G. Early exercise testing and elective coronary artery bypass surgery after complicated myocardial infarction: effect on morbidity and mortality. Br Heart J 1984;52:413–417.

63. Singh AK, Rivera R, Cooper GN, Karlson KE. Early myocardial revascularization for postinfarction angina: results and long-term follow-up. J Am Coll Cardiol 1985;6:1121–1125.

64. Norris RM, Agnew TR, Brandt PW, et al. Coronary surgery after recurrent myocardial infarction: progress of a trial comparing surgical with nonsurgical management for asymptomatic patients with advanced coronary disease. Circulation 1981;63:785–792.

65. Norris RM, Barnaby PF, Brandt P, et al. Prognosis after recovery from first acute myocardial infarction: determinants of reinfarction and sudden death. Am J Cardiol 1984;53:408–413.

66. De Feyter PJ, Serruys PW, Soward A, van Den Brand M, Bos E, Hugenholtz PG. Coronary angioplasty for early postinfarction unstable angina. Circulation 1986;74:1365–1370.

67. Ellestad MH, Wan MK. Predictive implications of stress testing: follow-up of 2700 subjects after maximum treadmill stress testing. Circulation 1975;51:363–369.

68. Falcone C, De Servi S, Poma E, et al. Clinical significance of exercise-induced silent myocardial ischemia in patients with coronary artery disease. J Am Coll Cardiol 1987;9:295–299.

69. Weiner DA, Ryan TJ, McCabe C, et al. Significance of silent myocardial ischemia during exercise testing in patients with coronary artery disease. Am J Cardiol 1987;59:725–729.

70. Multiple Risk Factor Intervention Trial Research Group. Exercise electrocardiogram and coronary heart disease mortality in the Multiple Risk Factor Intervention Trial. Am J Cardiol 1985;55:16–24.

71. Kannel WB, Abbott RD. Incidence and prognosis of unrecognized myocardial infarction: an update on the Framingham Study. N Engl J Med 1984;311:1144–1147.

72. Beller GA. Role of nuclear cardiology in evaluating the total ischemic burden in coronary artery disease. Am J Cardiol 1987;59:31C–38C.

27

The Patient with Known or Suspect Coronary Heart Disease: Unstable Ischemic Syndromes

Sheldon Goldberg, M.D.
Michael Savage, M.D.

INTRODUCTION

Clinically, coronary artery disease (CAD) may present in two distinct manners. As the atherosclerotic lesion gradually enlarges and progressively occludes the vessel lumen, coronary blood flow through the lesion may be inadequate during periods of increased myocardial oxygen consumption. These patients often present with signs and/or symptoms of transient ischemia that are usually relatively stable (e.g., exertional angina pectoris). Alternatively, a relatively abrupt change in the biology of an atherosclerotic lesion may occur, leading to an acute reduction in coronary flow. This abrupt reduction in perfusion can be mediated by a variety of intracoronary events that may be interrelated, including plaque rupture, intraluminal thrombus, and coronary vasospasm (1). Patients with these "complicated" atherosclerotic lesions typically present with one of the unstable ischemic syndromes (e.g., unstable angina, non Q wave infarction, or Q-wave myocardial infarction). These acute ischemic events are a major cause of morbidity and mortality in patients with cardiac disease. The purpose of this chapter is to review the role of diagnostic and interventional cardiac catheterization in the management of patients with these unstable coronary syndromes.

UNSTABLE ANGINA

General Considerations

The medical literature on unstable angina is somewhat confused by inconsistencies in the nomenclature and definition of the syndrome. Historically, the syndrome of unstable angina has been discussed using a variety of names, including crescendo angina, accelerating angina, status anginosus, preinfarction angina, and acute coronary insufficiency. The term intermediate coronary syndrome has also been used to designate unstable angina pectoris as the clinical and pathoanatomic link between chronic stable angina and acute myocardial infarction (2). Few have improved upon Paul Wood's description of the syndrome: "Characteristically. . .the onset of acute coronary insufficiency is sudden, a state of normal health, or of relatively mild angina of effort, with or without a previous history of cardiac infarction, changing abruptly to one of almost total incapacity. Although the pain is usually provoked by all the familiar triggers, including changes of temperature, a meal, getting into bed at night, or getting up in the morning, as well as by trivial effort and excitement, it may also occur spontaneously when the patient is sitting quietly in a chair reading the paper, or may wake him repeatedly from sleep. . .An ischemic electrocardiogram taken during an attack of pain confirms the diagnosis of angina pectoris. . .[but] a diagnosis of acute coronary insufficiency denies evidence of cardiac infarction" (3). Recognizing that the diagnosis of unstable angina pectoris encompasses a heterogeneous population of patients, more recent authors have classified patients according to specific subgroups. The most commonly used classification attempts to identify three types of unstable angina: (*a*) new onset exertional angina, (*b*) crescendo angina (i.e., prior chronic stable angina with a relatively recent increase in the frequency or severity of ischemic symptoms), and (*c*) angina at rest (4).

Recognition of these different subsets of patients with unstable angina may be important for decision-making, since prognosis may be influenced by initial clinical presentation. Patients with rest angina have a poorer long-term outcome than patients with recent onset or progressive exertional angina (5). In addition, the presence of relatively prolonged (>15 min) angina associated with ischemic-type ST-T wave ECG changes and persistence of angina despite intensive medical therapy are associated with a high risk of subsequent myocardial infarction (6, 7).

Electrocardiograms (ECG) obtained during a spontaneous episode of angina typically demonstrate transient deviations of the ST segments and/or T waves. Of 288 patients with unstable angina associated with ECG changes enrolled prospectively by the National Cooperative Study Group, ST segment elevation was observed in 27% of patients, ST depression in 61% of patients, and T wave inversion alone in 12% (8). Although ischemic changes on the ECG usually normalize shortly after the relief of angina, ECG abnormalities may occasionally persist for several hours or even days with no evidence of myocardial infarction by serum enzyme analyses. The direction of ST segment shift occurring during angina does not show a high degree of correlation with the extent of CAD subsequently assessed by coronary angiography (9). While transient ST segment elevation was frequently observed in unstable angina patients with disease of the right and left anterior descending coronary arteries (78 and 48%, respectively), ST segment elevation was only rarely seen (9%) in patients with disease of the left cir-

cumflex coronary artery (10). Studies from our laboratory suggest that regional transmural myocardial ischemia associated with left circumflex occlusion is not frequently accompanied by ST segment elevation, but rather, may be associated with ST segment depression alone or without ST segment shift at all (Fig. 27.1) (11). Therefore, the presence or absence of ST segment elevation in association with spontaneous angina seems to be determined not only by the degree of myocardial ischemia but also by the location of the coronary artery obstruction. The absence of ECG change during chest pain suggests that symptoms are not due to myocardial ischemia, or that ischemia involves the posterior left ventricular wall.

In the future, continuous ECG monitoring may play an increasingly important role in management of patients with unstable angina. Several groups have now demonstrated that silent ischemia detected by this type of monitoring is prevalent in patients with unstable angina and that the presence of silent ischemia despite antianginal medication that prevents recurrent angina predicts an increased likelihood of adverse clinical events (12, 13).

Intensive medical therapy should be initiated in all unstable angina patients upon hospital admission. β-blockers, calcium antagonists, and nitrates should be used in combination and dosed as tolerated. In addition, we routinely use intravenous heparin for patients with rest angina associated with ischemic ECG changes. Several randomized double-blind trials demonstrated a significant reduction in the incidence of myocardial infarction with the use of intravenous heparin. Transmural myocardial infarction developed in 15% of 114 patients following a 1-week course without heparin in comparison to an infarction rate of only 3% in 100 patients treated with 5000 units of intravenous heparin every 6 hr (14). The benefit of oral aspirin in unstable angina over 3 to 24 months of follow-up has also been demonstrated by controlled clinical trials (15, 16). The usefulness of aspirin (325 mg, twice daily), heparin (1000 units/hr), and both in combination was examined in a controlled trial involving 479 unstable angina patients (17). The incidence of myocardial infarction was reduced in all treatment groups compared with placebo.

Role of the Catheterization Laboratory in Unstable Angina Pectoris

While the optimal timing and indications for cardiac catheterization in patients with unstable angina have not been evaluated by controlled clinical trials, general principles can be outlined. In patients with recurrent angina on maximal medical therapy, cardiac catheterization should be undertaken without delay with the goal of assessing the patient for potential revascularization with coronary angioplasty (PTCA) or coronary artery bypass graft (CABG) surgery. We also recommend cardiac catheterization for most patients with unstable angina whose symptoms initially improve after intensification of medical therapy. Within 3 months of clinical presentation, acute myocardial infarction and/or death will occur in approximately 20% of patients (7). In light of the variable course of these patients and the high incidence of untoward cardiac events soon after symptom onset, evaluation of coronary anatomy by cardiac catheterization prior to hospital discharge is extremely valuable in the management of these patients. Patients with rest angina associated with ST or T wave changes are at particularly high risk and should undergo early evaluation for possible revascularization. Patients with a pattern of crescendo angina have a relatively high incidence of left main and triple-vessel CAD, and therefore cardiac catheterization should be performed to identify these candidates for CABG (18). In patients with new onset exertional angina, it may be reasonable to initially defer cardiac catheterization if there are no ischemic changes on the resting ECG and if symptoms are controlled after institution of medical therapy. Exercise testing can be used to assess risk and help guide the need for further invasive testing. Patients with angina at a low exercise workload, marked ischemic changes, or exercise induced hypotension would warrant coronary angiography. On the other hand, in our view, exercise stress testing is contraindicated in patients presenting with rest angina and ECG evidence of ischemia. Exercise testing in these patients rarely mitigates the need for cardiac catheterization, unnecessarily delays more definitive evaluation, and exposes the patient to unnecessary additional risk (Fig. 27.2). In such patients, it is preferable to undertake cardiac catheterization after initial intensification of medical therapy.

Approach to the Patient in the Cardiac Catheterization Laboratory

The critical importance of adequate antiischemic medical therapy in preparation for cardiac catheterization cannot be overemphasized. Angiography may precipitate acute ischemia and myocardial dysfunction in these unstable patients. Meticulous attention must be paid towards optimal stabilization of the patient beforehand. Concurrent factors that increase myocardial oxygen demand, such as infection, fever, anemia, congestive heart failure, and arrhythmias, should be identified and treated. Pharmacologic therapy, using multiple antianginal drugs, is recommended to minimize oxygen demands, which can be estimated clinically by the heart rate–blood pressure product. Oral or parental β-blockade should be used to achieve a resting heart rate of approximately 60 bpm, both to reduce the potential for aggravating myocardial ischemia during the procedure and to allow optimal cineangiographic assessment of coronary anatomy that is not possible at rapid heart rates.

The clinical status of the patient on entry to the catheterization suite dictates the sequence of the cardiac catheterization procedure and the approach to data acquisition. The most important immediate concern is whether the patient is having ongoing myocardial ischemia. Continuous monitoring of the ECG should be performed to assess for development of arrhythmias or ischemic ST-T wave changes. This is best done by means of a multichannel recorder with the capability of monitoring several leads simultaneously. We have found it most useful to monitor an inferior lead (lead II) and a precordial lead (V_2 or V_4). Alternatively, other leads can be used if they have shown more pronounced changes in a previous 12-lead ECG. In patients with persistent angina on entry to the catheterization laboratory, initial attempts at stabilization should be made by administration of nasal oxygen, intravenous β-blockade, intravenous nitroglycerin, and adequate analgesia. In patients with ongoing ischemia refractory to these intensive pharmacologic maneuvers, insertion of an intraaortic balloon pump

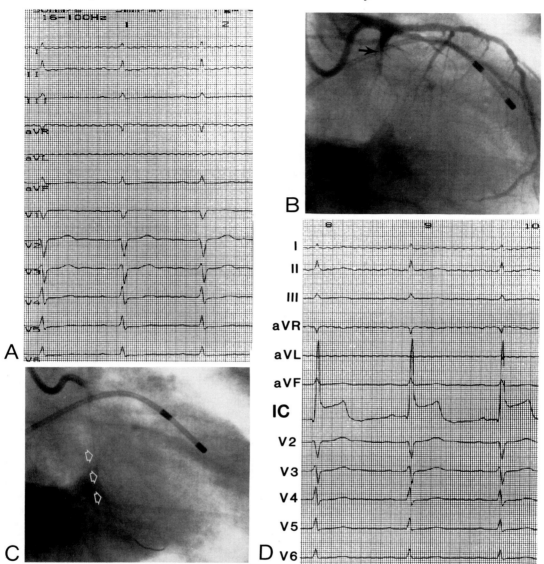

Figure 27.1. The relative insensitivity of the surface ECG in detecting posterior wall ischemia due to left circumflex occlusion and utility of the intracoronary ECG. *A,* The ECG recorded during angina shows no ischemic changes. *B,* The left coronary angiogram (RAO projection) obtained during pain shows total occlusion of the left circumflex coronary artery. *C,* Emergency PTCA was performed, and a regional electrogram was recorded from the guidewire (*arrows*), which was connected to the V₁ lead of the ECG. *D,* Epicardial electrogram recorded from the intracoronary (*IC*) guidewire overlying the posterior left ventricle. There is marked ST elevation in the intracoronary lead despite the absence of ST shifts on the surface ECG (see next page). *E,* Left coronary angiogram after PTCA showing restoration of antegrade flow in the left circumflex coronary artery. *F,* Surface and intracoronary ECG after PTCA showing resolution of the acute injury current on the intracoronary recording.

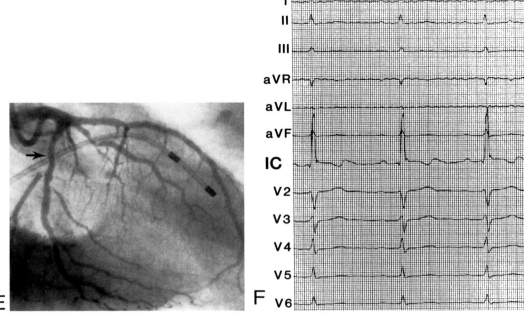

Figure 27.1 *E* and *F.*

should be considered. Intraaortic balloon counterpulsation should be initiated prior to coronary angiography in patients with ongoing angina associated with hemodynamic compromise (i.e., congestive heart failure or hypotension) or marked ischemic type shifts in the ST segments (Fig. 27.3). Obviously, the decision to use the intraaortic balloon pump in this setting must be individualized. For example, if left main or severe multivessel coronary disease is likely, and the patient is suspected to be a candidate for coronary artery bypass surgery, balloon pump insertion will be useful to stabilize the patient and allow safe performance of the diagnostic catheterization procedure and subsequent surgical revascularization. Alternatively, if the patient is hemodynamically stable and single-vessel disease is likely on a clinical basis, once can proceed expeditiously with PTCA and immediate coronary angioplasty, thus averting the risks associated with the intraaortic balloon pump. Another group of patients in which coronary angiography should be undertaken first is those with a history of variant angina. Spontaneous coronary spasm should be suspected in this group of patients. Selective administration of intracoronary nitroglyc-

erin into the involved artery, followed by repeat angiography, will be both diagnostic and therapeutic if spasm is present (19).

Cardiac catheterization in patients with unstable angina may be done by means of either the brachial or femoral approaches. The approach used is best determined by the experience of the individual operator. We feel that the femoral approach provides a slight margin of safety in that immediate vascular access for intraaortic balloon counterpulsation is available should abrupt hemodynamic deterioration occur during the procedure. However, lack of control with preformed catheters falling into the left main coronary artery is a disadvantage that may be disastrous. Selection of type of angiographic contrast agent must also be individualized. Injection of ionic contrast material during coronary angiography results in important electrical and hemodynamic changes. These include slowing of the heart rate, prolongation of the QT interval, depression of myocardial contractility and systemic blood pressure, and elevation of left ventricular end-diastolic pressure. These effects may be particularly deleterious in the unstable patient obscuring changes due to ischemia and contribute to the increasing risk of the

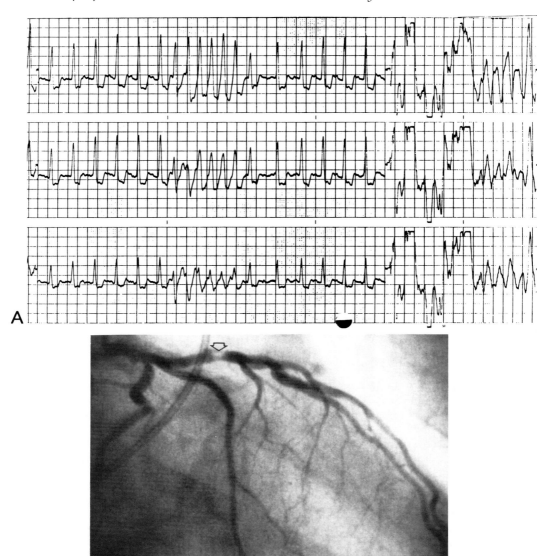

Figure 27.2. The danger of exercise testing in a patient with new onset rest angina. *A,* Treadmill exercise test demonstrating marked ST depression and ventricular fibrillation, which necessitated multiple electrical countershocks. *B,* Left coronary angiogram (RAO projection) subsequently showed a critical stenosis of the proximal left anterior descending coronary artery (*arrow*).

procedure. The newer nonionic and low-osmolar contrast agents allow cardiac catheterization to be performed in a more physiologic manner in unstable patients. Compared with standard ionic and high-osmolar contrast agents, the newer agents have significantly

less electrical and mechanical depressant effects (20). We use these agents routinely in patients with unstable angina and one or more of the following: ongoing ischemia at the time of the cardiac catheterization procedure, suspected critical left main disease, aortic

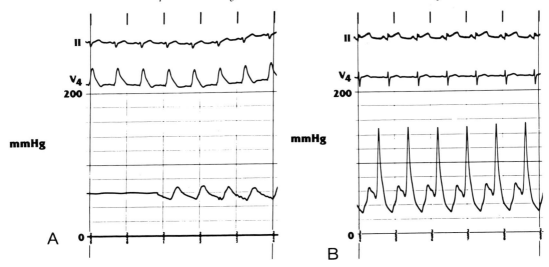

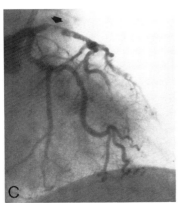

Figure 27.3. Usefulness of the intraaortic balloon pump during emergency cardiac catheterization of a patient with an unstable ischemic syndrome. *A,* Surface ECGs and arterial pressure showing marked ST elevation and profound hypotension. *B,* Relief of acute injury current in lead V_4 and improved arterial pressure by intraaortic balloon counterpulsation. *C,* The coronary angiogram was then safely obtained and demonstrated subtotal occlusion of the proximal left anterior descending artery with preserved, but sluggish, antegrade flow.

stenosis, congestive heart failure, and bradyarrhythmias (see also Chapter 10). The availability of biplane x-ray has also been useful for unstable angina patients since the contrast load is effectively reduced by one-half.

We use a 8 Fr vascular sheath in the femoral vein, through which a 7 Fr Zucker catheter is advanced for measurement of right heart pressures. The bipolar electrodes at the tip allow this catheter to also function as a temporary pacemaker when positioned within the right atrium or right ventricle. Right heart pressures are particularly useful in the setting of hypotension, congestive heart failure, prior myocardial infarction, or pulmonary hypertension. The ability to measure right heart and pulmonary vascular pressures also allows assessment of hemodynamic effects of acute ischemia. An abrupt rise in pulmonary artery and pulmonary-capillary wedge pressures in the patient with transient ischemia implies acute ischemic left ventricular dysfunction or acute mitral insufficiency due to papillary muscle dysfunction (Fig. 27.4). For patients in whom right heart pressures are not recorded, a 6 Fr bipolar pacing catheter is inserted into the right atrium or right ventricle via the venous sheath. A 8 Fr sheath is then inserted into the femoral artery and 5000 units of intravenous sodium heparin are administered. In patients with unstable angina and resting ischemic ECG changes already receiving intravenous heparin, the infusion should not be stopped beforehand but is continued up to the time of catheterization. We have observed several patients who developed acute coronary thrombosis and myocardial infarction before cardiac catheterization when intravenous heparin was discontinued 6 hr prior to the planned procedure (Fig. 27.5).

Ideally, left ventriculography is performed

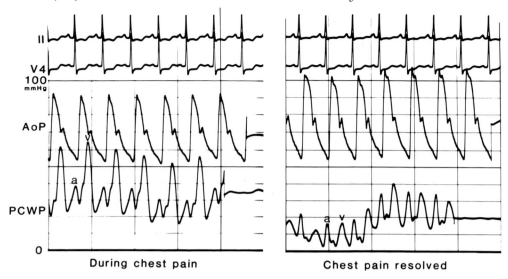

Figure 27.4. Acute mitral regurgitation due to ischemic papillary muscle dysfunction in a patient with unstable angina and critical stenosis of the left circumflex coronary artery. During angina (*left*), marked ST segment depression is accompanied by arterial hypotension (*AoP*) and large V waves in the pulmonary-capillary wedge pressure (*PCWP*) tracing. After relief of angina (*right*), there is improvement in the hemodynamics and ECG.

prior to coronary angiography in order to assess left ventricular hemodynamics, systolic function, and mitral valve competence. This is usually well tolerated in patients who have been stable for 24 to 48 hr prior to the procedure. On the other hand, left ventriculography in itself may precipitate myocardial ischemia. Therefore, left ventriculography should be deferred until after coronary angiography in patients with active myocardial ischemia or if there is persistent marked elevation of left ventricular end-diastolic pressure (>20 mm Hg) despite nitroglycerin. In patients with ongoing ischemia, it is often best to defer left ventriculography altogether unless the information is essential for planning therapy and cannot be obtained by noninvasive technique (e.g., suspected mitral insufficiency or aneurysm). Again, nonionic or low-osmolar contrast agents are particularly useful in this setting.

We feel that the left coronary artery should be visualized first. Attention should be directed towards assessing the left main coronary artery since this is the most threatening location for coronary obstruction. Significant left main stenosis will be present in 10 to 15% of patients with unstable angina. Critical stenosis at the left main ostium is often

first signaled by dampening of the pressure waveform on entry of the catheter tip into the ostium (Fig. 27.6). This finding will be observed with preformed end-hole catheters, such as Judkins or Amplatz catheters, but may not be seen with side-hole catheters, such as the multipurpose or Sones catheters. When ostial stenosis is suspected, test injections of contrast material should be avoided, as repeated injections are hazardous in this circumstance. Initial injection should be performed with cinefilming so that, should a critical ostial lesion be confirmed, the risk of repeated contrast injections can be averted. The patient with unstable angina and critical left main coronary artery disease is one of the most high-risk combinations encountered in the laboratory. Although diagnostic catheterization is usually done with relatively low risk of mortality, risk is substantial in patients with left main coronary stenosis (21) (see Chapter 3). When left main coronary stenosis is suspected, it is of utmost importance to take precautions to prevent bradycardia and hypotension that may lead to further hypoperfusion and cardiogenic shock.

Clinical features that suggest high likelihood of left main obstruction include any of

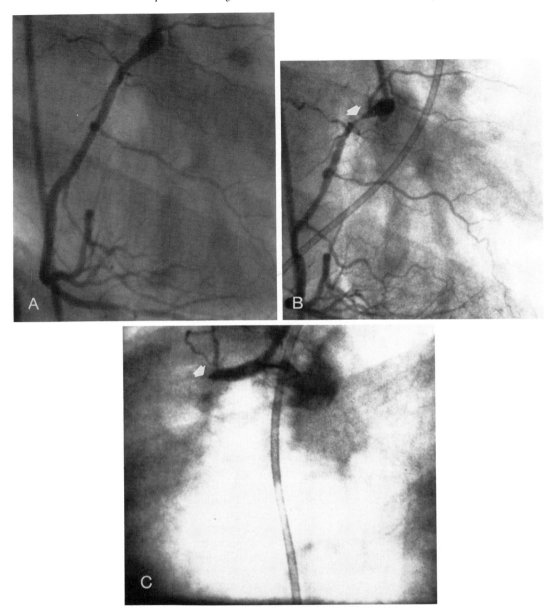

Figure 27.5. Progression of coronary atherosclerosis associated with onset of unstable angina, as shown by serial angiograms over a 3-year period. *A,* Initial right coronary angiogram shows no significant disease. *B,* Repeat angiogram 3 years later, after the development of unstable angina, shows a severe stenosis of the proximal right coronary artery (*arrow*). *C,* Acute thrombotic occlusion of the right coronary artery after discontinuation of intravenous heparin infusion prior to planned elective PTCA.

the following: history of crescendo symptoms superimposed upon chronic stable angina, ST segment depression in both inferior and anterior ECG leads simultaneously, and calcification of the left main coronary artery on fluoroscopy (22). In addition, prior exercise stress testing accompanied by marked ST segment depression at a low workload or hypotension is associated with an increased incidence of left main obstruction. Under these conditions, several steps should be taken routinely prior to left coronary angiography

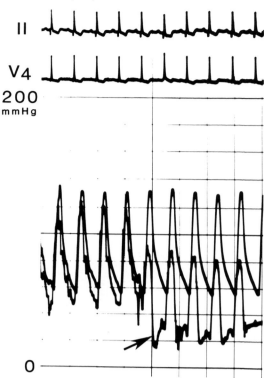

II

V4

200
mmHg

0

Figure 27.6 Importance of continuous pressure monitoring during catheter entry into coronary ostium in a patient with unstable angina. Simultaneous pressure recordings from the femoral artery sheath and diagnostic catheter are shown during catheter engagement of the left coronary artery. The presence of a critical stenosis of the left main ostium is signaled by the dampening and ventricularization of the pressure waveform on entry of the catheter tip into the ostium (*arrow*).

to help maintain hemodynamic stability during the procedure. Selective coronary angiography should be undertaken before ventriculography, and nonionic low-osmolar contrast agents should be used. Volume loading is used to reduce the likelihood of hypotension, and a pacing catheter is placed at the right ventricular apex to prevent bradycardia during coronary angiography. Injections into the left coronary artery should be limited to the minimum number sufficient for diagnostic purposes (ideally, one). In all cases, the initial angiographic projections utilized should be those that best delineate the left main coronary artery without overlap or foreshortening, the shallow right anterior oblique (RAO) view (0 to 15°), and/or the 30 to 45° left anterior

oblique (LAO) view with 30° of cranial angulation (Fig. 27.7). If a critical proximal stenosis is excluded, sufficient diagnostic information should be available for clinical decision-making with these views alone. Unless the severity of a given stenosis is in doubt, additional injections are extraneous and may cause otherwise avoidable complications. If critical left main coronary artery stenosis is excluded, additional views can then be safely undertaken in order to best delineate the remaining coronary anatomy.

Coronary Angiographic Findings

When patients with unstable angina are considered regardless of subgroup, coronary angiography demonstrates a distribution of single-, double-, and triple-vessel disease similar to that seen in patients with chronic stable angina (23). As in the case of chronic stable angina, the left anterior descending coronary artery is the most commonly affected vessel in unstable angina. The incidence of significant left main obstruction, however, is approximately 15% in patients with unstable angina, and this is much higher than with stable angina patients (22, 24, 25). Approximately 5 to 10% of patients clinically diagnosed with unstable angina have normal coronary angiography. Coronary spasm is presumed to play a role in the development of angina in some, if not many, of these patients (23).

As previously noted, the term "unstable angina" encompasses a relatively heterogeneous group of patients with distinct subgroups. The expected angiographic findings and extent of coronary disease vary depending upon the patient's history and presentation. Patients with crescendo angina usually have severe left main and/or multivessel coronary artery disease. Crescendo angina refers to a pattern of new rest pain or increasing frequency or severity of exertional pain superimposed upon previously stable symptoms that have been present for more than 3 months in duration. More than one-half of patients presenting for angiographic evaluation with unstable angina have a crescendo angina pattern (26). Crescendo angina is associated with significant left main disease in more than 20% of patients, and triple- or double-vessel disease (without critical left main obstruction) in more than 60%, while single-vessel disease is seen in about 10%. In contrast, single-vessel

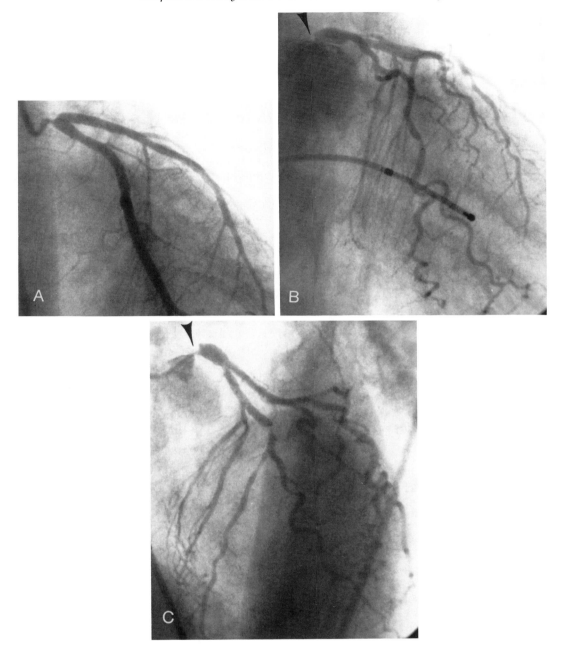

Figure 27.7. Importance of proper angiographic views to demonstrate left main coronary artery disease in unstable patients. *A,* The shallow RAO projection showing a "high-grade" ostial stenosis. *B,* The shallow RAO angiogram from another patient with critical left main disease; the proximal left coronary is not well seen due to contrast in the aortic sinus and superimposed soft tissue densities. *C,* Same patient shown in *B* using the shallow LAO projection with cranial angulation demonstrates severe stenosis of the left main coronary artery (*arrow*), as well as proximal left anterior descending stenosis.

disease is present in approximately one-half of all patients with unstable angina of <90 days' duration (24). The incidence of significant left main and triple-vessel disease is much lower in patients with unstable angina of recent onset, as compared with those with crescendo angina (26). These observations have important clinical implications in terms of assessing patients as potential candidates for revascularization procedure. Patients with crescendo angina will tend to have significant left main or multivessel coronary disease best managed by CABG. Patients with new onset angina will frequently have single-vessel disease amenable to PTCA. An additional and important subgroup of patients is those presenting with the clinical syndrome of variant angina, i.e., angina occurring exclusively at rest and associated with transient ST segment elevation. Although normal or near normal coronary anatomy is a frequent finding in this population, severe fixed atherosclerotic stenoses are associated with coronary spasm in up to two-thirds of patients presenting with variant angina (23). Moreover, patients with variant angina associated with severe (>70%) "fixed" coronary atherosclerotic obstruction have a worse prognosis than those without severe fixed obstructions. Coronary angioplasty has been used successfully in those patients with variant angina and severe fixed atherosclerotic lesions (27) (Fig. 27.8). Coronary angiography, therefore, should be routinely performed to define the underlying anatomy and to determine appropriate therapy in patients presenting with this clinical syndrome (28, 29).

The pathophysiologic mechanisms responsible for unstable angina have been the subject of several recent reviews (1, 30, 31). Serial coronary angiographic studies have demonstrated that the development of unstable angina is usually associated with recent worsening of coronary stenosis severity (Fig. 27.5)(29). Evidence has accumulated to indicate unstable rest angina is a dynamic process associated with abrupt reductions in coronary blood flow. Development of unstable angina appears invariably associated with an acute change in coronary anatomy due to one or more of the following mechanisms: plaque rupture, coronary thrombosis, and coronary spasm (32) (Fig. 27.9-27.11). It is important to emphasize that more than one of the above mechanisms may contribute to development of angina in a given individual patient.

In patients with unstable angina, the morphology of coronary artery lesions has been qualitatively assessed (Fig. 27.12) (33). The "angina-producing" lesion took the form of an eccentric stenosis associated with a sharp overhanging edge or irregular borders in over 70% of patients with unstable angina. This finding is seen infrequently in patients with stable angina. These observations suggest that unstable angina is frequently associated with a "complicated" eccentric (type II, Fig. 27.9) lesion. Previous histopathologic studies indicate that these complicated stenoses correlate with the presence of ruptured atherosclerotic plaques and/or partially occlusive thrombi (34). These complicated lesions appear to be the pathophysiologic trigger responsible for acute unstable ischemic syndromes.

Treatment of Unstable Angina with Interventional Cardiac Catheterization

Percutaneous transluminal coronary angioplasty is an increasingly important tool in the treatment of unstable angina pectoris. In one report, 44% of 360 consecutive patients hospitalized with unstable angina were candidates for PTCA (35). Ideally, patients should have discreet single-vessel CAD and symptoms that are refractory to maximal medical therapy. We also offer PTCA to patients with severe (>90%) stenosis involving a proximal major epicardial vessel because of the propensity of such lesions to progress to complete occlusion (36, 37). According to an early report from the National Heart, Lung and Blood Institute PTCA registry, results of coronary angioplasty in the treatment of single-vessel CAD were comparable in the presence of either stable or unstable angina (38). Immediate angiographic success rates of PTCA were 63% in 214 patients with stable angina and 61% in 442 patients with unstable angina. In-hospital mortality rates were 0.5 and 0.9% for the two groups, respectively. After 18 months of follow-up in the unstable angina group, the incidence of mortality was 2.6%, and the incidence of myocardial infarction was 9.5%. Procedural success rates have since improved with the introduction of steerable guidewire catheter systems. In one report, emergency

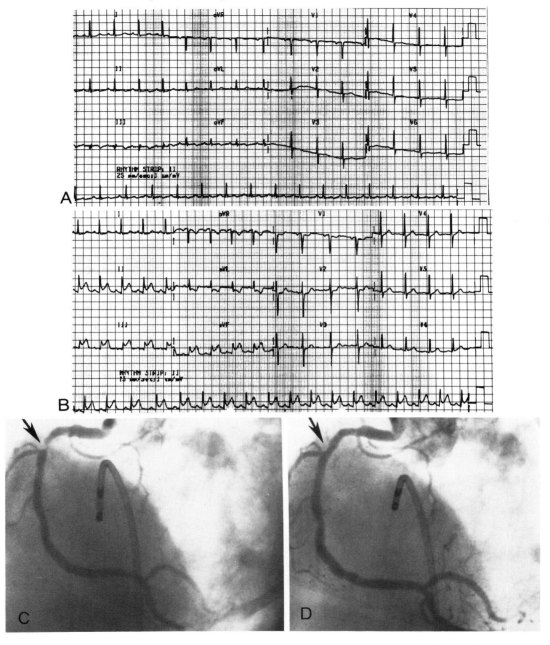

Figure 27.8.   A patient with variant angina associated with severe atherosclerotic disease and treatment with PTCA. *A* and *B,* Serial ECGs before and during rest angina. Note the transient ST elevation in inferior leads. *C,* Right coronary angiogram showing a complex lesion of the proximal right coronary artery persisting after nitroglycerin. *D,* Right coronary angiogram after PTCA.

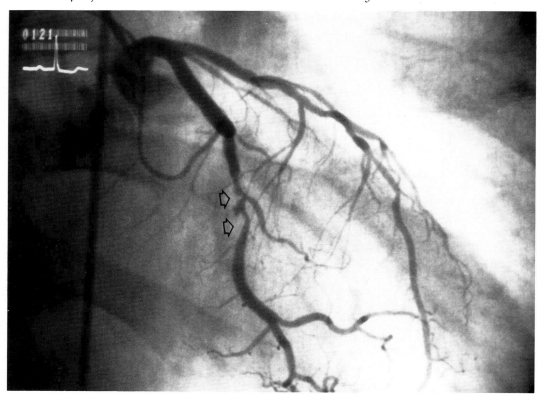

Figure 27.9. Angiographic features of plaque rupture, intraluminal thrombus, and coronary spasm, underlying unstable ischemic syndromes. Ulcerated plaque (*arrows*) in left circumflex coronary artery in a patient with unstable angina.

PTCA was successful in 56 of 60 patients (93%) with unstable angina pectoris refractory to maximal medical therapy (39). Although there were no procedural deaths, acute coronary occlusions occurred in four patients (7%), resulting in acute myocardial infarction despite emergency CABG. After a minimum follow-up of 6 months, there was one death and a restenosis rate of 28%. Improved functional status after sustained successful PTCA was demonstrated by a near normal exercise capacity and absence of ischemia demonstrated by thallium scintigraphy in 80% of patients.

Single-vessel PTCA of the angina-producing artery or "culprit lesion" may be suitable for selected patients with unstable angina and multivessel disease (Fig. 27.13) (40). This approach, however, is limited by the frequent recurrence of angina due to incomplete revascularization (41). Therefore, we advocate PTCA in patients with multivessel disease

only when dilation can achieve revascularization comparable with CABG.

We have also found interventional cardiac catheterization techniques to be useful in treatment of unstable ischemic syndromes following coronary bypass surgery (42). Myocardial ischemia occurring early after coronary bypass surgery is typically caused by graft thrombosis resulting from a mechanical graft problem, while late ischemic events are caused by progressive atherosclerotic stenosis with or without plaque rupture (Fig. 27.14). Cardiac catheterization is essential in order to define the underlying anatomic substrate, which is often complex in the postoperative setting. A variety of interventional catheterization strategies may be useful, depending upon the specific angiographic findings. In patients with acute graft thrombosis, reperfusion and amelioration of ischemia can be achieved with selective streptokinase infusion into the involved graft. In patients with unstable

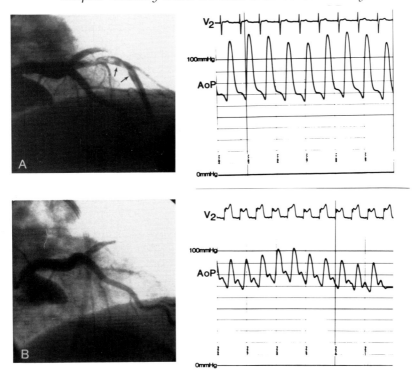

Figure 27.10. Angiographic features of plaque rupture, intraluminal thrombus, and coronary spasm, underlying unstable ischemic syndromes. *A,* Baseline coronary angiogram, ECG, and aortic pressure (AOP) recordings in a patient with unstable angina. Note a large thrombus is present within the proximal left anterior descending artery (*arrow*). *B,* Repeat angiogram and ECG during chest pain in the same patient, showing total acute occlusion of the left anterior descending coronary artery associated with marked ST segment elevation and hypotension.

angina due to atherosclerotic disease in the bypass graft, transluminal angioplasty may be an effective alternative to surgical revascularization. In other patients with bypass graft occlusions not amenable to PTCA, dilation may be undertaken within the diseased native coronary artery.

In general, the procedure in patients with unstable angina is similar to that of elective PTCA undertaken in patients with stable symptoms (see Chapter 15). However, it is our impression that these vessels are more reactive in terms of development of coronary spasm and thrombosis, and special safeguards against these untoward events are warranted. To reduce the potential for coronary spasm during PTCA, all of our patients are pretreated with high doses of calcium antagonists, as well as intracoronary nitroglycerin, immediately prior to dilation. Intraluminal filling defects consistent with coronary artery thrombus are detected angio-graphically in 6 to 37% of patients with unstable angina (43-45). Angiographically detectable coronary thrombi are particularly common in patients with recurrent rest angina when they are studied within hours of a rest angina episode (45). More recently, intraoperative observations made with the use of a flexible fiberoptic angioscope indicate that coronary mural thrombus is present in virtually all patients with unstable rest angina, even when thrombi are unsuspected on coronary angiography (46). Intracoronary thrombus assessed angiographically has been identified as an important risk factor associated with unsuccessful PTCA and with acute coronary occlusion during dilation (47, 48). Preliminary data suggest that prolonged heparin infusion prior to PTCA in patients with unstable angina may improve the immediate outcome of PTCA and reduce acute closure rates (49).

The potential role of thrombolytic therapy

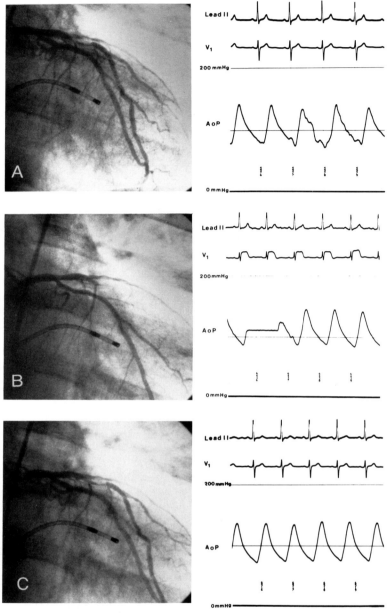

Figure 27.11 Angiographic features of rupture, intraluminal thrombus, and coronary spasm. *A–C,* Coronary spasm (elicited by ergonovine) superimposed on a severe atherosclerotic stenosis in a patient with rest angina. *A,* Control. *B,* Ergonovine. *C,* IC TNG, . (From Goldberg S. Coronary artery spasm and thrombosis. Philadelphia: FA Davis, 1983.)

in management of unstable myocardial ischemia requires further evaluation. Vetrovec et al. reported partial or complete coronary thrombolysis in 10 of 13 ischemia-related vessels following infusion of intracoronary streptokinase (mean dose 187,000 ± 22,000 IU) (50).

In contrast, Ambrose et al. found no significant changes after intracoronary streptokinase (mean dose 177,000 ± 80,000 IU) in 36 consecutive catheterized patients with unstable angina or subendocardial infarction (51). Randomized, placebo-controlled study

CONCENTRIC LESIONS

ECCENTRIC LESIONS

Type I

or

Type II

or

MULTIPLE IRREGULARITIES

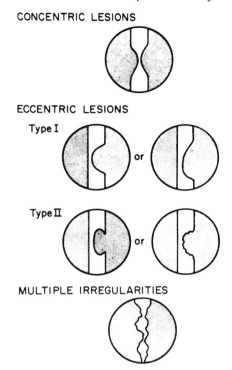

Figure 27.12. One suggested angiographic classification of lesion morphology. In patients with unstable angina, the ischemia-producing artery often has the appearance of an eccentric type II lesion with irregular borders and/or sharp overhanging edges. Similar findings have been noted in non-Q-wave infarction. (From Ambrose JA, Winters SL, Arora RR, et al. Angiographic evolution of coronary morphology in unstable angina. J Am Coll Cardiol 1986;7:472-478.)

suggests that intravenous administration of recombinant tissue plasminogen activator (rtPA) may be useful in the treatment of unstable angina (52). Unstable angina persisted in 6 of 11 patients after placebo infusion, as compared with only 1 of 12 patients after rtPA (1.75 mg/kg over 12 hr). Coronary angiography performed after the infusion demonstrated subocclusive thrombus in 8 of 11 patients receiving placebo but in none of the patients receiving rtPA. While these preliminary findings are promising, larger controlled trials will be necessary to better evaluate the benefits and risks of thrombolytic therapy, heparin and aspirin alone, and in combination for patients with unstable angina.

ACUTE MYOCARDIAL INFARCTION

General Considerations

The concept that coronary artery thrombi are involved in the pathogenesis of acute myocardial infarction was first suggested by Herrick in 1912 (53). In subsequent decades, the cause of acute myocardial infarction was widely debated until 1980, when DeWood et al. demonstrated conclusively by coronary angiography that patients with evolving myocardial infarction had thrombus (54) (Fig. 27.15). Acute myocardial infarction was associated with total occlusion of the infarction-related artery in nearly 90% of patients who underwent coronary angiography within 6 hr of symptom onset. Coronary thrombi were retrieved in 52 of 59 patients who underwent emergency CABG surgery. In contrast, in patients catheterized more than 12 hr after symptom onset, the incidence of complete coronary artery occlusion decreased to 65%, presumably due to spontaneous lysis by the patient's intrinsic fibrinolytic system. Myocardial necrosis is a dynamic process that begins approximately 20 min after occlusion of an epicardial coronary artery and is generally completed at 6 hr after interruption of coronary flow in animal models; therefore, effective reperfusion treatment of acute myocardial infarction should begin as early as possible.

In 1981, Rentrop et al. reported that intracoronary streptokinase given during evolving transmural infarction was associated with reperfusion of the infarction-related artery in 75% of treated patients (55). Subsequently, the efficacy of intracoronary streptokinase in recanalizing acutely occluded coronary arteries was reported to be between 62 and 85% (56–64). The rate of reperfusion was increased in patients with persistent ischemic discomfort (64) and in subgroups of patients who were treated relatively early after symptom onset (64, 65). Reperfusion was usually reestablished within 30 min of intracoronary drug infusion, with greater efficacy reported by some authors who used subselective techniques (57).

Since the goal of reestablishing antegrade coronary flow during acute myocardial infarction is to salvage myocardium in the region supplied by the affected coronary artery, end points for measuring the efficacy of coronary

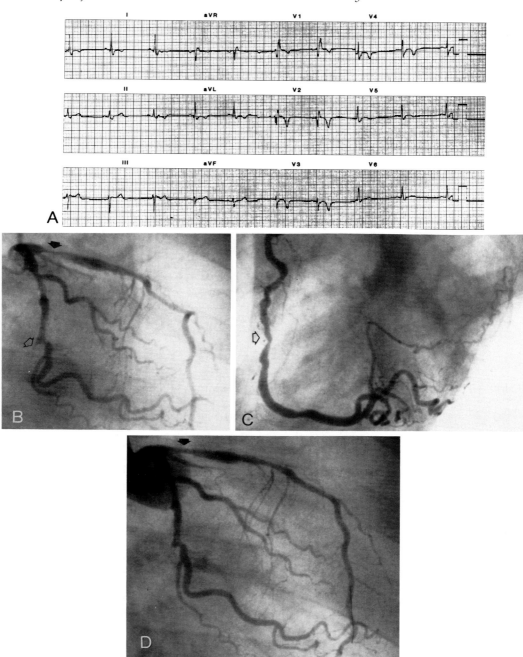

Figure 27.13. Single-vessel angioplasty of the "culprit lesion" in a patient with new onset unstable angina and multivessel disease. *A*, ECG shows anterior lead ST wave changes which implicate the left anterior descending artery as the culprit vessel. *B* and *C*, Left and right coronary angiograms, respectively, demonstrating multivessel involvement (*arrows*). *D*, PTCA (*arrow*) of the proximal left anterior descending coronary artery stenosis was performed with resolution of angina.

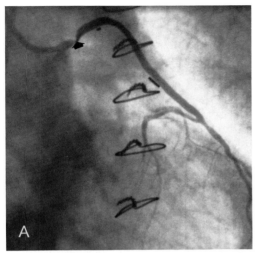

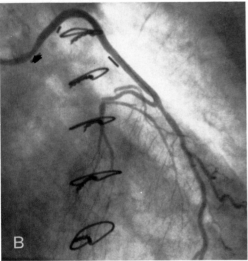

Figure 27.14. Vein graft angiograms in patient with unstable angina developing 8 years after coronary bypass surgery. *A,* Severe stenosis near aortic anastomosis (*arrow*). *B,* Results after PTCA of stenosis (*arrow*).

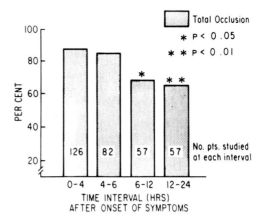

Figure 27.15. Incidence of coronary artery occlusion during the early hours of acute myocardial infarction. (From DeWood MA, Spores J, Notske R, et al. Prevalence of total coronary occlusion during the early hours of transmural myocardial infarction. N Engl J Med 1980;303:897-902.)

thrombolysis include changes in left ventricular function, as well as mortality. Assessment of left ventricular function after intracoronary thrombolysis showed only modest improvement (58) or no significant benefit (59-61). These findings were probably due to relatively late drug administration because of logistics problems involved with intracoronary administration of thrombolytic agents. Effects of intracoronary streptokinase on mortality were reported in the Western Washington Randomized Trial (59, 66). When intracoro-

nary streptokinase was administered within 12 hr of symptom onset, the 30-day mortality was reduced from 11.2% in patients treated with placebo to 3.7% in patients treated with intracoronary streptokinase. Although this difference in mortality was no longer statistically significant at 1 year, the treated patients had a 44% lower mortality rate when compared with the placebo group. Those who were reperfused had significant reduction in mortality, as compared with those who were not reperfused when the infarction was located in the anterior region.

Because of the delays inherent in transporting patients to the catheterization laboratory to give intracoronary thrombolysis, the effects of **intravenous lytic agents** were examined in patients with acute myocardial infarction. This therapy could be started earlier in the course of the infarction. If intravenous treatment proved effective in achieving coronary reperfusion, the overall effects on myocardial salvage and mortality might be expected to be superior to intracoronary drug delivery. The results of various randomized trials with the use of intravenous streptokinase showed reperfusion rates that were substantially lower than those achieved with intracoronary streptokinase. Recanalization varied between 31 and 55% (67, 68). Most trials that reported higher reperfusion rates lacked pretreatment angiography and, therefore, included patients with subtotal occlusion of the infarction-related artery. Despite the lower rate of coronary reperfusion with intravenous streptokinase, some studies have shown improvement in left ventricular function (69). The results of trials with the use of mortality as an end point with this form of treatment are somewhat conflicting. The Intravenous Streptokinase in Acute Myocardial Infarction Trial (ISAM) and the Western Washington IV Streptokinase Trial failed to demonstrate improved overall survival in treated patients (70, 71). In contrast, the GISSI study (72), which included 11,712 patients randomized to either placebo or intravenous streptokinase, demonstrated an 18% reduction in in-hospital mortality in the treated group. Of note, the salutory effect of intravenous streptokinase in mortality was more pronounced in the subgroup of patients treated very early after symptom onset (72). This benefit persisted at 1 year. A similar benefit was demonstrated by ISIS-2, a randomized trial involving 17,187 patients with suspected acute myocardial infarction (73).

Thus, it would appear that early clot lysis by means of intravenous thrombolytic agents was limited by relatively low reperfusion rates reported with intravenous streptokinase administration. In order to increase coronary recanalization rates, investigators began using more potent specific lytic agents, the most notable being tissue plasminogen activator (rtPA). The results of studies on this relatively fibrin-specific, short half-life thrombolytic agent demonstrated substantially higher coronary reperfusion rates, as compared with those of intravenous streptokinase. When a coronary angiogram taken 90 min postadministration was used as the end point, successful reperfusion was present in 62 to 75% of patients treated with intravenous rtPA (67, 68, 74, 75).

An important problem that remained following successful coronary thrombolysis was presence of high-grade residual coronary stenosis of the infarction-related artery (69). Significant residual coronary stenosis in the infarction-related artery might limit improvement in myocardial function. In addition, severe residual stenosis in the infarction-related artery was associated with a significant rate of reocclusion and reinfarction (74, 76-78). This prompted investigators to study the effects of PTCA on the infarction-related artery.

Coronary angioplasty could be used either as primary treatment for totally occluded infarction-related arteries (79-81) or in conjunction with thrombolytic agents (72, 75, 77, 79, 82, 83). If used in the latter situation, PTCA could be performed immediately after or during thrombolysis, or the procedure could be performed in a delayed, elective manner (74, 75). When PTCA was used as a primary treatment, marked improvement in luminal diameter was accompanied by significant improvement in left ventricular ejection fraction (80). In one study, when PTCA was compared directly with intracoronary streptokinase infusion, the rates of coronary recanalization were similar in both treatment groups, as were the times to achieve reperfusion. However, in patients treated with primary PTCA, the residual coronary stenosis was significantly less (43 ± 31%) than in the group treated with intracoronary streptokinase (83 ± 17%). Ventricular function was superior in the PTCA-treated patients. Serial left ventriculograms revealed that both the change in ejection fraction and regional wall motion at 7 to 10 days showed significantly greater improvement in the group treated with primary PTCA (Fig. 27.16).

If PTCA was used in conjunction with thrombolysis, the timing of PTCA remained an important concern. This issue was addressed in the Thrombolysis and Angioplasty in Myocardial Infarction trial (TAMI). The efficacy of immediate vs. delayed, elective PTCA after coronary thrombolysis with intravenous rtPA was compared. When a 5-hr infusion of rtPA was administered approximately 3 hr after symptom onset to 386 patients with acute evolving anterior wall myocardial infarction, the patency of the infarction-related artery was demonstrated in 288 patients (75%) at 90 min. One hundred and ninety-seven patients were randomized to either immediate angioplasty or delayed elective PTCA at 7 to 10 days. The 91 patients who could not be randomized were excluded because of the presence of predefined angiographic criteria, including the presence of a multivessel and left main coronary artery disease. Of the 197 randomized patients, 99 were assigned to immediate angioplasty, and 98 patients were assigned to delayed elective angioplasty. The rates of reocclusion were

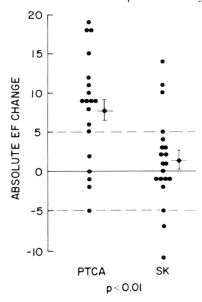

Figure 27.16. Comparative effects of intra-coronary streptokinase (*SK*) vs. primary coronary angioplasty (*PTCA*) on global left ventricular ejection fraction (*EF*) in patients with acute myocardial infarction. (From O'Neill W, Timmis GC, Bourdillon PD, et al. A prospective randomized clinical trial of intracoronary streptokinase versus coronary angioplasty for acute myocardial infarction. N Engl J Med 1986; 314:812–818.)

similar in both groups (11% vs. 13%), and neither group exhibited a significant improvement in global left ventricular function. The moderate improvement in regional wall motion was similar for both treatment groups. However, the rate of emergency coronary angioplasty because of recurrent ischemia or infarction was significantly higher for the patients assigned to the delayed PTCA strategy. The crossover rate for emergency PTCA was 16% for the delayed elective angioplasty group, while only 5% of the patients assigned to immediate PTCA required repeat emergency angioplasty (Table 27.1).

Of particular note was substantial reduction in stenosis severity in 14% of patients assigned to the elective delayed PTCA strategy; this was most likely due to continued clot lysis and obviated the need for angioplasty in this important subgroup. These findings, when taken together, suggest that one suitable treatment strategy for patients with evolving myocardial infarction might be early adminis-

tration of intravenous rtPA, continued heparinization, and delayed elective PTCA if needed. These patients would require close observation for signs of recurrent ischemia with the option for moving ahead with emergent revascularization if necessary.

Modes of Clinical Presentation

The invasive cardiologist may be asked to evaluate and treat patients who fall into several distinct clinical settings:
1. In the acute phase of evolving myocardial infarction;
2. In a stable state in the first week after the patient has received thrombolytic therapy;
3. During recurrent myocardial ischemia after thrombolytic treatment has already been administered.

Patients Presenting in the First 6 Hours of Acute Myocardial Infarction

A rapid and complete assessment of the hemodynamic status of such patients should be carried out. Critical historical elements include the patient's age, the time of onset of symptoms to presentation, and whether there is continued ischemic discomfort. The patient should be screened for specific contraindications to thrombolytic treatment (Table 27.2). In addition, we ascertain whether there is a prior history suggesting CAD, the duration of any prior angina symptoms, and whether prior coronary bypass surgery or angioplasty has been performed. On physical examination, the blood pressure, heart rate, and status of the neck veins are quickly assessed, as is the heart for the presence of any murmurs, gallops, or rubs. Of particular importance are the peripheral pulses, if urgent invasive procedures are contemplated.

The ECG is scrutinized for rhythm disturbances, repolarization abnormalities, and the status of the QRS complex. In addition to ST segment elevation, a common finding that may be present is the acute growth in R wave amplitude in the same leads that demonstrate ST segment elevation (76). The time course for R wave loss and the development of pathologic Q waves may be quite variable, and we do not consider the presence of Q waves per se as a contraindication for acute intervention. An additional important finding is the presence of persistent ST segment depression in the precordial leads, which is accompanied by chest

Table 27.1.
Clinical Outcome in the TAMI Trial: Immediate vs. Delayed Angioplasty [a]

Outcome	% of patients		
	Immediate PTCA (n = 99)	Elective PTCA (n = 98)	p
Death	4	1	0.37
Emergency CABG	7	2 [b]	0.17
Reocclusion	11	13	0.67
Emergency PTCA	5	16	0.01
CABG before day 7	4	2	0.68
CABG after day 7	4	11	0.07

[a] From Topol EJ, Califf RM, George BS, et al. A randomized trial of immediate versus delayed elective angioplasty after intravenous tissue plasminogen activator in acute myocardial infarction. N Engl J Med 1987;317:581-588.
[b] One patient who was assigned to receive elective PTCA required both emergency PTCA and emergency CABG.

Table 27.2.
Contraindications to Thrombolytic Therapy

History of coagulopathy or bleeding diathesis
Active peptic ulcer disease or internal bleeding
Prior cerebrovascular accident
Intracranial neoplasm
Severe uncontrolled hypertension
Recent surgery, invasive procedure, or trauma
Cardiopulmonary resuscitation
Pregnancy
Diabetic hemorrhagic retinopathy

pain of >30 min in duration. Since the majority of acute myocardial infarction interventional trials have required the presence of ST segment elevation, the distribution of the infarction-related arteries has been divided approximately equally between the left anterior descending and the right coronary arteries, which together account for 85 to 90% of cases. Recent evidence indicates that persistent ST depression in the precordial leads may also be a marker of acute posterior infarction due to circumflex coronary artery occlusion (11, 84). The decision to attempt reperfusion by urgent catheterization is made on the basis of a combination of clinical factors, including the duration of symptoms for <6 hr, persistent discomfort accompanied by continued injury current, and the hemodynamic status of the patient. We feel that the majority of patients with cardiogenic shock should undergo urgent catheterization.

If the decision is made to attempt coronary reperfusion, the choice must be quickly made among several treatment options:

1. The patient may be taken directly to the catheterization suite for diagnostic study and possible urgent revascularization.
2. Intravenous thrombolytic agents may be administered; the patient can then be admitted to the coronary care unit, and catheterization can be performed on an elective basis.
3. Intravenous thrombolytic agents can be administered, followed by a "period of observation" watching for clinical signs of reperfusion.
4. Intravenous thrombolytic agents may be administered and the patient taken for urgent catheterization to precisely define left ventricular function and coronary anatomy. Decisions regarding the method and timing of PTCA or CABG surgery are made on the basis of the catheterization findings.

We favor option 1 when catheterization facilities are available and specific contraindications to thrombolytic treatment exist. The decision as to whether to perform revascularization by PTCA or coronary bypass surgery is made on the basis of specific angiographic criteria. It should be pointed out that emergency PTCA in acute myocardial infarction may have certain advantages in properly equipped tertiary care facilities (see Chapter 5). For example, in a study performed by Rothbaum et al. (81), 151 patients with evolving acute myocardial infarction underwent emergency coronary angioplasty as primary treatment. PTCA was successful in 132 (87%) of patients. Following urgent PTCA, the mean residual stenosis severity was 29%, and the population included 18 patients with cardiogenic shock (12%). The in-hospital mortality for the entire group was 9%, with 7 of 13 deaths occurring in patients presenting with cardiogenic shock or intractable ventricular tachyarrhythmias. The hospital mortality was 5% in patients with successful angioplasty vs. 37% in those who had unsuccessful attempts.

Primary PTCA has the potential advantage of a lower incidence of generalized bleeding complications. In addition, primary PTCA may be associated with a lower incidence of intramyocardial hemorrhage compared with that associated with thrombolytic therapy(85).

Option 2 has been a routine strategy of many hospitals with active interventional programs. The reasons for this are severalfold. The information gained from urgent diagnostic catheterization is crucial to identify patients with persistent occlusion of the infarction-related artery. Since only 62 to 75% of patients receiving rtPA and a lesser percentage of those receiving streptokinase achieve reperfusion, a substantial number of patients have persistent occlusion of the infarction-related artery who could possibly benefit from salvage PTCA (Fig. 27.17). In addition, coronary angiography would identify those high-risk groups of patients who should be candidates for urgent CABG surgery. An additional factor favoring immediate angiography is that current noninvasive methods are relatively insensitive to assess reperfusion following thrombolytic therapy (86, 87). As has been pointed out by others, chest pain and ST segment changes accurately predict vessel patency in only 25% of patients and vessel occlusion in only 44% of patients (80).

Despite the potential advantages of urgent

catheterization, several recent prospective studies have failed to demonstrate definite overall clinical benefit for immediate coronary arteriography and angioplasty following intravenous thrombolysis. The Thrombolysis in Myocardial Infarction (TIMI) II A Study evaluated whether immediate cardiac catheterization with adjunctive PTCA confers an advantage over the same procedures performed electively 18 to 48 hours after admission (88). All patients were treated with intravenous rtPA within 4 hours of the onset of acute myocardial infarction. Of 195 patients randomized to the immediate intervention group, PTCA was attempted in 141 patients and was successful in 84%. Of 194 patients randomized to the delayed catheterization group, PTCA was attempted in 107 patients and was successful in 93%. There were no differences between the immediate and delayed intervention groups in predischarge left ventricular ejection fraction (50.3 vs. 49.0%) reinfarction (6.7 vs. 4.1%), or early mortality (7.2 vs. 5.7%). Immediate catheterization was associated with an increased frequency of both bleeding requiring transfusion (20.0 vs. 7.2%) and coronary artery bypass surgery (16.4 vs. 7.7%). The TAMI trial similarly reported an increased need for emergency bypass surgery in patients undergoing immediate rather than delayed angioplasty (74). The European Cooperative Study Group also failed to demonstrate any additional clinical benefit of immediate PTCA following intravenous rtPA administration (89). In this randomized trial of 367 patients with acute myocardial infarction treated with rtPA, 14-day mortality was higher in the group treated with immediate PTCA (7%) than in the group treated with a conservative, noninvasive strategy (3%). Based on the results of these studies, emergency coronary arteriography and angioplasty following intravenous thrombolytic therapy appear unwarranted as a routine measure and may be associated with a higher rate of complications. On the other hand, emergency interventional catheterization might be beneficial for certain patients (e.g., patients with extensive anterior infarction and/or acute cardiogenic shock), and the role of invasive therapies in the management of these high-risk subgroups requires further systematic evaluation. Patients with hemodynamic compromise and ongoing evidence of ischemia in particular may benefit from option 2, since it presents many important advantages in managing these critically ill patients: assessment of right heart hemodynamics, adjunctive support with intraaortic balloon counterpulsation, and use of salvage angioplasty in selected patients.

Option 3 seems somewhat problematic in that the various clinical markers of reperfusion (relief of chest pain, rapid devolution of ST segments, reperfusion arrhythmias) are too insensitive to accurately predict the status of the infarction-related artery (86, 87).

Option 4 seems most suitable for the community hospital setting when there is no immediate access to a catheterization facility. Thus, intravenous thrombolytic agents can be rapidly administered, and the patient can be transferred in an elective fashion for diagnostic catheterization and subsequent revascularization as necessary. Option 4 is also an appropriate strategy in centers with catheterization laboratories if the patient has no contraindication to thrombolytic therapy and if the hemodynamic status appears stable. When a conservative "wait-and-see" strategy is selected postthrombolysis, one should anticipate a 15 to 20% rate of intercurrent ischemic events necessitating emergency revascularization (74). The role of routine cardiac catheterization and elective angiography in the clinically stable patient who has received intravenous thrombolytic therapy remains controversial. There is general agreement that myocardial revascularization is indicated for patients with objective evidence of ischemia on the predischarge low-level stress test. In the absence of postinfarction angina or a positive predischarge stress test, the preliminary results of the TIMI II-B study indicate that cardiac catheterization and coronary angioplasty may not be necessary as a routine strategy (90).

Specific Approach to the Patient

After the diagnosis of acute myocardial infarction has been established, we administer intravenous rtPA in the emergency department according to recommended dosage schedules. The patient is taken to the catheterization suite, where a 7 Fr sheath is placed in the femoral vein, and a 9 Fr long sheath is placed in the femoral artery. A pacing catheter is placed in the right atrium or ventricle, and

the patient is given 5000 units of sodium heparin intravenously. Arterial pressure is constantly monitored through the sidearm of the arterial sheath. A pigtail catheter is then placed in the left ventricle, taking care to avoid ventricular irritability, which is more pronounced in this setting. Baseline hemodynamic data are recorded. Contrast left ventriculography is performed using nonionic contrast agents to help prevent hemodynamic compromise. We use biplane ventriculography with injection rates of 12 to 15 ml/sec for total volumes of 42 to 45 ml. We then perform selective cineangiography, visualizing the suspected noninfarction-related vessel first. This approach has the advantage of documenting the presence or absence of collateral flow to the infarction-related artery. We then perform the angiogram of the infarction-related vessel obtaining paired orthogonal views that best demonstrate the anatomy and the perfusion status of the infarction-related artery.

Angiographic Findings

If a patient is taken directly to the catheterization suite in the first 6 hr of acute myocardial infarction without prior administration of thrombolytic agents, the infarction-related artery will demonstrate total occlusion in approximately 90% of cases. Although coronary spasm may be associated with coronary occlusion in some individuals, intracoronary administration of nitroglycerin only occasionally restores antegrade flow. The ECG is carefully monitored for changes in the level of ST segment elevation and arrhythmias (we routinely monitor three ECG leads, two reflecting the infarction zone and the third the contralateral myocardial zone). Both a decrease in the ST segment and an abrupt increase in ST elevation have been described in conjunction with reperfusion (82). Dysrhythmias that occur include accelerated idioventricular rhythm (Fig. 27.18), ventricular tachycardia and fibrillation, sinus bradycardia and asystole. Moreover, hypotension during reperfusion of the inferoposterior left ventricular wall (Bezold-Jarisch reflex) may occur (91). At the time of these events we immediately repeated the angiogram to recheck the perfusion status of the infarction-related artery.

Perfusion status of the infarction-related artery is classified according to the TIMI criteria shown in Table 27.3. If TIMI grades 0 or 1

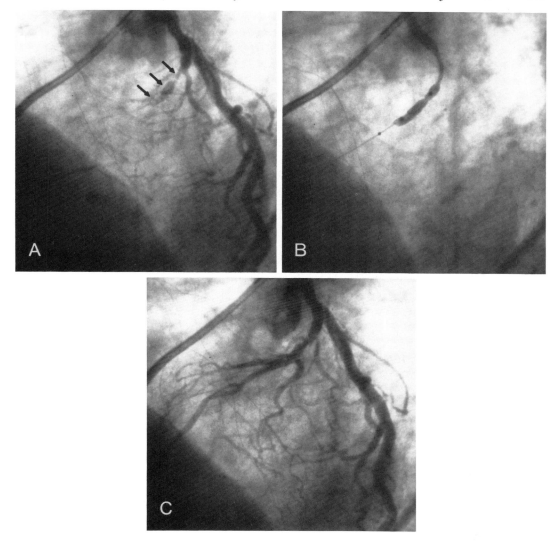

Figure 27.17. Salvage angioplasty following failed thrombolysis in a patient with acute anterior myocardial infarction. *A,* Persistent occlusion of the left anterior descending coronary artery is present (*arrows*) despite a 90-min infusion of intravenous rtPA. *B,* Balloon inflation in the totally occluded segment. *C,* Restoration of LAD patency and antegrade flow following angioplasty.

perfusion is present, the cardiologist should consider performing salvage PTCA in order to acutely restore antegrade flow (Fig. 27.17). In patients who exhibit grades 0 to 1 perfusion of the infarction-related artery and who have severe diffuse multivessel and/or left main coronary involvement, a strong case can be made for urgent CABG surgery. If TIMI grade 2 or 3 perfusion is demonstrated in the infarction-related artery in conjunction with a stenosis greater than 70% in severity, several treatment options exist: If patients have left main or triple-vessel disease, we recommend semiurgent bypass grafting. Usually this procedure can be delayed until the next day. If single-vessel or double-vessel disease is present with lesions deemed suitable for PTCA, urgent PTCA of the infarction-related artery may be undertaken (Fig. 27.19), or alternatively the catheterization procedure may be terminated and the patient may return to the coronary care unit with follow-up catheterization planned to reassess the status of the infarction-related artery several days

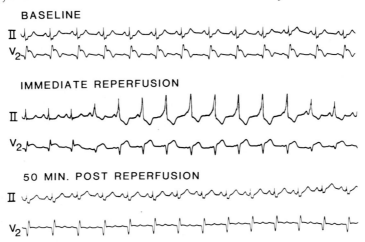

Figure 27.18. Reperfusion arrhythmias during thrombolytic treatment in a patient with evolving myocardial infarction. *Top,* Baseline ECG tracing showing ST elevation in lead V$_2$. *Middle,* The ECG following 7 min of streptokinase infusion showing accelerated idioventricular rhythm. *Lower,* The ECG 50 min after successful thrombolysis, showing resolution of the ST elevation and arrhythmia. (From Goldberg S, Greenspon AJ, Urban PL, et al. Reperfusion arrhythmia: a marker of restoration of antegrade flow during intracoronary thrombolysis for acute myocardial infarction. Am Heart J 1983;105:26-32.)

later. The former approach has the advantage of achieving a more complete revascularization at one sitting. The latter approach has the advantage of allowing for continued clot lysis, perhaps avoiding the need for PTCA, as occurs in 10 to 15% of patients. In addition, acute PTCA may be associated with greater vessel reactivity and a resultant increased need for emergency CABG. Mortality in patients subject to acute PTCA tended to be higher in the TAMI study (74).

PTCA Procedure

If the patient is a candidate for PTCA, the diagnostic catheter is exchanged for a suitable guide catheter, and an additional 5000 units of heparin are administered. A flexible guidewire is carefully passed through the occlusion. At this point it is not usual for the arrhythmias described above to occur, especially if patients have grade 0 or 1 perfusion prior to the attempted PTCA. The patient is stabilized, and the operator proceeds with the dilation. At this point, a vigorous guide catheter contrast injection is performed in an attempt to outline the course of the distal vessel. The balloon is then carefully placed in the occlusion or stenosis with the use of translesional pressure monitoring, if available. We perform the first inflation generally for 1 to 2

min, slowly increasing the pressure in the balloon until it is 1 to 2 atm above the popping pressure of the stenosis. After we deflate the balloon, we recheck the pressure gradient, and if this has been substantially reduced, we recheck flow and then perform a half exchange (i.e., the balloon dilation catheter is removed from the guide catheter while the guidewire (300 cm) is left in place in the distal infarction-related artery). The guide catheter injection is then repeated, which usually results in excellent visualization of the infarction-related artery. If a satisfactory hemodynamic and angiographic result is obtained, we observe the vessel for approximately 15 to 30 min, specifically watching for signs of abrupt reclosure. If this occurs, we recross the stenosis and repeat the inflation, attempting to perform prolonged inflations to enhance plaque molding and "tack down" intimal disruptions.

Patients Presenting in a Stable State after Administration of Thrombolytic Agents

With the increasingly widespread use of intravenous thrombolytic agents, a greater percentage of patients will be receiving these agents in the community setting. Subsequent transfer will then be undertaken so that diagnostic catheterization can be performed. The major-

Table 27.3.
Definitions of Perfusion Status Used in the TIMI Trial

Grade		Definition
0	No Perfusion:	There is no antegrade flow beyond the point of occlusion.
1	Penetration without perfusion:	Contrast material passes beyond area of obstruction but "hangs up" and fails to opacify entire coronary bed distal to obstruction for duration of cineangiographic filming sequence.
2	Partial perfusion:	Contrast material passes across obstruction and opacifies coronary bed distal to obstruction. However, rate of entry of contrast material into vessel distal to obstruction or its rate of clearance from distal bed (or both) are perceptibly slower than its entry into or clearance from comparable areas not perfused by previously occluded vessel, e.g., the opposite coronary artery or coronary bed proximal to obstruction.
3	Complete perfusion:	Antegrade flow into bed distal to obstruction occurs as promptly as antegrade flow into bed proximal to obstruction, and clearance of contrast material from the involved bed is as rapid as clearance from an uninvolved bed in same vessel or opposite artery.

ity of such patients will demonstrate pathologic Q waves, along with enzymatic evidence of myocardial necrosis. Historically, we attempt to ascertain information regarding chest pain, ST segment changes, and reperfusion arrhythmias in the perithrombolysis phase. In addition, we attempt to identify whether serial serum CK values reflect an early peak and washout (i.e., less than 16 hr after onset of symptoms) suggesting reperfusion.

The catheterization findings in these patients will most likely show an akinetic region of myocardium supplied by the infarction-related artery. The infarction-related artery may be totally occluded, or more likely it will be patent with a high-grade residual stenosis. Patients with left main and triple-vessel CAD should be referred for CABG surgery.

We generally perform PTCA on candidates with suitable angiographic anatomy, realizing that it is difficult to ascertain the amount of salvageable myocardium supplied by the infarction-related artery. At the time of PTCA, we note whether recurrent ischemia and ST segment change occur with balloon dilation. These findings may contribute important markers of myocardial salvage, although direct evidence for this hypothesis is currently lacking.

Patients Presenting with Recurrent Infarction

Patients recently treated with thrombolytic agents who do not undergo cardiac catheterization constitute a group at risk for reocclu-

sion and reinfarction (92). The rate of coronary reocclusion postadministration of thrombolytic agents varies between 10 to 40% (74, 76-78), with the majority of reocclusions occurring in the first 48 hr after treatment. Emergency PTCA (either with or without repeat infusion of rtPA) is generally undertaken in such patients. However, the prospect for myocardial salvage diminishes significantly once reinfarction has occurred. For this reason, patients receiving rtPA in the community hospital setting should generally be transferred within 24 to 48 hr to a center with the capability of providing timely diagnostic and therapeutic cardiac catheterization.

POSTINFARCTION ANGINA

General Considerations

The appearance of angina within the first few days or weeks after myocardial infarction is a disturbing occurrence and is common even in patients without prior thrombolytic treatment (93). Early postinfarction angina often heralds recurrent infarction and has been associated with a relatively grim prognosis. In one series of 70 consecutive patients with postinfarction angina, a 56% mortality was observed after a follow-up period of only 6 months (94). Patients with ECG evidence of ischemia at a distance from the initial infarct zone were at particularly high risk with a 6-month mortality of 72%, as compared with a 33% mortality in patients with recurrent ischemia in the infarct zone. Patients with early postinfarction angina, therefore, warrant an aggressive

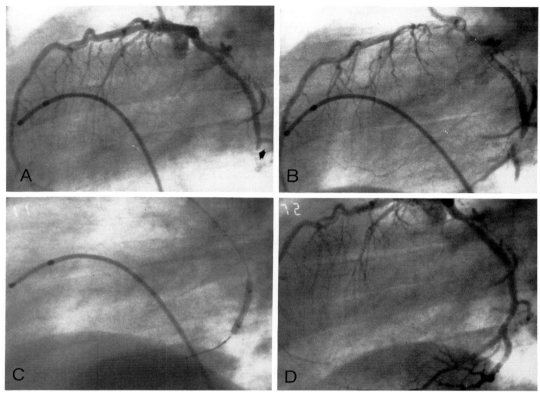

Figure 27.19. Sequential therapy with thrombolysis and PTCA for acute inferior myocardial infarction. A, Complete occlusion (*arrow*) of the left circumflex coronary artery (TIMI grade 0 perfusion). B, Improvement in antegrade perfusion (TIMI grade 2) following intravenous rtPA infusion. C and D, Reduction of residual high-grade left circumflex stenosis following PTCA with further improvement in perfusion (TIMI grade 3).

management approach with cardiac catheterization to identify potential candidates for percutaneous or surgical revascularization. Patients with subendocardial or non Q-wave infarction are especially likely to experience recurrent ischemia during the in-hospital period. Reinfarction occurred in 43% of 58 patients with non Q-wave infarction carefully studied by Marmor et al. (93). Non Q-wave myocardial infarction is a strong indication for cardiac catheterization predischarge. Given the high risk associated with this patient subset, we advocate the use of early interventional catheterization on a preemptive basis prior to recurrent angina and infarction.

Catheterization Laboratory

Coronary angiography in patients with early postinfarction angina due to ischemia within the infarction zone typically reveals a high-grade but nontotally occluded culprit lesion in the infarction-related artery (95). Total occlusion of the infarction vessel is a less common finding and, when present, usually is associated with collateral flow that allows for preserved myocardial viability within the infarction area. Because of the relatively high incidence of single-vessel disease in this setting, recurrent ischemia in the infarction zone can be frequently managed with PTCA. DeFeyter et al. reported a success rate of 89% in 53 patients with postinfarction angina treated by angioplasty (96). However, PTCA was complicated by an 11% rate of myocardial infarction and/or emergency bypass surgery. We have also reported the effective use of PTCA on the infarction-related artery in 54 patients with ischemia in the zone of prior infarction (91). PTCA was successful in 94% (33/35) of critical stenoses and in 58% (11/19) of total occlusions. Two patients (4%) required emergency surgery, but there were no new infarctions or deaths. After approximately 1 year of follow-up, there was only one reinfarction, and there were no deaths. Thus, PTCA was associated with an excellent long-term outcome in this unstable group of patients.

In patients with postinfarction angina due to ischemia at a distance, coronary angiography invariably reveals multivessel disease. Typically, the infarction-related artery is totally occluded while one or more contralateral vessels demonstrate a critical stenosis jeopardizing noninfarcted regions of myocardium. Early postinfarction ischemia at a distance from the infarction zone has been attributed to interruption of collateral flow from the occluded infarction-related artery to the territory of another diseased vessel (94). Unstable angina with ischemia at a distance may also emerge, after a clinically stable interval of several months or years following the initial infarction, due to interim progression of disease. PTCA of vessels contralateral to the infarcted region will be undertaken at potentially increased risk to the patient. In the presence of a prior infarction, abrupt closure of a contralateral vessel may result in severe left ventricular dysfunction and hemodynamic decompensation (97). Accordingly, most patients with postinfarction ischemia at a distance are best treated with coronary bypass surgery. However, our experience has demonstrated that with careful case selection, coronary angioplasty offers an effective therapeutic option for many of these patients (98). Selection criteria for use of angioplasty in this high risk population have been reviewed in detail elsewhere (99). These considerations include the likelihood of primary successful dilation based on lesion morphology, the expected outcome with alternative therapies, the total area of myocardium potentially at risk, and the capability of protecting ischemic myocardium potentially at risk and of protecting ischemic myocardium with intraaortic balloon counterpulsation. The status of collateral circulation is also an important consideration. If a stenosed contralateral vessel supplies collateral flow to the infarction-related vessel, initial dilation of the infarction-related artery should be performed first in order to reciprocally provide collateral protection during subsequent angioplasty of the contralateral vessel. Widespread application of PTCA in patients

with left ventricular dysfunction is currently restrained by the potential for unresolved vessel closure and by a limited ability to protect the acutely ischemic myocardium. Future technical innovations with the capability of better protecting the ischemic heart will further expand the use of interventional catheter techniques in high-risk patients with these acute coronary syndromes (100).

SUMMARY

In summary, cardiac catheterization plays an increasingly important role in the management of patients with unstable ischemic syndromes. This application has contributed to major advances in the diagnosis and treatment of these patients.

References

1. Gorlin R, Fuster V, Ambrose JA. Anatomic–physiologic links between acute coronary syndromes. Circulation 1986;74:6–9.
2. Scanlon PH. The intermediate coronary syndrome. Prog Cardiovasc Dis 1981;23:351–364.
3. Wood P. Acute and subacute coronary insufficiency. Br Med J 1961;1:1779–1782.
4. Conti CR, Brawley RK, Griffith LSC, et al. Unstable angina pectoris: morbidity and mortality in 57 consecutive patients evaluated angiographically. Am J Cardiol 1973;32:745–750.
5. Bertolasi CA, Tronge JE, Riccitelli MA, et al. Natural history of unstable angina with medical or surgical therapy. Chest 1976;70:596–605.
6. Sharma GVRK, Deupree R, Olson H, et al. Can the high risk unstable angina patient be identified? (abstr). J Am Coll Cardiol 1986;7:32A.
7. Gazes PC, Mobley ME, Faris HM, Duncan RC, Humphries GB. Preinfarctional (unstable) angina—a prospective study—ten year follow-up. Circulation 1973;48:331–337.
8. Russell RO, Moraski RE, Kouchoukos N, et al. Unstable angina pectoris: national cooperative study group to compare surgical and medical therapy. Am J Cardiol 1978;42:839–848.
9. Plotnick GD, Conti CR. Transient ST segment elevation in unstable angina: prognostic significance. Am J Med 1979;67:800–803.
10. Papapietro SE, Niess GS, Paine TD, et al. Transient electro-cardiographic changes in patients with unstable angina: relation to coronary arterial anatomy. Am J Cardiol 1980;46:28–33.
11. Berry C, Zalewski A, Savage M, et al. Is acute transmural ischemia always manifested by ST segment elevation? (abstr). Circulation 1987;76:IV123.
12. Nademanee K, Intarachot V, Josephson MA, Rieders D, Mody FV, Singh BN. Prognostic significance of silent myocardial ischemia in patients with unstable angina. J Am Coll Cardiol 1987;10:1–9.

13. Gottlieb SO, Weisfeldt ML, Ouyang P, Mellits D, Gerstenblith G. Silent ischemia predicts infarction and death during 2 year follow–up of unstable angina. J Am Coll Cardiol 1987;10:756–760.

14. Telford AM, Wilson C. Trial of heparin versus atenolol in prevention of myocardial infarction in intermediate coronary syndrome. Lancet 1981;1:1225–1228

15. Lewis HD, Davis JW, Archibald DG, et al. Protective effects of aspirin against acute myocardial infarction and death in men with unstable angina. Results of a Veterans Administration cooperative study. N Engl J Med 1983;309:396–403.

16. Cairns JA, Gent M, Singer J, et al. Aspirin, sulfinpyrazone, or both in unstable angina. Results of a Canadian multicenter trial. N Engl J Med 1985;313:1369–1375.

17. Theroux P, Ouimet H, McCans J, et al. Aspirin, heparin, or both to treat acute unstable angina. N Engl J Med 1988;319:1105–1111.

18. Luchi RJ, Scott SM, Deupree RH, and the Principal Investigators and Their Associates of Veterans Administration Cooperative Study No. 28. Comparison of medical and surgical treatment for unstable angina pectoris. Results of a Veterans Administration cooperative study. N Engl J Med 1987;316:977–984.

19. Buxton A, Goldberg S, Hirshfeld JW, et al. Refractory ergonovine–induced coronary vasospasm: importance of intracoronary nitroglycerin. Am J Cardiol 1980;46:329–334.

20. Gertz EW, Wisneski JA, Chiu D, Akin JR, Hu C. Clinical superiority of a new nonionic contrast agent (iopamidol) for cardiac angiography. J Am Coll Cardiol 1985;5:250–258.

21. Davis K, Kennedy JW, Kemp HG, Judkins MP, Gosselin AJ, Killip T. Complications of coronary arteriography from the Collaborative Study of Coronary Artery Surgery (CASS). Circulation 1979;59:1105–1112.

22. Plotnick GD, Greene HL, Carliner NH, Becker LC, Fisher ML. Clinical indicators of left main coronary artery disease in unstable angina. Ann Intern Med 1979;91:149–153.

23. Rutherford JD, Braunwald E, Cohn PF. Chronic ischemic heart disease. In: Braunwald E, ed. Heart disease. 3rd ed. Philadelphia: WB Saunders, 1988:1314–1378.

24. Victor MF, Likoff MJ, Mintz GS, Likoff W. Unstable angina pectoris of new onset: a prospective clinical and arteriographic study of 75 patients. Am J Cardiol 1981;47:228–232.

25. Alison HW, Russell RO, Mantle JA, Kouchoukos NT, Moraski RE, Rackley CE. Coronary anatomy and arteriography in patients with unstable angina pectoris. Am J Cardiol 1978;48:204–209.

26. Plotnick GD, Fisher ML, Carliner NH, Becker LC. Cardiac catheterization in patients with unstable angina: recent onset vs. crescendo pattern. JAMA 1980;244:574–576.

27. Corcos T, David PR, Bourassa MG, et al. Percutaneous transluminal coronary angioplasty for the treatment of variant angina. J Am Coll Cardiol 1985;5:1046–1054.

28. Bott–Silverman C, Heupler FA, Yiannikas J. Variant angina: comparison of patients with and without fixed severe coronary artery disease. Am J Cardiol 1984;54:1173–1175.

29. Moise A, Theroux P, Taeymans Y, et al. Unstable angina and progression of coronary atherosclerosis. N Engl J Med 1983;309:685–689.

30. Ambrose JA, Hjemdahl–Monsen CE. Arteriographic anatomy and mechanisms of myocardial ischemia in unstable angina. J Am Coll Cardiol 1987;9:1397–1402.

31. Forrester JS, Litvack F, Grundfest W, Hickey A. A perspective of coronary disease seen through the arteries of living man. Circulation 1987;75:505–513.

32. Goldberg S. Coronary artery spasm and thrombosis. Philadelphia: FA Davis, 1983.

33. Ambrose JA, Winters SL, Stern A, et al. Angiographic morphology and the pathogenesis of unstable angina pectoris. J Am Coll Cardiol 1985;5:609–616.

34. Levin DC, Fallon JT. Significance of the angiographic morphology of localized coronary stenoses: histopathologic correlations. Circulation 1982;66:316–320.

35. Rafflenbeul W, Smith LR, Rogers WJ, Mantle JA, Rackley CE, Russell RO. Quantitative coronary arteriography: coronary anatomy of patients with unstable angina pectoris reexamined 1 year after optimal medical therapy. Am J Cardiol 1979;43:699–707.

36. Neill WA, Wharton TP, Fluri–Lundeen J, Cohen IS. Acute coronary insufficiency: coronary occlusion after intermittent ischemic attacks. N Engl J Med 1980;302:1157–1162.

37. de Feyter PJ, Serruys PW, Suryapranata H, Beatt K, van den Brand M. Coronary angioplasty early after diagnosis of unstable angina. Am Heart J 1987;114:48–54.

38. Faxon DP, Detre KM, McCabe CH, et al. Role of percutaneous transluminal coronary angioplasty in the treatment of unstable angina: report from the National Heart, Lung, and Blood Institute Percutaneous Transluminal Coronary Angioplasty and Coronary Artery Surgery Study Registries. Am J Cardiol 1983;53:131C–135C.

39. de Feyter PJ, Serruys PW, van den Brand, et al. Emergency coronary angioplasty in refractory unstable angina. N Engl J Med 1985;313:342–346.

40. Wohlgelernter D, Cleman M, Highman HA, Zaret BL. Percutaneous transluminal coronary angioplasty of the "culprit lesion" for management of unstable angina pectoris in patients with multivessel coronary artery disease. Am J Cardiol 1986;58:460–464.

41. de Feyter PJ, Serruys PW, Arnold A, et al. Coronary angioplasty of the unstable angina–related vessel in patients with multivessel disease. Eur Heart J 1986;7:460–467.

42. Slysh S, Goldberg S, Dervan JP, Zalewski A. Unstable angina and evolving myocardial infarction following coronary bypass surgery: pathogenesis and treatment with interventional catheterization. Am Heart J 1985;109:744–752.

43. Vetrovec GW, Cowley MJ, Overton H, Richardson DW. Intracoronary thrombus in syndromes of unstable myocardial ischemia. Am Heart J 1981;102:1202–1208.

44. Bresnahan DR, Davis JL, Holmes DR, Smith HC. Angiographic occurrence and clinical correlates of intraluminal coronary artery thrombus: role of unstable angina. J Am Coll Cardiol 1985;6:285–289.
45. Capone G, Wolf NM, Meyer B, Meister SG. Frequency of intracoronary filling defects by angiography in angina pectoris at rest. Am J Cardiol 1985;56:403–406.
46. Sherman CT, Litvack F, Grundfest W, et al. Coronary angioscopy in patients with unstable angina pectoris. N Engl J Med 1986;315:913–919.
47. Savage M, Goldberg S, Hirshfeld J, et al. for the M–HEART Study Group. Determinants of primary angioplasty success: a report from the Multihospital Atlantic Restenosis Trial (M–HEART) (abstr). Cathet Cardiovasc Diagn, in press, 1989.
48. Mabin TA, Holmes DR, Smith HC, et al. Intracoronary thrombus: role in coronary occlusion complicating percutaneous transluminal coronary angioplasty. J Am Coll Cardiol 1985;5:198–202.
49. Lukas MA, Deutsch E, Laskey WK. Beneficial effect of heparin on PTCA outcome in unstable angina (abstr). J Am Coll Cardiol 1988;11:132A.
50. Vetrovec GW, Leinbach RC, Gold HK, Cowley MJ. Intracoronary thrombolysis in syndromes of unstable ischemia: angiographic and clinical results. Am Heart J 1982;104:946–952.
51. Ambrose JA, Hjemdah–Monsen C, Borrico S, et al. Quantitative and qualitative effects of intracoronary streptokinase in unstable angina and non–Q wave infarction. J Am Coll Cardiol 1987;9:1156–1165.
52. Gold HK, Johns JA, Leinbach RC, et al. A randomized, blinded, placebo–controlled trial of recombinant human tissue–type plasminogen activator in patients with unstable angina pectoris. Circulation 1987;75:1192–1199.
53. Herrick JB. Clinical features of sudden obstruction of the coronary arteries. JAMA 1912;59:2015–2020.
54. DeWood MA, Spores J, Notske R, et al. Prevalence of total coronary occlusion during the early hours of transmural myocardial infarction. N Engl J Med 1980;303:897–902.
55. Rentrop KP, Blanke H, Karoch KR, Kaiser H, Kostering H, Leitz K. Selective intracoronary thrombolysis in acute myocardial infarction and unstable angina pectoris. Circulation 1981;63:307–317.
56. Mathey DG, Kuck KH, Tilsner V, Krebber HJ, Bleifeld W. Nonsurgical coronary artery recanalization in acute transmural myocardial infarction. Circulation 1981;63:489–497.
57. Ganz W, Ninomiya K, Hashida J, et al. Intracoronary thrombolysis in acute myocardial infarction: experimental background and clinical experience. Am Heart J 1981;102:1145–1149.
58. Anderson JL, Marshall HW, Bray BE, et al. A randomized trial of intra–coronary streptokinase in the treatment of acute myocardial infarction. N Engl J Med 1983;308:1312–1318.
59. Kennedy JW, Ritchie JL, Davis KB, Fritz JK. Western Washington randomized trial of intracoronary streptokinase in acute myocardial infarction. N Engl J Med 1983;309:1477–1482.
60. Khaja F, Walton JA, Brymer JF, et al. Intracoronary fibrinolytic therapy on acute myocardial infarction. N Engl J Med 1983;308:1305–1311.
61. Rentrop KP, Feit F, Blanke H, et al. Effects of intracoronary streptokinase and intracoronary nitroglycerin infusion on coronary angiographic patterns and mortality in patients with acute myocardial infarction. N Engl J Med 1984;311:1457–1463.
62. Simoons ML, van de Brand M, DeZwaans C, et al. Improved survival after early thrombolysis in acute myocardial infarction. Lancet 1985;2:578–581.
63. Raizner AE, Tortoledo FA, Verani MS, et al. Intracoronary thrombolytic therapy in acute myocardial infarction: a prospective, randomized, controlled trial. Am J Cardiol 1985;55:301–308.
64. Kennedy JW, Gensini GG, Timmis GC, Maynard C. Acute myocardial infarction treated with intracoronary streptokinase: a report of the Society for Cardiac Angiography. Am J Cardiol 1985;55:871–877.
65. Weinstein J. Treatment of myocardial infarction with intracoronary streptokinase: efficacy and safety data from 209 United States cases in the Hoechst–Roussel registry. Am Heart J 1982;104:894–898.
66. Kennedy JW, Ritchie JL, Davis KB, Stadius ML, Maynard C, Fritz J. Western Washington intracoronary streptokinase trial follow–up. N Engl J Med 1985;312:1073–1078.
67. Verstraete M, Bory M, Collen D, et al. Randomized trial of intravenous recombinant tissue–type plasminogen activator versus intravenous streptokinase myocardial infarction. Lancet 1985; 1:842–847.
68. Sheehan FH, Braunwald E, Canner P, et al. The effect of intravenous thrombolytic therapy on left ventricular function: a report on tissue–type plasminogen activator and streptokinase from thrombolysis in myocardial infarction (TIMI Phase I) trial. Circulation 1987;75:817–829.
69. White HD, Norris RM, Bown MA, et al. Effect of intravenous streptokinase on left ventricular function and early survival after acute myocardial infarction. N Engl J Med 1987;317:850–855.
70. I.S.A.M. Study Group. A prospective trial of intravenous streptokinase in acute myocardial infarction (I.S.A.M.) N Engl J Med 1986;314:1465–1471.
71. Kennedy JW. Streptokinase for the treatment of acute myocardial infarction: a brief review of randomized trials. J Am Coll Cardiol 1987;5:28B–32B.
72. Gruppo Italiano Per Lo Studio Della Streptochinasi Nell' Infarto Miocardico (GISSI). Effectiveness of intravenous thrombolytic treatment in acute myocardial infarction. Lancet 1986;1:397–401.
73. ISIS-2 (Second International Study of Infarct Survival) Collaborative Group. Randomized trial of intravenous streptokinase, oral aspirin, or both or neither among 17,187 cases of suspected acute myocardial infarction. Lancet 1988;2:545–549.
74. Topol EJ, Califf RM, George BS, et al. A randomized trial of immediate versus delayed elective angioplasty after intravenous tissue plasminogen activator in acute myocardial infarction. N Engl J Med 1987;317:581–588.
75. Guerci AD, Gerstenblith G, Brinker JA, et al. A randomized trial of intra–venous tissue plasminogen activator for acute myocardial infarction with

subsequent randomization to elective coronary angioplasty. N Engl J Med 1987;317:1613–1618.

76. Gold HK, Leinbach RC, Garabedian HD, et al. Acute coronary reocclusion after thrombolysis with recombinant human tissue–type plasminogen activator: prevention by a maintenance infusion. Circulation 1986;73:347–352.

77. Chesebro JH, Knatterud G, Roberts R, et al. Thrombolysis in myocardial infarction (TIMI) trial. Phase I. A comparison between intravenous tissue plasminogen activator and intravenous streptokinase. Circulation 1987;76:142–154.

78. Topol EJ, O'Neill WW, Langburd AB, et al. A randomized, placebo–controlled trial of intravenous recombinant tissue–type plasminogen activator and emergency coronary angioplasty in patients with acute myocardial infarction. Circulation 1987;75:420–428.

79. Hartzler GO, Rutherford BD, McConahay DR, et al. Percutaneous transluminal coronary angioplasty with and without thrombolytic therapy for treatment of acute myocardial infarction. Am Heart J 1983:106:965–973.

80. O'Neill W, Timmis GC, Bourdillon PD, et al. A prospective randomized clinical trial of intracoronary streptokinase versus coronary angioplasty for acute myocardial infarction. N Engl J Med 1986;314:812–818.

81. Rothbaum DA, Linnemeier TJ, Landin RJ, et al. Emergency percutaneous transluminal coronary angioplasty in acute myocardial infarction: a 3 year experience. J Am Coll Cardiol 1987;10:264–272.

82. Meyer J, Merx W, Schmitz H, et al. Percutaneous transluminal coronary angioplasty immediately after intracoronary streptolysis of transmural myocardial infarction. Circulation 1982;66:905–913.

83. Serruys PW, Wijns W, van den Brand M, et al. Is transluminal coronary angioplasty mandatory after successful thrombolysis? Br Heart J 1983;50:257–265.

84. Boden WE, Kleiger RE, Gibson RS, et al. Electrocardiographic evolution of posterior acute myocardial infarction: importance of early precordial ST–segment depression. Am J Cardiol 1987;59:782–787.

85. Waller BF, Rothbaum DA, Pinkerton CA, et al. Status of the myocardium and infarct–related coronary artery in 19 necropsy patients with acute recanalization using pharmacologic (streptokinase, r–tissue plasminogen activator), mechanical (percutaneous transluminal coronary angioplasty) or combined types of reperfusion therapy. J Am Coll Cardiol 1987;9:785–801.

86. Miller FC, Krucoff MW, Satler LF, et al. Ventricular arrhythmias during reperfusion. Am Heart J 1986;112:928–931.

87. Califf RM, O'Neill WW, Stack RS, et al. Failure of simple clinical measurements to predict perfusion status after intravenous thrombolysis. Ann Intern Med 1988;108:658–662.

88. The TIMI Research Group. Immediate vs delayed catheterization and angioplasty following thrombolytic therapy for acute myocardial infarction: TIMI II A results. JAMA 1988;260:2849–2858.

89. Simoons ML, Betriu A, Col J, et al. (for The European Cooperative Study Group for Recombinant Tissue-Type Plasminogen Activator [rtPA]). Thrombolysis with tissue plasminogen activator in acute myocardial infarction: No additional benefit from immediate percutaneous coronary angioplasty. Lancet 1988;1:197–202.

90. Braunwald E. Comparison of invasive and conservative strategies following intravenous tissue plasminogen activator in acute myocardial infarction: results of the thrombolysis in myocardial infarction trial by the TIMI Study Group. N Engl J Med 1989, (in press).

91. Goldberg S, Greenspon AJ, Urban PL, et al. Reperfusion arrhythmia: a marker of restoration of antegrade flow during intracoronary thrombolysis for acute myocardial infarction. Am Heart J 1983;105:26–32.

92. Schroder R, Neuhaus KL, Leizorovicz A, Linderer T, Tebbe U for the ISAM Study Group. A prospective placebo controlled double–blind multicenter trial of intravenous streptokinase in acute myocardial infarction (ISAM): long–term mortality and morbidity. J Am Coll Cardiol 1987;9:197–203.

93. Marmor A, Sobel BE, Roberts R. Factors presaging early recurrent myocardial infarction ("extension"). Am J Cardiol 1981;48:603–610.

94. Schuster EH, Bulkley BH. Early post–infarction angina. Ischemia at a distance and ischemia in the infarct zone. N Engl J Med 1981;305:1101–1105.

95. Hopkins J, Savage M, Zalewski A, Dervan JP, Goldberg S. Recurrent ischemia in the zone of prior myocardial infarction: results of coronary angioplasty of the infarct–related artery. Am Heart J 1988;115:14–19.

96. DeFeyter PJ, Serruys PW, Soward A, Van Den Brand M, Bos E, Hugenholtz PG. Coronary angioplasty for early postinfarction unstable angina. Circulation 1986;74:1365–1370.

97. Murphy DA, Craver JM, Jones EL, King SB, Curling PE, Douglas JS. Hemodynamic deterioration after coronary angioplasty in the presence of previous left ventricular infarction. Am J Cardiol 1984;54:448–450.

98. Savage MP, Dervan JP, Zalewski A, Hopkins J, Goldberg S. Percutaneous transluminal coronary angioplasty in patients with prior myocardial infarction: angioplasty at a distance from the prior infarct zone. Am Heart J 1987;114:1102–1110.

99. Savage M, Goldberg S. Coronary angioplasty in the high risk patient. In: Goldberg S, ed. Cardiovascular Clinics: Coronary angioplasty. Philadephia: FA Davis, 1988.

100. Zalewski A, Savage M, Goldberg S. Protection of the ischemic myocardium during percutaneous transluminal coronary angioplasty. Am J Cardiol 1988;61:54G–60G.

28

The Patient with Valvular Heart Disease

Michael E. Assey, M.D.
Bruce W. Usher, M.D.
Blase A. Carabello, M.D.
James F. Spann, Jr., M.D.

INTRODUCTION

For most symptomatic patients with valvular heart disease, cardiac catheterization is critical in clinical decision-making. At catheterization, the primary valve lesion is confirmed and quantified, other valve lesions and important changes in the pulmonary vasculature are defined, associated coronary artery disease is demonstrated, and left ventricular function is evaluated. Proper patient management requires an understanding of the pathophysiology and natural history of valvular heart disease and the integration of data generated from noninvasive techniques as well as the cardiac catheterization.

When the history and physical examination suggest valvular heart disease, the physician must make several decisions. Establishing the proper etiology is important in advising as to the need for bacterial endocarditis or antistreptococcal prophylaxis, as well as the need for cardiac catheterization. Answers to such questions are greatly facilitated by current noninvasive techniques including standard echocardiography, combined Doppler echocardiography, Doppler color flow imaging, and radionuclide studies. These techniques are helpful in confirming the suspected diagnosis, establishing etiology in many instances and allowing repetitive evaluations of cardiac chamber size, wall thickness,

valve area, and ventricular function (Table 28.1).

When the decision to proceed with cardiac catheterization is made, the noninvasive evaluation provides the catheterizing physician with valuable information prior to the procedure. This knowledge can reduce radiation exposure and decrease the volume of contrast material administered, which is particularly important in patients with renal insufficiency or decompensated congestive heart failure.

Throughout this chapter, the complementary nature of certain noninvasive techniques and cardiac catheterization is emphasized, providing a realistic and optimal approach to patient management. For each valvular lesion, a similar format is followed. Initially, there is a brief discussion of etiology, clinical presentation, and pathophysiology. Following this, a precatheterization noninvasive assessment is presented, emphasizing information that is helpful in deciding when to proceed with cardiac catheterization. The typical catheterization findings are then presented, with a discussion as to how these data are used in clinical decision-making. All of these data are then integrated and synthesized, culminating in specific recommendations. Approaching the various valvular lesions in isolation may provide clarity at the expense of realism, since combined valvular lesions are often the most problematic for the practitioner. Accordingly, a

Table 28.1.
Role of Echo-Doppler in the Assessment of
Valvular Heart Disease

Diagnosis
Etiology
Chamber size
Ventricular ejection fraction
Ventricular hypertrophy
Estimate pressure gradients across stenotic
   valves
Estimate valve areas (aortic, mitral, pulmonic)
Estimate intracardiac pressures
   LVEDP[a] in aortic insufficiency
   RV peak systolic pressure in tricuspid
      insufficiency

---

[a] LVEDP, left ventricular end-diastolic pressure;
   RV, right ventricular.

discussion of some of the commonly occurring combined lesions is included at appropriate points in the chapter.

AORTIC STENOSIS

Clinical Presentation and Pathophysiology

Obstruction to left ventricular outflow may be supravalvular, valvular, or subvalvular. Valvular aortic stenosis may be acquired or congenital. The congenitally bicuspid aortic valve is found in up to 2% of all adults, with half of these showing some degree of aortic stenosis by age 50 (1, 2). Rheumatic aortic stenosis, characterized by commissural fusion, is often associated with some degree of aortic insufficiency and usually involves the mitral valve as well. In the degenerative form of acquired aortic stenosis, years of wear on an anatomically normal valve result in fibrosis and immobility of the leaflets. Calcium deposition occurs at the bases of the cusps, but the commissures are spared. This type of aortic stenosis, frequent in the elderly, is not usually associated with significant aortic insufficiency, unless bacterial endocarditis supervenes. Thus, it is particularly amenable to valvuloplasty. It may also be associated with conduction abnormalities, calcification of the mitral annulus, and coronary artery calcification.

The fixed obstruction to left ventricular outflow resulting from valvular aortic stenosis increases left ventricular systolic wall stress

causing parallel replication of sarcomeres and concentric left ventricular hypertrophy (3). When such a pressure overload develops gradually, the hypertrophy can provide adequate compensation that maintains left ventricular ejection performance (4). Ejection fraction in adults with compensated aortic stenosis is usually normal or only slightly depressed (5, 6). In congenital aortic stenosis, the hypertrophy, and perhaps hyperplasia as well, result in supernormal cardiac ejection parameters (7, 8). Left ventricular hypertrophy, however, often leads to abnormal diastolic stiffness (9, 10). As a result, left ventricular diastolic filling pressures are usually elevated even in compensated aortic stenosis. Some chamber stiffness may be secondary to myocardial ischemia. Both chamber stiffness and hypertrophy regress following removal of the pressure overload (11, 12).

In each of the three common forms of acquired aortic valve stenosis, a long latency period is observed prior to the onset of symptoms. Symptoms include those related to congestive heart failure, angina pectoris, and syncope. These generally occur when the valve is narrowed to an area of 0.7 cm^2 or less, although symptoms may occur in patients with somewhat larger valve areas when other valve lesions or coronary artery disease are present (13–15). The development of symptoms is an extremely important point in the natural history of valvular aortic stenosis. Mortality may reach 50% in the ensuing 4 years, with a particularly poor prognosis for those patients with symptoms of congestive heart failure (16, 17). Patients with aortic stenosis and left ventricular failure are characterized by dilation and reduced shortening of that chamber. However, this abnormal hemodynamic pattern may be entirely due to "afterload mismatch" and not represent depressed myocardial contractility (18). On the other hand, Spann and colleagues found that for any level of afterload (stress), patients with aortic stenosis and congestive heart failure had underlying contractile impairment (6). Ejection fraction has been shown to return to normal following aortic valve replacement even in the face of severely depressed preoperative ejection fraction (12, 19). Thus, no symptomatic patient is denied catheterization and treatment (valve replacement or valvuloplasty) because of a low ejection fraction, although surgical risk increases significantly as the ejection fraction falls. Because left ventricular ejection fraction generally improves following valve replacement or valvuloplasty for aortic stenosis, asymptomatic patients are not usually treated in hopes of preventing irreversible left ventricular dysfunction. The management of the asymptomatic patient with aortic stenosis is discussed below.

Precardiac Catheterization Noninvasive Assessment

Patients with left ventricular outflow murmurs, particularly those with systemic hypertension and resulting left ventricular hypertrophy on electrocardiogram, are frequently sent to the noninvasive laboratory to exclude or confirm the presence of left ventricular outflow tract obstruction. Doppler echocardiography is utilized to localize the obstruction to subvalvular, valvular, or supravalvular, and to quantitate the severity. Abnormalities of the aortic valve, such as aortic sclerosis, calcific aortic stenosis, and congenital aortic stenosis (Fig. 28.1), can usually be differentiated from the normal aortic valve by two-dimensional echocardiography. This information is important in deciding when a patient with an outflow murmur needs bacterial endocarditis prophylaxis.

Doppler echocardiography represents a major advance in assessing the severity of the aortic valve gradient as well as detecting concomitant mitral, pulmonic, and tricuspid involvement. Several studies have demonstrated a good correlation between transvalvular gradient measured at cardiac catheterization and the estimated gradient calculated in the noninvasive laboratory by Doppler technique utilizing the modified Bernoulli equation (20, 21). In our laboratory, we found a fair correlation ($r = 0.86$) between the peak-to-peak gradient obtained at catheterization and the Doppler-derived gradient (Fig. 28.2). One should not really expect the cardiac catheterization **peak-to-peak** systolic pressure gradient to be the same as the **peak instantaneous** gradient derived from Doppler echocardiography. As illustrated in Figure 28.3, there is a clear temporal inequality between peak left ventricular and peak aortic pressure.

It should be noted that the Doppler-derived gradient represents the peak instantaneous gradient calculated from the peak instantaneous blood flow velocity across the valve. When we compared the peak instantaneous gradient obtained at catheterization, using high-fidelity micromanometer catheters, with the peak instantaneous Doppler gradient, an excellent correlation was found (Fig. 28.4). In reality, instantaneous gradients are not routinely assessed in most catheterization laboratories, and therefore the Doppler-derived gradient may be significantly higher than the gradient reported from the catheterization laboratory, particularly when peak-to-peak gradient is estimated by superimposing temporally disparate events. However, the mean Doppler gradient is comparable to the mean planimetered gradient determined at catheterization. Thus, we primarily rely on the mean Doppler gradient in our noninvasive assessment of aortic stenosis severity.

Since the pressure gradient is flow-dependent, the severity of aortic stenosis is optimally determined by measurement of valve area (see Chapter 23). Aortic valve area can be estimated noninvasively by combining Doppler and imaging echocardiographic techniques utilizing the continuity equation (22). This technique is particularly valuable in assessing the potential significance of aortic stenosis when the transvalvular mean Doppler gradient is less than 50 mm Hg or when the patient has associated aortic insufficiency. A low valve gradient, resulting from a decreased cardiac output, may still indicate severe aortic stenosis and can be uncovered by this technique. When high-quality studies are obtained, an aortic valve area >0.9 cm^2 is said to exclude severe aortic stenosis (23, 24). An aortic valve area <0.60 cm^2 indicates severe aortic stenosis. Many patients, of course, have aortic valve areas between these levels. Since further discrimination of significance between these levels is not technically possible, cardiac catheterization is usually necessary. Catheterization is also needed when high-quality echo/Doppler studies cannot be obtained.

The information obtained in the noninvasive laboratory may have a bearing on the technical aspects of the catheterization procedure.

Although some may feel a reduced need to enter the left ventricle in selected cases where severe aortic stenosis is suggested by Doppler study, the variability in quality of Doppler studies observed in some patients and some

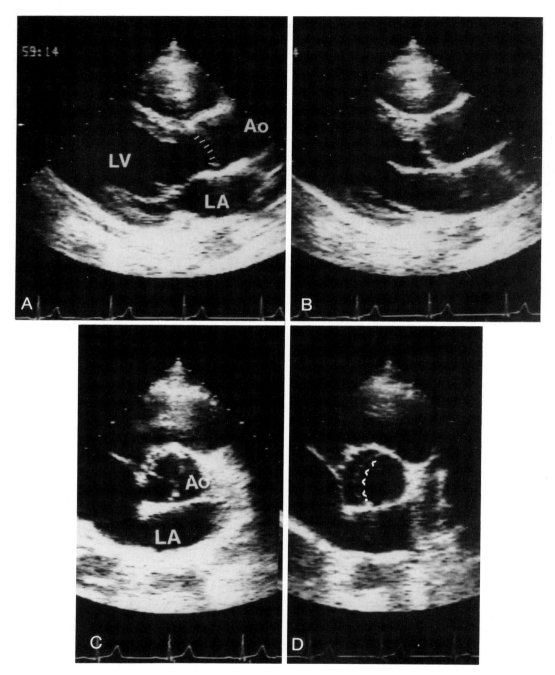

Figure 28.1. Two-dimensional echocardiogram of a congenital bicuspid aortic valve. *A,* Parasternal long-axis view during systole, and *B,* parasternal long-axis view during diastole demonstrate doming of the valve during systole. *C,* Parasternal short-axis view during systole, and *D,* parasternal short-axis view during diastole demonstrate deformity of the valve during systole. *Ao,* aorta; *LA,* left atrium; *LV,* left ventricle.

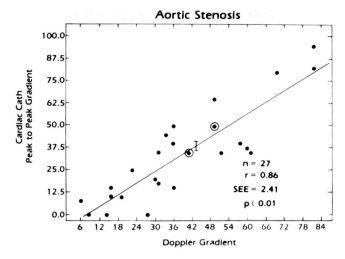

Figure 28.2. Correlation of peak-to-peak aortic valve gradients determined at cardiac catheterization with Doppler-derived peak instantaneous gradients. (Data from the Medical University of South Carolina).

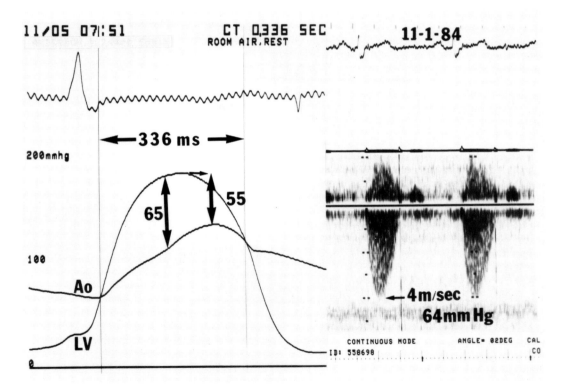

Figure 28.3. Micromanometer recordings of left ventricular (*LV*) and ascending aortic (Ao) pressures demonstrating discrepancy between peak-to-peak and peak instantaneous pressures. Doppler velocity envelope demonstrating correlation of Doppler-derived peak instantaneous gradient with peak instantaneous gradient determined by micromanometer catheter measurements.

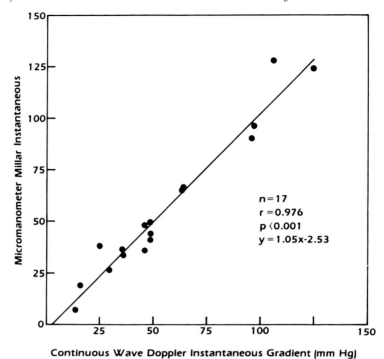

Continuous Wave Doppler Instantaneous Gradient (mm Hg)

Figure 28.4. Correlation of instantaneous peak aortic valve gradient determined at cardiac catheterization using micromanometer catheter technique (*vertical axis*) with Doppler-derived estimated peak instantaneous gradient (*horizontal axis*). (Data from the Medical University of South Carolina).

practice settings makes this an undesirable approach. Should mitral insufficiency be detected by Doppler or physical examination, it is essential to enter the left ventricle and perform a ventriculogram to quantify the severity of the mitral insufficiency. Also, physical examination alone may fail to detect the mitral insufficiency murmur masked by a harsh aortic stenosis murmur. At times the aortic stenosis murmur has a higher pitch at the cardiac apex, mimicking the murmur of mitral insufficiency (Gallivardin effect).

The availability of nonsurgical valvuloplasty has further expanded the role of Doppler echocardiography in aortic stenosis management. In patients undergoing valvuloplasty, preprocedure and postprocedure gradient measurements allow for serial follow-up with proper identification of restenosis and changes in left ventricular function.

Information Obtained at the Time of Cardiac Catheterization

Cardiac catheterization of a patient with known or suspected valvular aortic stenosis is

performed to confirm and quantify the severity of the stenosis, demonstrate associated valvular lesions, evaluate ventricular function, and define the coronary anatomy. Patients with angina often have coronary artery disease as well. Generally speaking, two-thirds of aortic stenosis patients have angina, and in half of these significant coronary atherosclerosis is demonstrated by coronary angiography (25). There is general agreement that it is not possible to identify by currently available noninvasive studies which of these patients has significant coronary artery disease. Although somewhat controversial (26–28), when significant coronary disease is identified, we generally recommend combined aortic valve replacement and coronary artery bypass surgery. We feel that this combined procedure can be performed without increasing the surgical risk and that substantial morbidity may result if severe coronary artery disease is not revascularized. Recently, favorable results have also been reported when combining balloon valvuloplasty and coronary angioplasty (29).

The catheterization protocol typically begins with obtaining venous access and

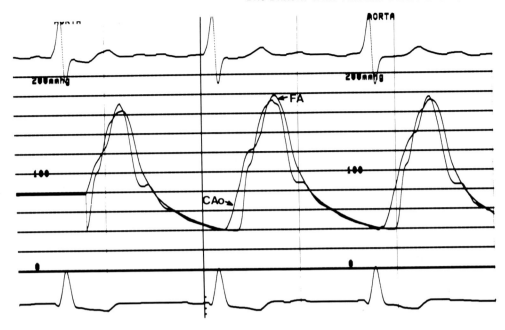

Figure 28.5. Simultaneous central aortic (*CAo*) and femoral artery (*FA*) pressure tracings in a patient with valvular aortic stenosis and chronic atrial fibrillation. The femoral artery pressure overshoots the central aortic systolic pressure but the diastolic and mean pressures are similar.

placement of the right heart catheter. When the right atrium is reached, the mean pressure may be normal or elevated with variable types of waveforms. The patient with aortic stenosis and biventricular heart failure may demonstrate an elevated right atrial mean pressure with an abnormally high V wave secondary to functional tricuspid insufficiency. A prominent A wave in the right atrial tracing suggests reduced right ventricular compliance secondary to pulmonary hypertension or bulging of the hypertrophied interventricular septum towards the right ventricle. Right ventricular and pulmonary artery pressures are measured in the usual fashion, and the pulmonary artery catheter is left in proper position for later determination of cardiac output simultaneously with transaortic valve gradient.

Left heart catheterization is performed from the brachial or femoral approaches. Some physicians prefer the transseptal approach. The left heart catheter is advanced to the ascending aorta just above the aortic valve, and a measurement of central aortic pressure is made. We generally perform this maneuver with the catheter advanced through a sheath in the femoral artery, allowing for simulta-neous evaluation of central aortic and femoral artery pressure curves through a sideport in the sheath. The femoral artery pressure curve will be somewhat time delayed and damp-ened with a systolic pressure over-shoot, although the mean and diastolic pressures are generally similar in the central aorta and femoral artery tracings (Fig. 28.5). If they are not, a transducer malfunction should be suspected. Alternatively, there may be a true biological gradient, resulting from a vascular stenosis between the central aorta and the femoral artery.

The left heart catheter is advanced in retro-grade fashion across the aortic valve for measurement of left ventricular pressures. The type of catheter used is variable and may include a micromanometer single- or double-tipped catheter, a pigtail catheter (straightened out and directioned with a straight guidewire), a multipurpose catheter, a left Amplatz catheter, or a brachial A-2 catheter, which provides a large proximal bore with distal tapering in size and multiple side holes. Whenever multiple side holes are present, catheter position is critical, as straddling of the valve orifice may produce an erroneous gradient. Measurement of left ventricular systolic

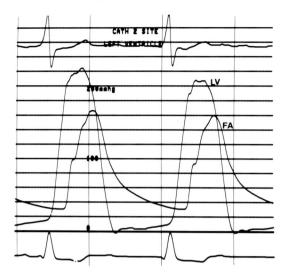

Figure 28.6. Simultaneous left ventricular (*LV*) and femoral artery (*FA*) pressures, the latter measured through the side-arm of a femoral sheath. Planimetry of this unaltered left ventricular-femoral artery gradient will overestimate the true transvalvular gradient.

pressure at fast paper speed is made, and left ventricular filling pressures are recorded on the appropriate scale.

The transvalvular gradient may then be measured in a number of ways. Simultaneous left ventricular and femoral artery pressures may be used to determine the aortic valve gradient. Folland et al. (30) have shown the potential for error when using this technique to measure the aortic valve gradient. As can be seen from Figure 28.6, planimetry of the unaltered left ventricular-femoral artery gradient will overestimate the actual transvalvular gradient. However, temporal alignment of these waveforms by shifting the femoral artery waveform to the left will result in an underestimate of the valve gradient. Averaging the results of the aligned and nonaligned planimetered gradients may approximate the true left ventricular-central aortic (transvalvular) gradient. This is a less acceptable technique compared with direct measurement of the central aortic pressure. Pullback of the ventriculography catheter across the valve will sequentially record left ventricular and central aortic pressures. Although not simultaneous, this is generally adequate to determine the gradient in patients with sinus rhythm.

Planimetry is performed after superimposing the left ventricular and central aortic pressure waves obtained at fast paper speed. An increase in peripheral (brachial or femoral) systolic pressure of 5 mm Hg or more during withdrawal of the catheter across the narrowed orifice is associated with severe stenosis. Fifteen of 20 (75%) patients demonstrating this finding had an aortic valve area, calculated by the Gorlin formula, of ≤0.6 cm^2, while none of 22 patients with an aortic valve area ≥0.7 cm^2 demonstrated this sign (31).

Alternatively, high-fidelity, simultaneous left ventricular and central aortic pressures can be recorded through a double-tipped micromanometer catheter (Fig. 28.3). When properly positioned, one transducer is in the left ventricle and the second is in the ascending aorta. The use of micromanometer catheters, while somewhat cumbersome, avoids over-damping and catheter whip artifacts, which may be critical when the gradient is small. When the gradient across the aortic valve is low, significant aortic stenosis may still be possible because of a low cardiac output. In this setting, it is best to record simultaneous left ventricular and central aortic pressures either using a double-tipped micromanometer catheter or by inserting a second catheter through an alternate arterial route.

Cardiac output determination is made at the same time that the pressure gradient is recorded. Aortic valve area can then be calculated by the Gorlin formula (Chapter 24). The basic concept of the Gorlin formula is that the pressure gradient across the aortic valve must be viewed in light of the fraction of cardiac output passing through the valve. In essence, it states that if an accurately determined cardiac output is related to an accurately determined gradient by an accurate formula, one can calculate aortic valve area. In 1951 when the Gorlins described their formula (32), they had no data to validate aortic valve calculations or the constants used in the equation, since at that time it was considered highly dangerous to cross the aortic valve. Thus, it is not surprising that several limitations of the Gorlin formula in the calculation of aortic valve area have been described. Most importantly, Cannon and colleagues, using valves with fixed orifices, demonstrated that the calculated area increased with cardiac output even though true area did not change. By knowing actual flow and gradient, Cannon et al. recalculated the constants in the Gorlin equation (33). They found that the constant K was not a constant at all but varied directly with the square root of the mean pressure gradient. Mathematically this is described as $AVA = CO/(K' MPG)(MPG)$, where AVA = aortic valve area, CO = cardiac output, and MPG = the mean pressure gradient from the original Gorlin formula. This new equation is then simplified to $AVA = CO/K' MPG$.

Currently, the new constant for the Gorlin equation has yet to be worked out. Thus, the old formula continues to be used. In light of the new revelations about the formula, it must be recognized that at low outputs the Gorlin formula will underestimate aortic valve area, and at high outputs it will overestimate aortic valve area. These constraints may seriously hinder its use in accurately assessing the severity of aortic stenosis in humans. The most serious consequence is in the patient with a low transvalvular gradient and a low cardiac output. In such cases, the Gorlin formula is likely to predict that the aortic valve area is "critical" when only moderate aortic stenosis exists. Clinical judgment, reflecting the sum of the patient's history, physical examination, echo-Doppler studies, and fluoroscopy to detect the amount of calcium in the valve, is an important adjunct to the Gorlin formula in assessing the severity of stenosis.

To allow for a quick intraprocedural calculation, Hakki et al. (34) have suggested that valve area may be estimated from the cardiac output divided by the square root of the pressure gradient. This ratio ignores the systolic ejection period. It is justifiable, however, because in the resting state, the product of heart rate, ejection or filling period, and Gorlin constant is usually close to 1. However, the systolic ejection period, like the diastolic filling period, may change significantly when heart rates change, and this has prompted a further modification of the formula by Angel et al. (35). When heart rate exceeds 90 bpm in aortic stenosis, Hakki's derived valve area estimated by the Hakki equation should be further decreased, dividing by 1.35.

In our laboratory, left ventriculography is performed in a modified fashion for patient safety. This includes the use of nonionic contrast agents which are less likely to produce potentially deleterious hemodynamic changes (see Chapter 10). Patients with well-compensated aortic stenosis have small, thick-walled left ventricles that can be adequately opacified, without creating ventricular ectopy, with lower than usual contrast volume (~25 to 30 cc) and injection rate. The patient with very high pulmonary-capillary wedge pressure (>20 mm Hg) may be pretreated with diuretics and other preload reducing agents to minimize the risk of precipitating acute pulmonary edema. Ventriculography is necessary if coexistent mitral insufficiency or ventricular aneurysm is suspected. When severe aortic stenosis is found, and aortic insufficiency is neither heard nor demonstrated by Doppler, aortography is not essential unless desired by the operating surgeon. Aortography is performed when supravalvular or subvalvular aortic stenosis is suspected. In the left anterior oblique view, a jet of negative contrast with domed rigid valve leaflets and poststenotic dilation of the central aorta may be seen in bicuspid valves.

Data Evaluation and Recommendations

Symptomatic patients with an aortic valve area <0.7cm^2 are offered surgery or valvuloplasty. The decision as to which of these techniques is preferred is fully discussed in an earlier chapter (Chapter 17). At present, we reserve valvuloplasty for symptomatic patients who are not surgical candidates. This may be based on an unacceptably high surgical risk, excessive noncardiac morbidity, or patient refusal to undergo surgery. Significant aortic insufficiency or severe coronary atherosclerosis requiring revascularization are general contraindications to valvuloplasty. Since the long-term success rate of aortic valvuloplasty is currently not well-defined, we use frequent (3 to 6 months) follow-up with Doppler echocardiography as a supplement to our postvalvuloplasty clinical evaluation. It is important to realize, however, that significant restenosis may occur without an increase in postvalvuloplasty gradient if the cardiac output has decreased.

As noted previously, the vast majority of patients with aortic stenosis and congestive heart failure will experience significant improvement in left ventricular performance following valve replacement or valvuloplasty

(12, 19). No patient is refused surgery (36, 37) or valvuloplasty (38) on the basis of a low ejection fraction. It is hoped that the low ejection fraction is due to the afterload mismatch of aortic stenosis rather than depressed contractility, and that ejection fraction will improve following valvuloplasty or valve replacement. It must be realized, however, that many patients with low left ventricular ejection fractions and low aortic valve gradients will not improve following surgery or valvuloplasty (39). In such patients, left ventricular wall stress is likely to be low, in which case afterload cannot be significantly reduced by valve replacement or valvuloplasty. Recent reports indicate that some patients with low ejection fraction and low gradients may improve, and it has even been suggested that such patients should undergo valvuloplasty as a test of myocardial contractility reserve. Aortic valve replacement would be indicated if significant improvement in ejection fraction is noted following the valvuloplasty (40).

Occasionally, noninvasive studies uncover a significant gradient (exceeding 50 mm Hg) in a totally asymptomatic patient. The management of such a patient is controversial. Recently, 51 asymptomatic aortic stenosis patients, all with Doppler-derived peak systolic aortic valve gradients exceeding 50 mm Hg (range 50 to 132 mm Hg) were compared with 39 symptomatic patients (41). Asymptomatic patients were statistically significantly younger, had higher left ventricular ejection fractions, and were less likely to have a left ventricular strain pattern or left atrial enlargement. During follow-up (17 ± 9 months) 21 of the 51 asymptomatic patients became symptomatic, with dyspnea being the most common initial complaint. Only two of the 51 initially asymptomatic patients died. Importantly, both deaths were preceded by the development of angina pectoris or congestive heart failure. This study supports a conservative approach, albeit with close follow-up, of the asymptomatic aortic stenosis patient.

At present, the recommendation for cardiac catheterization in such asymptomatic patients is controversial. Patients should be carefully instructed concerning bacterial endocarditis prophylaxis and what specific symptoms to watch for, in an effort to minimize the chance of unrecognized aortic stenosis symptoms. Serial Doppler studies may be useful in the follow-up of a patient with nonspecific or atypical symptoms. When characteristic symptoms do develop, cardiac catheterization is performed promptly. Inherent in this approach is the risk that an asymptomatic aortic stenosis patient will present with sudden cardiac death. This risk is very low, however, and must be weighed against a similar risk for valve replacement.

Aortic stenosis may coexist with mitral stenosis. When the mitral stenosis is severe, the clinical findings of aortic stenosis, particularly the murmur length and intensity, may change. The cardiac output is usually quite low, resulting in a small aortic valve gradient. Precatheterization echo/Doppler studies help prevent an underestimation of aortic stenosis severity in the face of this combined valvular lesion.

When aortic stenosis is accompanied by mitral insufficiency, the physical findings expected to be associated with either lesion in isolation may change. For example, the classic carotid upstroke of significant aortic stenosis (pulsus parvus et tardus) may be "normalized" by coexistent mitral insufficiency. The relative importance of two systolic murmurs may be difficult to analyze at the bedside. Precatheterization echocardiography with Doppler studies are important in planning catheterization strategy in patients with this mixed lesion. Hemodynamically, the left ventricle may be dilated more with the mixed lesion than with isolated aortic stenosis.

In summary, symptomatic patients with aortic stenosis should undergo cardiac catheterization. In asymptomatic patients, a conservative approach is generally followed, even when noninvasive studies (specifically echocardiography with Doppler) reveal a significant aortic valve gradient. Obviously, these patients need bacterial endocarditis prophylaxis and close clinical follow-up as previously emphasized. When symptomatic patients are found to have an aortic valve area less than 0.7 cm^2, aortic valve replacement or balloon valvuloplasty is indicated. Concomitant coronary artery disease or associated valvular lesions may require earlier intervention.

AORTIC INSUFFICIENCY

Clinical Presentation and Pathophysiology

There are multiple etiologies of aortic insufficiency including disorders that affect the valve itself (rheumatic heart disease, congenitally bicuspid aortic valve, myxomatous degeneration of the valve, infective endocarditis) as well as those etiologies that primarily affect the supporting aortic root and annulus (hypertension, trauma, dissection, aortic root aneurysm secondary to cystic medial necrosis). It is important to establish the etiology because both the approach to cardiac catheterization and timing of surgical intervention as well as surgical results are directly related to the etiology. For example, rheumatic aortic insufficiency generally presents as a well compensated, chronic left ventricular volume overload. Acute aortic insufficiency secondary to infective endocarditis may result in major valve disruption and torrential aortic insufficiency constituting a surgical emergency affecting the timing and type of cardiac catheterization. Indeed, proper identification and management of acute aortic insufficiency is so important that it is discussed separately in this chapter.

Like mitral insufficiency, chronic aortic insufficiency imparts a volume overload on the left ventricle resulting in increased end-diastolic volume and increased end-diastolic stress compensated by eccentric left ventricular hypertrophy. However, the higher systemic systolic blood pressure, intraventricular pressures, and ventricular radius all increase both peak and end-systolic wall stress. This situation mimics the mechanics of a left ventricular pressure overload. In part, this may explain why the natural history of left ventricular function in aortic insufficiency differs from the pure volume overload of mitral insufficiency. Wisenbaugh and colleagues (42) studied ventricular mechanics in nine patients with severe aortic insufficiency and eight patients with severe mitral insufficiency. Compared with normal subjects, both groups showed reduced ejection performance. While preload (estimated as end-diastolic stress) was comparably elevated in both groups with regurgitation, afterload (estimated as mean systolic stress) was markedly elevated in aortic insufficiency and normal in mitral insufficiency. In aortic insufficiency, this excessive afterload contributed to poor pump performance, while the more favorable loading condition for mitral insufficiency masked underlying contractile dysfunction.

Chronic, slowly progressing, and compensated aortic insufficiency is associated with marked left ventricular dilation and eccentric hypertrophy, resulting in the largest left ventricular mass seen among the valvular lesions. This increased left ventricular size can accommodate the volume overload without increasing intraventricular pressures that would tend to cause an increase in pulmonary venous pressures. The enhanced run-off from the central circulation into the dilated, compliant left ventricle contributes to the widening of aortic pulse pressure and the classical peripheral pulse findings of chronic, compensated aortic insufficiency (43). When aortic insufficiency decompensates or occurs acutely, these peripheral findings may be absent.

Precardiac Catheterization Noninvasive Assessment of Chronic Aortic Insufficiency

Echocardiography is useful in establishing the etiology of the aortic insufficiency and assessing aortic root pathology. An estimate of global left ventricular systolic function can be made and coronary artery disease inferred by the presence of regional wall motion abnormalities. Semiquantification of the severity of aortic insufficiency can be made from the **pulsed Doppler** interrogation of the left ventricle (Fig. 28.7). With this technique, the depth of the regurgitant jet detected in the left ventricle correlates with the angiographic severity of aortic insufficiency (44). Because the regurgitant jet can be eccentric and/or wide, Doppler color flow imaging allows a better noninvasive assessment of severity and closer correlation with angiography (45). With this technique, grading of the aortic insufficiency severity is made by comparing the area of the regurgitant jet in the short-axis view with the area of the left ventricular outflow tract in that same view (Fig. 28.8). Perry et al. found that the thickness of the regurgitant stream, relative to

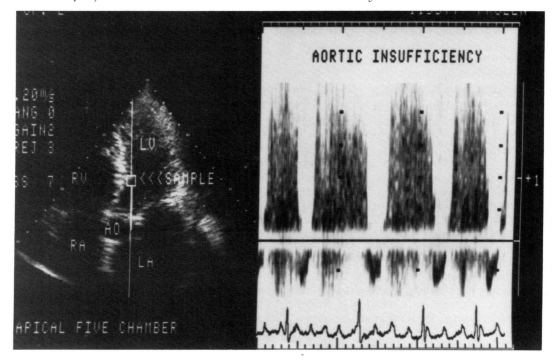

Figure 28.7. Doppler echocardiogram utilizing conventional pulsed wave Doppler to detect aortic insufficiency from apical five-chamber view. *RV,* right ventricle; *RA,* right atrium; *LV,* left ventricle; *LA,* left atrium; *Ao,* aorta.

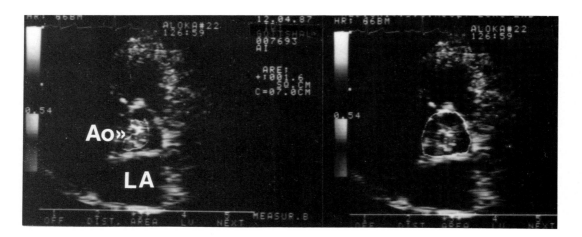

Figure 28.8. Doppler color flow imaging in the parasternal short-axis view demonstrating aortic insufficiency. The severity of insufficiency is estimated by determining the ratio of the area of the Doppler color signal during diastole to the area of the left ventricular outflow. *LA,* left atrium; *Ao,* aorta.

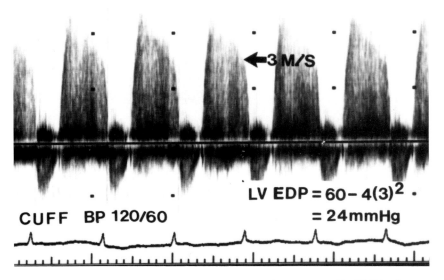

$$LVEDP = DBP - 4(V_{max})^2 \text{ (CW DOPPLER)}$$

AORTIC INSUFFICIENCY

←3 M/S

$$LV\ EDP = 60 - 4(3)^2$$
$$= 24\,mmHg$$

CUFF BP 120/60

Figure 28.9. Doppler estimate of left ventricular end-diastolic pressure (*LVEDP*) in the presence of aortic insufficiency. *DBP*, diastolic blood pressure; *M/S*, meters/second.

the area of the left ventricular outflow tract, recorded just below the aortic valve, correlated well with angiographic severity (46).

Continuous wave Doppler flow pattern of aortic insufficiency allows for an analysis of the rate of decay of the velocity profile (pressure or velocity half-time) and gives an indirect assessment of the severity of insufficiency (47). When aortic insufficiency is severe, the gradient during diastole between the aorta and the left ventricle dissipates early in diastole, yielding a more rapid decline in the flow velocity of the aortic insufficiency. This finding may be particularly beneficial when mitral stenosis coexists with aortic insufficiency since the mitral stenosis itself produces a high-velocity diastolic jet that can complicate mapping during pulsed Doppler evaluation.

We have found that when the continuous wave Doppler velocity envelope provides a sharp end-diastolic point, the left ventricular end-diastolic pressure can be estimated if the aortic diastolic pressure (obtained indirectly by cuff) is simultaneously determined (Fig. 28.9).

Information Obtained at Time of Cardiac Catheterization for Chronic Aortic Insufficiency

Right-sided cardiac pressures are generally normal in chronic, compensated aortic insufficiency. Cardiac output measurements are made close to the time of left ventriculography, allowing for calculation of the regurgitant fraction. Regurgitant fraction is the difference between angiographic and forward cardiac output divided by the angiographic cardiac output. Prior to entering the left ventricle, it is important to measure and record central aortic pressure, since the normal discrepancy between central aortic and peripheral systolic pressures (brachial or femoral) is exaggerated in the setting of aortic insufficiency.

Left ventricular end-diastolic pressure

Figure 28.10. Aortogram, performed in the 45° left anterior oblique view in a patient with malfunctioning St. Jude prosthesis. Injection of contrast material through the pigtail catheter resulted in progressive opacification of a dilated left ventricle indicating "4 +" aortic insufficiency. *Ao,* ascending aorta; *LV,* left ventricle.

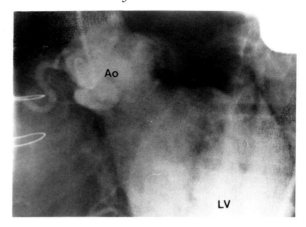

varies, depending on the severity of aortic insufficiency, compliance of the left ventricle, degree of ventricular hypertrophy, and associated coronary artery disease. The actual degree of aortic insufficiency is determined by the pressure differential between the aortic diastolic and left ventricular diastolic pressure, the length of diastole, and the size of the regurgitant orifice.

The amount of contrast agent entering the left ventricle during aortic root injection allows for a qualitative assessment of severity. Since the left ventricle in aortic insufficiency is often markedly enlarged, failure to inject enough contrast at a rapid enough rate may result in an underestimate of the amount of aortic insufficiency. Although several grading systems have been proposed, we prefer the following. In mild (1 +) aortic insufficiency, the contrast from the aortic root fails to reach the left ventricular apex, and the ventricle is cleared of contrast material with each beat. Moderate (2 +) aortic insufficiency opacifies the entire left ventricular chamber, but the degree of opacification of the left ventricle is less than the aortic root. Moderately severe (3 +) aortic insufficiency occurs when opacification of the entire left ventricle is equal to that of the aorta. Severe (4 +) aortic insufficiency indicates total opacification of the left ventricular cavity on the first or second heart beat following injection of contrast material into the aorta, with progressive opacification during the injection (Fig. 28.10).

There is relatively poor correlation be-

tween noninvasive studies (e.g., pulsed Doppler), qualitative angiographic assessment of contrast reflux, and calculated regurgitant fraction. This discrepancy results from several factors. There may be at least a 10% variation in accuracy when forward cardiac output is computed by the thermodilution method. The amount of contrast material refluxing into the left ventricle varies with catheter position, volume of contrast material injected, and rate of contrast injection. The size of the aortic root (which may be massive in annulo-aortic ectasia or ascending aortic aneurysm) and the size of the left ventricular cavity also affects the degree of opacification by a given amount of contrast material. Finally, the forcefulness of global left ventricular contractility and/or the presence of associated mitral insufficiency will affect the qualitative assessment by cineangiography. Left ventricular hypokinesis reduces the rate of contrast clearance, favoring progressive opacification of the left ventricle. When mitral insufficiency is present, contrast material escapes into the left atrium, decreasing the rate and degree of opacification of the left ventricle during aortic injection. Cineangiography in the 30° right anterior oblique view allows measurement of left ventricular volumes and ejection fraction from an aortic injection when moderately severe or severe aortic insufficiency is present. It has been our impression that the degree of regurgitation in the right anterior oblique view appears qualitatively less than a similar degree of regurgitation in the left anterior oblique view.

Table 28.2.
Predictors of a Suboptimal Response to Aortic Valve Replacement
for Chronic Aortic Insufficiency

	Value	Reference
Echocardiography		
LV[a] shortening fraction	<0.27	49
End-diastolic dimension index	>38 mm/m^2	50
End-systolic dimension	>55 mm	49
End-systolic dimension index	>26 mm/m^2	50
Ratio LV diastolic radius to thickness	>3.8	50
Cardiac catheterization		
Subnormal LV ejection fraction	<0.50	52
Reduced cardiac index	<2.2 liters/m^2	51
Elevated PCW pressure	>12 mm Hg	51
Large LV end-systolic volume	>90 cc/m^2	53,54
Large LV end-diastolic volume	>180 cc/m^2	54
Ratio of regurgitant to end-diastolic volume	<0.25	55

[a] LV, left ventricular; PCW, pulmonary-capillary wedge.

Data Evaluation and Recommendations for Chronic Aortic Insufficiency

Controversy exists regarding the appropriate timing of cardiac catheterization and surgery for patients with chronic aortic insufficiency. Clearly, patients with moderate or severe symptoms due to this valvular lesion need cardiac catheterization and most likely aortic valve replacement. Asymptomatic or mildly symptomatic patients pose a problem as to the timing of catheterization and surgery, since previously reported determinants of a poor surgical outcome appear less reliable in the modern surgical era. Table 28.2 lists many of the frequently quoted noninvasive and invasive indicators of suboptimal surgical outcome in patients with chronic aortic insufficiency (48–55). Ten of these indicators were applied to 14 patients with isolated aortic insufficiency (3+ or 4+) and an ejection fraction <55%. Despite the fact that there were 82 (58%) of a possible 140 predictors of negative outcome preoperatively, no patient died. All but two patients had a decrease in symptoms and an increase in ejection fraction into the normal range after operation (48). Such results suggest that, while these indicators are useful guidelines in the management of chronic aortic insufficiency, they should not of themselves supersede clinical judgment in determining the timing of catheterization and/or surgery.

In contrast to mitral insufficiency, patients with aortic insufficiency who have a below normal ejection fraction or increased end-systolic dimensions and volumes may still improve following valve replacement in the modern surgical era.

Aortic insufficiency frequently coexists with aortic stenosis and other valvular lesions (56). Severe aortic stenosis and aortic insufficiency cannot by definition coexist. However, the combination of a moderate degree of both lesions can cause symptoms and impaired ventricular function. This might require surgery that otherwise would not be needed if lesions of the same severity were present in isolation in different patients. When aortic insufficiency occurs with severe mitral stenosis, the wide pulse pressure responsible for the typical peripheral pulse changes of isolated aortic insufficiency are usually absent. Echocardiography with Doppler will aid the physical examination when this combination is suspected. Hemodynamically, the mitral stenosis will attenuate the left ventricular volume overload expected of isolated aortic insufficiency. The use of end-systolic stress/volume relationships are useful in assessing left ventricular contractility in this setting (57).

When aortic insufficiency coexists with mitral insufficiency, the etiology may be rheumatic, combined prolapse of both valves, or dilation of annuli from various types of connective tissue diseases. Mitral insufficiency may also be functional in the setting of

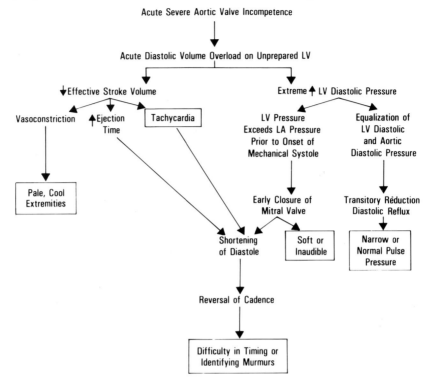

Figure 28.11. Pathophysiology and clinical correlates in acute aortic insufficiency. Note explanations for potential difficulty in timing the murmur of aortic insufficiency. *LA,* left atrial; *LV,* left ventricular.

aortic insufficiency with left ventricular dilation. Separate contrast material injections into the aorta and the left ventricle are usually needed to assess severity. When this is done, sufficient time should be allowed to elapse between injections for the hemodynamic effects of the initial contrast injection to dissipate.

ACUTE AORTIC INSUFFICIENCY

Clinical Presentation and Pathophysiology

This valvular lesion represents a true surgical emergency even in a patient with apparently mild congestive heart failure. It generally occurs as a complication of infective endocarditis, aortic root trauma, or dissection and must be promptly identified and appropriately treated if cardiovascular collapse is to be avoided. Unlike chronic aortic insufficiency,

there is no dilated left ventricle to accommodate the sudden increase in left ventricular diastolic volume. Left ventricular filling pressure rises severely and prematurely during each diastole. As a result, the mitral valve is prematurely closed prior to the onset of left ventricular systole (58). This premature closure of the mitral valve protects the left atrium and pulmonary vascular bed from increased volume and pressure but causes a severe increase in left ventricular wall stress. The increased ventricular diastolic wall stress can cause subendocardial ischemia, myocardial infarction, and lethal ventricular arrhythmias. On physical examination, the premature closure of the mitral valve diminishes the first heart sound. The combination of tachycardia and a soft first heart sound makes timing of the murmur difficult (Fig. 28.11). Many an experienced clinician has confused the short diastolic murmur of acute aortic insufficiency with murmurs of other etiologies.

Precardiac Catheterization Noninvasive Assessment of Acute Aortic Insufficiency

The M-mode echocardiogram of a patient with acute aortic insufficiency who developed premature closure of the mitral valve while receiving antibiotics for aortic valve endocarditis appears in Fig. 28.12. Early mitral closure occurred when left ventricular pressure exceeded left atrial (pulmonary-capillary wedge) pressure (Fig. 28.13). Vasodilator therapy with sodium nitroprusside attenuated the hemodynamic abnormality. The fall in peripheral resistance, produced by this potent systemic vasodilator, reduced the volume of aortic diastolic regurgitation decreasing the prematurity of mitral valve closure. Pepine and colleagues (59) have demonstrated similar hemodynamic improvement and loss of premature mitral valve closure when administering nitroprusside in chronic aortic insufficiency.

In acute aortic insufficiency, echocardiographic or angiographic detection of a vegetation on the aortic valve establishes the diagnosis of endocarditis, as does detection of a flail leaflet in the proper clinical setting. In some instances, associated myocardial or annular abscess can be detected. Doppler color flow imaging is helpful in establishing the presence or absence of a left to right shunt from a fistulous tract. When the surgical emergency of acute aortic insufficiency is due to dissection of the aorta, two-dimensional echocardiography may be useful in detecting the dissection and determining its extent (Fig. 28.14).

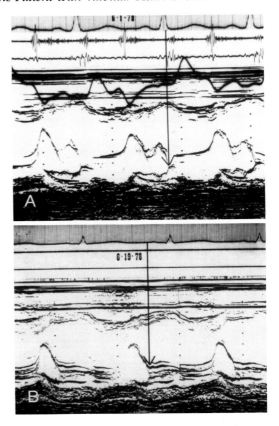

Figure 28.12. M-mode echocardiogram demonstrating mitral valve closure point in a patient with acute aortic insufficiency secondary to bacterial endocarditis. *A,* Mitral valve closure point is normal (*arrow*) on admission. *B,* Early closure of the mitral valve detected 18 days later while receiving antibiotic therapy. (From Assey ME. Echocardiography in diagnosis and managing aortic valve endocarditis. South Med J 1981;74:561.)

Information Obtained at the Time of Cardiac Catheterization for Acute Aortic Insufficiency

Patients with acute aortic insufficiency may be too ill to undergo emergency catheterization and contrast injection without pretreatment with systemic vasodilator drugs. If aortic valve echocardiography demonstrates a large vegetation, particularly with a flail aortic valve, it may be best not to cross the aortic valve at the time of cardiac catheterization due to the risk

of embolization. Other laboratories, however, have not found the risk of embolization to be increased by catheterization. When the left ventricle is not entered but a left ventriculogram is considered necessary, adequate opacification of the left ventricle may be obtained by injection of contrast material into the aortic root, in the presence of severe aortic insufficiency.

Right heart cardiac catheterization is important, particularly if a left to right intracardiac shunt is suspected. Such a shunt may be the result of endocarditis with abscess and fistula formation. In acute aortic

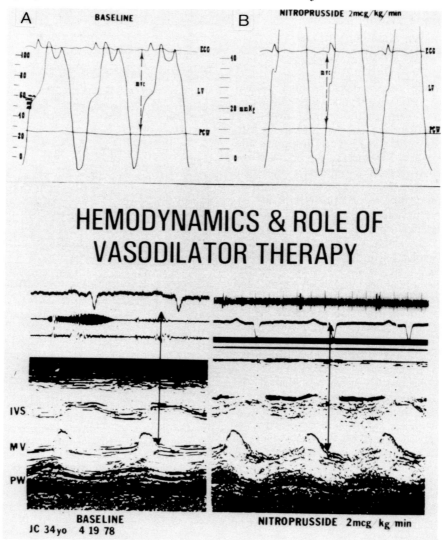

Figure 28.13. Simultaneous intracardiac pressure recordings (*top*) and M-mode echocardiograms (*bottom*) obtained in the cardiac catheterization laboratory in a patient with acute aortic insufficiency. *A*, Left ventricular end-diastolic pressure (*LVEDP*) is 60 mm Hg with a simultaneous pulmonary-capillary wedge pressure (*PCW*) of 26 mm Hg. The LVEDP exceeds the PCW in early diastole, well before the onset of the QRS complex of the electrocardiogram (*ECG*) with resulting early closure of the mitral valve. *B*, During infusion of nitroprusside, the *LVEDP* decreased to approximately 30 mm Hg and the *PCW* to 12 to 14 mm Hg. The *LVEDP* exceeds the *PCW* later in diastole, resulting in a shift in the mitral valve closure point to later in diastole at the onset of the QRS complex.

insufficiency, the left ventricular pressure tracing shows a very high left ventricular end-diastolic pressure (which is the limiting factor to further regurgitation from the central aorta), striking late diastolic rise (earlier diastasis which shortens the acute aortic in-

sufficiency murmur), a left ventricular end-diastolic pressure that exceeds pulmonary-capillary wedge pressure early in diastole, and loss of the usual distinct A wave seen in chronic ventricular hypertrophy (Fig. 28.13).

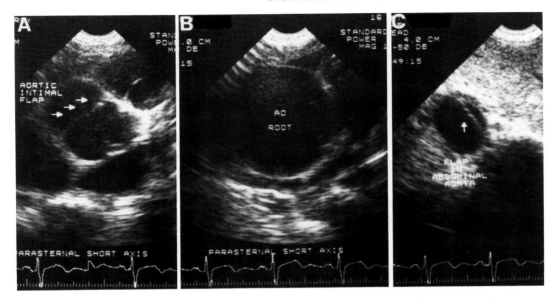

Figure 28.14. Two-dimensional echocardiogram of a patient with an aortic dissection. *A*, Parasternal short-axis view at the level of the aortic valve. *B*, Parasternal short-axis view of the ascending aorta demonstrating dilated aorta. *C*, Short-axis view of abdominal aorta. *Ao*, aorta.

Data Evaluation and Recommendations for Acute Aortic Insufficiency

Since this situation represents a surgical emergency, immediate cardiothoracic surgical consultation is needed prior to catheterization in any patient presenting with acute aortic insufficiency. High-quality noninvasive studies, in the proper clinical setting, accurately define the cause and complications of the acute aortic insufficiency and may obviate cardiac catheterization. Invasive studies are required if coronary anatomy must be determined. Invasive studies are also needed when noninvasive studies indicate intracardiac abscess formation with possible fistulous tracts or if there is need to define the anatomy of aortic root dissection. Although these patients are critically ill, complete cardiac catheterization while on vasodilators provides detailed information for the surgeon and will maximize the chances of operative success. In fact, since aortic insufficiency is already established noninvasively, the catheterization itself should focus on other possible lesions (associated valve lesions, coronary artery disease, etc.) that might change the surgical approach.

MITRAL STENOSIS

Clinical Presentation and Pathophysiology

In most cases, obstruction to left ventricular inflow at the level of the mitral valve results from rheumatic inflammation. As a result, mitral stenosis frequently coexists with mitral insufficiency or rheumatic involvement of other valves. Other rare causes of left ventricular inflow obstruction include congenital mitral stenosis, severe mitral annular calcification, cor triatriatum, and obstruction of the mitral orifice due to a ball valve thrombus or left atrial myxoma. Although a left atrial to left ventricular gradient may develop when the mitral valve area is reduced to 2 cm^2, symptoms (dyspnea, hemoptysis, low output) do not develop until the mitral valve area reaches approximately 1 cm^2, which is 20 to 25% of normal size. At this level of stenosis, when the tachycardia of exercise or rapid atrial fibrillation shortens the diastolic filling period, the obligatory increase in transvalvular gradient frequently produces acute dyspnea causing the patient to seek medical evaluation.

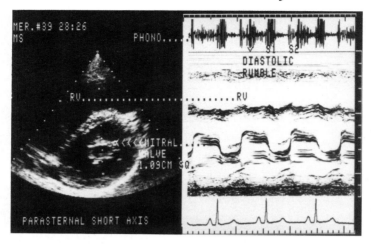

Figure 28.15. M-mode and two-dimensional echocardiogram of patient with mitral stenosis. The mitral valve area is determined by planimetering the mitral valve orifice in the parasternal short-axis view of the two-dimensional echocardiogram. The mitral valve area is 1.09 cm2. *RV,* right ventricle.

Precardiac Catheterization Noninvasive Assessment

The patient with suspected mitral stenosis should undergo noninvasive assessment with Doppler echocardiography in order to confirm the diagnosis and rule out other causes of obstruction at the mitral valve level (myxoma, annular calcification, etc.). The Doppler echocardiographic evaluation will provide data regarding the hemodynamic severity of the mitral stenosis, left atrial size, detection of left atrial masses, mitral insufficiency, and associated involvement of other valves.

The reliability of conventional echocardiography and Doppler echocardiography is now so refined in the case of mitral stenosis that some patients undergo surgery without a preceding cardiac catheterization. Generally this applies to patients under the age of 35, particularly women, not felt to need coronary angiography. In such patients, however, right heart catheterization may still be performed to measure pulmonary artery pressures and calculate pulmonary vascular resistance to aid in risk stratification. As demonstrated in Figure 28.15, planimetry of the mitral valve area from the two-dimensional echocardiographic short-axis view provides excellent correlation with the mitral valve area (Fig. 28.16) calculated from catheterization data by the Gorlin formula (Chapter 24). Equally good correlation has been obtained with Doppler-derived

mitral valve area using the pressure half-time technique (Fig. 28.17), which we have found to be reliable (Fig. 28.18). It may be superior to the calculation of mitral valve area by planimetry in patients who have undergone prior mitral valve commissurotomy. In such cases, the mitral valve orifice is often very distorted and difficult to planimeter, and obstruction may be secondary to thickening and fibrosis of the subvalvular apparatus. In patients with associated mitral insufficiency and atrial fibrillation, measurement of mitral valve area by Doppler pressure half-time may be more reliable than the valve area determined at catheterization, due to the beat-to-beat variability in diastolic flow.

Optimal noninvasive evaluation requires the application of multiple techniques, particularly when mitral stenosis coexists with other lesions. For example, a recent study (60) suggested that the estimate of mitral valve area by Doppler pressure half-time was less reliable than the continuity equation when aortic insufficiency was present. However, when mitral stenosis was associated with mitral insufficiency, the continuity equation overestimated the mitral valve area, as compared with cardiac catheterization measurement of mitral valve area.

In addition to screening patients with rheumatic heart disease, these noninvasive techniques have been useful in predicting which patients can be treated with

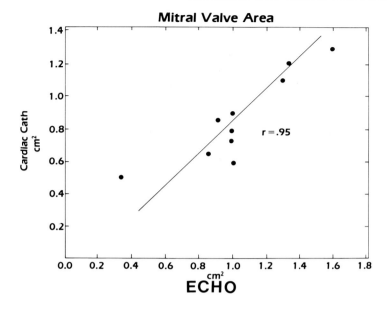

Figure 28.16. Correlation of the mitral valve area determined by planimetry from the two-dimensional echocardiogram with that obtained at cardiac catheterization using the Gorlin formula. (Data from the Medical University of South Carolina).

commissurotomy rather than valve replacement (61). This is an important consideration when timing surgical intervention in patients with mild or moderate symptoms. Pulmonary hypertension may complicate the natural history of mitral stenosis, but in the presence of tricuspid insufficiency (Fig. 28.19), Doppler echocardiography can provide an estimate of right ventricular systolic pressure (Fig. 28.20) (62). In the absence of pulmonic stenosis, it will also estimate pulmonary artery systolic pressure. The noninvasive demonstration of mitral stenosis may also permit valvuloplasty in selected patients without a separate diagnostic cardiac catheterization. Echocardiography with Doppler is used to follow patients after balloon valvuloplasty or following surgical commissurotomy in order to detect restenosis.

Information Obtained at the Time of Cardiac Catheterization

Symptomatic patients with mitral stenosis, in whom noninvasive evaluation confirms significant valvular obstruction, are referred for cardiac catheterization. The degree of mitral stenosis can be quantitated, other valvular lesions evaluated, and the pulmonary vascular resistance measured. In addition, cineangiographic and fluoroscopic assessment of the mitral valve aid in the decision as to whether or not a patient requires mitral valve replacement or can be treated with operative repair of the mitral valve. Left ventricular function can be evaluated and coronary angiography performed. When high-quality, reliable noninvasive data is available, the major indication for cardiac catheterization of mitral stenosis patients at our institution is the need to demonstrate the coronary anatomy.

The catheterization protocol generally begins with the measurement of right heart pressures. If associated tricuspid insufficiency is present, right atrial mean pressure will be elevated and a prominent V wave may be seen. Alternatively, if obstruction to right ventricular inflow is present secondary to associated tricuspid stenosis, right atrial mean pressure will be elevated, and a prominent right atrial A wave (larger than the corresponding right ventricular A wave) will be seen in patients without atrial fibrillation. As the catheter is advanced, right ventricular and pulmonary artery pressures are measured

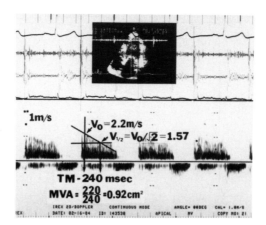

Figure 28.17. Doppler echocardiogram of patient with mitral stenosis. The mitral valve area is calculated from the Doppler diastolic velocity envelope by the pressure half-time technique. *MVA*, mitral valve area; V_0, peak velocity; $V_{1/2}$, half of the peak velocity; *TM*, time from onset of diastolic Doppler signal to $V_{1/2}$. 220 msec is the known TM for 1 cm² valve area.

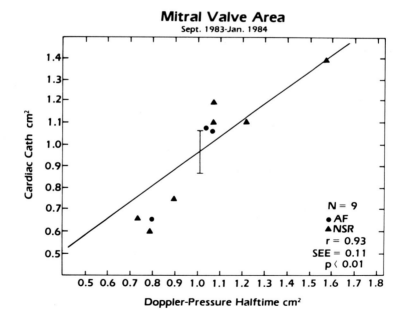

Figure 28.18. Correlation of the mitral valve area determined by the Doppler pressure half-time method with that obtained at cardiac catheterization using the Gorlin formula. *AF*, atrial fibrillation; *NSR*, normal sinus rhythm. (Data from the Medical University of South Carolina.)

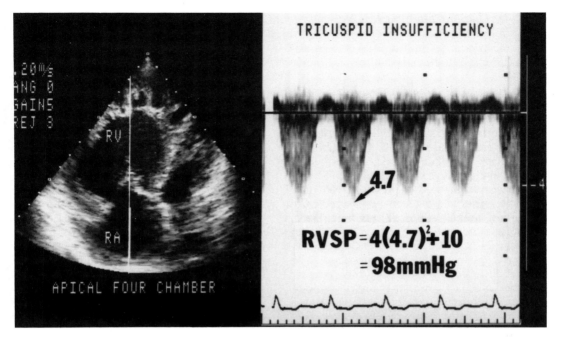

Figure 28.19. Estimation of right ventricular systolic pressure in patient with tricuspid insufficiency. The *left-hand panel* demonstrates Doppler echocardiogram sampling in the apical four-chamber view. Using this conventional pulsed Doppler and sampling in the right atrium, tricuspid insufficiency is detected. The *right-hand panel* demonstrates continuous wave Doppler echocardiogram in a patient with tricuspid insufficiency. The peak right ventricular pressure (*RVSP*) is estimated from the Doppler-derived pressure gradient across the tricuspid valve in systole added to 10 (an estimate of right atrium (*RA*) pressure). *RV,* right ventricle.

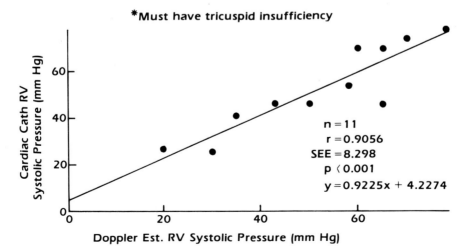

Figure 28.20. Correlation of the Doppler-derived estimate of peak right ventricular (*RV*) pressure with that measured at cardiac catheterization. V_{max}, maximum Doppler velocity during systole. *RA,* right atrial. (Data from the Medical University of South Carolina.)

and recorded, permitting the diagnosis of associated tricuspid and/or pulmonic stenosis.

In order to obtain an accurate transmitral gradient, simultaneous measurement of left atrial (or phasic, nondamped pulmonary-capillary wedge) pressure and left ventricular diastolic pressure are needed. Many laboratories utilize a balloon-tipped, flow-directed pulmonary artery catheter to estimate pulmonary-capillary wedge pressure from pulmonary artery occlusion pressure. The important limitations resulting from use of balloon-tipped catheters are addressed in Chapter 24. It is important that a true pulmonary-capillary wedge pressure be recorded. Documentation that the pressure recorded is in fact a true pulmonary-capillary wedge pressure is made by demonstrating a high oxygen saturation when blood is drawn from that position (arterial oxygen saturation exceeds 95% or is equal to that of systemic arterial specimen). Furthermore, the pulmonary-capillary wedge pressure is distinguished from a damped pulmonary artery pressure by a decrease in mean pressure when the balloon is inflated. While the normal pulmonary-capillary wedge pressure demonstrates a V wave greater than the A wave, this pattern is reversed in mitral stenosis with sinus rhythm. The pulmonary-capillary A wave is much larger than the A wave present on the left ventricular diastolic pressure curve in mitral stenosis.

If the pulmonary-capillary wedge pressure is used as an indirect measure of left atrial pressure, a realignment will be required when planimetry of the mitral valve pressure gradient is done. The pulmonary-capillary wedge pressure is a damped, phase-delayed left atrial pressure, and it should be shifted (to the left) to allow the descent of the V wave to be superimposed on the descent of the left ventricular diastolic pressure tracing. Pulmonary-capillary wedge pressure may not accurately estimate left atrial mean pressure in the face of associated mitral insufficiency, pulmonary venous obstruction, cor triatriatum, or with a prosthetic mitral valve (63).

To properly calculate the mitral valve area using the Gorlin equation, cardiac output must be determined while recording the valve gradient. Diastolic filling period and heart rate are also measured although, as suggested

by Hakki et al. (34) and explained above, intraprocedural estimation of mitral valve area can be made without exact knowledge of these parameters. This quick calculation is helpful when deciding the need for hemodynamic measurement during exercise. Generally, exercise is performed when there is a small resting gradient (<5 mm Hg), but the use of exercise in mitral stenosis has been decreased by the echo/Doppler precatheterization determination of mitral valve area. Invasive exercise study may, however, offer valuable information relating exertional symptoms to hemodynamic abnormalities, especially in patients with coexistent pulmonary disease or those with histories that are difficult to interpret. Left ventriculography is performed to exclude regional wall motion abnormalities and associated mitral insufficiency. In appropriate age groups, coronary arteriography is necessary to exclude coronary artery disease.

Data Evaluation and Recommendations

Because of excellent noninvasive techniques, it is rare that catheterization provides surprising information in patients with isolated mitral stenosis. In all patients with chest pain or other findings suggesting ischemia as well as in all men over 35 and women over 40 years of age, coronary angiography is recommended. Obviously, a review of coronary angiography and a decision as to the need for concomitant coronary artery bypass surgery is important, as is a discussion with the surgeon as to whether or not the patient can be treated with valve repair rather than valve replacement. Today, nonoperative balloon valvuloplasty is a rational option in patients who refuse operation or are not good candidates for surgery.

Consideration should be given to the degree of pulmonary hypertension and pulmonary vascular resistance. If they are out of proportion to the degree of mitral obstruction, primary pulmonary vascular disease, chronic lung disease, and recurrent pulmonary emboli (perhaps from a chronically fibrillating right atrium or dilated right ventricle) should be considered. When marked pulmonary hypertension and elevated pulmonary vascular resistance are due to severe mitral stenosis, the pulmonary hemodynamic abnormalities are expected to improve postoperatively (64,

65). However, it may be necessary for the surgeon to decide intraoperatively which patient will require tricuspid repair, since the ultimate reduction in pulmonary hypertension may not occur immediately after the mitral obstruction is alleviated. Intraoperative Doppler echocardiography has been used to help decide when to perform tricuspid valvuloplasty (66).

It has been suggested that a chronically deprived preload or smoldering, subclinical rheumatic myocarditis may cause reduced left ventricular contractility in mitral stenosis. However, left ventricular ejection fraction is usually normal or only slightly reduced. When ejection fraction is decreased, it is often associated with decreased end-systolic wall thickness as well as increased peripheral vascular resistance, in which case the resultant increase in afterload may reduce left ventricular systolic performance (67).

MITRAL INSUFFICIENCY

Clinical Presentation and Pathophysiology

The mitral valve is anatomically a complex structure with six component parts including the left atrium, annulus, leaflets, chordae, papillary muscles, and left ventricular free wall (68). Malfunction of any component can result in mitral insufficiency. The left atrial endocardium is continuous with the posterior mitral leaflet. As left atrial size increases, tension is transmitted to this leaflet, producing mitral insufficiency. Accordingly, when mitral insufficiency from any cause results in left atrial enlargement, this will further increase the degree of regurgitation. The mitral annulus is a dynamic structure that can produce mitral insufficiency when it dilates or does not contract adequately during systole. Functional mitral insufficiency can result from left ventricular and annular dilation, or when the annulus calcifies and loses its systolic contraction. Mitral annular calcification occurs most often as an elderly (degenerative) form and in long-standing left ventricular pressure overload (hypertension, aortic stenosis). Mitral annular calcification is also seen in various metabolic disorders including diabetes,

Marfan's syndrome, and chronic renal failure with secondary hyperparathyroidism.

Because of its almost rectangular shape, the posterior mitral leaflet is subjected to more tension during left ventricular emptying and therefore is more often affected by changes in the fibrous skeleton of the heart. The anterior mitral leaflet has no fibrous support, being an extension of the posterior aortic wall. The proximity of the anterior mitral leaflet to the aortic valve and supporting structures, however, predisposes it to secondary involvement from aortic valve endocarditis.

Rupture of one or more chorda tendineae may cause acute or chronic mitral insufficiency. The chorda may rupture due to chronic degenerative changes in the elderly, fibrocalcific changes secondary to pressure overloads, myxomatous degeneration as part of the mitral valve prolapse syndrome, or as a complication of bacterial endocarditis.

The anterolateral and posteromedial papillary muscles are frequently involved in acute and chronic mitral insufficiency. Each papillary muscle supports both mitral leaflets. If there is rupture of the belly or the head of either papillary muscle, massive mitral insufficiency is produced causing shock or fulminate pulmonary edema. This condition is usually rapidly fatal without emergency surgical intervention. Rupture of a secondary or tertiary chorda causes subacute mitral insufficiency, which is better tolerated. The base of the papillary muscles is attached to the free wall of the left ventricle and this connection is frequently affected in ischemic heart disease. This may occur in patients with coronary artery disease who have low ejection fractions and high left ventricular filling pressures. Acute or chronic ischemia of the left ventricular free wall results in regional wall motion abnormalities, preventing proper apposition of the papillary muscles with resultant mitral insufficiency. Primary myocardial disease, typified by the dilated, congestive cardiomyopathy, results in a spherically shaped ventricle, causing similar malposition of the papillary muscles and a varying degree of mitral insufficiency.

Mitral insufficiency is a classic volume overload of the left ventricle. Acutely, this results in increased sarcomere length and left ventricular size (Frank-Starling compensation). Chronically, eccentric left ventricular hypertrophy is an important compensatory mechanism (69–71). The degree of mitral insufficiency depends on the size of the regurgitant orifice, duration of the systolic ejection period, the gradient between the left ventricle and left atrium during ejection, and the relative impedances of the aorta and left atrium (72).

Chronic, compensated mitral insufficiency is not associated with increased left ventricular wall stress. Indeed, it may be reduced because the left ventricular stroke volume can empty into a low pressure left atrium (70). While this escape valve prevents excessive left ventricular wall stress, it complicates the assessment of left ventricular systolic function. Chronic mitral insufficiency affects cardiac pump function in opposing ways. The long-standing volume overload eventually results in reduced myocardial contractile function and cardiac failure. On the other hand, the presence of a low pressure left atrium escape valve prevents an increase in left ventricular systolic wall stress or afterload, at least early in the course of this valve lesion. As a result, ejection phase indices of left ventricular systolic function, which are sensitive to changes in afterload such as the ejection fraction, are unreliable in this setting (73, 74). In mitral insufficiency, the ejection fraction is increased or normal until very late in the course of the disease. When there is a minimal decrease in ejection fraction, there is usually extensive reduction in myocardial contractility (75). The patient with reduced or marginal global left ventricular ejection fraction may significantly worsen after mitral valve replacement as left ventricular wall stress increases (12, 76, 77).

Precardiac Catheterization Noninvasive Assessment

Two-dimensional echocardiography allows a visual assessment of each of the six components of the mitral valve apparatus, thereby helping to establish etiology. Left atrial size can be determined, which aids in establishing whether the mitral insufficiency is acute or chronic. Associated valvular lesions can be identified and overall left ventricular ejection fraction estimated. The presence of regional wall motion abnormalities suggests concomitant coronary artery disease.

Doppler echocardiography is particularly helpful in identifying acute mitral insufficiency, in which case emergent therapy is required even before cardiac catheterization can be performed. Following an acute myocardial infarction, the sudden development of pulmonary edema may indicate a mechanical complication such as rupture of a chorda tendineae. Echocardiography can demonstrate the flail mitral leaflet and the paradox of a well-maintained left ventricular ejection fraction despite pulmonary edema. This information may lead to hemodynamic monitoring and institution of vasodilator therapy or intraaortic balloon counter pulsation prior to cardiac catheterization. Even in the absence of echocardiographically demonstrated flail leaflet, Doppler assessment can provide clues as to the acuteness of the mitral insufficiency (Fig. 28.21).

In a more general sense, Doppler echocardiography is useful in semiquantitation of the degree of mitral insufficiency. The pulsed Doppler method allows an interrogation of the atrial side of the mitral valve. When a high velocity systolic flow jet is detected, the probe is moved progressively posterior in the left atrium to determine the extent of mitral insufficiency (Fig. 28.22). The further back in the left atrium that the mitral insufficiency jet is detected, the greater the degree of mitral insufficiency suggested. Multiple views are explored to map the extent of mitral insufficiency in three dimensions. The technique is limited, however, by the eccentricity or broad nature of some regurgitant jets and the varying geometry of the left atrium. For example, if a severe degree of regurgitation is moving in a very broad front and into a large left atrium, the degree of mitral insufficiency may be detected much less posteriorly than expected. In general, mitral insufficiency can be accurately classified using this technique, and moderately severe or severe mitral insufficiency is rarely missed (78). The most promising results have come from Doppler color flow imaging by comparing the area of the regurgitant color Doppler signal with the area of the left atrium in orthogonal views (Fig. 28.23). Correlation coefficients as high as 0.87 have been found between Doppler and angiographic estimates of severity (79).

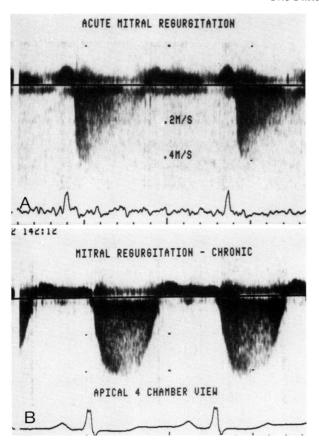

Figure 28.21. Conventional continuous wave, Doppler-obtained velocity envelopes, demonstrating the difference between acute (*A*) and chronic (*B*) mitral insufficiency.

Information Obtained at the Time of Cardiac Catheterization

An elevation of the mean right atrial pressure suggests right-sided volume overload from congestive heart failure, tricuspid insufficiency, or very rarely, coincidental pericardial disease. The presence of tricuspid insufficiency may indicate significant pulmonary hypertension from long-standing mitral insufficiency and a need for tricuspid valve replacement or repair at the time of mitral valve surgery. Right atrial mean pressure may also be elevated in tricuspid stenosis, which may accompany rheumatic mitral valve disease. In this setting, the elevated mean pressure will be associated with a large right atrial A wave in contrast to tricuspid insufficiency which is associated with a large V wave or C-V (regurgitant) wave. Right ventricular systolic pressure is documented, and if elevated, pulmonary hypertension or associated pulmonic

stenosis is suspected. Advancing the catheter across the pulmonic valve will differentiate these two etiologies. Accurate measurement of pulmonary artery pressure is important.

If acute mitral insufficiency is present, the regurgitant V wave may be transmitted back through a small left atrium across the pulmonary vascular bed into the pulmonary arteries. In that situation, the V wave may be present in the pulmonary artery pressure tracing. The demonstration of such a wave interrupting the normal diastolic descent of the pulmonary artery wave form strongly suggests acute and chronic mitral insufficiency (80). However, this finding is frequently absent when mitral insufficiency is severe.

The height of the V wave in the pulmonary wedge pressure tracing is not always helpful in determining the severity of chronic mitral insufficiency. In this setting, a large, compliant left atrium can absorb a tremendous regur-

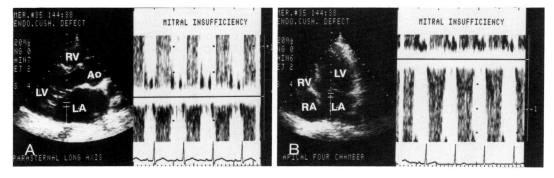

Figure 28.22. Doppler echocardiogram using conventional pulsed wave Doppler to detect mitral insufficiency. *A,* Parasternal long axis view. *B,* Apical four-chamber view. *Ao,* aorta; *LA,* left atrium; *LV,* left ventricle; *RA,* right atrium; *RV,* right ventricle.

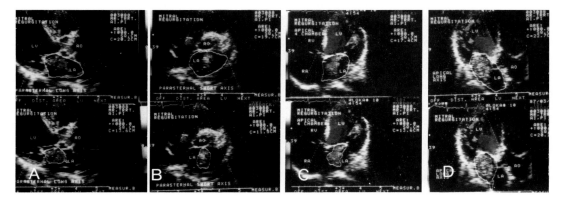

Figure 28.23. Doppler color flow imaging demonstrating mitral insufficiency. The severity of the mitral insufficiency is estimated by determining the ratio of the area of the Doppler signal in the left atrium to the area of the left atrium obtained from four orthogonal views. *A,* Parasternal long-axis view. *B,* Parasternal short-axis view. *C,* Apical four-chamber view. *D,* Apical long-axis view. *Ao,* aorta; *LA,* left atrium; *LV,* left ventricle; *RA,* right atrium; *RV,* right ventricle.

gitant jet without a significant increase in left atrial (pulmonary-capillary wedge) V wave. In a study of 37 patients with angiographically proven severe mitral insufficiency, 16 (43%) had large V waves, and in 12 (32%) the V wave was trivial (81). Pichard et al. evaluated multiple hemodynamic and echocardiographic variables in groups of patients with and without mitral insufficiency and found that only the slope of the ascent of the V wave distinguished the two groups (82). The size of the V wave is a function of not only regurgitant volume, but also the left atrial size and compliance, and the left atrial pressure-volume relationship prior to the onset of systole, among other factors. Other causes of large V waves in the absence of mitral insufficiency waves include ventricular septal defect, congestive heart failure, and very rarely, mitral obstruction (including mitral stenosis).

With the pulmonary artery catheter in place, systemic arterial pressure is recorded and a ventriculography catheter advanced into the left ventricle. Simultaneous left ventricular and pulmonary-capillary wedge pressures are recorded, looking for a transmitral gradient. With severe mitral insufficiency, transmitral flow is so severely increased that even a nor-

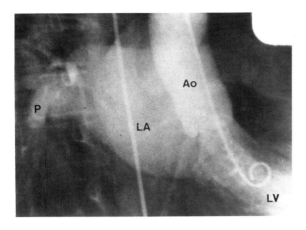

Figure 28.24. 30° right anterior oblique view of a left ventriculogram showing reflux of contrast material through a dilated left atrium (*LA*) into pulmonary veins (*P*). *Ao*, ascending aorta; *LV*, left ventricle.

mal valve area is relatively stenotic. In contrast to mitral stenosis, there will be no significant mid- or late-diastolic gradient, and the mean transmitral gradient is trivial. For practical purposes, this should not be a problem of discrimination in the catheterization laboratory, since precatheterization echocardiography is quite accurate in excluding associated mitral stenosis. As soon as the mitral valve gradient is obtained, pulmonary and systemic pressures are again measured, and cardiac output determinations are made. Pulmonary and systemic vascular resistances can now be computed and the mitral valve area calculated.

Left ventriculography is performed in a biplane (30° right anterior oblique; 60° left anterior oblique) or monoplane mode (30° right anterior oblique projection). In these views, an accurate estimation of the degree of contrast material regurgitated into the left atrium and ventricular volume measurements can be made. Through an appropriate ventriculography catheter, sufficient contrast agent must be injected to fully opacify the left ventricle at a rate of injection that does not cause significant ventricular ectopy. Ectopic beats should not be used in the determination of ventricular volumes or qualitative assessment of wall motion in order to avoid postextrasystolic potentiation of contractility. Also, the presence of premature ventricular beats, particularly in runs, can cause reflux of the contrast agent into the left atrium, resulting in pseudomitral insufficiency, or can increase the degree of mitral insufficiency, causing an overestimate of the actual severity.

Reflux of contrast material into the left atrium that results in faint opacification of the atrium, clearing with each beat, is judged 1 +, and correlates roughly with a regurgitant fraction of <20%. If cardiac rates are different at the time of ventriculography and forward cardiac output determination, comparative stroke volumes should be used in determining the regurgitant fraction.

When the regurgitant jet opacifies the left atrium and does not clear with each beat, but is less than the opacification of the left ventricle, a grade of 2 + is applied. This generally indicates moderate mitral insufficiency and a regurgitant fraction of 20 to 40%. A designation of 3 + mitral insufficiency indicates that the opacification of the left atrium is equal to that of the left ventricle, and calculated regurgitant fractions typically range from 40 to 60%. Finally, 4 + or severe mitral insufficiency is present when the entire left atrium opacifies with a single beat, progressively opacifies, or when the contrast agent refluxes back into the pulmonary veins (Fig. 28.24). In such cases, a regurgitant fraction of greater than 60% will be calculated.

Several technical factors may cause a discrepancy between the qualitative assessment of the degree of mitral insufficiency and the calculated regurgitant fraction (see Chapter 24). If the blood pressure is different at the time of forward cardiac output measurement than at the time of ventriculography, calculation of regurgitant fraction is not reliable. Arrhythmias, such as atrial fibrillation, left atrial dilation, and inaccurate cardiac output determinations, are also sources of discrepancy. The angiographic cardiac output of the left ventricle may be responsible for the discrepancy if the patient also has associated

Table 28.3.
Predictors of a Suboptimal Response to Mitral Valve Replacement for Chronic Mitral Insufficiency

	Value	Reference
Echocardiography		
LV^a shortening fraction	<0.32	84
End-diastolic dimension index	>40 mm/m^2	84
End-systolic dimension	>50 mm	76
End-systolic dimension index	>26 mm/m^2	84
Cardiac catheterization		
Subnormal LV ejection fraction	≤0.55	83
Elevated LV end-diastolic pressure	>12 mm Hg	86
Large LV end-systolic volume	>60 cc/m^2	85
Large LV end-diastolic volume	>220 cc/m^2	87
LV end-systolic stress/volume ratio	<2.5	77

^{a} LV, left ventricular.

aortic insufficiency. In this case, the total angiographic cardiac output will reflect both aortic and mitral insufficiency and the calculated regurgitant fraction will be an overestimate of the actual degree of mitral insufficiency. Finally, the inherent errors in valve area calculation and cardiac output computation are potential sources of discrepancy.

Data Evaluation and Recommendations

In chronic mitral insufficiency, patients may be asymptomatic despite a significant reduction in left ventricular contractile function. Noninvasive techniques including echocardiography, Doppler color flow imaging, and radionuclear studies are useful adjuncts to patient history and physical diagnosis in assessing left ventricular function. Normalization of what should be supernormal left ventricular systolic function would support cardiac catheterization even in an asymptomatic patient. Exercise treadmill testing is at times useful in convincing a patient who denies symptoms that in fact his or her cardiovascular fitness is subnormal.

Because of the low-pressure, low-impedance left atrium, patients with mitral insufficiency may have normal appearing systolic performance despite reduced myocardial contractility. When the insufficient mitral valve is made competent at the time of surgery, the underlying reduced contractility may be unmasked. Accordingly, considerable research has been aimed at determining at what point patients with mitral insufficiency

fail to improve left ventricular function following mitral valve replacement (Table 28.3). A normal or subnormal preoperative global left ventricular ejection fraction usually predicts a suboptimal surgical result (83). This may also be true for patients with above normal ejection fractions, which are artificially maintained by the low systolic wall stress. Using echocardiography, Zile et al. have shown that mitral insufficiency patients with an end-systolic left ventricular internal diameter >26 mm/m^2, an end-diastolic dimension >40 mm/m^2, or shortening fraction <32% had a suboptimal response to mitral valve replacement (84). Borow et al. found that a left ventricular end-systolic volume <60 cc/m^2 resulted in postoperative New York Heart Association class I or II, but that patients with left ventricular end-systolic volumes >60 cc/m^2 frequently were class III or IV following valve replacement (54).

The use of end-systolic stress/end-systolic volume **ratio** has allowed good discrimination of surgical outcome in patients with chronic mitral insufficiency. This index, which is relatively independent of preload and adjustable for afterload, is a better estimate of myocardial contractility in altered loading states such as mitral insufficiency (73). A ratio of <2.5 was associated with a poor surgical result, even in the face of a normal ejection fraction. Mitral valve replacement was successful with a good postoperative functional state when the ratio exceeded 2.5 (77).

Patients with mitral insufficiency who are symptomatic should undergo cardiac catheterization. A recommendation for surgery is based on a full review of all data with major emphasis on left ventricular contractile performance. If associated coronary artery disease is demonstrated, coronary artery bypass surgery should be performed at the time of mitral valve replacement or repair.

Asymptomatic mitral insufficiency patients with reduced left ventricular systolic function by noninvasive studies should undergo catheterization. Patients in whom serial noninvasive studies indicate decreasing left ventricular systolic function even in the absence of symptoms should undergo cardiac catheterization. Noninvasive and cardiac catheterization data, particularly end-systolic parameters of left ventricular function, are useful adjuncts to clinical judgment when recommending mitral valve replacement or repair in such patients (85). In general, a recommendation for surgery occurs earlier than symptoms might direct, due to the realization that valve replacement or repair is less successful once myocardial contractility has decreased (86).

TRICUSPID STENOSIS

Obstruction to tricuspid inflow occurs in rheumatic heart disease virtually always with associated mitral valve involvement and occasionally secondary to prosthetic valve dysfunction, in which case the prosthesis has been placed for tricuspid insufficiency. As the frequency of rheumatic heart disease has decreased and surgeons have utilized tricuspid valvoplasty to repair tricuspid insufficiency, the incidence of tricuspid stenosis has steadily declined.

Elevated right atrial filling pressures and low cardiac output are the hemodynamic hallmarks of tricuspid stenosis. Unlike tricuspid insufficiency, which is characterized by an elevated mean pressure and large V or regurgitant wave, tricuspid stenosis manifests a large right atrial A wave as long as the patient is in sinus rhythm. Atrial fibrillation frequently develops, making exact measurement of transvalvular gradient and tricuspid valve area difficult. The gradient across the tricuspid valve is usually determined at the time of pullback of a catheter from the right ventricle to the right atrium, or by simultaneous measurement of right atrial and right ventricular pressure.

The performance of precatheterization echo/Doppler studies will greatly facilitate the catheterization evaluation of patients with suspected rheumatic heart disease by uncovering a lesion such as tricuspid stenosis. At times, the tricuspid valve area can be better estimated noninvasively because of the atrial fibrillation and low holodiastolic gradient mentioned above. Consequently, a combined noninvasive and invasive evaluation is recommended. When cardiac catheterization and noninvasive data are combined, it is unlikely that the surgeon will be faced with an unexpected finding of significant tricuspid stenosis.

TRICUSPID INSUFFICIENCY

Most tricuspid insufficiency is functional, secondary to dilation of the tricuspid annulus as a result of right ventricular dilation, which itself is most often due to pulmonary hypertension. Any cause of left ventricular failure that results in chronic pulmonary hypertension can cause the right ventricle to dilate, with a variable degree of tricuspid insufficiency, even with an anatomically normal valve. Organic tricuspid insufficiency occurs with infective endocarditis or secondary to anterior chest trauma. In the latter case, the tricuspid insufficiency is due to right ventricular myocardial contusion and/or disruption of the tricuspid apparatus.

Noninvasive assessment is useful in quantitating the degree of tricuspid insufficiency, perhaps underestimated on physical examination because of more prominent left heart murmurs. Echocardiography excludes anatomical disruption of the valve and can demonstrate valvular vegetations. This information is helpful in planning catheterization, since catheter passage through the right heart could cause embolization of the vegetation. Pulsed Doppler mapping of the tricuspid insufficiency jet in the right atrium is done in a manner previously described for aortic and mitral insufficiency (Fig. 28.25). As was true with aortic and mitral insufficiency, quantitation of tricuspid insufficiency on the basis of color flow Doppler has yielded generally excellent correlation with angiographic assessment (87).

As mentioned earlier, the velocity shift across the tricuspid valve in tricuspid insufficiency allows an estimate of the right ventric-

Figure 28.25. Doppler echocardiogram in the apical four-chamber view. Using conventional pulsed wave Doppler and sampling in the right atrium, tricuspid insufficiency is detected. *RA,* right atrium; *RV,* right ventricle.

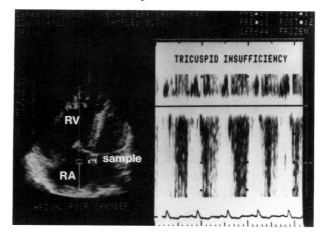

ular systolic pressure. The Doppler shift at that level is added to an estimation of right atrial mean pressure, made by an observation of neck veins (Fig. 28.19).

At the time of cardiac catheterization, tricuspid insufficiency is demonstrated by the presence of elevated right atrial mean pressures and a large V wave in the right atrial pressure tracing. As is true for mitral insufficiency, the height of the V wave is affected by the patient's rhythm, forcefulness of right ventricular contractility, and most importantly, the size of the right atrium.

When the V wave is two or three times greater than the right atrial mean pressure, severe tricuspid insufficiency probably exists. In this case, the right atrium is not enlarged and is unable to accommodate the regurgitant jet without a marked increase in pressure. The absence of a large V wave, however, in the face of a dilated right atrium, does not exclude severe tricuspid insufficiency. Patients with atrial fibrillation and moderate right ventricular volume overload may have a larger than normal V wave even without tricuspid insufficiency. This is distinguished from the regurgitant V wave of tricuspid insufficiency by its timing. The regurgitant wave occurs earlier and blends in with the later occurring antegrade V wave that is secondary to forward vena caval flow.

As the catheter is passed through the right ventricle and into the pulmonary vascular bed, one would expect to find pulmonary hypertension. When pulmonary hypertension is absent, primary tricuspid valve disease or associated complex congenital disorders

such as Ebstein's anomaly of the tricuspid valve are suggested. Pericardial disease may cause a similar elevation of right atrial pressure with normal pulmonary artery pressures. In the case of pericardial disease, however, the characteristic tricuspid insufficiency V wave would be absent, and right heart pressures would reveal equalization of diastolic pressures.

Cineangiography is performed in the right anterior oblique view with sufficient volume to opacify the dilated right heart chambers, but at a rate of injection that does not cause ventricular ectopy.

With the catheter placed across the tricuspid valve artifactual tricuspid insufficiency, secondary to a regurgitant orifice created by the catheter itself, will be present. For this reason, right ventricular angiography is not usually performed unless hemodynamic or noninvasive data conflict with the precatheterization clinical impression.

PULMONIC STENOSIS AND PULMONIC INSUFFICIENCY

These valvular lesions generally occur as part of complex congenital heart disease (Chapter 29) or in the case of pulmonary insufficiency, secondary to severe pulmonary hypertension. In the case of pulmonic stenosis, the obstruction may be valvular, subvalvular, or supravalvular, the last of which may be associated with pulmonary artery branch stenosis. It is often difficult to determine the exact position of the pulmonic stenosis at the time of

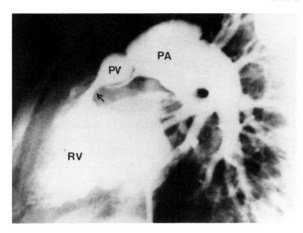

Figure 28.26. Right ventriculogram in a lateral projection of a 20-year-old woman with Noonan's syndrome. *Solid arrow* points to the narrowed right ventricular outflow tract (infundibular stenosis). Superior to the infundibular stenosis, a domed pulmonic valve (*PV*) with marked poststenotic dilation of the pulmonary artery (*PA*) is demonstrated. *RV,* right ventricle.

right heart catheter pullback; consequently, right ventricular angiography is performed in a view that delineates the right ventricular outflow tract, pulmonic valve, and (by way of pulmonary angiography) pulmonary branch stenosis. Figure 28.26 demonstrates pulmonic and infundibular stenosis in a 20-year-old patient with Noonan's syndrome. Doming of the pulmonic valve and poststenotic dilation of the pulmonary artery are well demonstrated.

Usually in severe pulmonary stenosis, right atrial filling pressures are elevated with a prominent A wave, especially when the right ventricular systolic pressure exceeds 60 mm Hg (Fig. 28.27*A*). An A wave will not be present, however, if atrial fibrillation has developed. The exact location of right ventricular outflow tract or pulmonary valvular obstruction is demonstrated by a slow pullback of an end-hole catheter with simultaneous fluoroscopy and pressure measurement (Fig. 28.27*B* and *C*). Cineangiography is usually performed in the anteroposterior and lateral (Fig. 28.27*D*) views.

Pulmonary insufficiency is generally secondary to pulmonary hypertension. The right ventricle must absorb the volume overload resulting from blood regurgitated back from the pulmonary vascular bed as well as that entering the right ventricle antegradely across the tricuspid valve. As a result, right ventricular dilation and a varying degree of right ventricular end-diastolic pressure elevation, depending on the compliance of that chamber, will be seen. Because of catheter-pro-

duced artifact, cineangiography is generally not useful in pulmonary insufficiency.

Estimation of pulmonary artery systolic pressure, semiquantitative assessment of the degree of pulmonary insufficiency, and anatomical evaluation of the pulmonic valve are facilitated by echo/Doppler studies (Fig. 28.28). Although pulmonary insufficiency is usually functional, we have seen cases of pulmonic valve endocarditis, secondary to intravenous drug abuse, resulting in significant pulmonic insufficiency.

SUMMARY

The evaluation of a patient with valvular heart disease begins with an accurate history and thorough physical examination. Following this, the physician typically orders one or more noninvasive studies, which usually confirm and help the diagnosis and help answer important management questions such as the need for bacterial endocarditis prophylaxis and the timing of invasive diagnostic and therapeutic procedures.

Throughout this chapter, we have emphasized that these noninvasive procedures complement and extend the information obtained at the time of cardiac catheterization. In the case of the chronic regurgitant lesions, for example, serial measurements of left ventricular systolic performance aid in the proper timing of both cardiac catheterization and valve replacement. In the acutely ill, decompensated patient with valvular heart disease, these noninvasive procedures are even more

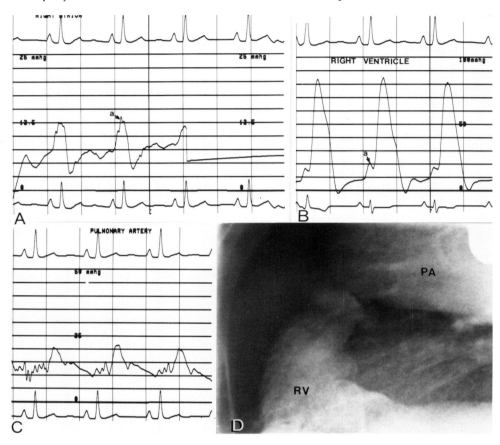

Figure 28.27. *A,* Right atrial phasic and mean tracing of a 56-year-old man with valvular pulmonic stenosis. Although the right atrial mean pressure is normal at 6 mm Hg, a prominent A wave is present (designated *a* at the *arrow*). *B,* Right ventricular tracing of the same patient in *A.* Right ventricular systolic pressure is markedly elevated at 66 mm Hg, with a prominent A wave (designated *a* at the *arrow*). *C,* Distal to the pulmonic valve, pulmonary artery pressures are normal (22/10 mm Hg), yielding a peak-to-peak gradient across the pulmonic valve of 45 mm Hg. *D,* Right ventricular angiogram in the lateral projection, of the same patient from *A, B,* and *C.* The infundibulum is not narrowed; however, the valve leaflets are domed and there is very severe poststenotic dilation of the pulmonary artery. *RV,* right ventricle; *PA,* pulmonary artery.

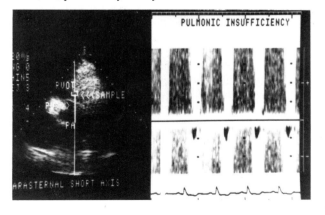

Figure 28.28. Doppler echocardiogram in the parasternal short-axis view. Using conventional pulsed wave Doppler and sampling in the right ventricular outflow tract, pulmonary insufficiency is detected. *PA,* pulmonary artery; *PV,* pulmonary valve; *RVOT,* right ventricular outflow tract.

important. Such patients do not tolerate prolonged catheterization procedures associated with the injection of large amounts of contrast agents. By appropriately utilizing these noninvasive techniques, the cardiac catheterization protocol can be modified to minimize risks, while at the same time, obtaining all of the information needed to make proper management decisions. It is the integration of these noninvasive and cardiac catheterization data that allow for optimal diagnosis and management of the patient with valvular heart disease.

We close this chapter with a word of caution. Despite impressive technological advances in both noninvasive and invasive techniques, clinical judgment remains of paramount importance. The patient with valvular heart disease is not optimally served by an undue reliance on any single noninvasive or invasive measurement. Finally, application of any of these techniques requires confidence in one's own noninvasive and invasive laboratories, emphasizing the need for ongoing quality control in these facilities.

References

1. Roberts WC. The congenitally bicuspid aortic valve—a study of 85 autopsy cases. Am J Cardiol 1970;26:72–79.
2. Finoglio JJ, McAllister HA, DeCastro CM, Davia JE, Cheitlin ME. Congenital bicuspid aortic valve after age 20. Am J Cardiol 1977;39:164–172.
3. Grossman W, Jones D, McLaurin LP. Wall stress and patterns of hypertrophy in the human left ventricle. J Clin Invest 1975;56:56–64.
4. Sasayama S, Ross J Jr, Franklin D, Bloor CM, Bishop S, Dilley RB. Adaptations of the left ventricle to chronic pressure overload. Circ Res 1976;38:172–180.
5. Gunther S, Grossman W. Determinants of ventricular function in pressure-overload hypertrophy in man. Circulation 1979;59:679–688.
6. Spann JF, Bove AA, Natarajan G, Kreulen T. Ventricular performance, pump function and compensatory mechanisms in patients with aortic stenosis. Circulation 1980;62:576–584.
7. Donner R, Carabello BA, Black I, Spann JF. Left ventricular wall stress in compensated aortic stenosis in children. Am J Cardiol 1983;51:946–951.
8. Assey ME, Wisenbaugh T, Spann JF Jr, Gillette PC, Carabello BA. Unexpected persistence into adulthood of low wall stress in congenital aortic stenosis: Is there a fundamental difference in hypertrophy response to a pressure overload present from birth rather than acquired? Circulation 1987;75:973–979.
9. Murakami T, Hess OM, Gage JE, Grimm J, Krayenbuehl HP. Diastolic filling dynamics in patients with aortic stenosis. Circulation 1986;73:1162–1170.
10. Peterson KL, Tauji J, Johnson A, DiDonna J, LeWintere M. Diastolic left ventricular pressure-volume and stress-strain relationships in patients with valvular aortic stenosis and left ventricular hypertrophy. Circulation 1978;58:77–89.
11. Pantely G, Morton M, Rahimtoola SH. Effects of successful, uncomplicated valve replacement on ventricular hypertrophy, volume and performance in aortic stenosis and in aortic competence. J Thorac Cardiovasc Surg 1978;75:383–391.
12. Kennedy JW, Doces J, Stewart DK. Left ventricular function before and following aortic valve replacement. Circulation 1977;56:944–950.
13. Frank S, Johnson A, Ross J Jr. Natural history of valvular aortic stenosis. Br Heart J 1973;35:41–49.
14. Morrow AG, Roberts WC, Ross J Jr, et al. Clinical staff conference. Obstruction to left ventricular outflow. Current concepts of management and operative treatment. Ann Intern Med 1968;69:1255–1261.
15. Tobin JR, Rahimtoola SH, Blundell PE, Swan HJC. Percentage of left ventricular stroke work loss, a simple hemodynamic concept for estimation of severity in valvular aortic stenosis. Circulation 1968;35:868–879.
16. Ross J Jr, Braunwald E. The influence of corrective operations on natural history of aortic stenosis. Circulation 1968;37:V61–V66.
17. Chizner MA, Pearle DL, deLeon AC. The natural history of aortic stenosis in adults. Am Heart J 1980;99:419–424.
18. Ross J Jr. Afterload mismatch and preload reserve: a conceptual framework for the analysis of ventricular function. Prog Cardiovasc Dis 1976;18:255–261.
19. Croke RP, Pifane R, Sullivan H, Gunnar R, Loeb H. Reversal of advanced left ventricular dysfunction following aortic valve replacement for aortic stenosis. Ann Thorac Surg 1977;24:38–43.
20. Hatle L, Angelsen B. Doppler ultrasound in cardiology - physical principals and clinical applications. 2nd ed. Philadelphia: Lea and Febiger, 1985:22.
21. Handshoe R, DeMaria AN. Doppler assessment of intracardiac pressures. Echocardiography 1985;2:127–139.
22. Richards KL, Cannon SR, Miller JF, Crawford MH. Calculation of aortic valve area by Doppler echocardiography: a direct application of the continuity equation. Circulation 1986;73:964–969.
23. Oh JK, Tajik AJ, Taliercio CP, Holmes DR, Reader GS, Seward JB. Prediction of severity of aortic stenosis by simple Doppler velocity measurements: correlation with catheterization in 100 patients (abstr). J Am Coll Cardiol 1987;9:236A.
24. Peller OG, Wallerson DC, Devereux RB. Role of Doppler and imaging echocardiography in selection of patients for cardiac valvular surgery. Am Heart J 1987;114:1445–1460.
25. Hakki AH, Kimbiris D, Iskandrian AS, Segal BL, Mintz GS, Bemis CE. Angina pectoris and coronary artery disease in patients with severe aortic valvular disease. Am Heart J 1980;100:441–449.
26. Richardson JV, Kouchoukos NT, Wright JO, Karp, RB. Combined aortic valve replacement and

myocardial revascularization: results in 220 patients. Circulation 1979;59:75–83.

27. Kirklin JW, Barratt-Boyes BG. Aortic valve disease. In: Cardiac surgery. New York: John Wiley & Sons, 1986:374–420.

28. Bonow RO, Kent KM, Rosing DR, et al. Aortic valve replacement without myocardial revascularization in patients with combined aortic valvular stenosis and coronary artery disease. Circulation 1981;63:243–251.

29. McKay RG, Safian RD, Berman AD, et al. Combined percutaneous aortic valvuloplasty and transluminal coronary angioplasty in adult patients with calcific aortic stenosis and coronary artery disease. Circulation 1987;76:1298–1306.

30. Folland ED, Parisi AF, Carbone C. Is peripheral arterial pressure a reliable substitute for ascending aortic pressure when measuring aortic valve gradients? J Am Coll Cardiol 1984;4:1207–1214.

31. Carabello BA, Barry WH, Grossman W. Changes in arterial pressure during left heart pullback in patients with aortic stenosis: A sign of severe aortic stenosis. Am J Cardiol 1979;44:424–430.

32. Gorlin R, Gorlin SG. Hydraulic formula for calculation of stenotic mitral valve, other cardiac valves and central circulatory shunts. Am Heart J 1951;41:1-19.

33. Cannon SR, Richards KL, Crawford M. Hydraulic estimation of stenotic orifice area: a correction of the Gorlin formula. Circulation 1985;71:1170–1178.

34. Hakki AH, Iskandrian AS, Bemis CE, et al. A simplified valve formula for the calculation of stenotic cardiac valve areas. Circulation 1981;63:1050-1056.

35. Angel J, Soler-Soler J, Anivarro I, Domingo E. Hemodynamic evaluation of stenotic cardiac valves: II. Modification of the simplified valve formula for mitral and aortic valve areas calculation. Cathet Cardiovasc Diagn 1985;11:127–138.

36. Henry WL, Bonow RO, Borer JS, et al. Evaluation of aortic valve replacement in patients with valvular aortic stenosis. Circulation 1980;61:814–825.

37. Smith N, McAnulty JH, Rahimtoola SH. Severe aortic stenosis with impaired left ventricular function and clinical heart failure: results of valve replacement. Circulation 1978;58:255–264.

38. McKay RG, Safian RD, Lock JE, et al. Assessment of left ventricular and aortic valve function after aortic balloon valvuloplasty in adult patients with critical aortic stenosis. Circulation 1987;75:192–200.

39 Carabello BA, Green LH, Grossman W, et al. Hemodynamic determinants of prognosis of aortic valve replacement in critical aortic stenosis and advanced congestive heart failure. Circulation 1980;62:42–48.

40. Wyman RM, Berman AD, Saffian et al. Balloon aortic valvuloplasty in patients with critical aortic stenosis and a low gradient (abstr). Circulation 1987;76:IV–75.

41. Kelly TA, Rothbart RM, Cooper CM, Kaiser DL, Smucker ML, Gibson RS. Comparison of outcome of asymptomatic to symptomatic patients older than 20 years of age with valvular aortic stenosis. Am J Cardiol 1988;61:123–130.

42. Wisenbaugh T, Spann JF, Carabello BA. Differences in myocardial performance and load between patients with similar amounts of chronic aortic ver-

sus chronic mitral regurgitation. J Am Coll Cardiol 1984;3:916–923.

43. Sapira JD. Quincke, de Musset, Duroziez, Hill: Some aortic regurgitations. South Med J 1981; 74:459–467.

44. Matsuo H, Morita T, Senda S, Kitabatake A, Chihara K, Sakurai Y. Noninvasive visualization and estimation of severity of aortic regurgitation by multigated pulsed Doppler technique. In: Spencer MP, ed. Cardiac Doppler diagnosis. Boston: Martinus-Nijhoff, 1983:281.

45. Kitabatake A, Masuyama T, Asao M, et al. Color visualization of two dimensional distribution of intracardiac flow abnormalities by multigate Doppler technique. In: Spencer MP, ed. Cardiac Doppler diagnosis. Boston: Martinus-Nijhoff, 1983: 309.

46. Perry GJ, Helmcke F, Nanda NC, Byard C, Soto B. Evaluation of aortic insufficiency by Doppler color flow mapping. J Am Coll Cardiol 1987;9:952–959.

47. Teague SM, Heinsimer JA, Anderson JL, et al. Quantification of aortic regurgitation utilizing continuous wave Doppler ultrasound. J Am Coll Cardiol 1986;8:592–599.

48. Carabello BA, Usher BW, Hendrix GH, Assey ME, Crawford FA, Leman RB. Predictors of outcome for aortic valve replacement in patients with aortic regurgitation and left ventricular dysfunction: a change in the measuring stick. J Am Coll Cardiol 1987;10:991–997.

49. Henry WL, Bonow RO, Borer JS, et al. Observations on the optimum time for operative intervention for aortic regurgitation. I. Evaluation of the results of aortic valve replacement in symptomatic patients. Circulation 1980;61:471–483.

50. Gaasch WH, Carroll JD, Levine HJ, Criscitiello MG. Chronic aortic regurgitation: prognostic value of left ventricular end-systolic dimension and end-diastolic radius/thickness ratio. J Am Coll Cardiol 1983;1:775–782.

51. Samuels DA, Curfman GD, Friedlich AL, Buckley MJ, Austen WG. Valve replacement for aortic regurgitation: long-term follow-up with factors influencing the results. Circulation 1979;60:647–654.

52. Forman R, Firth BG, Barnard MS. Prognostic significance of preoperative left ventricular ejection fraction and valve lesion in patients with aortic valve replacement. Am J Cardiol 1980;45:1120–1125.

53. Carabello BA, Williams H, Gash AK, et al. Hemodynamic predictors of outcome in patients undergoing valve replacement. Circulation 1986;74:1309–1316.

54. Borow KM, Green LH, Mann T, et al. End-systolic volume as a predictor of postoperative left ventricular performance in volume overload from valvular regurgitation. Am J Med 1980;68:655–663.

55. Levine HJ, Gaasch WH. Ratio of regurgitant volume to end-diastolic volume: a major determinant of ventricular response to surgical correction of chronic volume overload. Am J Cardiol 1983;52:406–410.

56. Schattenberg TT, Titus JL, Parkin TW. Clinical findings in acquired aortic valve stenosis. Effect of disease of other valves. Am Heart J 1967;73:322–326.

57. Gash AK, Carabello BA, Kent RL, Frazier JA, Spann

JF. Left ventricular performance in patients with coexistent mitral stenosis and aortic insufficiency. J Am Coll Cardiol 1984;3:703–705.

58. Botvinick EH, Schiller NB, Wickramasekaran R, Klausner SC, Gertz E. Echocardiographic determination of mitral valve closure in severe aortic insufficiency: its clinical implications. Circulation 1975;51:836–847.

59. Pepine CJ, Nichols WW, Curry RC, Conti CR. Reversal of premature mitral valve closure by nitroprusside in severe aortic insufficiency: beat to beat pressure-flow and echocardiographic relationships (abstr). Am J Cardiol 1976;37:161A.

60. Nakatani S, Masuyama T, Kodama K, Kitabatake A, Fujii K, Kamada T. Value and limitations of Doppler echocardiography in the quantification of stenotic mitral valve area: comparison of the pressure half-time and the continuity equation methods. Circulation 1988;77:78–85.

61. Erzengin F, Williams G, Rao S, Watson D. Closed or open mitral valvotomy or valve replacement? J Cardiovasc Ultrason 1985;4:253–258.

62. Yock PG, Popp RL. Noninvasive estimation of right ventricular systolic pressure by Doppler ultrasound in patients with tricuspid regurgitation. Circulation 1984;70:657–662.

63. Schoenfeld, MH, Palacios IF, Hutter AM Jr, Jacoby SS, Block PC. Underestimation of prosthetic mitral valve areas: role of transseptal catheterization in avoiding unnecessary repeat mitral valve surgery. J Am Coll Cardiol 1985;5:1387–1392.

64. Dalen JE, Matloff JM, Evans GL, et al. Early reduction of pulmonary vascular resistance after mitral valve replacement. N Engl J Med 1967;277:387–394.

65. Braunwald E, Braunwald NS, Ross J Jr, Morrow AG. Effects of mitral valve replacement on the pulmonary vascular dynamics of patients with pulmonary hypertension. N Engl J Med 1965; 273:509–518.

66. Messina AG, Yao FS, Isom OW, Illner P, Artusio JF, Devereux RB. Atrioventricular valve annuloplasty. Assessment by transesophageal echocardiographic Doppler and contrast studies (abstr). Clin Res 1987;35:305A.

67. Gash AK, Carabello BA, Cepin D, et al. Left ventricular ejection performance and systolic muscle function in patients with mitral stenosis. Circulation 1983;67:148–154.

68. Roberts WC, Perloff JK. Mitral valve disease: a clinicopathologic survey of the conditions causing the mitral valve to function abnormally. Ann Intern Med 1972;77:939–975.

69. Ross J Jr. Adaptations of the left ventricle to chronic volume overload. Circ Res 1974;35:II64–II70.

70. Eckberg DL, Gault JH, Bouchard RL, Karliner JS, Ross J Jr. Mechanics of left ventricular contraction in chronic severe mitral regurgitation. Circulation 1973;47:1252–1259.

71. Urschel CW, Covell JW, Sonnenblick EH, Ross J Jr, Braunwald E. Myocardial mechanics in aortic and mitral valvular regurgitation. The concept of instantaneous impedance as a determinant of the performance of the intact heart. J Clin Invest 1968;47:867–872.

72. Yoran C, Yellin EL, Becker RM, Gabbay S, Frater RW, Sonnenblick EH. Dynamic aspects of acute mitral regurgitation: effects of ventricular volume, pressure and contractility on the effective regurgitant orifice area. Circulation 1979;60:170–176.

73. Carabello BA, Spann JF. The uses and limitations of end systolic indexes of left ventricular function. Circulation 1984;69:1058–1064.

74. Sagawa K. The end systolic pressure volume relation of the ventricle: definition, modifications and clinical use. Circulation 1981;63:1223–1227.

75. Gault JH, Ross J Jr, Braunwald E. Contractile state of the left ventricle in man: instantaneous tension-velocity-length relationships in patients with and without disease of the left ventricular myocardium. Circ Res 1968;22:451–463.

76. Schuler G, Peterson KL, Johnson A, et al. Temporal response of left ventricular performance to mitral valve surgery. Circulation 1979;59:1218–1231.

77. Carabello BA, Nolan SP, McGuire LB. Assessment of preoperative left ventricular function in patients with mitral regurgitation: value of the end systolic wall stress-end systolic volume ratio. Circulation 1981;64:1212–1217.

78. Abbasi AS, Allen MW, DeCristofaro D, Ungar I. Detection and estimation of the degree of mitral regurgitation by range-gated pulsed Doppler echocardiography. Circulation 1980;61:143–147.

79. Miyatake K, Izumi S, Okamoto M, et al. Semiquantitative grading of severity of mitral regurgitation by real time two dimensional Doppler flow imaging technique. J Am Coll Cardiol 1986;7:82–88.

80. Carley JE, Wong BYS, Pugh DM, Dunn M. Clinical significance of the V wave in the main pulmonary artery. Am J Cardiol 1977;39:982–985.

81. Fuchs RM, Heuser RR, Yin FC, Brinker JA. Limitations of pulmonary wedge V waves in diagnosing mitral regurgitation. Am J Cardiol 1982;49:849–853.

82. Pichard AD, Kay R, Smith H, Rentrop P, Holt J, Gorlin R. Large V waves in the pulmonary wedge pressure tracing in the absence of mitral regurgitation. Am J Cardiol 1982;50:1044–1050.

83. Gaasch WH, Levine HJ, Zile MR. Chronic aortic and mitral regurgitation: mechanical consequences of the lesion and the results of surgical correction. In: Gaasch WH, Levine HJ, eds. The ventricle: basic and clinical aspects. Boston: Martinus-Nijhoff, 1985:237.

84. Zile MR, Gaasch WH, Carroll JD, Levine HJ. Chronic mitral regurgitation: predictive value of preoperative echocardiographic indexes of left ventricular function and wall stress. J Am Coll Cardiol 1984;3:235–242.

85. Vokonas PS, Gorlin R, Cohn PF, Herman MV, Sonnenblick EH. Dynamic geometry of the left ventricle in mitral regurgitation. Circulation 1973;48:786–796.

86. Salomon NW, Stinson EB, Griepp RB, Shumway NE. Surgical treatment of degenerative mitral regurgitation. Am J Cardiol 1976;38:463–468.

87. Suzuki Y, Kambara H, Kadota K, et al. Detection and evaluation of tricuspid regurgitation using a real time, two dimensional, color coded, Doppler flow imaging system: comparison with contrast two dimensional echocardiography and right ventriculography. Am J Cardiol 1986;57:811–815.

29

Cardiac Catheterization and the Patient with Congenital Heart Disease

C. Richard Conti, M.D.

INTRODUCTION

This chapter will focus on the clinical and catheter laboratory aspects of adolescent and adult patients with congenital heart disease. The discussion of the anatomy, physiology, and clinical management of the complex malformations in neonates is a subject too vast to be covered in a single chapter, and the interested cardiologist should consult textbooks on the subject (1–4). What follows will be a general approach to the diagnosis of known or suspected congenital heart disease using an algorithm based on the answers to several questions. The questions include: (*a*) Did the patient have heart surgery or an interventional catheterization procedure? (*b*) Is the patient cyanotic? (*c*) Is the pulmonary vascularity increased? (*d*) Is pulmonary hypertension present? and (*e*) Is this a right- or left-sided abnormality? The role of the cardiac catheterization laboratory will then be addressed using some common examples of patients with congenital heart disease.

Patients with congenital heart disease are becoming increasingly important to the adult cardiologist and internist. Of course, the vast majority of these patients are diagnosed and treated by pediatric cardiologists, since most patients are evaluated early in childhood. However, management guidelines appropriate for children do not necessarily apply to adults. Furthermore, pediatric cardiologists are much less familiar with the long-term follow-up care of many of these conditions because early

surgery has dramatically reduced their frequency or altered their course until other diseases, like coronary artery disease, become manifest. Occasionally, patients with undiagnosed or untreated congenital heart disease are seen initially by adult cardiologists. These are mostly acyanotic patients who have had either no symptoms or trivial symptoms beginning in adolescence or early adulthood, e.g., uncomplicated atrial septal defect. In the near future, however, adult cardiologists will be referred patients, with simple or complex congenital heart disease who may have undergone either palliative or definitive procedures to correct the defect. As adults the major thrust of catheter investigation is likely to be coronary angiography, but assessment of ventricular function, pulmonary vascular resistance, residual shunts, and cardiac anatomy will become increasingly important as these patients age. Thus, it is important for the adult cardiologist to be familiar with the anatomy and physiology of the congenital malformation, especially postoperative anatomy. It is also important to note that timely information relative to these patients in adulthood is difficult to obtain.

GENERAL APPROACH TO THE DIAGNOSIS OF CONGENITAL HEART DISEASE

Patients with congenital heart disease generally come to the attention of the physician because of an abnormal physical finding or laboratory test. Symptoms are important but rarely give clues to the diagnosis. Most commonly, patients present with a heart murmur (e.g., continuous murmur, patent ductus arteriosus), or other physical abnormalities, such as hypertension in the upper extremities (e.g., coarctation of the aorta), ECG abnormalities (e.g., pulmonic stenosis, atrial septal defect), chest x-ray abnormalities (e.g., cardiac enlargement, Ebstein's anomaly), unusual cardiac configuration (e.g., dextrocardia), increased pulmonary vascularity (e.g., atrial septal defect), or cyanosis, usually seen with clubbing and polycythemias in patients with right to left shunts (e.g., tetralogy of Fallot).

The combined use of the physical examination, electrocardiogram, and chest x-ray usually leads to the correct diagnosis in patients with single congenital heart defects. The echocardiogram and Doppler evaluation usually provide confirmation of the clinical impression.

The chest x-ray is of great importance for diagnosis of congenital heart disease, as it gives information on chamber enlargement and pulmonary vascularity. Of course, the Doppler echocardiogram gives much more precise information about cardiac chamber enlargement, shunts, and valve abnormalities. Cardiac catheterization and angiography are no longer required for precise definition of cardiac anatomy in many instances. Although this procedure is done in order to provide quantitative information about the defects and their physiologic significance, it is the only way to obtain information about the state of the coronary arteries, especially in older adults.

Indications for cardiac catheterization in these adults with known or suspect congenital heart disease cannot be generalized and must be case-specific. However, if information, necessary for diagnosis and management cannot be obtained by noninvasive means (e.g., ECG, cardiac ultrasound, magnetic resonance imaging (MRI)), then diagnostic hemodynamic and angiographic investigation is warranted. An example of this would be to determine pulmonary vascular resistance in an adult patient with a left to right shunt or one with slight cyanosis. Another example is the older patient who develops chest discomfort on exertion with or without mitral valve insufficiency.

SPECIFIC APPROACH TO THE DIAGNOSIS OF CONGENITAL HEART DISEASE IN THE ADULT

The diagram illustrated in Figure 29.1 is an example of an algorithm that can be used to approach the differential diagnosis of congenital heart disease. It does not allow the physician to make a specific diagnosis. Obviously, physical exam, ECG, chest x-ray, echocardiography, and possible cardiac catheterization will be necessary to arrive at a precise diagnosis. In the next sections of this chapter, use of this algorithm to arrive at a group of diagnoses will be illustrated. Specific clinical and laboratory findings of each diagnosis will be discussed, as well as indications for catheterization, expected findings, and techniques.

PREOPERATIVE: ACYANOTIC PATIENT

Increased Pulmonary Blood Flow

Atrial Septal Defect

The older patient with a significant shunt due to an atrial septal defect may relate the history of recurrent pulmonic infections, palpitations, or even symptoms of heart failure. Atrial fibrillation may occur as a result of dilation of the right atrium. Because of increased flow across the tricuspid valve, a diastolic rumble may be audible. Fixed splitting of the second heart sound, incomplete right bundle branch block, right axis deviation, or right ventricular hypertrophy and increased pulmonary vascularity are key features that lead to the diagnosis of this condition. Echocardiography can demonstrate the location of atrial septal defect in many instances, as well as quantify the size of the dilated right ventricle and show paradoxical septal motion. Doppler study is also useful to assess valve dysfunction. In many instances, mitral valve prolapse is found in patients with **secundum atrial septal defect.**

In the primum type of atrial septal defect (defects much lower in the septum involving tricuspid and mitral valve and ventricular septum), a major difference is that the ECG shows left axis deviation. Other clinical and laboratory features may be identical to a secundum atrial septal defect, but the A-V valves may

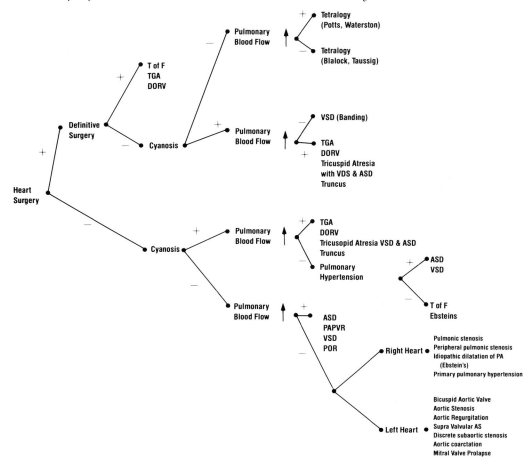

Figure 29.1. An example of an algorithm that can be used to approach the differential diagnosis of congenital heart disease. *AS,* aortic stenosis; *ASD,* atrial septal defect; *DORV,* double outlet right ventricle; *PAPVR,* partial anomalous pulmonary venous return; *PDA,* patent ductus arteriosus; *RV,* right ventricle; *T of F,* tetralogy of Fallot; *TGA,* transposition of the great arteries; *VSD,* ventricular septal defect.

have a "cleft" that results in mitral or tricuspid insufficiency.

Catheterization to assess shunt size and pulmonary vascular resistance is most easily accomplished from the right femoral vein. The catheter introduced in this fashion into the atrium usually crosses the atrial septal defect quite easily and enters the left atrium. Left heart catheterization via the arterial approach is indicated if coronary artery or aortic disease is suspected. Figure 29.2 illustrates the basic anatomic and hemodynamic findings for a typical secundum atrial septal defect.

Because of the the left-to-right shunt oxygen saturation is increased in the right atrium, as compared with that in the superior vena cava. When the shunt is large, fluo-

roscopy of the pulmonary vessels will reveal "hilar dance" due to increased pulmonary blood flow and a wide pulse pressure in the pulmonary circulation. Estimation of the shunt size is determined by oximetry, as outlined in Chapter 20. When the ratio of left-to-right shunt is greater than 2 to 1, levophase filming of pulmonary angiography in the adult often will reveal early appearance of contrast in the right atrium. However, because of the large heart size, high flow, and dilution of the contrast material, it may not be well visualized. The best projection is the 30° left anterior oblique (LAO) with 20° cephalad angulation. If the shunt is large, pulmonary artery (PA) pressure may be slightly increased, and in some instances a pressure

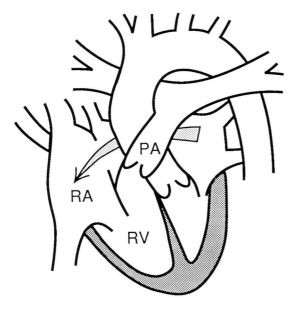

Figure 29.2. Secundum atrial septal defect. Basic anatomy and catheterization findings for an uncomplicated secundum type atrial septal defect. Oxygen saturation: increased in RA, RV, and PA. Pressure: increased or unchanged in RA, RV, and PA. Volume: increased in RA, and RV. Pulmonary resistance: increased or normal. *PA,* pulmonary artery; *RA,* right atrium; *RV,* right ventricle.

difference can be measured across the pulmonary valve secondary to high flow. In adults over the age of 40 years coexistence of coronary artery disease should be considered, and coronary angiography is indicated.

Treatment of this condition in the symptomatic patient is surgical. A simple secundum atrial septal defect repair can usually be accomplished at low risk, but risk increases as the patient ages, principally due to associated coronary artery disease. Repair of an ostium primum defect is more troublesome to the surgeon because of problems with the AV valve and conduction system. Heart block may result, and the patient may require a pacemaker.

Partial Anomalous Pulmonary Venous Return

This anatomic abnormality is the result of an ectopic venous return from either one lobe or the entire lung into the right atrium, or a systemic vein that increases pulmonary blood flow similar to that of atrial septal defect. This condition is almost always associated with an atrial septal defect, most commonly, a sinus venosus defect. A schematic diagram of such a situation and associated hemodynamic findings is given in Figure 29.3. When partial anomalous pulmonic venous return is associated with an atrial septal defect, the two conditions are often difficult to separate because the defect and anomalous drainage may be in close proximity. There are catheter techniques to help in this issue (see Chapter 20), but this is not usually of great concern to the surgeon, since these two defects can be identified at the time of surgery. When the defect is present without atrial septal defect, a selective right pulmonary angiogram performed in the shallow LAO position (20°) with slight cephalad angulation (20°) may reveal the defect. However, dilution of contrast material in

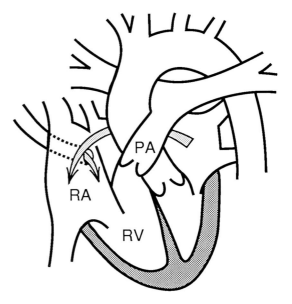

Figure 29.3 Diagram of basic anatomic and physiologic alterations in partial anomalous pulmonary venous return in association with a sinus venosus-type atrial septal defect. Oxygen saturation: increased in RA, RV, and PA. Pressure: normal. Volume: increased in RA and RV. Pulmonary resistance: normal. *PA,* pulmonary artery; *RA,* right atrium; *RV,* right ventricle.

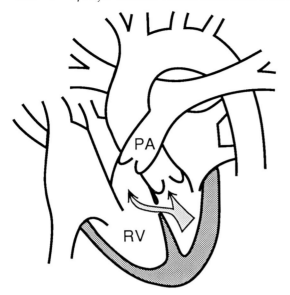

Figure 29.4 Anatomic and hemodynamic changes observed in uncomplicated ventricular septal defect, as described in the text. Oxygen saturation: increased in RV and PA. Pressure: increased or normal in RV and PA. Volume: increased or normal in RV. Pulmonary resistance usually normal. *PA,* pulmonary artery; *RA,* right atrium; *RV,* right ventricle.

adults sometimes makes visualization of the defect quite difficult. Selective indicator dilution curves from the right and left pulmonary arteries may identify a shunt from one side but not from the other. The key to catheterization diagnosis is to obtain blood oxygen samples from the superior vena cava above the site of possible entrance of the anomalous pulmonary vein and compare them with right atrium and pulmonary artery samples. Often if these patients are catheterized from the leg, the venous catheter will inadvertently enter the anomalous pulmonary vein. This is rapidly confirmed by measuring the O_2 saturation.

Ventricular Septal Defect

The most distinguishing feature of this lesion is a pansystolic murmur. This occurs when left ventricular systolic pressure is greater than right ventricular systolic pressure and the diastolic pressures are similar (Fig. 29.4). The murmur is of high frequency; it is loud and associated with a thrill that is easily palpable, especially if the ventricular septal defect is small (which usually is the case in the adult). When the left-to-right shunt is large, all pulmonary blood flow is increased, as in atrial septal defect, but since the shunt excludes the right atrium, the left atrium and left ventricle enlarge, instead of the right atrium and right ventricle. The clinical features of ventricular septal defect are related to the size of the defect. Patients with trivial ventricular septal defects are likely to be asymptomatic. Cardiac ultrasound may suggest the diagnosis by indicating left atrial and left ventricular enlargement. Color flow Doppler study may visually demonstrate the shunt. Treatment of this condition in the symptomatic patient is surgical. Subacute bacterial endocarditis prophylaxis should be used if the defect is not corrected.

Indications for cardiac catheterization are to assess pulmonary vascular resistance, valvular incompetence, and coronary arteries in adults who may be considered for surgery because of signs or symptoms relating to either myocardial ischemia or heart failure. The diagnosis is confirmed at cardiac catheterization by noting an oxygen step-up in the right ventricle. Left ventriculography in the steep LAO position (70°), with cephalad angulation will show a flow of contrast material from the left ventricle to the right ventricle. Aortography should be performed in these patients. On occasion, there will be aortic valve incompetence associated because the proximal septum forms a buttress for the right sinus of Valsalva. If a large septal defect is present, the right coronary cusp may prolapse into the right ventricle. A very large shunt, over time, may result in an increase in pulmonary vascular resistance, thus decreasing the left-to-right shunt and creating a right-to-left shunt and cyanosis (Eisenmenger reaction). Indications for cardiac catheterization at this stage are difficult to justify unless the diagnosis is in question. For chronic management of these adults with cyanotic congenital heart disease the reader is referred elsewhere (3, 4).

Patent Ductus Arteriosus

The characteristic abnormality of patent ductus arteriosus is a continuous systolic and diastolic murmur. This occurs because aortic

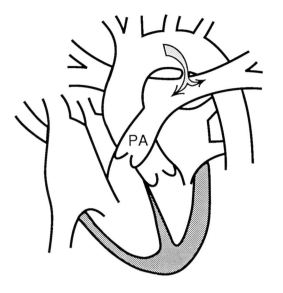

Figure 29.5 Patent ductus arteriosus. Isolated patent ductus arteriosus and associated hemodynamic findings, as described in the text. Oxygen saturation: increased in PA. Pressure: normal. Volume: normal. Pulmonary resistance: normal. *PA*, pulmonary artery.

some instances it is possible to catheterize the right ventricle in a retrograde fashion. Similarly, in adults one can cross the ductus from the pulmonary artery to the aorta, but this is not as easy as crossing from aorta to pulmonary artery. If one crosses the ductus from the pulmonary artery and enters the aorta, the catheter characteristically takes a course down the descending aorta. Many adult patients with patent ductus arteriosus are asymptomatic. Treatment of this condition is surgical in symptomatic patients. Recently, catheter occlusion techniques have been used in children and may have application in adults. Subacute bacterial endocarditis (SBE) prophylaxis should be used in all cases.

Normal Pulmonary Blood Flow (Right Heart)

Pulmonic Valve Stenosis

The clinical features of isolated pulmonary valve stenosis (Fig. 29.6) depend on the severity of the stenosis. Patients with this condition generally have a left parasternal lift, an

systolic and diastolic pressures are higher than pulmonary systolic and diastolic pressures. The electrocardiogram and chest x-ray are not specifically diagnostic of patent ductus arteriosus. Since the shunt involves only the aorta and pulmonary artery and excludes the right side of the heart, the left atrium, left ventricle, and aortic root can be dilated. However, gross enlargement is unusual in adults because shunts are usually small. Cardiac ultrasound can exclude other intracardiac problems, but in the older patient the quantitation of the shunt and state of the coronary arteries provide useful information to the cardiologist, who must make a decision about the appropriateness of surgery in such patients.

Diagnosis is confirmed by cardiac catheterization when a catheter (not a pigtail) is introduced from the femoral artery (Fig. 29.5). One can often cross the patent ductus arteriosus from the aorta to the pulmonary artery and detect a decline in pressure and in O₂ saturation, as compared with that in the aorta. When the catheter enters the ductus from the descending thoracic aorta, it may enter the left, main, or right pulmonary artery. In

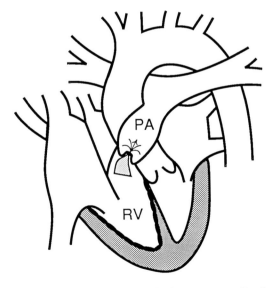

Figure 29.6 Pulmonic valvular stenosis. Findings in pulmonic valve stenosis as described in the text. Oxygen saturation: normal. Pressure: increased in RV, decreased in PA. Volume: increased or normal in RV. Pulmonary resistance: normal. *PA*, pulmonary artery; *RV*, right ventricle.

ejection systolic murmur that increases with inspiration, and a systolic ejection click that decreases with inspiration. If right ventricular hypertrophy is present (due to pressure overload), the right ventricle may be stiff and, as a result, diastolic pressure is elevated. In this situation, large A waves can be seen in the neck, and catheterization will show that the right atrial pressure is elevated. The ECG shows evidence of right ventricular hypertrophy and prominent P waves. The chest x-ray will show marked dilation of the main and left pulmonary artery (poststenotic dilation), and the pulmonary vascularity will be normal. The echocardiogram and Doppler study often confirm the clinical findings and provide an estimate of the severity of stenosis.

Catheterization of the pulmonary artery in these patients is easily accomplished from the arm. However, the pulmonary artery can be catheterized from the leg as well. Sometimes catheterization can be difficult because of the hypertrophied trabeculae in the right ventricle. In addition, because of the valvular pulmonary stenosis, the risk of perforating the outflow tract of the right ventricle with aggressive manipulation of the catheter is increased. Some have reported problems with hypotension when using balloon flotation catheters to cross the stenotic pulmonary valve. If a balloon flotation catheter is used, it should be inflated so that the catheter takes up the position just underneath the valve. The balloon should then be deflated, and the catheter advanced across the stenotic pulmonic valve.

Indications for cardiac catheterization relate to the symptom status of the patient and the status of the valve, coronary arteries, and the ventricles, in addition to the presence or absence of subvalvular or peripheral pulmonic stenosis. At the time of catheterization, it is important to obtain information about valve mobility. Often these data are used to confirm or reject information learned from the echo study. In addition, catheterization can exclude other associated defects (e.g., atrial septal defect) and determine the status of the subvalvular area. In some of these patients, infundibular stenosis can be a problem. Thus, careful pressure recording during pullback from the pulmonary artery to the right ventricle must be accomplished. A double-lumen flotation catheter permits simultaneous recordings of both pulmonary artery and right ventricular pressures. Angiography of the right ventricle in both posterior-anterior (PA) and lateral views (LAT) will help delineate the anatomy of the valve and infundibulum.

Subvalvular pulmonic stenosis is rare as an isolated lesion, but it may be associated with hypertrophic cardiomyopathy. Coarctation of the pulmonary arteries can occur and is referred to as peripheral pulmonic stenosis. It is usually the result of a maternal rubella infection during pregnancy and is usually bilateral. Auscultation of the lungs frequently will reveal systolic and sometimes continuous murmurs. When peripheral pulmonic stenosis is present, the main pulmonary artery pressure signal resembles right ventricular pressure, although diastolic pressure does not fall to 0. Once the catheter is advanced across the peripheral stenotic vessels, there is a marked fall in pressure, as there would be across any other stenotic lesion.

In recent years, catheter balloon pulmonary valvuloplasty has become an established treatment for congenital pulmonary valve stenosis (5). This procedure is discussed in detail in Chapter 17. Catheter balloon dilation has also been used for stenotic pulmonary arteries (6).

Idiopathic Dilation of the Pulmonary Artery

This is a benign condition but is associated with a loud systolic ejection murmur and click that varies with inspiration and is not associated with right ventricular hypertrophy. The most striking abnormality seen on x-ray or angiography of the pulmonary artery is marked dilation of the main pulmonary artery. This situation must be differentiated from atrial septal defect and pulmonic stenosis. Noninvasive evaluation with cardiac ultrasound and MRI can usually exclude any significant hemodynamic abnormality.

Ebstein's Anomaly

Patients with this condition who survive to adult life generally, but not always, have a mild abnormality of the tricuspid valve (Fig. 29.7). The tricuspid valve is downwardly displaced into the right ventricle. The condition has a wide spectrum from little to marked

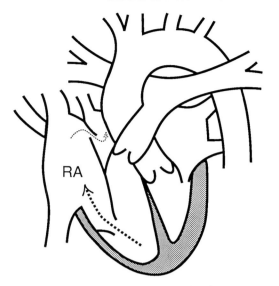

Figure 29.7 Ebstein's anomaly. Findings in Ebstein's anomaly, as described in the text. Oxygen saturation: normal. Pressure: normal or increased in RA. Volume: increased in RA. Pulmonary resistance: normal. *RA,* right atrium.

displacement. Tricuspid regurgitation is often present. The ECG may reveal the Wolff-Parkinson-White abnormality or occasionally P-R interval prolongation and right bundle branch block. The chest x-ray may be normal, but in many instances the right atrium is greatly enlarged. Patient's symptoms may vary from trivial to severe, depending on the presence or absence of arrhythmias, the presence or absence of atrial fibrillation, and the degree of tricuspid insufficiency. If a large cardiac silhouette is detected on chest x-ray in an asymptomatic person, Ebstein's anomaly should be suspected.

The diagnosis can be confirmed easily by two-dimensional cardiac ultrasound, which reveals an abnormally displaced and deformed tricuspid valve in what looks to be a hypoplastic right ventricle. Doppler ultrasound study provides useful information about the degree of tricuspid regurgitation.

Cardiac catheterization is indicated in the adult patient who has symptoms that may be relieved by surgical procedures, e.g., tricuspid valve replacement or reconstruction. Assessment of shunts, status of right and left ventricular function, and coronary arteries should be performed prior to any major surgical proce-

dure, including conduction system surgery. When these patients are catheterized, especially from the leg, one often crosses a patent foramen ovale. In some instances, this may lead to right-to-left shunting, causing a variable degree of cyanosis. Because the tricuspid valve is displaced into the ventricle, an "atrialized ventricular chamber" is created. Thus, there is ventricular muscle above the tricuspid valve. At catheterization the definitive diagnosis, in mild cases, is made by recording simultaneous pressure and intracardiac electrogram from an electrode catheter advanced from the arm. In the right atrium itself, an atrialized electrogram and right atrial pressure will be recorded. When the catheter is advanced toward but not across the tricuspid valve, atrial pressure will be recorded, accompanied by a ventricular electrogram in the atrialized portion of the right ventricle. If the catheter is advanced across the tricuspid valve, right ventricular pressure and ventricular electrograms are recorded. Thus, discontinuity between the electrical and pressure signals confirms the diagnosis.

Prognosis depends on the degrees of abnormalities. Arrhythmias should be treated in the usual fashion, but if they cannot be controlled, particularly if the Wolff-Parkinson-White syndrome results in refractory tachyarrhythmias, one should consider the possibility of cardiac surgery. If tricuspid incompetence is marked and the patient has severe symptoms because of this, one can consider replacing the tricuspid valve and revising the atrialized portion of the right ventricle.

Primary Pulmonary Hypertension

Primary pulmonary hypertension is a rapidly progressive disease, and patients with this condition often die during their adolescent or young adult years. However, adult cardiologists may see these patients on occasion. The hallmark of this condition is a loud pulmonic second sound, as well as a pulmonic ejection click. There may be some low grade murmurs during systole, and occasionally one can hear pulmonic insufficiency and secondary tricuspid insufficiency. Usually, there is marked elevation of both right ventricular systolic and diastolic pressures. Thus, large venous A waves in the neck can be appreciated. The ECG always shows right ventricular hypertrophy and right atrial enlargement. Chest x-ray will show large central pulmonary arteries with rapidly tapering peripheral vessels. Treatment of this condition is discouraging. Attempts have been made to use vasodilators of all kinds, including calcium antagonists, but the results are usually not satisfactory. In recent times, use of high-dose calcium antagonists has shown some encouraging results in some patients, but time will tell how effective these agents are. One must be aware that there are treatable causes of pulmonary hypertension, e.g., pulmonary venous obstruction, cor triatriatum, mitral valve stenosis, and left atrial myxoma; therefore, definitive evaluation is warranted.

Cardiac catheterization should be performed in all patients with the diagnosis of primary pulmonary hypertension. The goal is to measure pressure and cardiac output in a control state and then remeasure these same variables after interventions with various drugs, such as hydralazine, oxygen, calcium antagonists, and isoproterenol. It may be helpful to monitor pulmonary artery pressures for several hours to observe maximal effects. Two-dimensional echocardiography is useful to assess the left atrium and mitral valve as potential causes of pulmonary hypertension. Pulmonary venous obstruction is a difficult diagnosis to make but can be confirmed by obtaining simultaneous pulmonary-capillary wedge and left atrial pressures. If the wedge pressure is higher than the left atrial pressure, then the possibility of pulmonary venous obstruction exists.

Contrast material injection into the pulmonary artery in these patients with pulmonary hypertension is more hazardous than when given to patients without pulmonary hypertension. When it is important to perform pulmonary angiography to investigate possible thrombotic pulmonary disease, it is probably safest to use low osmolar contrast agents.

Normal Pulmonary Blood Flow (Left Heart)

Bicuspid Aortic Valve

This common form of congenital heart disease usually results in survival to adulthood, because there is often no severe hemodynamic impairment. As a result, few patients have any symptoms. On physical exam an early systolic click and short midsystolic murmur at the second right intercostal space is often heard. Echocardiography reveals an eccentric closure line of the aortic valve. Doppler study can be used to assess the gradient. The importance of this lesion is that patients may be prone to bacterial endocarditis, and they may develop increasingly severe aortic stenosis and/or aortic regurgitation as they age. Unless these secondary phenomena occur, there is no indication for cardiac catheterization unless one suspects an associated coarctation of the aorta.

Aortic Stenosis

Aortic stenosis is often the result of a congenital malformation of the valve. For example, a bicuspid aortic valve often becomes calcified in later life and results in valvular aortic stenosis. Rheumatic processes can produce aortic stenosis but less commonly than the congenital variety. High pressure in the left ventricle results in hypertrophy of the left ventricular myocardium. If the valve is pliable and not calcified, it will protrude into the aorta and produce an ejection click and an eccentric jet of blood that may result in poststenotic dilation. The aortic pulse pressure is narrow and slow rising, which is reflected by a slow rising and small carotid pulse (see Chapters 24 and 28).

Most patients with symptoms from severe aortic stenosis have pressure differences across the valve >50 mm Hg and an aortic valve area <1 cm^2. The ECG usually shows signs of left ventricular hypertrophy. The chest x-ray may appear to be normal, with the exception of some dilation of the ascending aorta. Cardiac ultrasound will confirm the presence of a hypertrophied left ventricle and a thickened echo-dense, poorly mobile aortic valve.

Cardiac catheterization and angiography are usually performed in all patients who are candidates for cardiac surgery to assess the degree of aortic stenosis and possible involvement of other valves; to assess left ventricular performance; and to evaluate the coronary circulation (see Chapter 6). It is accepted clinical practice to perform coronary angiography in patients over 40 years of age with aortic stenosis when they come to catheterization. Many of these patients have coronary atherosclerosis, and if surgical procedures are contemplated, knowing the status of the coronary arteries is important to the cardiac surgeon.

Many patients with aortic stenosis are now being subjected to catheter balloon aortic valvuloplasty (5). Indications for and details of this technique are discussed in Chapter 17.

Supravalvular Aortic Stenosis

Supravalvular aortic stenosis is an uncommon condition and may be familial. It has been associated with hypercalcemia during pregnancy. Patients with this condition may be mentally retarded. Because of supravalvular obstruction, there is a loud aortic second sound but no ejection click. The echocardiogram may demonstrate a narrowing of the aorta above the valve, but this is not easy to demonstrate in most instances. Cardiac catheterization should be performed in these patients to assess the pressure difference from left ventricle to aorta, as well as the location of the stenosis and the degree of involvement of other vessels. Catheterization can be accomplished easily from the arm or from the leg. Aortic angiography reveals a normal size aortic root and the extent and location of the obstruction. In these patients, it is important to remember that peripheral pulmonic stenosis is often present. Thus, pulmonary artery catheterization should be performed and pulmonary angiography should be done when a pressure gradient is noted. Treatment of symptomatic patients is surgical.

Aortic Insufficiency

A bicuspid aortic valve may produce isolated aortic insufficiency. In contrast to aortic stenosis, aortic insufficiency can be tolerated for many years. Physical findings are those of a widened pulse pressure and include bounding pulses, systolic ejection flow murmur, and a diastolic regurgitant murmur along the lower external border. There is usually left ventricular hypertrophy on the ECG. The indication for cardiac catheterization in these patients is to properly define ventricular function, anatomy, associated valve lesions, and status of the coronary arteries. Aortic root angiography and coronary angiography should be performed. Aortic root injection is ideally performed in LAO and right anterior oblique (RAO) projections, but if only one projection can be performed, the LAO is preferable.

Discrete Subvalvular Aortic Stenosis

Occasionally, patients with discrete subvalvular stenosis tolerate adolescence and first present as adults. Often, these patients have no symptoms, but examination will generally show a slow carotid upstroke, no ejection click, and a systolic murmur during ejection along the lower left sternal border. Occasionally, aortic and/or mitral regurgitation may be associated with this abnormality. Echocardiogram should reveal early closure of the aortic valve and a discrete membrane-like structure in the left ventricular outflow tract.

Cardiac catheterization is indicated in these patients to properly define the pressure changes across the left ventricular outflow constriction and to define the location of the lesion. Left ventriculography should be performed, and the best view to evaluate this is 70° LAO with 20° cranial angulation. In addition, the aortic valve leaflets themselves may be traumatized by the turbulence and the status of the coronary arteries should be known. Thus, ascending aortic and coronary angiography should be performed. Aortic insufficiency and/or mitral insufficiency may be associated with these discrete membranes. Symptomatic patients with significant left ventricular hypertension should be considered for surgical therapy. Catheter balloon dilation of the subaortic membrane has been attempted, but experience is limited (5).

Coarctation of the Aorta

Coarctation of the aorta usually is found just distal to the ductus arteriosus (postductal coarctation). Most adult patients have few symptoms. However, an occasional patient may have intermittent claudication due to decreased blood flow to the lower extremities. There is usually systemic hypertension in the upper extremity, although this may be mild and is generally how patients come to medical attention. Patients often have a bicuspid aortic valve, and an ejection click and aortic insufficiency may be audible. Because of the abnormal aortic valve, an ejection murmur may be heard in the aortic area as well. Decreased and delayed femoral pulses are the rule. The ECG may show left ventricular hypertrophy.

The classic chest x-ray shows rib notching because of the dilated collateral blood vessels (intercostal and internal mammary arteries) from the proximal to the distal aorta. A "three-sign" (aortic "knob" and left subclavian artery) may be present. This three-sign is due to the dilation of the aorta proximal to the coarctation that usually occurs just distal to the ductus arteriosus. Aortic rupture and subarachnoid hemorrhage can occur but are rare, except during pregnancy. SBE is also a known complication. A bicuspid aortic valve may be associated with coarctation of the aorta.

Cardiac catheterization should be performed if correction is contemplated (see Chapters 14 and 33). In these adult patients it is important to assess the status of the aortic valve, the coronary arteries, and the pressure difference across the coarctation, as well as the precise location of the coarctation. Catheterization via the femoral artery can be accomplished in the majority of cases. Angiography usually localizes the coarctation site. Sometimes the narrowing of the aorta occurs without any pressure differential across the apparent obstruction. This may be the result of the extensive collateral circulation to the lower extremities. These patient may not have upper extremity hypertension. This condition must be differentiated from pseudocoarctation (see Chapter 33).

Many patients obtain relief of systemic hypertension after repair of a coarctation although reports are now showing a number of patients with exercise-induced hypertension. If hypertension recurs, restudy of the coarctation site is warranted because of the possibility of persistent obstruction or recoarctation.

Catheter balloon dilation of aortic coarctation has been successfully performed, as well as recoarctation following surgery, and is discussed in Chapter 33 (5).

Mitral Valve Prolapse

Although mitral valve prolapse is not often considered as a congenital heart disease, it probably begins at or near birth. Fortunately, this condition is usually benign. There are no characteristic symptoms, ECG changes, or chest x-ray abnormalities. On physical exam, the mitral valve prolapse is characterized by a click followed by a late systolic murmur if mitral incompetence is present. The ECG occasionally shows nonspecific abnormality, even in patients with mitral incompetence. Cardiac ultrasound is the definitive diagnostic test for mitral valve prolapse. Since the condition has been associated with many symptoms (some of which have nothing to do with mitral valve prolapse), the physician must treat the symptoms accordingly (e.g., palpitations, chest pain, tachycardia). Often, these symptoms bring the patient to the attention of the catheterizing cardiologist, who then performs coronary angiography, most commonly with normal coronary arteries being found. The major indication for cardiac catheterization and angiography is preoperative assessment, in order to provide quantitative information about the degree of mitral insufficiency, the left ventricular function, the presence or absence of other valve abnormalities, and the presence or absence of coronary disease.

Hypertrophic Cardiomyopathy

This condition is discussed in detail in Chapter 31.

PREOPERATIVE-CYANOTIC

Increased Pulmonary Blood Flow

Transposition of the Great Arteries

For the patient to survive into adulthood, transposition of the great arteries (Fig. 29.8) has to be associated with other cardiac abnormalities. In this congenital anomaly, the aorta arises anteriorly from the right ventricle and the pulmonary artery posteriorly from the left ventricle. For the patient to survive, a ventricular septal defect or atrial septal defect has to be present so that oxygen saturated blood can be distributed to the systemic circulation. If pulmonary stenosis is not present, an Eisenmenger situation is created. In the presence of pulmonary stenosis and a ventricular septal defect, many of these patient can survive into adulthood.

There is another type of transposition of the great arteries called "corrected transposition" that is compatible with adult survival. Basically, these patients can survive without any associated defects because of the situation known as "ventricular inversion." In these patients, the left atrium empties across a

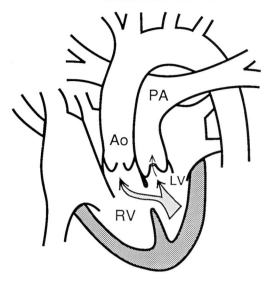

Figure 29.8 Transposition of the great vessels with pulmonary valve stenosis and ventricular septal defect. Findings in transposition of the great vessels with pulmonary valve stenosis and ventricular septal defect. Oxygen saturation: decreased in RV, LV, and Ao. Pressure: increased in RV, decreased in PA. Volume: increased in RV. Pulmonary resistance: usually normal. *Ao,* aorta; *LV,* left ventricle; *PA,* pulmonary artery; *RV,* right ventricle.

tricuspid valve into an anatomic right ventricle and then into the aorta. The right atrium empties across a mitral valve into an anatomic left ventricle and then into the pulmonary artery. The peripheral circulation is, therefore, normally saturated because of ventricular inversion. Because the AV valves follow the ventricle, the tricuspid valve is located on the left side of the heart. The common anomaly associated with corrected transposition is Ebstein's malformation of the tricuspid valve. Thus, the "physiologic" left ventricle (anatomic right ventricle) can regurgitate blood into the anatomic left atrium. Other associated problems with corrected transposition include dextrocardia, congenital heart block, and ventricular septal defect.

During catheterization of these patients an attempt should be made to enter all chambers and great vessels in order to obtain pressures and oxygen saturations. Coronary angiography in these patients is usually of less importance unless one finds abnormal distribution of the major epicardial vessels. This becomes very important to the cardiac surgeon who must perform a ventriculotomy in some of these patients.

Surgical procedures available for treatment of transposition of the great arteries include palliative, as well as "definitive," procedures. Palliative procedures for transposition include pulmonary artery banding to decrease pulmonary blood flow in a patient without pulmonic stenosis and a ventricular septal defect, creation of an atrial septal defect with either catheter balloon (Rashkind) or blade septotomy, or closed heart surgical incision of the atrial septum (Blalock-Hanlon). This procedure, when done in a patient without an intraventricular or intraatrial shunt, creates a pathway for oxygenated blood to flow into the right atrium, the right ventricle, and thus to the aorta.

An older method of increasing oxygenation of the right atrium and aortic blood is accomplished by anastomosing a right pulmonary vein to the right atrium (Baffes procedure). Another procedure in which blood is routed from the pulmonary veins through the tricuspid valve to the right ventricle and vena cava blood is routed through the mitral valve to the left ventricle results in oxygenated blood in the aorta. Variations of this operation ("Mustard's" or "Senning's") are accomplished by using baffles in the atria.

Definitive treatment for transposition of the great arteries includes closure of the ventricular septal defect (if present), with the septal defect patch fashioned to connect left ventricle to the aorta in combination with an extracardiac conduit from the right ventricle to the pulmonary artery with or without a pulmonary valve (Rastelli procedure). A second operation involves closing of the ventricular septal defect, combined with the Mustard/Senning procedure. A third operation involves separation of the aorta and pulmonary arteries and realignment to the appropriate ventricle (Jatene procedure). This operation requires that the coronary arteries be reanastomosed to the translocated aorta.

Double Outlet Right Ventricle with Pulmonic Stenosis

This congenital condition is a severe variation of tetralogy of Fallot. Patients have similar physical findings. Correction of this defect is more difficult than correcting the usual tetralogy of Fallot. It involves closure of the ventricular septal defect with the patch fashioned to connect the left ventricle to the aorta, as well as resection of the infundibular pulmonic stenosis or pulmonary valvulotomy.

Tricuspid Atresia

To survive into adulthood, these patients must have two septal defects: an atrial septal defect, so that unoxygenated blood can mix with the oxygenated blood in the left atrium, and a ventricular septal defect, so that partially oxygenated blood can enter the pulmonary circulation. If pulmonic stenosis is present, a procedure can be done to increase pulmonary blood flow by connecting the right atrium to the pulmonary artery (Fontan procedure). A similar procedure devised earlier by Glenn involves connecting the superior vena cava to the right pulmonary artery.

Truncus Arteriosus

The "pulmonary arteries" take their origin from the aorta, or truncus. A ventricular septal defect must be present. If pulmonary hypertension has been established and if pulmonary vascular resistance is fixed, there is no operative procedure to correct this defect. However, if pulmonary vascular resistance is low and the left and right pulmonary arteries are large, it is possible to use an extracardiac conduit (Fontan procedure) from the right ventricle to the pulmonary arteries to establish proper blood flow to the pulmonary circulation.

Normal Pulmonary Blood Flow and Pulmonary Hypertension

This condition is generally referred to as the "Eisenmenger reaction." If pulmonary vascular resistance is fixed, there is no operative procedure to correct the condition. Eisenmenger reactions may be seen in the adult patient with an atrial or ventricular septal defect or patent ductus arteriosus or, rarely, an atrial septal defect. It is usually the result of a large left-to-right shunt in childhood associated with the development of pulmonary hypertension. Once vascular resistance is fixed, the left-to-right shunt decreases markedly, and in many instances right-to-left shunting may occur.

Cardiac catheterization is indicated in these patients to assess pulmonary vascular resistance. Pulmonary vascular reactivity can be tested with agents such as oxygen, isoproterenol, hydralazine, and high-dose calcium antagonists. If pulmonary vascular resistance can be decreased and a left-to-right shunt persists, surgical correction may be possible but at very high risk. Heart and lung transplantation may be the only hope for many of these patients.

Normal/Decreased Pulmonary Blood Flow and Pulmonary Pressure

Tetralogy of Fallot

Physiologic abnormalities of tetralogy of Fallot are due to the presence of a ventricular septal defect associated with right ventricular outflow obstruction. As a result of these two defects, the right ventricle hypertrophies, and the patient is cyanotic because unoxygenated right ventricular blood is shunted directly into the aorta. The degree of cyanosis is directly related to the degree of pulmonary stenosis. It is unusual for an adult cardiologist to see a patient with tetralogy of Fallot who has not undergone palliative surgery. However, patients do survive undetected into adulthood because of a delicate balance between the size of the ventricular septal defect and the degree of pulmonary stenosis. Some patients become cyanotic only with exercise.

Cardiac catheterization and angiography are indicated in these patients because all patients have the potential for definitive treatment.

Palliative procedures include the Blalock-Taussig subclavian to pulmonary artery anastomosis, the "Potts" descending aorta to left pulmonary artery anastomosis, and the "Waterston-Cooley" ascending aorta to right pulmonary artery anastomosis. All of these procedures increase pulmonary blood flow and oxygenation of aortic blood. Patients who have undergone "palliative" systemic to pulmonic shunts often have problems as they grow into adults. Typically, the Blalock-Taussig shunts thrombose or fail to provide adequate flow to the pulmonary artery. Catheter balloon dilation of Blalock-Taussig shunts has been done to delay operation requiring a conduit (7). In contrast, the Potts and Waterston-Cooley shunts may overload the lung and create significant pulmonary congestion and pulmonary hypertension. Of course, the degree of shunting determines the eventual outcome. Definitive procedures for this abnormality include closure of the ventricular septal defect and resection of the outflow tract of the right ventricle. In addition, the left-to-right shunt (palliative procedures) should be closed in most instances. In the case of the Blalock-Taussig shunt, balloon embolization has been tried and has proven to be feasible.

Ebstein's Anomaly

This congenital malformation has been previously discussed.

POSTOPERATIVE ASSESSMENT OF PATIENTS AFTER "DEFINITIVE" SURGERY: NO CYANOSIS

Typical patients in this category include those with tetralogy of Fallot, transposition of the great arteries, and double outlet right ventricle. If definitive surgery is complete, there should be no residual intracardiac shunts, but there may be some residual stenosis of the pulmonary artery when it is present prior to surgery. The anatomy of the heart may not appear to be normal on angiography because of the complex nature of the corrective surgery. Intracardiac pressure should be normal or slightly elevated (e.g., right ventricle) or slightly decreased (e.g., pulmonary artery).

POSTOPERATIVE ASSESSMENT OF PATIENTS AFTER PALLIATIVE SURGERY

The different types of palliative procedures have been described previously in this chapter under the specific congenital conditions.
1. Cyanotic with increased pulmonary blood flow: These patients have undergone procedures but right-to-left and left-to-right shunts have persisted, e.g., transposition of the great arteries, double outlet right ventricle, tricuspid atresia with ventricular septal defect, and truncus arteriosus.
2. Cyanotic with normal or decreased pulmonary blood flow: The typical example of this category is the patient with a large ventricular septal defect with too much pulmonary artery banding, resulting in a right-to-left shunt.
3. No cyanosis but increased pulmonary blood flow: An example of this category is the patient with tetralogy of Fallot after a Potts aortopulmonary shunt.
4. No cyanosis with normal or near normal pulmonary blood flow: The classic example in this category is the patient with tetralogy of Fallot after a Blalock-Taussig shunt.

FOLLOW-UP OF PATIENTS WHO HAVE HAD PALLIATIVE CATHETER-BASED INTERVENTION

Balloon Valvuloplasty

Results of balloon valvuloplasty are discussed in Chapter 17.

Closure of Left-to-Right Shunts by Interventional Catheterization

Blalock-Taussig shunts have been embolized with balloons. Thus, the procedure is feasible (5). However, the number of procedures performed is quite small, and enthusiasm for the procedure should be tempered since surgical closure is quite easy and is generally done when a definitive correction of the tetralogy of Fallot is performed.

Nonoperative Closure of Atrial Septal Defects

Experience with this technique is very limited, although the enthusiasts claim that the prosthetic devices work quite well (5). However, it must be remembered that surgical closure of an atrial septal defect is a relatively benign procedure by cardiac surgical standards, and the long-term results of the surgical procedure are of proven benefit. There are no long-term studies of prosthetic devices inserted by means of catheter techniques into the atrial septum.

References

1. Perloff JK. The clinical recognition of congenital heart disease. 3rd ed. Philadelphia: WB Saunders, 1987.
2. Roberts WC. Adult congenital heart disease. Philadelphia: FA Davis, 1987.
3. Moss AJ, Adams FH, Emmanovialides GC, eds. Heart disease in infants, children and adolescents. 3rd ed. Baltimore: Williams & Wilkins, 1988.
4. Engle MA, Perloff JK, eds. Congenital heart disease after surgery: benefits, residua, sequale. New York: Yorke Medical Books, 1983.
5. Baker EJ. Valvuloplasty, angioplasty and embolotherapy in congenital heart disease (editorial review). Int J Cardiol 1986;139–145.
6. Lock JE, Castaneda-Zuniga WR, Fuhrman BP, Bass JL. Balloon dilation angioplasty of hypoplastic and stenotic pulmonary arteries. Circulation 1983;67:962–967.
7. Marx GR, Allen HD, Ovitt TW, Hanson W. Balloon dilation angioplasty of Blalock-Taussig shunts. Am J Cardiol 1988;62:824–827.

30

The Patient with Known or Suspect Arrhythmia

Alan Woelfel, M.D.
Leonard S. Gettes, M.D.

INTRODUCTION

Cardiac arrhythmias, particularly those which are life-threatening, occur most frequently in the setting of acute or chronic abnormalities of myocardial function. Some arrhythmias, such as those due to electrolyte disturbances or those occurring within 24 hr of an acute myocardial infarction (AMI), are secondary to a self-limited or reversible event and require no further study. However, when symptomatic arrhythmias are recurrent and unassociated with reversible factors, long-term antiarrhythmic therapy is indicated. In these situations, correct diagnosis of the arrhythmia is essential, and an understanding of the arrhythmia substrate, the factors giving rise to the substrate, and the effect of therapeutic modalities, particularly antiarrhythmic drugs, on this milieu is frequently helpful. Knowledge of these factors not only allows the physician to determine the most effective therapy but also lessens the likelihood of deleterious and potentially life-threatening effects of inappropriate treatment.

Many **noninvasive techniques,** such as echocardiography, nuclear ventriculography, and ambulatory, exercise, and high-frequency electrocardiography, are capable of yielding information pertinent to the correct diagnosis of an arrhythmia and its underlying electrophysiologic and myocardial substrate. However, information provided by these techniques is often incomplete and inadequate for appropriate therapeutic decisions. In these situations, **invasive studies** employing intracardiac catheter techniques are indicated. In this chapter we will focus on use of these techniques in patients with disturbances of cardiac rhythm.

CORONARY ANGIOGRAPHY AND CONTRAST VENTRICULOGRAPHY

In many situations, the specific cardiac diseases responsible for arrhythmias are apparent from clinical findings and the results of noninvasive studies. However, in some cases coronary angiography and/or contrast ventriculography may be required to adequately characterize the disease substrate that is associated with the arrhythmias and thereby provide direction for rational therapy. This principle is particularly evident in patients with sustained ventricular tachycardia (VT) or ventricular fibrillation in the setting of coronary artery disease (CAD). Findings of one or more critical coronary artery stenoses and minimal ventricular dysfunction at cardiac catheterization in a given patient strongly implicate acute ischemia in the pathogenesis of the arrhythmia. Severe left ventricular dysfunction without myocardium jeopardized by coronary stenoses suggests that the arrhythmia arises from fixed scar tissue. In patients with ventricular tachyarrhythmia due to acute myocardial ischemia, VT is usually not inducible at electrophysiologic study, and coronary artery bypass grafting or antiischemic medical therapy prevents recurrent arrhythmia (1).

523

Therapy directed primarily at the arrhythmia is neither needed nor likely to be effective in such patients. In contrast, in patients without acute ischemia, electrophysiologic testing usually reveals inducible VT that requires definitive antiarrhythmic treatment, rather than antiischemic therapy.

Cardiac catheterization is helpful in other situations as well. In patients with left ventricular dysfunction and nonsustained VT, distinction between ischemic and nonischemic cardiomyopathy by coronary angiography influences arrhythmia management, because electrophysiologic study is useful only in the setting of previous myocardial infarction (see below). Contrast right ventriculography may be the only method of establishing the correct diagnosis in patients with VT due to right ventricular dysplasia, which may be treated by surgery developed specifically for this disorder (2). In patients with arrhythmias due to coronary artery spasm, coronary angiography determines whether spasm is occurring in the setting of normal or diseased coronary arteries and thus dictates whether surgical or medical therapy is most appropriate.

Cardiac catheterization also plays a major role in determining suitability for arrhythmia surgery in patients with recurrent sustained VT. The best candidates for surgery are those with discrete aneurysms from prior infarction, and contrast ventriculography is required to accurately define the location and extent of the aneurysm. In addition, coronary angiography determines whether coronary artery bypass grafting is needed at the time of aneurysmectomy and endocardial resection.

Thus, cardiac catheterization is frequently complementary to the principal invasive method for arrhythmia evaluation, the intracardiac electrophysiologic study. In the sections which follow, we will review techniques for invasive electrophysiologic studies and define their use (*a*) to diagnose documented arrhythmias, (*b*) to determine electrophysiologic mechanisms of arrhythmias, (*c*) to determine whether undocumented arrhythmias are the cause of unexplained symptoms, and (*d*) to predict the occurrence of arrhythmias in patients judged to be at high risk for this event. We will also discuss the use of electrophysiologic techniques to document drug efficacy and predict adverse drug effects. Finally, we will discuss the use of electrical techniques in providing nonpharmacologic therapy to terminate and prevent tachyarrhythmias.

INTRACARDIAC ELECTROPHYSIOLOGY STUDY TECHNIQUE

General Comments

Intracardiac electrical data are obtained with multielectrode catheters that can be placed at any intracardiac site in order to pace the heart and/or record local electrical activity. The catheters are generally placed percutaneously by means of the modified Seldinger technique, using the femoral vein. This is more convenient than the cephalic vein and does not carry the risk of pneumothorax or hemothorax from jugular or subclavian venipuncture. In some cases, the desired pacing/recording site may dictate the approach used. Recording the His bundle potential from the superior aspect of the tricuspid annulus is most easily achieved via a femoral approach, while the coronary sinus is most easily entered by an approach from the left subclavian vein. Arterial puncture is required only when left ventricular recording or stimulation is performed or when invasive monitoring of arterial pressure is desired. Single-plane fluoroscopy is usually adequate to guide catheter placement, but biplane fluoroscopy is required for mapping procedures that require recording from many precisely localized sites.

Once the catheters are in place, the local electrical signals are amplified and filtered, and they are displayed along with several surface ECG leads on an oscilloscope. Hard copies are made by a physiologic recorder (photographic or electrostatic) with the frequency response and variable paper speed needed to accurately duplicate intracardiac electrical signals (Fig 30.1). For cardiac pacing and arrhythmia induction or termination, a stimulator is required that can (*a*) provide a constant current output variable over a range of outputs, (*b*) pace at a constant rate over a range of cycle lengths, and (*c*) accurately introduce multiple premature stimuli over a wide range of programmable intervals ("programmed stimulation").

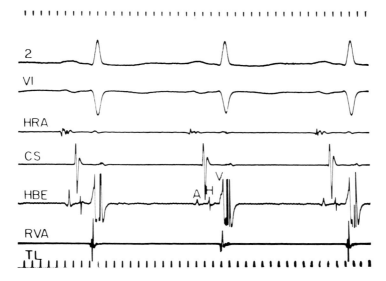

Figure 30.1. Representative tracing from an intracardiac electrophysiologic study. Shown are electro-cardiographic leads II (2) and V_1 (*V1*), and intracardiac electrograms from the high right atrium (*HRA*), coronary sinus (*CS*), His bundle (*HBE*), and right ventricular apex (*RVA*). The His bundle potential (*H*) is seen as a high-frequency deflection between the atrial (*A*) and ventricular (*V*) electrical activity on the HBE recorded from the superior aspect of the tricuspid annulus. Time lines (TL) = 50 msec.

Risks

An intracardiac electrophysiologic study is not without risk (see Chapter 3), but the most comprehensive report on the safety of this procedure (3) found major complications to be rare (see Table 3.4). It is hoped that adherence to standards for personnel training and equipment set forth by the Committee on Electro-cardiography and Cardiac Electrophysiology (4) will help minimize the risks of this procedure as its application becomes more widespread. However, as with all catheterization procedures the risks and benefits of intracardiac electrophysiologic study must be carefully assessed prior to its performance in each potential candidate.

Diagnostic Uses of Electrophysiologic Study When Arrhythmia Has Been Documented

Determination of the Etiology of Wide-Complex Tachycardia

Tachycardias with a QRS duration >120 msec and an abnormal QRS morphology may represent either VT, supraventricular tachycardia (SVT) with bundle branch block, or anterograde conduction over an accessory atrioventricular (AV) pathway. It is crucial that distinction between VT and SVT be made with certainty, because these arrhythmias differ markedly with respect to prognosis and therapy. Correct diagnosis may be inferred in some cases from a 12-lead electrocardiogram if available (5). However, frequently electrophysiologic study is required for definitive arrhythmia identification. It is our feeling that this procedure is indicated in virtually all patients in whom any doubt exists concerning the correct diagnosis (6).

Usually, the origin of wide-complex tachycardia may be determined by simultaneously recording electrical activity from the right atrium and His bundle during either a spontaneous tachycardia episode or an episode induced by programmed stimulation. Presence of AV dissociation (independent electrical activity of atrium and ventricle) is virtually diagnostic of VT (Fig. 30.2), while demonstration of a His potential prior to each ventricular electrogram implies that the rhythm is SVT with aberrant conduction (Fig. 30.3). When these recordings are nondiagnostic (i.e., when a 1:1 AV relation is present but a His bundle potential cannot be recorded),

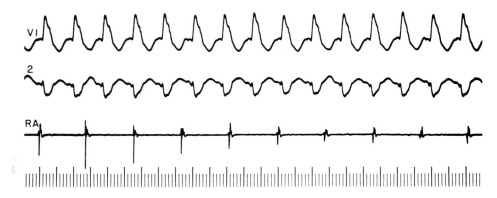

Figure 30.2. Wide-complex tachycardia of **ventricular origin** recorded in leads V_1 (*V1*) and II (*2*). The right atrial electrogram (*RA*) demonstrates that atrial activity is independent of ventricular activity (AV dissociation) and confirms that this arrhythmia is of ventricular origin. Time lines = 40 msec.

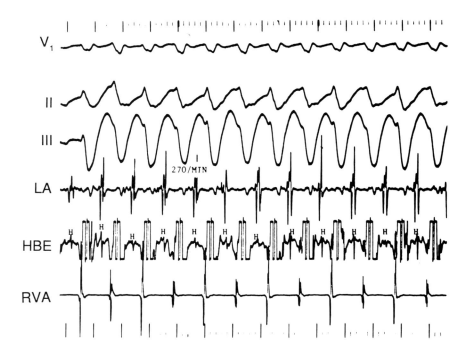

Figure 30.3. Wide-complex tachycardia of **supraventricular origin** recorded in leads V_1, II, and III (*top three*). The left atrial (*LA*) electrogram demonstrates a 1:1 relation between atrium and ventricle, and the His bundle electrogram (*HBE*) demonstrates a His potential (*H*) prior to each ventricular electrogram. The rhythm was atrial flutter with 1:1 AV conduction and right bundle branch block. *RVA*, right ventricular apex.

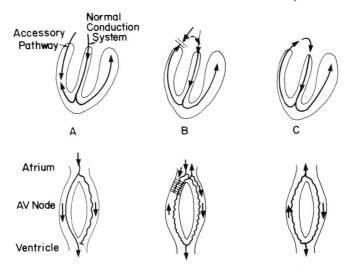

Figure 30.4. Mechanisms of AV reciprocating tachycardia. (*Top*): AV reentry due to **accessory pathway.** *A,* in sinus rhythm, impulses conduct anterograde in both accessory and normal conduction system pathways. The amount of ventricle depolarized via the accessory pathway determines the degree of pre-excitation seen on the surface electrocardiogram. *B,* A critically timed premature atrial impulse blocks anterograde in the accessory pathway, conducts over the normal pathway, and "reenters" the accessory pathway from the retrograde direction. *C,* Direction of impulse circulation in AV reentrant SVT. (*Bottom*): AV nodal reentry due to **dual AV nodal pathways.** *A,* In sinus rhythm, impulses conduct anterograde in both AV nodal pathways. Slow conduction in the abnormal pathway (*wavy lines*) is not expressed on the surface electrocardiogram. *B,* A critically timed premature atrial impulse blocks anterograde in the normal pathway, conducts slowly over the abnormal pathway, and "reenters" the normal pathway from the retrograde direction. *C,* Direction of impulse circulation in AV nodal reentrant SVT.

more comprehensive study is required to establish a definitive diagnosis (see below).

Determination of the Pathogenesis of Supraventricular Tachycardia

SVT may be subdivided into the following types: (*a*) AV reciprocating tachycardia, (*b*) sinus node reentrant tachycardia, (*c*) ectopic atrial tachycardia, and (*d*) atrial flutter. As is the case with wide-complex tachycardia, the type of SVT sometimes may be determined from careful analysis of a 12-lead electrocardiogram (7). However, these tachycardias are most reliably distinguished by invasive study, which enables the electrophysiologist to identify the electrical substrate predisposing to a specific type of tachycardia, determine the mode of tachycardia initiation, and record intracardiac electrical events during tachycardia.

AV reciprocating tachycardia is responsible for the majority of cases of paroxysmal SVT. This arrhythmia is due to continuous circula-

tion of an electrical impulse over a circuit composed of two limbs: (*a*) a portion of the normal AV conduction system, and (*b*) an abnormal conduction pathway. The two forms of AV reciprocating tachycardia are distinguished by the type of abnormal pathway present. In patients with AV reentry, an accessory pathway connects the atria and ventricles and thus bypasses the normal conduction system. Accessory pathways capable of anterograde conduction generally produce ventricular preexcitation evident on the surface electrocardiogram (Wolff-Parkinson-White syndrome), while those capable only of retrograde conduction are identifiable only by electrophysiologic study. In patients with AV nodal reentry, an abnormal conduction pathway detectable only by invasive study is located within or immediately adjacent to the AV node ("dual" AV nodal pathways). Both types of reciprocating tachycardia may be initiated by critically timed atrial or ventricular premature stimuli which block in one limb of the tachy-

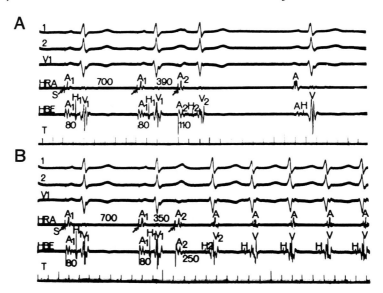

Figure 30.5. Demonstration of dual AV nodal pathways and induction of AV nodal reentrant SVT. *A*, After atrial pacing (A_1) at a cycle length of 700 msec, an atrial premature stimulus at an interval of 390 msec produces minimal prolongation of the AH interval from 80 to 110 msec. *B*, A slightly more premature stimulus at an interval of 350 msec produces marked AH prolongation to 250 msec, reflecting block of the impulse in the normal pathway and slow conduction in the abnormal pathway. The impulse then conducts retrograde over the normal pathway and continuously circulates in the AV node, giving rise to AV nodal reentrant SVT. Note the simultaneous atrial and ventricular activation during SVT. *1, 2,* and *V1* are leads II, III and V₁, respectively; *A*, atrial; *H*, His bundle potential; *HBE*, His bundle electrogram; *HRA*, high right atrium. *S*, atrial pacing spike; Time lines (*T*) = 10 msec.

cardia circuit, conduct over the alternate limb, and then "reenter" the blocked limb from the opposite direction (Fig. 30.4). AV reentry and AV nodal reentry may be distinguished at electrophysiologic study by several features:

1. Response to premature atrial stimulation. Abrupt, marked prolongation of AV nodal conduction time in response to a critically timed stimulus implies the presence of dual AV nodal pathways (8) and reflects block of the stimulus in the normal pathway and slow conduction over the abnormal pathway (Fig. 30.5).
2. Response to ventricular pacing. A constant retrograde VA conduction time at different paced rates implies that retrograde conduction bypasses the AV node via an accessory pathway.
3. Timing of local electrical activation. The atria and ventricles are activated nearly simultaneously in AV nodal reentry (Fig. 30.5) and are activated sequentially in AV reentry (9).
4. Retrograde atrial activation sequence. The pattern of retrograde atrial activation is normal in AV nodal reentry and is abnormal in AV reentry when the accessory pathway is free wall in location.
5. Response to a ventricular premature stimulus delivered during reciprocating tachycardia at a time when the His' bundle is refractory. Conduction of the premature stimulus to the atrium occurs only when an accessory pathway is present.

The substrate for sinus node reentrant tachycardia is presumed to be dual pathways in the sinus node, but existence of these pathways cannot be demonstrated by electrophysiologic testing. During tachycardia, atrial activation precedes the QRS complex, and the anterograde activation sequence of the atrium is normal. Sinus node reentry is thus morphologically identical to physiologic sinus tachycardia and is diagnosed by its paroxysmal initiation and termination by atrial stimulation (10).

Ectopic atrial tachycardia probably is a

mixture of arrhythmias due to intraatrial reentry and arrhythmias due to enhanced automaticity of an ectopic atrial focus (11). The former are inducible by atrial premature stimuli, while the latter are not. In both types of ectopic atrial tachycardia, the atrial electrogram precedes the QRS complex, and the anterograde atrial activation sequence (which originates from either ectopic focus or area of reentry) is abnormal.

Atrial flutter is likely due to reentry within the atrium (12) and may be induced by one or more atrial premature stimuli or by rapid atrial pacing. Occasionally it may be difficult to distinguish from other types of SVT on the surface ECG, but short atrial cycle length, usual presence of 2:1 or higher-grade AV block, and absence of the electrical substrate of other types of SVT make it readily identifiable by electrophysiologic study.

The mechanism underlying SVT determines eligibility of a given patient for treatment with surgery, catheter ablation, or antitachycardia pacing. For this reason, definitive documentation of the SVT mechanism by electrophysiologic study is essential when nonpharmacologic therapy is contemplated. When only drug therapy is envisioned, this documentation may not be essential. It has been suggested that in patients with reciprocating tachycardia, determination of the "weak link" of the tachycardia circuit by invasive testing may improve the likelihood of selecting an effective drug (13). However, this hypothesis has not been proven, and effective agents for SVT usually can be identified without detailed knowledge of the specific arrhythmia mechanism.

Determination of the Mechanism of Ventricular Tachycardia

Mechanisms of VT, in contrast to those of SVT, are poorly understood and cannot be definitively determined by electrophysiologic study. The majority of VT is felt to be due to reentry, although triggered activity or enhanced automaticity may occur in certain patients (14). It is generally agreed that VT due to enhanced automaticity cannot be induced by programmed stimulation, but inability to reproduce clinical VT by programmed stimulation in a given patient does not necessarily implicate this mechanism. Induction and termination of VT by premature stimulation is consistent with reentry, but these characteristics are theoretically consistent with triggered activity as well. Criteria have been proposed for separating reentry from triggered activity by electrophysiologic study (15), but until their validity has been established, use of this procedure for determining the mechanism of VT remains investigational.

Identification of the Site of Atrioventricular Block

Historically, recording of the His bundle potential to localize abnormalities of AV conduction was one of the first uses of the catheter in modern electrophysiology (16). Recording the His potential permits AV block to be localized to either within the AV node or distal to the AV node, based on whether the blocked atrial impulse is followed by a His bundle deflection (Fig. 30.6). In asymptomatic patients with second degree or third degree AV block, the site of block generally determines whether pacemaker implantation is warranted. Most patients with block in the AV node may be safely followed without pacing, while patients with block distal to the AV node require permanent pacing to prevent subsequent syncope or even sudden death (17). The site of block frequently may be inferred from the morphology of the QRS complex and responses of AV conduction to autonomic maneuvers, but recording of the His potential is necessary when these are inconclusive. In addition, when AV block is intermittent, increasing the atrial rate with pacing may be necessary to reproduce the block and permit its localization. Symptomatic patients with high-grade AV block require permanent pacing, regardless of the site of block, and do not require electrophysiologic study.

In patients with bifascicular block on the surface electrocardiogram (right bundle branch block and left anterior or posterior hemiblock, or left bundle branch block) and a history of syncope or near syncope, electrophysiologic study is indicated if noninvasive studies do not reveal the cause of symptoms. Marked prolongation of the interval between

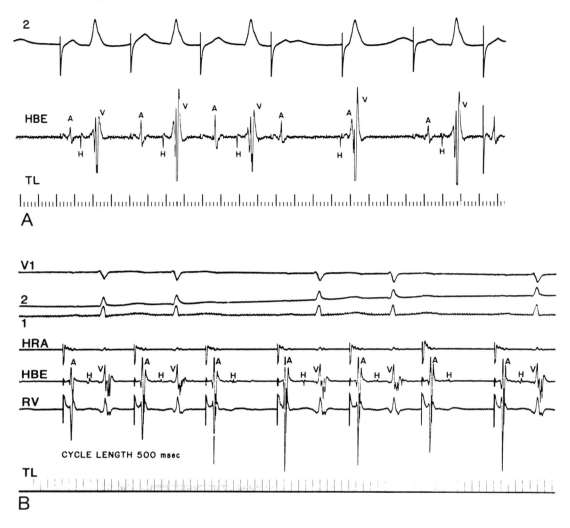

Figure 30.6. His bundle recordings during AV block. *A*, Block within the AV node. The atrial (*A*) electrogram is not followed by a His potential (*H*). *B*, Block distal to the AV node. Each atrial (*A*) electrogram is followed by a His potential (*H*). *1*, *2*, and *V1* are leads I, II and V₁, respectively; *HBE*, His bundle electrogram; *HRA*, high right atrium; *RV*, right ventricle; *TL*, time lines.

the His potential and ventricular activation (His-ventricular interval) during sinus rhythm or block distal to the His potential in response to atrial pacing suggests that AV block may be responsible for symptoms and that permanent pacemaker implantation is warranted. However, programmed ventricular stimulation should also be performed in an attempt to induce VT (see below), because this arrhythmia may be responsible for symptoms in many of these patients (18, 19).

Evaluation of Severity of Sinus Node Disease

Dysfunction of the sinus node may be due either to abnormal impulse formation (depressed automaticity) within the sinus node or abnormal impulse conduction from sinus node to atrium (sinoatrial block). Abnormal sinus node automaticity may be manifest at electrophysiologic study by a prolonged escape interval following cessation of over-

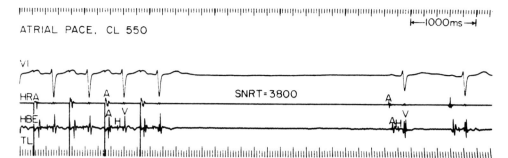

Figure 30.7. Sinus node recovery time (*SNRT*) determination. Following cessation of atrial pacing at a cycle length (*CL*) of 550 msec, a prolonged interval precedes the next sinus impulse. The SNRT is the duration of the interval between P waves or atrial depolarization immediately following atrial pacing. *A*, atrial; *H*, His bundle potential; *HBE*, His bundle electrogram; *HRA*, high right atrium; *TL*, time lines; *V*, ventricular; *V1*, surface lead V$_1$.

drive atrial pacing (i.e., sinus node recovery time) (Fig. 30.7), while abnormal sinoatrial conduction may be reflected in prolongation of the time required for an atrial premature beat to penetrate the sinus node (i.e., sinoatrial conduction time).

Unfortunately, sinus node recovery time and sinoatrial conduction time have not proven as reliable in assessing sinus node function as had been hoped, and their utility in selecting patients for permanent pacemaker implantation has been limited. These indices are usually normal in patients without sinus node disease and, thus, prolonged values are reasonably specific for sinus node dysfunction. However, they are prolonged in only 18 to 75% of patients with ECG documented sinus node dysfunction (20–23), and the type of abnormality identified during testing frequently may not correlate well with the symptomatic rhythm disturbance present (24). Given the imperfect sensitivity of sinus node recovery time and sinoatrial conduction time, it is not surprising that normal values have not obviated the eventual need for pacing in some patients (25). Although permanent pacemakers implanted on the basis of abnormal sinus node function indices have generally produced relief of symptoms, both in patients with neurologic symptoms without a clear relation to documented bradycardia (25) and in patients with syncope of unknown etiology and no evidence of bradycardia (26–28), the spontaneous variability of episodic syncope and dizziness limits the significance of these findings.

It is conceivable that refinements of invasive sinus node testing may improve the clinical utility of this technique. These refinements include (*a*) determination of sinus node recovery time corrected for heart rate and sinoatrial conduction time both before and after total autonomic blockade to distinguish intrinsic sinus node dysfunction from that mediated by extrinsic autonomic influence (29), (*b*) measurement of the sinus node-effective refractory period (30), and (*c*) direct recording of the sinus node electrogram (31). However, given current limitations of electrophysiologic study of sinus node function, invasive sinus node testing should be reserved for symptomatic patients in whom the relation between bradycardia and symptoms is unclear and in whom prolonged monitoring is judged to be unsafe or has proven nonproductive. Electrophysiologic study is not necessary in patients with a noninvasively documented relation between symptoms and sinus node dysfunction and is not indicated in asymptomatic patients with incidental sinus bradycardia.

Diagnostic Uses of Electrophysiologic Study When Arrhythmia Is Suspected but Undocumented

The utility of electrophysiologic study in evaluation of documented arrhythmias has led to its use in patients with syncope, near syncope, or palpitations in whom arrhythmias are suspected but cannot be documented non-

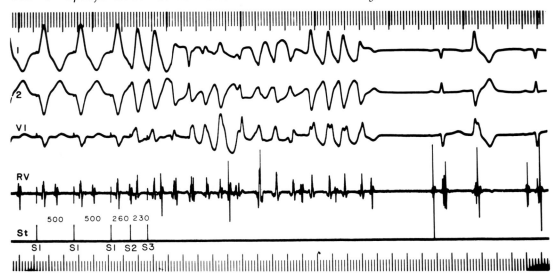

Figure 30.8. Induction of polymorphic ventricular tachycardia. Two ventricular premature stimuli (S_2, S_3) produce VT that continually changes morphology. Contrast with the uniform morphology of VT in Figure 30.10B. *1, 2, V1* are leads I, II, and V_1, respectively. *RV*, right ventricular electrogram; *St*, stimulus 1, 2, and 3, respectively.

invasively. Specifically, abnormalities of sinus node dysfunction and AV conduction are sought, and programmed stimulation is used in an attempt to induce clinically relevant ventricular and supraventricular tachyarrhythmias. This approach can potentially provide a diagnosis and enable rational therapy to be instituted.

Electrophysiologic study has been studied most systematically in patients with syncope of unknown etiology. The incidence of abnormal electrophysiologic findings in such patients has ranged from 18 to 69% (26-28), and the abnormality most commonly detected has been inducible VT. Treatment based on the results of electrophysiologic testing has generally been effective in preventing recurrent syncope, and symptoms often have resolved spontaneously in patients with normal studies. Although encouraging, these results must be evaluated in the context of several issues. First, the incidence of abnormal electrophysiologic findings is higher in patients with heart disease than in those without. There is no consensus on definitions of normal responses to sinus node testing and atrial pacing (32) (Fig. 30.7), and the implications of a prolonged His'-ventricular (HV) interval and induction of polymorphic VT or ventricular fibrillation are uncertain (Fig. 30.8). There is

also no guarantee that even a definitive abnormality is actually responsible for the patient's symptoms, and frequent spontaneous resolution of syncope without treatment makes it difficult to judge the effectiveness of therapy instituted on the basis of electrophysiologic study results. Finally, arrhythmias occasionally may not be inducible by programmed stimulation even when they have been clinically documented, and thus a negative electrophysiologic study does not necessarily imply that symptoms are not due to arrhythmia. For these reasons, invasive electrophysiologic testing should be restricted to patients in whom suspicion of arrhythmia is high, and the results of testing must be interpreted with care.

Diagnostic Uses of Electrophysiologic Study When Arrhythmia Has Not Yet Occurred

The concept of anticipating untoward clinical events and preventing their occurrence with therapy is inherently attractive. To this end, the ability of invasive electrophysiologic testing to predict the development of serious arrhythmic events in patients judged to be at risk has been examined in the clinical situations that follow.

Atrioventricular Block

In asymptomatic patients with bifascicular block, several investigators have recorded HV intervals and performed atrial pacing in an attempt to identify patients destined to subsequently develop high-grade AV block. The incidence of progression to complete AV block has been low in such patients, and a prolonged HV interval has not proven to be an independent predictor of this event (33, 34). Block distal to the His bundle during atrial pacing has been reported to be relatively specific for subsequent symptomatic AV block (35), but this finding is infrequent in asymptomatic patients. In addition, mortality in patients with bifascicular block is due primarily to myocardial failure and ventricular tachyarrhythmias, rather than to AV block, and prophylactic pacemaker insertion in such patients has not improved survival (36). For these reasons, electrophysiologic study currently is not indicated in patients with asymptomatic bifascicular block.

Wolff-Parkinson-White Syndrome

In some patients with Wolff-Parkinson-White syndrome, the accessory pathway is capable of exceptionally rapid anterograde AV conduction. In these patients, the ventricular response to paroxysmal atrial fibrillation may be sufficiently rapid to produce ventricular fibrillation and sudden cardiac death. Because the risk of ventricular fibrillation is confined to patients with R-R intervals of ≤250 msec during atrial fibrillation (37), induction of atrial fibrillation at electrophysiologic study and determination of the minimum resulting R-R interval identify those patients in whom prophylactic therapy is warranted (Fig. 30.9). Although the percentage of patients with a minimum R-R interval ≤250 msec who would later develop ventricular fibrillation is not known, all such patients probably should receive definitive treatment. Induction of atrial fibrillation to identify rapidly conducting accessory AV pathways is thus indicated in Wolff-Parkinson-White syndrome patients who have symptomatic tachyarrhythmias, even if atrial fibrillation has not occurred clinically (38). However, the incidence of ventricular fibrillation as the initial manifestation of this syndrome is probably too low to justify electrophysiologic study in asymptomatic patients (39).

Ventricular Tachycardia

Nonsustained VT is a frequent incidental finding in asymptomatic patients with cardiomyopathy and may constitute a marker for risk of subsequent sustained ventricular tachyarrhythmia and/or sudden cardiac death. Several investigators have tested the hypothesis that induction of sustained VT by programmed stimulation may identify those patients at highest risk for subsequent clinical sustained arrhythmia who would benefit from prophylactic antiarrhythmic therapy. Results have been encouraging in patients with nonsustained VT in the setting of ischemic cardiomyopathy, with better arrhythmia-free survival reported in patients treated on the basis of the results of electrophysiologic study than in those in whom the results of electrophysiologic study were ignored (40). In contrast, electrophysiologic study has not proven valuable in patients with nonischemic cardiomyopathy (41, 42).

A similar rationale has led to use of electrophysiologic study early after AMI to determine if VT induction identifies patients who subsequently die suddenly from ventricular tachyarrhythmia. Results of this approach have varied widely (43–49), probably reflecting differences in stimulation protocols and patient populations. However, trends evident in these reports suggest that the induction of VT is relatively nonspecific in unselected survivors of AMI but may be much more specific in those with ventricular ectopy and poor ventricular function, and sudden cardiac death is rare in patients without inducible VT, provided a sufficiently aggressive stimulation protocol is employed. On the basis of these results, it is conceivable that future studies will establish the clinical utility of programmed stimulation in specific subgroups of survivors of myocardial infarction.

Therapeutic Uses of Electrophysiologic Study

Determination of the Efficacy of Antiarrhythmic Therapy

Assessment of the effectiveness of empirical antiarrhythmic therapy is complicated by the

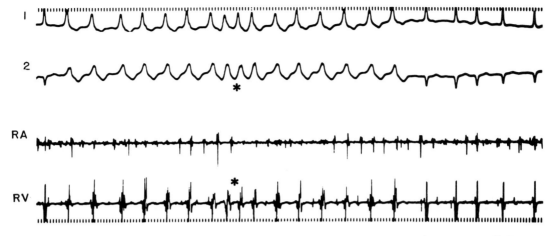

Figure 30.9. Induced atrial fibrillation in Wolff-Parkinson-White syndrome. The minimum R-R interval between preexcited beats (*) is approximately 170 msec, indicating that the patient is at risk for ventricular fibrillation. *1* and *2* are leads I and II, respectively; *RA,* right atrial electrogram; *RV,* right ventricular electrogram. Time lines = 40 msec.

fact that the tachyarrhythmias are often paroxysmal and unpredictable. Between episodes, there may be no way to determine the effectiveness of antiarrhythmic therapy, other than to await a spontaneous recurrence. Electrophysiologic study provides a potential solution to this problem by providing a tool with which to evaluate the effect of antiarrhythmic treatment. Because most supraventricular and ventricular tachyarrhythmias are inducible by programmed electrical stimulation, responses to therapy may be quickly determined by attempting to reinduce the arrhythmia after treatment. This approach may be used to evaluate the effectiveness of both pharmacologic agents and nonpharmacologic ablative procedures. Rationale for assessment of therapy by programmed stimulation rests on the assumptions that the induced tachycardia is identical to the spontaneous clinical tachycardia and the clinical response to therapy will parallel the response observed in the laboratory. Provided these assumptions are judged by the electrophysiologist to be valid in a given patient, this approach may substantially improve the safety, efficiency, and effectiveness of the therapeutic process.

Supraventricular Tachycardia

Invasive electrophysiologic testing is a useful means of selecting an effective drug in patients with SVT in whom empiric therapy has been ineffective. Provided SVT is inducible by programmed stimulation in the absence of therapy, different antiarrhythmic drugs may be administered, and stimulation may be repeated until an agent or combination of agents that prevents arrhythmia induction is identified. This approach may spare the patient multiple empiric trials of drugs that later prove ineffective, a process that can be time-consuming, inconvenient, and frustrating. Although variability of autonomic tone occasionally may make laboratory and clinical responses to drugs discordant, the efficacy of agents selected by programmed stimulation is high (50, 51).

In patients with Wolff-Parkinson-White syndrome who are at risk of ventricular fibrillation from a rapidly conducting accessory pathway, it is important to prove conclusively that prophylactic therapy is effective. This is accomplished by electrophysiologic study to document suppression of inducible atrial fibrillation or prolongation of the minimum R-R interval to ≥250 msec if drug therapy is chosen (52), or successful ablation of the accessory pathway if surgery or catheter fulguration is employed.

Ventricular Tachycardia

The rationale and procedure for serial drug testing by programmed stimulation in VT are the same as in SVT, but its use is much more controversial. The arrhythmias induced at electrophysiologic study in patients with VT are frequently hemodynamically unstable and may require emergent cardioversion. Thus, some investigators prefer to assess drug efficacy noninvasively using ventricular ectopy on ambulatory monitoring or treadmill testing as a therapeutic marker (53). However, up to 25% of patients will not have sufficient ventricular ectopy during noninvasive studies for the response to antiarrhythmic drugs to be interpretable (54), and noninvasive techniques may be less accurate than invasive electrophysiologic study in predicting drug efficacy (55, 56). These limitations of noninvasive techniques have led to widespread acceptance of serial programmed stimulation in treatment of patients with sustained VT or ventricular fibrillation.

Despite acceptance of this approach, a number of unresolved issues remain concerning the performance of programmed stimulation and the interpretation of results (57):

1. Stimulation protocol. The optimal method for employing premature stimuli to induce VT has not been determined. Consequently, stimulation protocols have varied considerably with respect to the number of premature stimuli delivered, current strength of stimulation, number and location of stimulation sites, and use of isoproterenol to facilitate VT induction. Although individual variations between laboratories remain, most protocols in current use consist of three or fewer premature stimuli given at 2 to 4 times diastolic threshold current at two right ventricular sites. Left ventricular stimulation and isoproterenol infusion are not routinely employed.

2. Significance of induced arrhythmias. The most appropriate marker to use in judging effectiveness of antiarrhythmic drugs by programmed stimulation is sustained monomorphic VT. This is true even if the presenting clinical arrhythmia is ventricular fibrillation rather than VT, because a period of monomorphic VT frequently precedes onset of ventricular fibrillation. The morphology of induced VT need not necessarily match that of the clinical VT, because most morphologies of induced VT ultimately prove to be clinically relevant (58). Nonsustained monomorphic VT induced by stimulation is a less desirable marker upon which to base selection of therapy when a sustained arrhythmia cannot be induced. However, the minimum duration of nonsustained VT required to be a valid marker has not yet been established. Polymorphic VT (Fig. 30.8) and

ventricular fibrillation are nonspecific responses to programmed stimulation and can be induced in patients with normal hearts and with no history of arrhythmia. They are probably irrelevant in patients whose clinical arrhythmia is monomorphic VT, and their validity as therapeutic markers, even in patients whose clinical arrhythmia is polymorphic VT or ventricular fibrillation, is controversial. Inability to induce VT by programmed stimulation in the absence of therapy does not imply the absence of risk of recurrent arrhythmia but does mean that this technique cannot be used to guide therapy.

3. Criteria for predicting drug efficacy. There is general agreement that complete suppression of inducible monomorphic VT best predicts clinical drug efficacy and should be the goal of serial drug testing with programmed stimulation. In patients with inducible sustained VT, subsequent induction of only nonsustained VT may constitute an adequate response to therapy, but the duration of nonsustained VT considered acceptable varies considerably (Fig. 30.10). Conversion of rapid, hemodynamically unstable VT to slower VT that is well-tolerated may predict that VT would not be lethal if it recurred, but the accuracy of this prediction is uncertain. Given the variability of VT induction parameters in the absence of therapy (59–61), greater difficulty of VT induction is probably not significant only if the number of stimuli required to induce VT after therapy increases by two. It must be emphasized that all criteria for predicting drug efficacy depend on reproducible baseline induction of VT. If electrophysiologic study is either not performed or does not reliably induce VT in the absence of antiarrhythmic drugs, the findings following drug administration have no basis for comparison and thus cannot be meaningfully interpreted.

Despite differences in methodology used, previous studies have consistently found suppression of inducible VT to be a reliable predictor of arrhythmia-free survival (62–65). Some patients with persistently inducible VT on therapy may not experience subsequent arrhythmia (66), particularly those treated with amiodarone (67, 68). However, the potential for fatal recurrences remains considerably higher in patients with persistently inducible VT than in those whose inducible arrhythmia is suppressed (66). For these reasons, we feel that invasive electrophysiologic testing is the method of choice for selecting

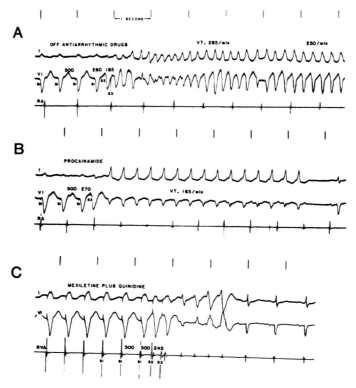

Figure 30.10. Serial programmed stimulation to assess antiarrhythmic drug efficacy. *A,* In the absence of antiarrhythmic drugs, two ventricular premature stimuli (S_2, S_3) delivered after ventricular pacing (S_1) induce a brief period of polymorphic VT, followed by sustained monomorphic VT at 250 bpm. *B,* After administration of procainamide, a single premature stimulus (S_1) induces 15 beats of slower, nonsustained VT. *C,* After administration of mexiletine plus quinidine, two ventricular premature stimuli (S_2, S_3) induce only four repetitive ventricular beats. The patient remained free of VT on this regimen. *1* and *V1,* leads I and V_1, respectively. *RA,* right atrial; *RVA,* right ventricular apex. Time lines = 1 sec.

therapy in patients with sustained VT or ventricular fibrillation. When drug therapy does not suppress inducible VT, alternative treatment such as surgery, catheter ablation, or defibrillator implantation should be strongly considered.

Identification of Adverse Drug Effects

Sinus Node/Atrioventricular Conduction Abnormalities

Sinus node conduction system abnormalities that are asymptomatic may be exacerbated by drug therapy required for coexistent conditions. In patients with sinus bradycardia, therapy of concomitant angina pectoris or paroxysmal atrial tachyarrhythmias may further depress sinus node function and precipi-

tate symptomatic bradycardia. In patients with intraventricular conduction disturbances, antiarrhythmic drug therapy for concomitant VT may further impair distal AV conduction and provoke symptomatic high-grade AV block. In these instances, electrophysiologic study may identify adverse effects of therapy before they are expressed clinically and, thus, enable alternative drug selection or prophylactic pacing to prevent the occurrence of symptoms.

Ventricular Tachycardia

Antiarrhythmic drugs have the potential to exacerbate, as well as suppress, ventricular arrhythmias. Proarrhythmic drug effects are expressed clinically as more frequent and/or more sustained arrhythmias and may be either confirmed retrospectively or anticipated prospectively by electrophysiologic study. In patients who were taking an antiarrhythmic drug at the time of their initial episode of VT or cardiac arrest, absence of inducible VT after rechallenge with the drug strongly implicates the agent itself as the cause of the clinical event. Therapy of such patients may be limited to withholding the offending agent. Proarrhythmic drug effects may also include findings by programmed stimulation that arrhythmia is more sustained, is faster and more poorly tolerated, or is substantially easier to induce by fewer premature stimuli after administration of a particular agent. These results are generally considered unacceptable, and alternative therapy is used.

Guidance of Arrhythmia Surgery

Curative surgical procedures for tachyarrhythmias depend on accurate localization of the arrhythmia substrate or focus of origin so that the arrhythmogenic tissue can be selectively ablated without damage to normal myocardium. This localization is accomplished by mapping, which involves recording electrical signals from multiple sites throughout the heart to determine the sequence of cardiac electrical activation. Although most precise when performed intraoperatively by positioning the recording electrodes under direct visualization, intracardiac mapping using a catheter and biplane fluoroscopy may provide reasonably accurate information. Preoperative catheter mapping is useful for several reasons. (*a*) It helps to direct intraoperative mapping to the area of most interest. (*b*) It may dictate the operative approach to be used. (*c*) It may be the only guide for the surgical procedure if the tachyarrhythmia is not inducible intraoperatively.

Supraventricular Tachycardia

AV reentrant SVT can be permanently prevented by surgical division of the accessory pathway (69). Although the approximate location of the pathway may be determined noninvasively, catheter mapping is mandatory to confirm its location if surgery is contemplated. The atrial insertion of the accessory pathway is located at the area of earliest retrograde atrial activation, which is identified by mapping both the left and right AV grooves (Fig. 30.11). This is accomplished on the left by

recording at multiple sites from a catheter within the coronary sinus, and on the right by fluoroscopically positioning the catheter in multiple sites about the tricuspid annulus (70). Preferably, mapping is performed during reciprocating tachycardia when retrograde atrial activation occurs exclusively over the accessory pathway. However, when reciprocating tachycardia cannot be induced, mapping during ventricular pacing at a rate that produces retrograde ventriculoatrial (VA) block in the normal pathway but preserves retrograde conduction over the accessory pathway may be adequate.

In ectopic atrial tachycardia, the site of earliest atrial activation during the tachycardia, representing the area of reentry or enhanced automaticity, is sought by fluoroscopically positioning a catheter in multiple sites throughout the body and appendage of each atrium. Surgical resection or cryoablation of this area may prevent further tachycardia episodes.

Ventricular Tachycardia

Surgical ablation of the myocardial region showing the earliest electrical activation during VT may permanently prevent recurrence of this arrhythmia (71, 72). The area ablated is presumed either to represent the site of origin of VT or to contain the arrhythmogenic substrate. This site is generally found in the subendocardium at the margin of a previous myocardial infarction and is best localized by precise mapping performed intraoperatively under direct visualization. However, VT may not be inducible in the operating room in as many as 25% of cases (72). In these instances, a preoperative catheter map is helpful in guiding the ablation, especially if a diffuse scar, rather than a discrete aneurysm, is present. Three types of catheter mapping procedures have been utilized for this purpose: VT mapping, sinus rhythm mapping, and pace-mapping. VT mapping involves determination of the electrical activation sequence during VT in order to identify the area of earliest activation presumed to represent the site of VT origin. This technique is the one most commonly used, and results have generally correlated well with those obtained intraoperatively (73). In sinus rhythm mapping, sites of late activation and low amplitude electrograms likely to

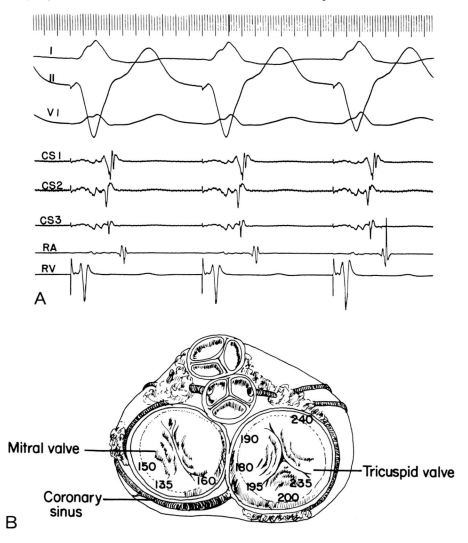

Figure 30.11 Atrial activation sequence during ventricular pacing in a patient with a left free wall accessory pathway. *A,* Electrogram recordings from the high right atrium (*RA*) and three adjacent sites in the coronary sinus (*CS, 1, 2, 3*). Earliest activation occurs in the midportion of the coronary sinus. *RA,* right atrial electrogram; *RV,* right ventricular electrogram. *B,* Complete map of retrograde atrial activation sequence in the same patient as in *A.* Shown are the V-A conduction times in milliseconds at each site about the left and right AV grooves. Earliest activation occurs in the left lateral free wall, indicating the site of the atrial insertion of the accessory pathway. This location was subsequently confirmed during successful surgical division of the accessory pathway.

comprise the arrhythmogenic substrate are located during sinus rhythm. Pace-mapping involves pacing throughout the ventricles until a QRS morphology identical to that during VT is obtained, the site at which pacing produces this morphology approximates the site of VT origin. Sinus rhythm

mapping and pace-mapping do not require VT induction but are probably not as reliable as VT mapping. All three catheter techniques require considerable skill to manipulate the catheter to multiple sites within both ventricles and to accurately assess catheter position.

Termination or Prevention of Tachyarrhythmias

Most paroxysmal tachyarrhythmias can be terminated by delivering one or more appropriately timed premature stimuli. This principle is most frequently utilized during electrophysiologic studies when episodes of induced SVT and VT are terminated by pacing techniques that obviate the need for electrical cardioversion or drug administration. The same principle has been employed to terminate spontaneously occurring tachyarrhythmias, both on a short-term basis by use of a temporary pacing catheter and on a long-term basis by implantation of a permanent "antitachycardia" pacemaker. Antitachycardia pacemakers consist of a permanent atrial or ventricular pacing lead and a pulse generator that can be programmed to deliver different types of pacing and/or premature stimulation. All potential pacemaker recipients require extensive electrophysiologic testing prior to implantation to verify that the arrhythmia can be readily terminated by programmed stimulation and to determine the optimal termination parameters. These parameters are then programmed into the pulse generator and used to terminate spontaneous occurrences of tachycardia. The device is either automatically activated when an algorithm designed to detect a tachyarrhythmia is satisfied, or it is manually activated by the patient or a physician. Appropriate candidates for antitachycardia pacemakers are patients with frequent episodes of tachycardia despite drug therapy who are not candidates for surgical therapy.

Antitachycardia pacemakers have been used successfully both in patients with SVT and patients with VT. A recent review of their use in over 200 patients with each disorder reported favorable results in all but 3 to 4% of implants (74). Long-term efficacy was reasonably good, and reported complications were minimal. In SVT, automatic operation or manual activation by the patient frequently obviates the need to present to a physician for arrhythmia termination. This substantial benefit cannot be realized in VT because of the potential for programmed stimulation to accelerate VT or produce ventricular fibrillation. Unfortunately, acceleration of VT cannot be predicted by laboratory testing. It may occur clinically despite uniformly effective arrhythmia termination by pacing in the laboratory. For this reason, automatic antitachycardia pacemakers should not be employed in patients with VT. Nonautomatic devices may be used but should be activated only by medical personnel having facilities for providing rescue in the event of VT acceleration. Devices with the capacity to provide antitachycardia pacing and defibrillation in a single unit are currently under development and may substantially increase the application of automatic pacing therapy to VT.

Pacing therapy may also be used to prevent tachyarrhythmias in specific situations. In patients whose tachyarrhythmia is initiated by an escape rhythm during marked bradycardia, a simple demand pacemaker is adequate treatment. In cases of the long QT syndrome, either drug-induced or congenital, pacing may prevent polymorphic VT, presumably by decreasing the dispersion of refractoriness thought to be responsible for this arrhythmia (75, 76). In patients with AV reciprocating tachycardia, simultaneously pacing the atrium and ventricle to produce continual refractoriness of both limbs of the reentry circuit may prevent initiation of the tachycardia (77). Atrial or ventricular pacing at rates faster than that of the sinus rate ("overdrive" pacing) may occasionally reduce the frequency of premature beats that initiate SVT or VT and thus decrease the incidence of the sustained tachyarrhythmia. The latter techniques require careful evaluation by temporary pacing before a permanent device is implanted.

Permanent Ablation of Tachyarrhythmias

Use of the catheter to localize the origin or substrate of tachyarrhythmias has been logically extended to selective ablation of those areas in order to permanently eliminate the tachycardia. Several forms of energy may be delivered through a catheter to ablate myocardial tissue, including laser (78) and radiofrequency (79) energy. However, the technique most extensively used to date has been electrical fulguration, which involves delivery of a direct current shock from a conventional defibrillator between a skin pad electrode and one or more catheter electrodes appropriately positioned within the heart. The mechanism of tissue injury produced by this method remains uncertain, and the optimal energy level and mode of delivery have not yet been determined. Potential complications include myocardial perforation, depression of ventricular function, coronary artery spasm, and transient ventricular arrhythmias. Arrhythmias to which catheter fulguration has been applied are discussed below.

Supraventricular Tachycardia

Ablation of the His bundle is a valuable therapeutic option for refractory supraventricular tachyarrhythmias. In cases of atrial flutter/fibrillation or AV nodal reentrant SVT, His bundle ablation prevents the transmission of supraventricular impulses to the ventricle by completely interrupting the normal AV conduction pathway. In AV reentrant SVT involving an accessory pathway, His bundle ablation eliminates a necessary limb of the reentry circuit and thus prevents the arrhythmia entirely. This procedure was initially performed by direct visualization during open heart surgery. However, ablation may also be achieved by fulguration with a catheter positioned to record the His bundle deflection (80). Catheter ablation has been successful in 73% of the 501 patients reported to the international registry (81), with no fatalities and few complications consisting of hypotension, ventricular arrhythmias, and cardiac tamponade. Because it yields equally effective results with lower morbidity and less cost than surgery, the catheter technique has become clinically accepted and is preferable to surgical His bundle ablation in patients with highly symptomatic drug-resistant SVT. The primary disadvantage of His bundle ablation (with either method) is that it renders patients permanently pacemaker-dependent, which particularly limits its utility in younger patients.

The potential for catheter ablation of accessory pathways in patients with refractory AV reentrant SVT is currently being evaluated. Results have been best in posteroseptal accessory pathways, which are located near the os of the coronary sinus, and thus, can be closely approached by a catheter placed in this structure. Fulguration has been successful in approximately 75% of patients with pathways in this location (M.M. Scheinman, personal communication) and has not produced serious complications. Unfortunately, catheter ablation has not proven acceptable for pathways in other locations. Results have been poor in the few reported right free wall pathway ablation attempts (82), perhaps due to difficulty in achieving adequate catheter position without a natural landmark. Although the coronary sinus offers a natural approach to left free wall pathways, low energy shocks delivered within it have not produced permanent pathway ablation, and high energy shocks have resulted in coronary sinus rupture requiring emergent pericardial drainage (83).

Catheter ablation has also been attempted in ectopic atrial tachycardia. The procedure has been successful in 8 of the 12 reported cases (82), suggesting that catheter ablation may become a useful therapeutic alternative in patients with ectopic atrial tachycardia refractory to drugs.

Ventricular Tachycardia

When the apparent site of origin of VT can be localized by endocardial catheter mapping, fulguration of that site using the mapping catheter may permanently abolish the arrhythmia. Catheter ablation has been moderately effective in published reports, eliminating VT in approximately one-third of patients, and rendering an additional one-third of patients responsive to drugs that were previously ineffective (82). Complications have included depression of ventricular function and cardiogenic shock. This procedure is an especially attractive alternative in patients with recurrent drug-resistant VT who are poor risks for surgical endocardial resection. However, mapping with sufficient precision for effective use of this approach is technically difficult, and multiple VT morphologies with multiple sites of origin may be impossible to map adequately. Only those patients whose tachycardias are sustained and hemodynamically tolerated well enough to permit detailed mapping are potential candidates for the procedure. The marginal risk-benefit ratio and the limited applicability of catheter ablation for VT continue to confine its performance to the realm of clinical investigation, although advances in catheter design and alternative ablation modes may ultimately improve its overall utility.

References

1. Morady F, DiCarlo L, Winston S, Davis JC, Scheinman MM. Clinical features and prognosis of patients with out of hospital cardiac arrest and a normal electrophysiologic study. J Am Coll Cardiol 1984;4:39–44.
2. Guiraudon G, Klein G, Gulamhusein S, et al. Total disconnection of the right ventricular free wall: surgical treatment of right ventricular tachycardia associated with right ventricular dysplasia. Circulation 1983;67:463–470.
3. Horowitz LN, Kay HR, Kutalek SP, et al. Risks and complications of clinical cardiac electrophysiologic studies: a prospective analysis of 1,000 patients. J Am Coll Cardiol 1987;9:1261–1268.
4. Gettes L, Zipes DP, Gillette PC, et al. Personnel and equipment required for electrophysiologci testing. Report of the Committee on Electrocardiography and Cardiac Electrophysiology, Council on Clinical Cardiology, American Heart Association. Circulation 1984;69:1219A–1221A.
5. Wellens HJJ, Bar FWHM, Lie KI. The value of the electrocardiogram in the differential diagnosis of a tachycardia and with a widened QRS complex. Am J Med 1978;64:27–33.
6. Gettes LS, Foster JR, Woelfel AK, Simpson RJ Jr. Use of electrophysiologic studies to establish the diagnosis, mechanism, and site of tachyarrhythmias. Circulation 1987;75:III116–118.
7. Bar FW, Brugada P, Dassen WRM, Wellens HJJ. Differential diagnosis of tachycardia with narrow QRS complex (shorter than 0.12 second). Am J Cardiol 1984;54:555–560.
8. Denes P, Wu D, Amat-y-Leon F, Dhingra R, Wyndham CR, Rosen KM. The determinants of atrioventricular re-entrance with premature atrial stimulation in patients with dual A-V nodal pathways. Circulation 1977;56:253–259.
9. Benditt DG, Pritchett ELC, Smith WM, Gallagher JJ. Ventriculoatrial intervals: diagnostic use in paroxysmal supraventricular tachycardia. Ann Intern Med 1979;91:161–166.
10. Gomes JA, Hariman RJ, Kang PS, Chowdry IH. Sustained symptomatic sinus node reentrant tachycardia: incidence, clinical significance, electrophysiologic observations and the effects of antiarrhythmic agents. J Am Coll Cardiol 1985;5:45–57.
11. Waldo AL. Mechanisms of atrial fibrillation, atrial flutter, and ectopic atrial tachycardia—a brief review. Circulation 1987;75:III37–40.
12. Inoue H, Matsuo H, Takayanagi K, Murao S. Clinical and experimental studies of the effects of extrastimulation and rapid pacing on atrial flutter: evidence of macroreentry with an excitable gap. Am J Cardiol 1981;48:623–631.
13. Ross DL, Farre J, Bar FWHM, et al. Spontaneous termination of circus movement tachycardia using an atrioventricular accessory pathway: incidence, site of block and mechanisms. Circulation 1981;63:1129–1139.
14. Sung RJ, Shapiro WA, Shen EN, Morady F, Davis J. Effects of verapamil on ventricular tachycardias possibly caused by reentry, automaticity, and triggered activity. J Clin Invest 1983;72:350–360.
15. Akhtar M, Tchou PJ, Jazayeri M. Mechanisms of clinical tachycardias. Am J Cardiol 1986;61:9A–19A.
16. Narula OS, Scherlag BJ, Samet P, Javier RP. Atrioventricular block: localization and classification by His bundle recordings. Am J Med 1971;50:146–165.
17. Rosen KM, Dhingra RC, Loeb H, Rahimtoola SH. Chronic heart block in adults: clinical and electrophysiological observations. Arch Intern Med 1973;131:663–672.
18. Ezri M, Lerman BB, Marchlinski FE, Buxton AE, Josephson ME. Electrophysiologic evaluation of syncope in patients with bifascicular block. Am Heart J 1983;106:693–697.
19. Morady F, Higgins J, Peters RW, et al. Electrophysiologic testing in bundle branch block and unexplained syncope. Am J Cardiol 1984;54:587–591.
20. Gupta PK, Lichstein E, Chadda KD, Badui E. Appraisal of sinus nodal recovery time in patients with sick sinus syndrome. Am J Cardiol 1974;34:265–270.
21. Reiffel JA, Ferrick K, Zimmerman W, et al. Electrophysiologic studies of the sinus node and atria. In: Dreifus LS, ed. Cardiovascular clinics: Cardiac arrhythmias: electrophysiologic techniques and management. Philadelphia: FA Davis, 1985:37–59.
22. Strauss HC, Bigger JT Jr, Saroff AL, Giardina EGV. Electrophysiologic evaluation of sinus node function in patients with sinus node dysfunction. Circulation 1976;56:763–776.
23. Breithardt G, Seipel L, Loogen F. Sinus node recovery time and calculated sino-atrial conduction time in normal subjects and patients with sinus node dysfunction. Circulation 1977;56:43–50.
24. Strauss HC, Grant AG, Scheinman MM, Wallace AG. The use of cardiac stimulation techniques to evaluate sinus node dysfunction. In: Little RC, ed. Physiology of atrial pacemakers. Mt. Kisco, NY: Futura, 1980:339–365.
25. Gann D, Tolentino R, Samet P. Electrophysiologic evaluation of elderly patients with sinus bradycardia. Ann Intern Med 1979;90:24–29.
26. Doherty JU, Pembrook–Rogers D, Grogan EW, et al. Electrophysiologic evaluation and follow-up characteristics of patients with recurrent unexplained syncope and presyncope. Am J Cardiol 1985;55:703–708.
27. Hess DS, Morady F, Scheinman MM. Electrophysiologic testing in the evaluation of patients with syncope of undetermined origin. Am J Cardiol 1982;50:1309–1315.
28. Gulamhusein S, Naccarelli GV, Ko PT, et al. Value and limitations of clinical electrophysiologic study in assessment of patients with unexplained syncope. Am J Med 1982;73:700–705.
29. Benditt DG, Benson DW Jr, Dunnigan A, Gornick CC, Scheinman MM. Drug therapy in sinus node dysfunction. In: Rapaport E, ed. Cardiology update. New York: Elsevier, 1984:79–102.
30. Kerr CR, Strauss HC. The measurement of sinus node refractoriness in man. Circulation 1983;68:1231–1237.
31. Reiffel JA, Gang E, Gliklich J, et al. The human sinus node electrogram: a transvenous catheter technique and a comparison of directly

measured and indirectly estimated sinoatrial conduction time in adults. Circulation 1980;62:1324–1334.

32. Woelfel A, Simpson RJ, Foster JR. Functional type I-like distal atrioventricular block induced by atrial pacing. Am J Cardiol 1984;54:1363–1366.

33. McAnulty JH, Rahimtoola SH, Murphy E, et al. Natural history of "high-risk" bundle-branch block. N Engl J Med 1982;307:137–143.

34. Dhingra RC, Palileo E, Strasburg B, et al. Significance of the HV interval in 517 patients with chronic bifascicular block. Circulation 1981; 64:1265–1271.

35. Dhingra RC, Wyndham C, Bauernfeind R, et al. Significance of block distal to His bundle induced by atrial pacing in patients with chronic bifascicular block. Circulation 1979;60:1455–1464.

36. Scheinman MM, Peters RW, Morady F, Sauve MJ, Malone P, Modin G. Electrophysiologic studies in patients with bundle branch block. PACE 1983;6:1157–1165.

37. Klein GJ, Bashore TM, Sellers TD, Pritchett ELC, Smith WM, Gallagher JJ. Ventricular fibrillation in the Wolff-Parkinson-White syndrome. N Engl J Med 1979;301:1080–1085.

38. Rinne C, Klein GJ, Sharma AD, Yee R, Milstein S, Rattes MF. Relation between clinical presentation and induced arrhythmias in the Wolff-Parkinson-White syndrome. Am J Cardiol 1987;60:576–579.

39. Milstein S, Sharma AD, Klein GJ. Electrophysiologic profile of asymptomatic Wolff-Parkinson-White pattern. Am J Cardiol 1986;57:1097–1100.

40. Buxton AE, Marchlinski FE, Flores BT, Miller JM, Doherty JU, Josephson ME. Nonsustained ventricular tachycardia in patients with coronary artery disease: role of electrophysiologic study. Circulation 1987;75:1178–1185.

41. Poll DS, Marchlinski FE, Buxton AE, Josephson ME. Usefulness of programmed stimulation in idiopathic dilated cardiomyopathy. Am J Cardiol 1986;58:992–997.

42. Das SK, Morady F, DiCarlo L, et al. Prognostic usefulness of programmed ventricular stimulation in idiopathic dilated cardiomyopathy without symptomatic ventricular arrhythmias. Am J Cardiol 1986;58:998–1000.

43. Roy D, Marchand E, Theroux P, Waters DD, Pelletier GB, Bourassa MG. Programmed ventricular stimulation in survivors of an acute myocaridal infarction. Am J Cardiol 1985;56:384–389.

44. Hamer A, Vohra J, Hunt D, Sloman G. Prediction of sudden death by electrophysiologic studies in high risk patients surviving acute myocardial infarction. Am J Cardiol 1982;50:223–229.

45. Marchlinski FE, Buxton AE, Waxman HL, Josephson ME. Identifying patients at risk of sudden death after myocardial infarction: value of the response to programmed stimulation, degree of ventricular ectopic activity, and severity of left ventricular dysfunction. Am J Cardiol 1983;52:1190–1196.

46. Denniss AT, Baaijens H, Cody DV, et al. Value of programmed stimulation and exercise testing in predicting one-year mortality after acute myocardial infarction. Am J Cardiol 1985;56:213–219.

47. Waspe LE, Seinfeld D, Ferrick A, Kim SG, Matos JA, Fisher JD. Prediction of sudden death and spontaneous ventricular tachycardia in survivors of complicated myocardial infarction: value of the response to programmed stimulation using a maximum of three ventricular extrastimuli. J Am Coll Cardiol 1985;5:1292–1301.

48. Bhandari AK, Rose JS, Kotlewski A, Rahimtoola SH, Wu D. Frequency and signficance of induced sustained ventricular tachycardia or fibrillation two weeks after acute myocardial infarction. Am J Cardiol 1985;56:737–742.

49. Santarelli P, Belloci F, Loperfido F, et al. Ventricular arrhythmia induced by programmed ventricular stimulation after acute myocardial infarction. Am J Cardiol 1985;55:2391–2394.

50. Bauernfeind RA, Wyndham CR, Dhingra RC, et al. Serial electrophysiologic testing of multiple drugs in patients with atrioventricular nodal reentrant paroxysmal tachycardia. Circulation 1980;62:1341–1349.

51. Wu D, Amat-y-Leon F, Simpson RJ, et al. Electrophysiologic studies with multiple drugs in patients with atrioventricular reentrant tachycardias utilizing an extranodal pathway. Circulation 1977;56:727–736.

52. Morady F, Sledge C, Shen E, Sung RJ, Gonzales R, Scheinman MM. Electrophysiologic testing in the management of patients with the Wolff-Parkinson-White syndrome and atrial fibrillation. Am J Cardiol 1983;51:1623–1628.

53. Lown B, Graboys TB. Management of patients with malignant ventricular arrhythmias. Am J Cardiol 1977;39:910–918.

54. Marchlinski FE, Buxton AE, Flores BT, Doherty JJ, Waxman HL, Josephson ME. Value of Holter monitoring in identifying risk for sustained ventricular arrhythmia recurrence on amiodarone. Am J Cardiol 1985;55:709–712.

55. Mitchell LB, Duff HJ, Manyari DE, Wyse DG. A randomized clinical trial for the noninvasive and invasive approaches to drug therapy of ventricular tachycardia. N Engl J Med 1987;317:1681–1687.

56. Kim SG, Felder SD, Figura I, Johnston DR, Waspe LE, Fisher JD. Comparison of programmed stimulation and Holter monitoring for predicting long-term efficacy of amiodarone used alone or in combination with a class 1A antiarrhythmic agent in patients with ventricular tachyarrhythmia. J Am Coll Cardiol 1987;9:398–404.

57. Mason JW, Anderson KP, Freedman RA. Techniques and criteria in electrophysiologic study of ventricular tachycardia. Circulation 1987;75:III125–130.

58. Miller JM, Kienzle MG, Harken AH, Josephson ME. Morphologically distinct sustained ventricular tachycardias in coronary artery disease: significance and surgical results. J Am Coll Cardiol 1984;4:1073–1079.

59. Garan H, Stavens CS, McGovern B, Kelly E, Ruskin JN. Reproducibility of ventricular tachycardia suppression by antiarrhythmic drug therapy during serial electrophysiologic testing in coronary artery disease. Am J Cardiol 1986;58:977–980.

60. Kudenchuk PJ, Kron J, Walance CG, et al. Reproducibility of arrhythmia induction with intracardiac electrophysiologic testing: patients with

clinical sustained ventricular tachyarrhythmias. J Am Coll Cardiol 1986;7:819–828.

61. McPherson CA, Rosenfeld LE, Batsford WP. Day-to-day reproducibility of responses to right ventricular programmed electrical stimulation: implications for serial drug testing. Am J Cardiol 1985;55:689–695.

62. Morady F, Scheinman MM, Hess DS, Sung RJ, Shen E, Shapiro W. Electrophysiologic testing in the management of survivors of out-of-hospital cardiac arrest. Am J Cardiol 1983;51:85–89.

63. Roy D, Waxman HL, Kienzle MG, Buxton AE, Marchlinski FE, Josephson ME. Clinical characteristic and long-term follow-up in 119 survivors of cardiac arrest; relation to inducibility at electrophysiologic testing. Am J Cardiol 1983;52:969–974.

64. Benditt DG, Benson DW, Klein GJ, Pritzker MR, Kreitt JM, Anderson RW. Prevention of recurrent sudden cardiac arrest: role of provocative electropharmacologic testing. J Am Coll Cardiol 1983;2:418–425.

65. Ruskin JN, DiMarco JP, Garan H. Out-of-hospital cardiac arrest: electrophysiologic observations and selection of long-term antiarrhythmic therapy. N Engl J Med 1980;303:607–613.

66. Mason JW, Winkle RA. Accuracy of the ventricular tachycardia-induction study for predicting long-term efficacy and inefficacy of antiarrhythmic drugs. N Engl J Med 1980;303:1073–1077.

67. Waxman HL, Groh WC, Marchlinski FE, et al. Amiodarone for control of sustained ventricular tachyarrhythmia: clinical and electrophysiologic effects in 51 patients. Am J Cardiol 1982;50:1066–1074.

68. Heger JJ, Prystowsky EN, Jackman WM, et al. Amiodarone: clinical efficacy and electrophysiology during long-term therapy for recurrent ventricular tachycardia or ventricular fibrillation. N Engl J Med 1981;305:539–545.

69. Sealy WC, Hattler BG, Blumenschein SD, Cobb FR. Surgical treatment of Wolff-Parkinson-White syndrome. Ann Thorac Surg 1969;8:1–11.

70. Gallagher JJ, Pritchett ELC, Benditt DG, et al. New catheter techniques for analysis of the sequence of retrograde atrial activation in man. Eur J Cardiol 1977;6:1–14.

71. Horowitz LN, Harken AH, Kastor JA, Josephson ME. Ventricular resection guided by epicardial and endocardial mapping for treatment of recurrent ventricular tachycardia. N Engl J Med 1980;302:589–593.

72. Haines DE, Lerman BB, Kron IL, DiMarco JP. Surgical ablation of ventricular tachycardia with sequential map-guided subendocardial resection: electrophysiologic assessment and long-term follow-up. Circulation 1988;77:131–141.

73. Josephson ME, Horowitz LN, Spielman SR, Greenspan AM, VandePol C, Harken AH. Comparison of endocardial catheter mapping with intraoperative mapping of ventricular tachycardia. Circulation 1980;61:395–404.

74. Fisher JD, Kim SG, Mercando AD. Electrical devices for treatment of arrhythmias. Am J Cardiol 1988;61:45A–57A.

75. Kay GN, Plumb VJ, Arciniegas JG, Henthorn RW, Waldo AL. Torsade de pointes: The long-short initiating sequence and other clincial features: observations in 32 patients. J Am Coll Cardiol 1983;5:806–817.

76. Eldar M, Griffin JC, Abbott JA, et al. Permanent cardiac pacing in patients with the long QT syndrome. J Am Coll Cardiol 1987;10:600–607.

77. Sung RJ, Styperek JL, Castellanos A. Complete abolition of the reentrant SVT zone using a new modality of cardiac pacing with simultaneous atrioventricular stimulation. Am J Cardiol 1980;45:72–78.

78. Lee BI, Gottdiener JS, Fletcher RD, Rodriguez ER, Ferrans VJ. Transcatheter ablation: comparison between laser photoablation and electrode shock ablation in the dog. Circulation 1985;71:579–586.

79. Huang SK, Jordan N, Graham A, et al. Closed-chest catheter dessication of atrioventricular junction using radiofrequency energy—a new method of catheter ablation (abstr). Circulation 1985;72:III-389.

80. Gallagher J, Svenson RH, Kasell JH, et al. Catheter technique for closed-chest ablation of the atrioventricular conduction system. N Engl J Med 1982;306:194–200.

81. Evans GT Jr, Scheinman MM, Fox C, Rodrigues M. Predictors of successful HIS bundle ablation: a report of the percutaneous cardiac mapping and ablation registry (abstr). J Am Coll Cardiol 1988;11:17A.

82. Fisher JD, Brodman R, Waspe LE, Kim SG. Nonsurgical electrical ablation (fulguration) of tachycardias. Circulation 1987;75:III194–199.

83. Fisher JD, Brodman R, Kim SG, et al. Attempted nonsurgical electrical ablation of accessory pathways via the coronary sinus in the Wolff-Parkinson-White syndrome. J Am Coll Cardiol 1984;4:685–694.

31

The Patient with Known or Suspect Cardiomyopathy

J. Michael Criley, M.D.
Robert J. Siegel, M.D.

INTRODUCTION

Heart muscle disease comprises a number of primary and secondary disorders, but may be conveniently classified into dilated, restrictive, and hypertrophic cardiomyopathy (1), based on morphologic and functional characteristics. Inherent in the diagnosis of cardiomyopathy is the absence of significant congenital, valvular, pericardial, or coronary vascular disease. These latter conditions have been well-characterized by hemodynamic and angiographic studies. In many instances these studies provide the investigator with sufficient information to undertake beneficial therapy.

Advances in our knowledge and treatment of the cardiomyopathies have made scant progress by comparison with the other cardiac disorders mentioned above. This lack of progress can be attributed to the nature of heart muscle disease. Unlike other forms of heart disease, there are no discrete mechanical defects or impediments that yield to catheterization's diagnostic and therapeutic potential. As a result, heart muscle diseases are truly "orphan diseases" and one of the last frontiers in cardiology.

JUSTIFICATION FOR CARDIAC CATHETERIZATION

The shortcomings of cardiac catheterization in the cardiomyopathies are further emphasized by the advances in noninvasive diagnostic techniques. It is now possible with a high degree of certainty to establish a categorical diagnosis in most patients with heart muscle disease by echocardiography and Doppler studies. Furthermore, bedside flotation-catheterization of the right heart provides almost as complete a hemodynamic characterization as a "formal" cardiac catheterization. One can therefore ask whether there is still a place for cardiac catheterization in suspected primary heart muscle disease. Is there enough potential benefit to the patient to outweigh the hazards and expense? We will first attempt to justify the need for continued hemodynamic-angiographic studies in selected patients with suspected cardiomyopathy and then outline our laboratories' approach to specific categories of heart muscle disease.

We feel that it is important to identify cardiac entities which may simulate heart muscle disease and in some instances have specific and effective alternate therapeutic options (Table 31.1). Specific case examples of several of these entities will be presented in the section pertaining to each category of cardiomyopathy.

GENERAL APPROACH TO CARDIAC CATHETERIZATION IN THE CARDIOMYOPATHIES

When a formal cardiac catheterization is to be performed (i.e., hemodynamic, angiographic, coronary angiographic, biopsy), we generally utilize the percutaneous transfemoral (modified Seldinger) approach because of its versatility. Transfemoral venous entry provides access to transseptal left heart catheterization which is often utilized in our studies of patients with hypertrophic cardiomyopathy (HCM). Similarly, we have adapted the transfemoral venous route to the performance of endomyocardial biopsy and have found the femoral artery more convenient for coronary arteriography and angioplasty.

Right heart catheterization is performed with a catheter designed to obtain an optimal pulmonary-capillary wedge (PCW) pressure, i.e., either a Goodale-Lubin or balloon flotation catheter. We have found the Swan-Ganz Paceport (Baxter Health Care, Edwards Division) catheter to be particularly useful for simultaneous recording of right atrial, right ventricular (via the Paceport lumen), and pulmonary artery or PCW pressure. Cardiac output is determined by indicator dilution technique, with either a calibrated indocyanine green (Cardiogreen) or thermal technique. When cardiac output is suspected to be abnormally low, we employ the direct Fick method to obtain more reliable data. We routinely obtain pulmonary artery, vena caval, and arterial oxygen saturation values to exclude intracardiac shunts and to assess the arteriovenous oxygen difference. Repeat determinations after provocative or therapeutic interventions can be anticipated in certain cases. To ensure reproducible data under these circumstances, a sufficient quantity of indicator should be on hand. For example, we combine the contents of several 10-ml vials of indocyanine green to allow sufficient indicator for calibration and repeat cardiac output determinations.

Left heart catheterization is usually performed by the retrograde technique unless there is the need for obtaining direct left atrial pressure or simultaneous pressure in the left ventricle and central aorta by utilizing the transseptal route. Because the "pigtail" catheter has multiple side holes which do not permit precise catheter withdrawal tracings, we prefer to employ a catheter with an end hole and "bird's-eye" side holes near the tip when there is a question of an intracavitary pressure gradient.

Endomyocardial biopsy is done principally in patients with dilated cardiomyopathy or restrictive cardiomyopathy; we have not found it to yield useful information in patients with hypertrophic cardiomyopathy. Biopsy is usually performed at the time of diagnostic catheterization but may also be performed as an independent procedure when serial studies are done. We have found the technique to have a low morbidity rate and have had no biopsy-related deaths in over 300 procedures. It is important to point out that the most crucial stage in the biopsy procedure is the handling and interpretation of the specimens. Accurate assessment requires individuals with considerable training and experience in myocardial histopathology. This expertise is not widely available. The transfemoral approach is used when right ventricular septal endomyocardial biopsy is combined with diagnostic cardiac catheterization (see Chapter 6). We believe that left heart samples add little to the diagnostic information obtained from right heart biopsies, with rare possible exceptions such as endomyocardial fibrosis or fibroelastosis principally affecting the left ventricle.

Angiography is performed to evaluate the status of the coronary arteries and left ventricle in all cases unless the former procedure is

Table 31.1.
Simulators Of Cardiomyopathy

1. Dilated cardiomyopathy simulators
   A. Chronic valvular disease
      1) Mitral regurgitation
      2) Aortic stenosis
      3) Aortic regurgitation
   B. Atherosclerotic coronary artery disease
      1) With infarction(s)
      2) With ischemic depression of left ventricular function
   C. Congenital heart disease
      1) Ebstein's anomaly
      2) Coronary anomalies
      3) Atrial septal defect
2. Restrictive cardiomyopathy simulators
   A. Constrictive pericarditis
   B. Acute valvular regurgitation
3. Hypertrophic cardiomyopathy simulators
   A. Discrete subaortic stenosis
   B. Aortic stenosis
   C. Hypertensive hypertrophic cardiomyopathy of the elderly
   D. Infiltrative diseases
      1) Glycogen storage disorders
      2) Lymphoma
      3) Amyloid

obviated by young age and/or the absence of symptoms or risk factors for ischemic heart disease. The benefit/risk ratio for coronary angiography and ventriculography is sufficiently high to justify their use except in rare circumstances (e.g., renal failure, severe allergy to contrast media, echocardiographic evidence of soft thrombus in the left ventricle). Coronary angiography may uncover an unsuspected and potentially reversible ischemic basis for dilated cardiomyopathy while left ventriculography remains the "reference standard" for evaluating regional wall motion and mitral valve competence.

Specialized research catheterization techniques have been utilized in some laboratories to record unique information in patients with cardiomyopathy which cannot be obtained by ordinary catheterization procedures. For example, Murgo and colleagues (2, 3) have used **multisensor catheters** containing two or three micromanometers and a flow velocity probe to study instantaneous pressure and blood flow signals; this technique is particularly well-suited to the study of patients with HCM (Fig. 31.1). A multipole **conductance catheter** can be used to estimate instantaneous ventricular volume while recording high-fidelity pressure with a 4 Fr micromanometer catheter advanced through the conductance catheter lumen. Pressure volume loops can be generated from the digitized

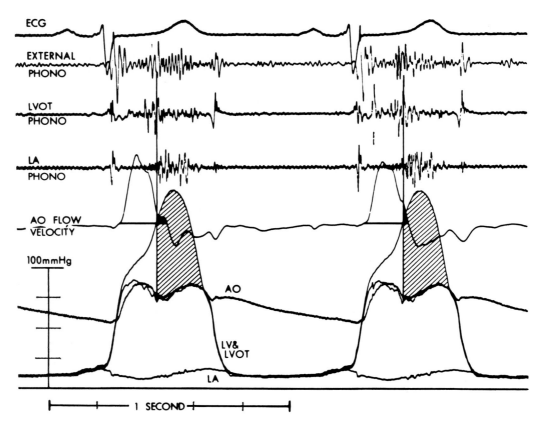

Figure 31.1. Multisensor recording of high-fidelity left heart pressures, aortic blood flow velocity, intracardiac phonocardiograms (*PHONO*) derived by filtering micromanometer pressure signals, and external phonocardiogram in a patient with hypertrophic cardiomyopathy. The midsystolic (*vertical line*) represents the time of systolic anterior motion-septal contact, following which there is an 80 mm Hg pressure gradient and very little forward flow. *AO,* aortic; *LA,* left atrial; *LV,* left ventricular; *LVOT,* left ventricular outflow tract. See text for details. (From Murgo JP, Miller JW. Hemodynamic, angiographic and echocardiographic evidence against impeded ejection in hypertrophic cardiomyopathy. In: Goodwin JR, ed. Heart muscle disease. Lancaster: MTP Press Limited, 1985.)

instantaneous pressure and volume signals by a microcomputer (Fig. 31.2). This technique is combined with abrupt alterations in venous return achieved by inflation and deflation of a vena caval balloon or atrial pacing. It is then possible to calculate the instantaneous end-systolic pressure/volume relationship over a wide range of volumes to estimate contractile function, as well as the diastolic pressure/volume relationships to assess diastolic properties of the ventricle (4).

SPECIFIC APPROACHES TO CARDIAC CATHETERIZATION IN PATIENTS WITH DIFFERENT CARDIOMYOPATHIES

Dilated Cardiomyopathy

Dilated cardiomyopathy (DCM) is defined by dilated ventricular chambers with poor systolic function without underlying coronary arterial or valvular disease (1) and cannot be considered a secure diagnosis until potentially reversible etiologic entities can be excluded (Table 31.1). End-stage dilated hearts

secondary to ischemic heart disease and/or chronic valvular disease can simulate primary DCM. Our approach, which is designed to exclude secondary causes of DCM, is outlined in Table 31.2.

It can be argued that, by the time the left ventricle is dilated and hypokinetic, regardless of the cause, determination of the etiology is a purely academic exercise since the condition is not reversible. It has been our experience that some reversibility of severely depressed ventricular function can be achieved by revascularization in "ischemic cardiomyopathy" if ongoing ischemia can be demonstrated. We therefore feel justified in the pursuit of the etiology even in the presence of poor left ventricular function. The following case will illustrate some of these points.

A 62-year-old farmer had progressive symptoms and signs of left and right heart failure for 1 month prior to admission for cardiac evaluation, but denied chest discomfort or anginal equivalent symptoms. Cardiac catheterization demonstrated

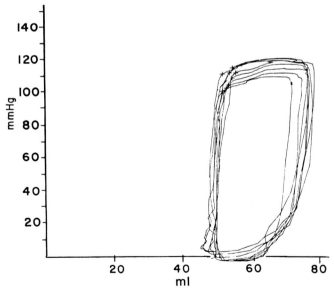

Figure 31.2. Pressure volume loops after release of positive intrathoracic pressure (Valsalva maneuver). Instantaneous volume is computed from conductance signals from a multipole catheter in the left ventricle, and the pressure derived from a micromanometer catheter. Eight pressure volume loops are generated as the venous return to the left ventricle increases. The slope of the right lower corner of the loops is a reflection of distensibility of the ventricle. See Ref. 4 for further details. (Used by permission from Peter C. D. Pelikan, M.D., Harbor-UCLA Medical Center).

global left ventricular dysfunction with an ejection fraction of 15%, severe pulmonary hypertension, moderate mitral regurgitation, and four-vessel coronary artery disease. Ambulatory electrocardiograms demonstrated frequent nonsustained ventricular tachycardia. The patient remained in class IV New York Heart Association (NYHA) status and was hospitalized repeatedly for cardiac decompensation despite diuretic, vasodilator, and antiarrhythmic therapy. He sustained a pulmonary embolism. Despite the clinical and laboratory presentation of DCM, he was evaluated for possible coronary revascularization in the hope that the depressed ventricular function was reversible. He only

Table 31.2.
Hemodynamic-Angiographic Study in Dilated Cardiomyopathy

1. Indications for study
   A. Cardiomegaly of unknown cause
   B. Stabilized hemodynamic status (e.g., not in overt failure)
   C. Absence of contraindications (e.g., hepatic congestion, coagulopathy, malignancy, mental instability)
2. Procedures
   A. Transfemoral venous right heart catheterization
      1) Establish level of pulmonary hypertension
      2) Measure cardiac output, mixed venous O_2 saturation
      3) Rule out tricuspid valve displacement (Ebstein's)
      4) Right ventricular endomyocardial biopsy for:
         a. Light microscopy
         b. Electron microscopy
         c. Immunohistochemistry
         d. Viral culture
   B. Transfemoral retrograde left heart catheterization
      1) Rule out aortic valve calcification, gradient
      2) Measure systemic vascular resistance (SVR)
      3) Left ventriculogram (nonionic contrast medium)
         a. Ejection fraction/wall motion
         b. Mitral regurgitation
         c. Repeat after arterial dilator if SVR elevated
      4) Coronary angiography

tolerated 3.3 min of treadmill exercise because of dyspnea and fatigue; the electrocardiogram and thallium-201 perfusion scan did not demonstrate evidence of ischemia; and there were no defects on the stress or redistribution thallium scan. A positron emission tomographic (PET) scan was then performed, which revealed decreased ^{13}N ammonia uptake (Fig. 31.3, *arrows*) and preserved or enhanced [18]F 2-deoxyglucose uptake, suggesting ischemic but viable myocardium.

The patient underwent four-vessel revascularization and had an uncomplicated recovery. His symptoms and signs of cardiac decompensation abated while taking quinidine and decreased doses of diuretics and vasodilators. There was a remarkable improvement in left ventricular functional parameters and diminution in pulmonary hypertension on echocardiography and Doppler study:

	Preoperative	Postoperative 1 month	1 year
Echo dimensions			
Left atrium (cm)	6.0	5.3	5.5
Left ventricular internal diameter			
Diastole (cm)	6.8	6.5	6.2
Systole (cm)	5.8	5.3	5.0
Doppler studies			
Mitral regurgitation	2–3+	2–3+	
Tricuspid regurgitation	3+	2+	
Estimated right ventricular systolic pressure (mm Hg)	70	23	

He continued to do well for 18 months until quinidine was discontinued because of gastrointestinal side effects. He died suddenly 2 weeks later.

This case was chosen to point out that ischemic cardiomyopathy may closely resemble DCM and is potentially reversible if viable but ischemic myocardium is present. The invasive study (cardiac catheterization with coronary angiography) provided the first evidence that he had coronary artery disease, and the PET scan demonstrated a metabolic pattern compatible with resting ischemia.

The useful diagnostic and therapeutic yield from performing endomyocardial biopsies in patients with DCM has been disappointingly low in comparison to coronary angiography. In over 12 years' experience with the procedure in DCM, the incidence of active inflammation has been under 3% in our laboratories, and we rarely uncover a condition that would change our clinical impression or suggest an alteration in therapy in a patient with DCM. When a population with recent onset DCM is subjected to biopsy, the yield for active myocarditis increases to about 10% (Fig. 31.4). Figure 31.5 demonstrates extensive fibrosis without active inflammation in a biopsy specimen from a patient with new onset cardiac decompensation. Although the extent of fibrosis is thought to have prognostic significance, it is difficult to assess "extent" on the basis of one or a few biopsy specimens. This patient remains stable 3 years after this biopsy was obtained.

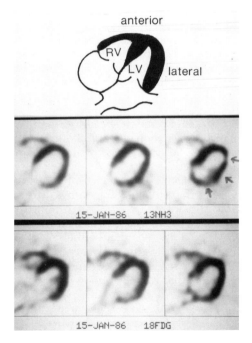

Figure 31.3. Cross-sectional cardiac PET images. The nitrogen-13-ammonia ($^{13}NH_3$) estimates regional myocardial blood flow and demonstrates reduced uptake in the anterolateral and posterior walls (*arrows*). Preserved fluorine-18-deoxyglucose (^{18}FDG) uptake is present in the anterolateral wall and septum, and reduced uptake is found in the inferoposterior walls. Postoperatively the anterolateral abnormalities normalized. (This study was performed in the laboratory of Henrich Schelbert, M.D., who kindly provided these images.)

The dismal prognosis associated with DCM has led many investigators to an aggressive effort to establish the presence of active myocardial inflammation in patients with recent onset DCM in the belief that myocarditis is potentially treatable. The premise that DCM is frequently the end-stage of myocarditis is widely believed but lacks substantiation and the supporting data currently available is tenuous (5, 6). The corollary to this premise, namely that myocarditis frequently leads to DCM, also lacks support. The mechanism by which a focal accumulation of lymphocytes might lead to severe myocardial depression also remains unexplained. We have found that myocardial immunoglobin deposition is very infrequent in patients with "clinical myocarditis" or new onset DCM. Furthermore, evidence that there is an effective treatment for established myocarditis is similarly lacking. When data from the world's literature is pooled (Table 31.3), it can be appreciated that only about 12% (on average) of patients with recent onset DCM have biopsy-proven myocarditis, and only 12.5% (on average) of patients with clinically suspected myocarditis will develop DCM. In regard to treatment, immunosuppression is associated with clinical improvement approximately 56% of the time, whereas spontaneous improvement is seen in approximately 48% of nonspecifically treated biopsy-proven myocarditis patients (7).

It is not our intent in the previous paragraph to spawn a nihilistic attitude about the

Table 31.3.
Myocarditis-Dilated Cardiomyopathy (DCM) Link and the Effect of Therapy: Summary of Pooled International Data[a] (See text for details)

12%	(range 0–67%) of 2223 patients with DCM developed biopsy-proven myocarditis.
12.5%	(range 0–30%) of 400 patients with clinically suspect myocarditis developed DCM.
56%	(range 0–100%) of 54 patients with biopsy-proven myocarditis improved with immunosuppressive therapy.
48%	(range 33–78%) of 33 patients with biopsy-proven myocarditis showed spontaneous improvement.

[a] Modified from O'Connell JB. The role of myocarditis in end-stage dilated cardiomyopathy. Tex Heart Inst J 1987;14:268–275.

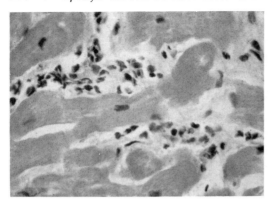

Figure 31.4. Myocarditis in DCM. High power photomicrograph of endomyocardial biopsy from a 72-year-old woman with new onset congestive heart failure and ventricular tachycardia demonstrates a mononuclear infiltrate and mild myocyte hypertrophy. Coagulation necrosis was evident on H and E stain.

validity of the myocarditis-DCM link or the likelihood that any effective treatment might emerge. It should be recognized that the current reference standard for myocarditis, i.e., endomyocardial biopsy, has significant limitations. One to five biopsy specimens cannot be considered statistically representative of the entire myocardium, and we lack sophisticated knowledge and methods to identify or exclude myocarditis with certainty from biopsy tissue.

New probes to establish the presence of myocarditis are being developed. A study by Bowles et al. (8) demonstrated Coxsackie-B-

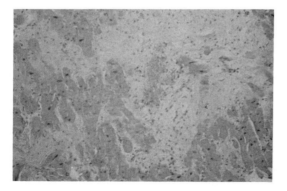

Figure 31.5. Extensive fibrosis in DCM. An endomyocardial biopsy from a 59-year-old woman with new onset dilated cardiomyopathy demonstrates myocyte hypertrophy and extensive interstitial fibrosis.

virus-specific RNA sequences in myocarditis and DCM, using cDNA-RNA hybridization techniques. The presence of viral-specific RNA sequences in acute myocarditis and chronic DCM suggests continuing viral replication. The significance, sensitivity, and specificity of these findings remain to be determined. It is hoped that cDNA probes will enhance our ability to detect viral-induced myocardial disease. It is anticipated that, as our ability to detect viral pathogens or altered autoimmunity improves, many current concepts about the cause of DCM will have to be revised radically or discarded.

Hypertrophic Cardiomyopathy

HCM is a primary heart muscle disorder characterized by disproportionate left ventricular hypertrophy in the absence of an identifiable underlying cause (e.g., aortic stenosis, hypertension) and without dilation of the ventricular cavities (1). The hypertrophy is usually asymmetrically distributed (LV > RV; interventricular septum > free wall; basal septum > apical septum), and the systolic function is usually well-preserved with an elevated ejection fraction. There is a specific form of HCM in which hypertrophy is confined to the apex, associated with giant negative T waves and a spade-shaped ventricle (9).

In the majority of instances, the diagnosis of HCM can be made with noninvasive evaluation, principally by physical examination, echocardiography, and Doppler ultrasonography (10) so that cardiac catheterization is rarely indicated for the sole purpose of establishing a diagnosis. Consequently, we do not perform cardiac catheterization in all patients with HCM, but reserve the procedure for those occasions when we believe that the findings will aid our therapeutic approach to the specific patient. At the same time, we believe that invasive studies should be designed to define the pathophysiology and enhance our understanding of the disease process. Our indications for and conduct of invasive studies in HCM are outlined in Table 31.4.

A cardiac muscle disorder that has many hemodynamic similarities to HCM has been described in elderly women with prior hypertension (11). These patients have elevated left ventricular filling pressures and well-preserved or enhanced systolic function. This

Table 31.4.
Hemodynamic-Angiographic Studies in
Hypertrophic Cardiomyopathy

1. Indications
   A. Signs/symptoms not responding to
      medical therapy
      1) Anginal chest pain
      2) Signs/symptoms of pulmonary
         congestion
      3) Syncope
      4) Refractory to medical management
         with β-blocker(s)
   B. "Malignant" personal or family history
      1) Sudden death in young first degree
         relatives
      2) Resuscitation from ventricular
         tachyarrhythmia
2. Procedures (without withdrawal of β-blocker)
   A. Right heart catheterization
      1) Assess pulmonary artery and
         capillary wedge pressures
      2) Establish or exclude right ventricular
         gradient
         a. Withdrawal recording from
            pulmonary artery through right
            ventricle (over guidewire to
            avoidarrhythmias)
         b. Withdrawal recording from apex to
            tricuspid valve
   B. Left heart catheterization (transseptal
      and retrograde)
      1) Resting (control) hemodynamic-
         angiographic-phonocardiographic
         evaluation: pressures, cardiac output,
         sounds, biplane left ventriculography
      2) Repeat above evaluation with
         appropriate perturbation(s)
         a. If resting LV^a filling pressure >25
            mm Hg, decrease filling pressure
            (calcium antagonist, nitrate)
         b. If resting intracavitary gradient
            >50 mm Hg
            i. Increase filling volume (raise
               legs, infusion) or
            ii. Increase aortic impedance
                (vasopressor) to diminish
                gradient
         c. If <50 mm Hg resting gradient
            i. Decrease filling volume
               (Valsalva maneuver, nitrates)
               and/or
            ii. Decrease aortic impedance
                and/or
            iii. Increase inotropic state to
                 provoke gradient
   C. Coronary angiography
   D. Electrophysiological evaluation (if indi-
      cated, usually done as a separate study)

---

^{a} LV, left ventricular.

condition can be distinguished from HCM by the concentric pattern of hypertrophy and the presence of an underlying cause for left ventricular hypertrophy. We have encountered a similar derangement of diastolic function in patients with mild aortic stenosis in lieu of hypertension and pathological left ventricular hypertrophy.

Our approach to the invasive study of HCM and hypertrophic hypertensive cardiomyopathy is designed to answer clinically relevant questions that pertain to the patient under study and to understand the pathophysiology of the various manifestations of the disease process (elevated filling pressure, pulse contours, ejection dynamics, intracavitary pressure gradient, mitral regurgitation, murmur, etc.) in that individual. If the patient has been taking a β-adrenergic blocking agent chronically, we usually continue the drug during the study in order to avoid possible complications from its withdrawal.

The abnormal diastolic function of the left ventricle may be the principal cause of symptoms in these patients and therefore should be a major focus of the hemodynamic-angiographic study (12). If the filling pressure is markedly elevated (>25 mm Hg), the response to a β-adrenergic or calcium channel blocking agent can be assessed. If the patient is already taking a β-blocking agent, nifedipine is given in preference to verapamil or diltiazem to avoid excessive heart rate depression. Nifedipine may be given in a sublingual suspension starting with 2.5 mg (1/4 capsule) and adding 2.5-mg increments, each 5 to 10 min for a total of 10 mg or until a favorable effect is achieved or hypotension occurs. If the patient becomes symptomatically hypotensive, any residual nifedipine should be irrigated out of the mouth, and the legs should be elevated until a fluid infusion is successful in restoring the blood pressure. We have found that an intravenous infusion of calcium chloride, 1 gm, can also reverse hypotension caused by calcium channel blocking drugs.

If the patient has not been taking a β-blocker, intravenous propranolol or verapamil may be administered in 1- to 2.5-mg increments until a lowering of the left ventricular filling pressure is achieved or an adverse effect occurs. Alternatively, the effects of sublingual nitrates on the filling pressure and cardiac output can yield useful data regarding the safety and effectiveness of this class of drug in the treatment of pulmonary congestive symptoms. If symptomatic hypotension occurs, it should be promptly countered with leg raising and volume expansion.

Although there has been considerable interest in dynamic intracavitary pressure gradients in HCM, our hemodynamic and angiographic studies have consistently demonstrated an intriguing paradox, namely that there is a positive correlation between the magnitudes of the pressure gradient and the ejection fraction. When groups of patients with HCM are compared, those with resting intracavitary gradients have the highest ejection fractions, and those without gradients, the lowest (13):

HCM Groups	LV Ejection Fraction
No gradient	73 ± 8%
Gradient with	
provocation only	83 ± 10%
Resting gradient	90 ± 8%

When the magnitude of an intracavitary gradient is increased or diminished, the numerical value of the ejection fraction changes in a corresponding manner. These findings are inconsistent with a "dynamic obstruction," which would be expected to impede ejection, diminish the ability to empty the ventricle, and lower the ejection fraction with increasing magnitude. Since dynamic gradients do not seem to adversely impair ventricular function, we do not believe that the pressure gradient ("obstruction") should be the primary focus of the hemodynamic evaluation in patients with HCM. When we encounter a resting intracavitary gradient or can readily provoke one, we repeat the hemo-dynamic-angiographic-phonocardiographic evaluation in order to determine if the gradient imposes a measurable impediment to ventricular function (13, 14).

Angiocardiography in HCM is technically difficult to perform and interpret. The small, irregular left ventricular cavity and irritable myocardium hamper efforts to obtain adequate opacification while avoiding premature beats and spurious mitral regurgitation. We have found that injections in the mitral valve region of the ventricle are better tolerated than injections in the trabecular submitral region (body) of the ventricle, especially if there is a resting pressure gradient, which is usually associated with systolic obliteration of the submitral ventricular cavity (Figs. 31.6 and 31.7). Injections into the submitral region of the ventricle frequently provoke ectopic beats and provide a distorted impression of the degree of mitral regurgitation and the dynamics of ventricular contraction. Contrast medium continuously injected into an obliterating chamber during systole will prevent the chamber from eliminating its contents and give the false impression that there is a substantial residual volume.

We do not perform biventriculography or simultaneous injections into both ventricles to define septal thickness; other techniques, such as echocardiography and magnetic resonance imaging, better define the septum and can be performed noninvasively. We have found that arrhythmias are difficult to avoid with simultaneous biventricular injections, and the details of the ventricles are better seen with separate selective injections.

The unique angiographic features of the left ventricle in HCM are best viewed in motion. The remarkable rate and degree of emptying of the craggy ventricle and the high velocity jet or spray of mitral regurgitation can best be observed in motion. The irregular ventricular outlines defeat precise quantitation of ventricle volume. The diastolic angiographic contour of the submitral cavity consists of a network of spicules representing contrast-filled intertrabecular recesses in the hypertrophied walls. As the ventricular walls thicken during systole, the recesses are obliterated centripetally yielding an exaggerated impression of the inward excursion of the ventricular endocardium shown in Figure 31.6. The aortic vestibule, the cylindrical region of the left ventricle between the mitral annulus and the aortic valve, is noncontractile and comprises the bulk of the residual volume or dead space at end systole. The vestibule may expand during systole and functionally serves as an extension of the aorta. The remaining portion of the end-systolic volume is confined to the mitral valve region, or inflow region, which contains the mitral apparatus consisting of elongated and thickened leaflets puckered and distorted by the exaggerated annular constriction and enlarged papillary muscles (Figs. 31.6 and 31.7). The irregular shape of the inflow region does not lend itself to volumetric assessment, and calculations are further compromised by the space-occupying valve apparatus within it.

Small pockets of contrast-laden blood, representing approximately 1 to 3 ml, may lie in the recesses on the ventricular aspect of the puckered posterior mitral valve leaflet, while the cavity of the contractile (submitral) region of the ventricle is frequently eliminated by midsystole. The thickened mitral leaflets may form a lucent line in midsystole and late systole, best seen in the left anterior oblique projection (Fig. 31.7), which is the angiographic analogue of echocardiographic systolic anterior motion. This lucent line can be seen to occur after the ventricle has ejected 80 to 90% of the stroke volume. It has been generally concluded that this abnormal mitral motion is responsible for the pressure gradient and obstructs the further egress of blood from the ventricle. Because we cannot demonstrate hindered flow (e.g., reduced rate and/or degree of emptying) in association with pressure gradients and systolic anterior motion

when the same ventricle is studied in the presence and absence of these phenomena (Fig. 31.8), we do not concur with this view. The reader is referred to more detailed discussions of the opposing arguments (10, 14, 15).

The following case will emphasize a tailored approach to several clinically relevant questions in a 26-year-old white male patient with HCM:

The patient's cardiac status was complicated by postendocarditic mitral regurgitation and immune-complex renal failure requiring hemodialysis. His brother had died suddenly in a high school gymnasium and was found to have HCM at autopsy, and the patient had undergone cardiac catheterization 5 years previously. The prior study revealed normal coronary arteries and an outflow tract gradient of 40 mm Hg, which was abolished after intravenous propranolol and sublingual nifedipine. He was discharged on these

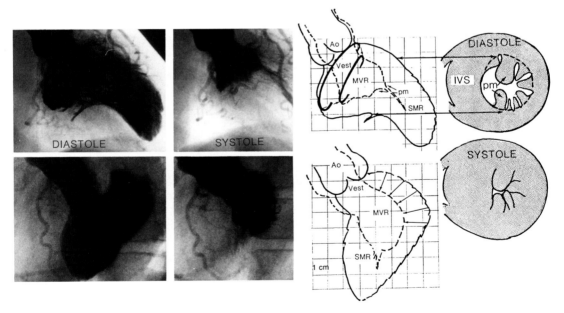

Figure 31.6. Left ventriculography in hypertrophic cardiomyopathy. The right anterior oblique end-diastolic and end-systolic frames are depicted on the *top row,* and the left anterior oblique on the *bottom.* The three regions of the ventricle, the aortic (*Ao*) vestibule (*Vest*), mitral valve region (*MVR*), and the submitral region (*SMR*) are indicated on the *silhouette diagrams.* The ejection fraction is 83%, and obliteration of the submitral cavity of the left ventricle is evident. The exaggerated mitral annular contraction and the descent of the annulus is depicted by *arrows* on the *superimposed silhouettes* on the *right.* Short-axis cross sections of the ventricle at the level of the papillary muscles (*pm*), based on echocardiograms, demonstrate the spiculated contour of the cavity and mechanism of cavitary obliteration (see text). *IVS,* interventricular septum.

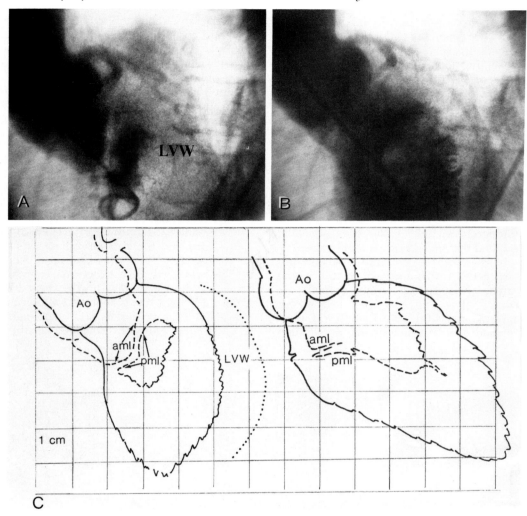

Figure 31.7. Left ventriculography in hypertrophic cardiomyopathy demonstrating the lucent line (systolic anterior motion). The exaggerated annular constriction and the obliterated submitral cavity can be appreciated. The lucent line, the angiographic analog of systolic anterior motion of the mitral valve, is comprised of a "sandwich" of anterior (*aml*) and posterior (*pml*) mitral leaflets. *Ao*, aortic; *LVW*, left ventricular wall.

medications but discontinued them because of side effects. He did well until developing, secondary to intravenous drug abuse, endocarditis (*Staphylococcus epidermidis*), which was successfully treated with 4 weeks of antibiotics but complicated by renal failure with anuria. He required hemodialysis 3 times a week. He gained 30 pounds and complained of abdominal distention and fatigue. He was taking propranolol, 20 mg t.i.d.

On cardiac examination he had jugular venous distention, full carotid pulses, and a surgical arteriovenous fistula in the left forearm with an overlying thrill and continuous murmur. The apical impulse was displaced laterally, and he had a palpable and audible 3rd heart sound over both ventricles. There was a III/VI long crescendo-decrescendo systolic murmur over the midprecordium, apex, and along the left sternal border. The murmur did not change appreciably with postural or Valsalva maneuvers. He had ascites and systolic hepatic pulsations.

Echocardiography demonstrated asym-

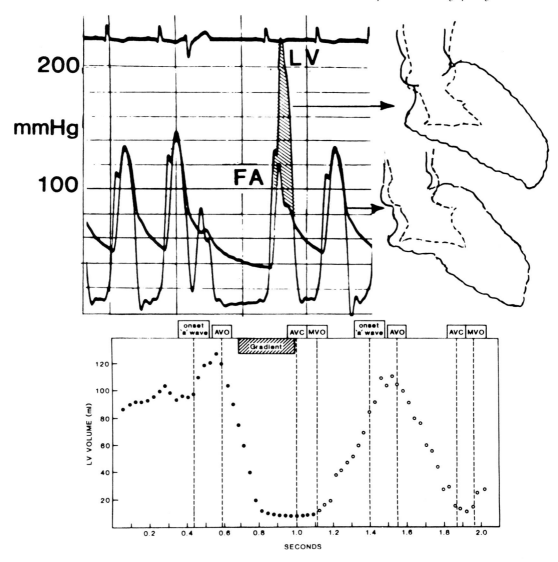

Figure 31.8. Left ventricular (*LV*) emptying with and without a pressure gradient in hypertrophic cardiomyopathy. Right anterior oblique left ventriculographic silhouettes during a postextrasystolic beat with a 110 mm Hg gradient (*top*) and a normal sinus beat without a gradient are depicted in the *right upper corner.* Frame-by-frame left ventricular volume calculations for these two beats demonstrate a larger ejection fraction and more rapid rate of emptying in the beat with the gradient. The duration of systole, the time between aortic valve opening (*AVO*) and aortic valve closure (*AVC*) is prolonged on the gradient beat, while the left ventricular emptying time (from aortic valve opening to minimal volume) is shorter in the gradient beat. The left ventricle continues to exert contractile force after the ventricle has reached its anatomic dead space. The exaggerated "a" wave kick increment in ventricular volume can be appreciated after the long diastolic pause on the gradient beat. *FA,* femoral artery; *MVO,* time of mitral valve opening.

metrical left ventricular hypertrophy with a septal thickness of 30 mm and a free wall thickness of 12 mm, left atrial dilation of 8.0 cm, systolic anterior motion of an elongated posterior mitral leaflet without septal contact, a defect in the midportion of the anterior leaflet, and flail chordae attached to the anterolateral papillary muscle. There was 3+ mitral and tricuspid regurgitation by Doppler interrogation.

Cardiac catheterization was performed in order to answer the following questions:

1. How severe was the mitral regurgitation (MR)?
2. Was the MR "functional" or structural?
3. Was the A-V fistula deleterious?
4. Was the diastolic left ventricular function impaired?
5. Was there a dynamic intracavitary gradient?
6. Was the patient a candidate for mitral valve replacement?
7. Was the patient a candidate for renal transplantation, or did his or her impaired cardiac status preclude this?

Prior to the procedure, the patient underwent vigorous hemodialysis to lower the blood volume in preparation for the obligatory volume load associated with the hemodynamic and angiographic study. Right heart, as well as transseptal and retrograde left heart, catheterization revealed severe pulmonary hypertension, tall left atrial V waves, elevated filling pressures in both ventricles, and a low cardiac index:

Site	Pressure in mm Hg	
	Phasic	Mean
Right atrium	a = 30 v = 30	24
Right ventricle	64/31	
Pulmonary artery	64/39	50
Left atrium	a = 20 v = 40	22
Left ventricle	80/30	
Aorta	76/59	65
Outflow gradient	peak 4	3
Cardiac output	3.1 liters/min	
Cardiac index	1.6 liters/min/m²	
Stroke volume	43 ml	
Pulmonary vascular resistance	9 Wood units	
Systemic vascular resistance	13 Wood units	

There was a trivial left ventricular pressure gradient at rest which did not increase with the Valsalva maneuver or postextrasystolic beats. Left ventriculography demonstrated a dilated ventricle with vigorous wall motion and 4+ mitral regurgitation. Hemodynamic and angiographic studies were repeated during manual occlusions of the A-V fistula (Fig. 31.9). Hemodynamic data with occlusion of the fistula:

Site	Pressure in mm Hg	
	Phasic	Mean
Left atrium	a = 22 v = 60	26
Left ventricle	82/8/30	
Aorta	78/60	66
Outflow gradient	peak 3	2
Cardiac output	2.5 liters/min	
Cardiac index	1.3 liters/min/m²	
Stroke volume	34 ml	
Systemic vascular resistance	18 Wood units	

There were deleterious hemodynamic and angiographic effects with occlusion of the shunt. Decrease in venous return was induced by a sustained Valsalva maneuver as well as a paroxysm of coughing (Fig. 31.10), and immediately after these maneuvers pressure recordings revealed a reduction in left heart filling pressures and the left atrial V waves. These perturbations were selected to assess the effects of alterations in aortic impedance and venous return on filling pressures, ventricular function, and mitral regurgitation.

It was concluded that the patient had:

1. Severe structural mitral regurgitation
2. Elevated filling pressures in right and left heart
   a. Dilated left ventricle suggesting unexpectedly increased distensibility for HCM
   b. Equal filling pressures in right and left heart suggesting pericardial restraint
3. Favorable effects from the A-V fistula
   a. Occlusion-reduced cardiac output
   b. Occlusion-increased regurgitant fraction
   c. Occlusion-increased left atrial pressure
4. Good left ventricular systolic function; no intracavitary gradient
5. Favorable indications for mitral valve replacement
6. No contraindication to renal transplantation

The patient underwent mitral valve replacement with a 29-mm St. Jude prosthesis and tricuspid annuloplasty. The pericardium was thickened. The chordae from the midportion of the anterior leaflet had ruptured, and there was extensive damage to the anterior mitral leaflet precluding repair. The patient had cardiac output determinations of 8 to 10 liters/min in the postoperative period. One year later (2 years prior to this writing) he had a successful cadaveric renal transplantation. His A-V fistula was maintained. He is currently free of symptoms on full activity and has good renal function.

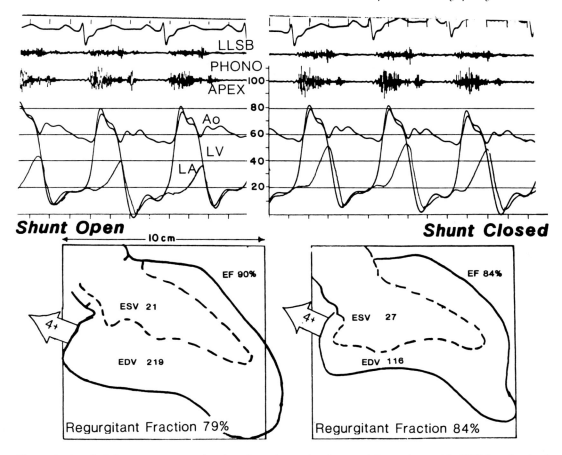

Figure 31.9. Left heart pressures (top) and angiography (bottom) in patient with HCM and mitral regurgitation; the effects of occlusion of peripheral A-V fistula (see text). *Ao*, aortic; *EDV*, end-diastolic volume in cubic centimeters; *EF*, ejection fraction; *ESV*, end-systolic volume in ml; *LA*, left atrial; *LLSB*, lower left sternal border; *LV*, left ventricular; *PHONO*, phonogram.

The next case will illustrate the potential confusion between HCM and discrete subaortic stenosis (DSAS):

> The patient was a 61-year-old female with exertional chest pain and a murmur. She had undergone prior catheterization at another hospital with a diagnosis of HCM, but on examination had a delayed carotid upstroke. With transseptal and retrograde catheters in the left ventricle and aorta (Fig. 31.11), a 40 mm Hg gradient was noted, and the central aortic pulse contour confirmed the clinical impression that the upstroke was delayed. Retrograde left ventricular catheterization demonstrated that the pressure drop occurred within the left ventricle. Angiography demonstrated a discrete subaortic constriction 2 cm below

> the aortic valve and an ejection fraction of 80%. The patient was given sublingual nitroglycerin for chest discomfort; shortly thereafter, she became hypotensive and the gradient had increased to 90 mm Hg. Her hypotension responded to leg elevation. When her blood pressure was stable, a Valsalva maneuver was performed, which markedly augmented the pressure gradient.

We surmised that the hypertrophic left ventricle with increased contractile force secondary to the DSAS had facilitated rapid and complete emptying after nitroglycerin administration, and the resulting augmentation was a result of the superimposition of a dynamic gradient due to cavitary obliteration. This phenomenon (superimposition of dynamic and

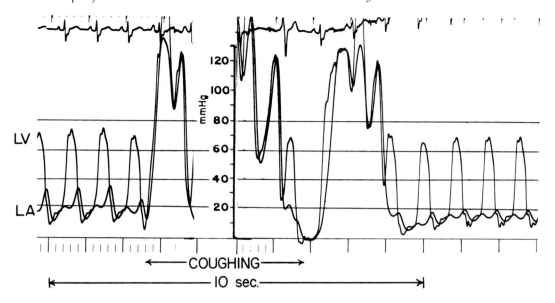

LV

LA

←—— COUGHING ——→

|←——————— 10 sec.————————→|

Figure 31.10. Left atrial (*LA*) and left ventricular (*LV*) pressures before and after a paroxysm of coughing in patient with HCM and mitral regurgitation. Immediately after the paroxysm, the left atrial V waves are reduced in magnitude (see text).

fixed gradients when the ventricle is induced to empty rapidly and excessively) can be provoked in patients and in experimental animals with administration of vasodilators or after replacement of a diseased aortic valve (16).

Restrictive Cardiomyopathy

The WHO/ISFC definition of restrictive cardiomyopathy (1) is, in our opinion, too restrictive in that it excludes amyloidosis, the most common cause of restrictive myocardial disease. We will therefore use our own definition, which is restrictive filling of one or both ventricles, often due to endocardial disease or infiltration of the myocardium and is characterized by small or partially obliterated ventricular cavities. Some causes of restrictive cardiomyopathy (RCM) are listed in Table 31.5.

The cardiovascular manifestations of collagen vascular disease can include an increased predisposition to both pericardial disease and myocardial restriction (17, 18). The cause of the restrictive physiology may in some cases be secondary to pulmonary hypertension and concomitant left ventricular dysfunction, in others be due to inflammatory infiltrates or have an unknown cause. In the past 6 years

we have seen more than a dozen patients with idiopathic RCM (19), six of whom went to surgery with either a tentative diagnosis of pericardial constriction or to "rule out pericardial constriction"; the pericardium was normal in all.

The clinical and hemodynamic findings in RCM simulate constrictive pericardial disease (see Chapter 32). The hemodynamic profile of elevated and equal left and right heart filling pressures (Fig. 31.12), with a diastolic dip and plateau ("square root sign"), and preserved ventricular systolic function in the absence of severe valvular regurgitation can be seen in both pericardial and myocardial disease. Thus, it may be difficult to differentiate the two on the basis of clinical and hemodynamic findings. Hemodynamic findings of both patients, as illustrated in Figure 31.12, have equal filling pressures in the left and right ventricles, and the pressures track together during respiration. It has been our experience that filling pressures can be dissociated in RCM with fluid loading or after injections of contrast media during angiography, whereas the filling pressures in constrictive pericarditis tend to track closely (Fig. 31.13) except when the blood volume is markedly depleted. Our approach to cardiac catheterization

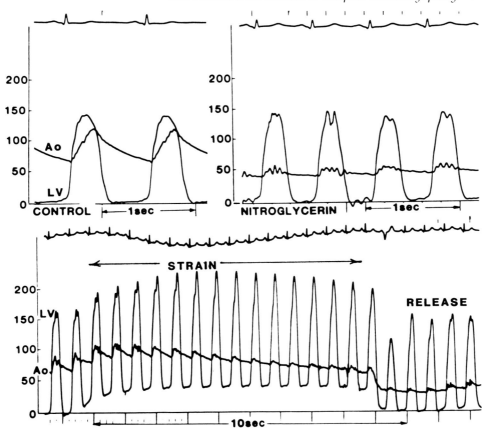

Figure 31.11. Left ventricular (*LV*) and aortic pressure (*Ao*) in patient with discrete subaortic stenosis with a superimposed "dynamic gradient" (see text).

studies in RCM is outlined in Table 31.6. This approach is designed to attempt to differentiate constrictive pericarditis from RCM, and the latter can often be detected by:

1. Pericardial calcification, often in the A-V grooves;
2. Thickened right atrial wall on right atriogram;
3. Equal filling pressures under various loading conditions;
4. Lack of specific biopsy findings.

It should be noted that an acute volume overload, such as acute mitral regurgitation, can lead to a square root sign and equal filling pressures in the ventricles. This is an indication of the restrictive role of the normal pericardium under these conditions (20).

Of the three types of cardiomyopathic processes, the diagnostic yield of endomyocardial biopsy is highest in RCM (21). We believe that every patient with clinical manifestations of restrictive myocardial or pericardial disease should undergo cardiac catheterization and biopsy unless there is a contraindication or an established diagnosis such as metastatic cancer or systemic amyloid. The relatively greater

Table 31.5.
Causes of Restrictive Cardiomyopathy

1. Infiltrative disorders
   A. Amyloidosis
   B. Hemochromatosis
   C. Neoplastic infiltration
   D. Glycogen storage disease
   E. Mucopolysaccharidosis
   F. Sarcoidosis
2. Collagen-vascular diseases
3. Endocardial diseases
   A. Endomyocardial fibrosis
      1) With eosinophilia
      2) Without eosinophilia
   B. Endocardial fibroelastosis
4. Idiopathic

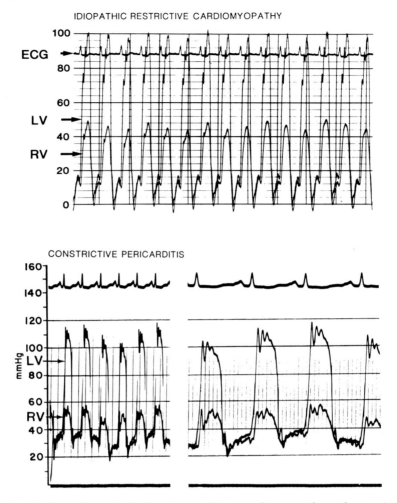

Figure 31.12. Similar hemodynamic findings in restrictive cardiomyopathy and constrictive pericarditis. Both patients exhibit equalization of diastolic pressures in the ventricles and a "dip and plateau" configuration. *LV,* left ventricle; *RV,* right ventricle.

frequency of abnormal biopsy findings reflects the infiltrative etiologies of this condition. In North America, most cases of restriction are due to amyloidosis (Fig. 31.14). Hemochromatosis (Fig. 31.15), sarcoidosis, and inflammatory etiologies, as well as endomyocardial fibrosis, are potentially treatable and possibly curable forms of RCM. While cardiac amyloidosis is associated with a dire prognosis with or without therapy, we feel a definitive diagnosis from a myocardial biopsy is justified to facilitate patient management. The following case will illustrate the

important role of biopsy in the diagnosis of cardiac vs. pericardial constriction.

A 61-year-old woman had ascites and recurrent pleural effusions for 15 years, treated with digitalis, diuretics, and vasodilators. She also had a history of thrombophlebitis, pulmonary emboli, and two cerebral vascular accidents and was taking coumadin. On examination she had jugular venous distention with rapid y descents, an S_3 gallop, murmurs of tricuspid and mitral regurgitation, a

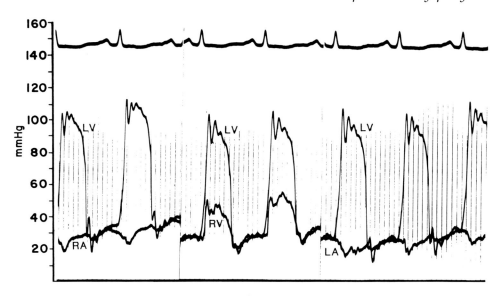

Figure 31.13. Diastolic pressure equalization in constrictive pericarditis. Pressures in the right atrium (*RA*), right ventricle (*RV*), and left atrium (*LA*) are recorded together with the left ventricle over a wide range of filling pressures.

pulsatile liver, and ascites. Pulmonary venous congestion, pleural effusions, and cardiac enlargement was present on chest x-ray; no calcification of the pericardium was seen. The echocardiogram demonstrated biatrial enlargement, normal ventricular size and contraction patterns, and enhanced endocardial signals. Doppler ultrasonography revealed severe 2 to 3 + mitral and tricuspid regurgitation.

Cardiac catheterization demonstrated pulmonary hypertension and equalization of diastolic pressures in the right and left heart. The coronary arteries were free of obstruction, and the left ventricle contracted well but had 3 + mitral regurgitation. A limited thoracotomy was performed to inspect the pericardium, which was normal. An endomyocardial biopsy was done later and revealed endomyocardial fibrosis with endocardial calcification (Fig. 31.16). The latter finding was demonstrated by computed tomography as well. Endocardial stripping was recommended.

Biopsy was not done in the case until after the thoracotomy but would have yielded the correct diagnosis of a potentially treatable con-

dition (22) and thereby the needless diagnostic thoracotomy would have been avoided (23).

Myocardial biopsy is also useful to exclude myocardial causes for a restrictive vs. constrictive disorder. This patient had multiple myeloma in remission and chronic severe coronary heart failure with anasarca. Hemodynamic study documented equalized left and right heart end-diastolic pressures, a computed tomography (CT) scan was equivocal for pericardial thickening, and because of the patient's myeloma, amyloid was considered to be the possible cause of coronary heart failure. The myocardial biopsy excluded amyloid. After ruling out RCM, a thoracotomy was performed with the hope that the patient had constrictive pericarditis, and the pericardium was found to be densely adherent to both ventricles. Three years after pericardial stripping, the patient is asymptomatic.

Unfortunately, a normal myocardial biopsy does not always ensure a diagnosis of constriction in all cases with the constrictive-restrictive hemodynamic profile. Ancillary tests, such as Doppler and radionuclide ventricular filling patterns used to differentiate restriction from constriction, need further validation. In our experience, CT (24) and magnetic resonance imaging are useful when marked pericardial thickening is identified; however, not all cases of constriction are identified by these imaging modalities. There is no single procedure that will clearly differentiate these two conditions with 100% certainty in every instance. Therefore, there is a justification for multiple procedures in difficult cases.

Another unfortunate feature of RCM is the lack of therapeutic efficacy of most pharmacological agents. Vasodilators and calcium channel blockers are particularly hazardous in patients with amyloidosis (25, 26).

CONCLUSIONS

This chapter has delineated our invasive laboratory approach to the diagnosis and hemodynamic characterization of patients with suspected myocardial disease. Case studies have been selected which highlight some of the important diagnostic and therapeutic challenges. We believe that cardiac catheterization and endomyocardial biopsy will continue to play an important role in furthering our understanding of this complex spectrum of diseases. With the widespread deployment of new techniques now in the developmental stages (multisensor catheters, conductance volume catheters, cDNA probes, histochemical processing of biopsy material) it is anticipated that invasive studies will yield more definitive information about the "last frontier" in cardiology.

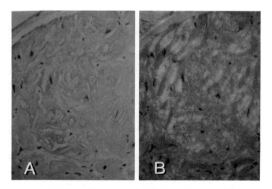

Figure 31.14. Amyloid in RCM. Congo red stain of right ventricular septal biopsy demonstrates amyloid deposition, which stains slightly darker than normal (*A*), and under polarizing light (*B*) the amyloid is birefringent and is more pale than the normal myocardial fibers. On direct viewing of the polarized histologic section, the apple green birefringence of the amyloid was seen.

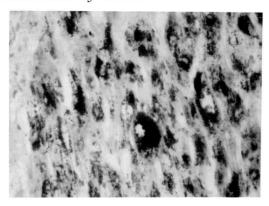

Figure 31.15. Hemochromatosis in RCM. An iron stain shows iron deposition as very dark granular staining in the myocardium of a patient who had received more than 100 blood transfusions due to thalassemia intermedia. These dark staining areas appeared blue on iron stain.

Table 31.6.
Catheterization Procedures in Restrictive Cardiomyopathy: Differentiation from Constrictive Pericarditis

1. Fluoroscopy to detect calcification
   A. Endocardium
   B. Pericardium
2. Simultaneous equisensitive pressure recordings with normal and exaggerated respirations, Valsalva maneuver, and leg raising
   A. Right atrium, right ventricle, pulmonary artery
   B. Right atrium and pulmonary-capillary wedge
   C. Right atrium and left ventricle
3. Angiography (if renal function permits)
   A. Frontal right atriogram
      1) Determine right atrial wall thickness
      2) Right ventricular filling pattern
      3) Left atrial size (levogram)
   B. Right anterior oblique right ventriculogram
      1) Tricuspid regurgitation
      2) Rule out Ebstein's anomaly, right ventricular dysplasia
   C. Right anterior oblique left ventriculogram
      1) Mitral regurgitation
      2) Distortion of left ventricular cavity
         a. Diastolic obliteration of apex (endomyocardial fibrosis)
         b. "Spade ventricle" (apical HCM)
4. Coronary angiography
   A. Obstructive lesions of amyloid
   B. Outer shell in constrictive pericarditis
5. Endomyocardial biopsy

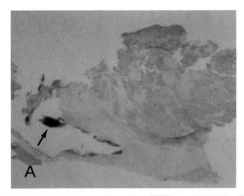

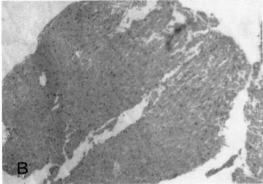

Figure 31.16. Endomyocardial fibrosis in RCM. Right ventricular septal endomyocardial biopsy reveals a markedly thickened and fibrous endocardium with calcification (*arrow*) under low power (*A*) as well as myocardial interstitial and replacement fibrosis (under high power (*B*).

ACKNOWLEDGMENTS

This project was supported by the Saint John's Heart Institute, Santa Monica, CA, and by an Investigative Group Support Award from the American Heart Association, Greater Los Angeles Affiliate. David Criley prepared the illustrations. The authors would like to thank Joseph P. Murgo, M.D., of the Ochsner Clinic, New Orleans, LA, for permission to use his original material for Figure 31.1, and Peter C. D. Pelikan, M.D., of Harbor-UCLA Medical Center for permission to use his original material for Figure 31.2.

References

1. Report of the WHO/ISFC Task Force on the definition and classification of cardiomyopathies. Br Heart J 1980;44:672–673.

2. Murgo JP, Alter BR, Dorethy JF, Altobelli SA, McGranahan GM Jr. Dynamics of left ventricular ejection in obstructive and nonobstructive hypertrophic cardiomyopathy. J Clin Invest 1980;66:1369–1382.

3. Murgo JP, Miller JW. Hemodynamic, angiographic and echocardiographic evidence against impeded ejection in hypertrophic cardiomyopathy. In: Goodwin JF, ed. Heart muscle disease. Lancaster: MTP Press Limited, 1985.

4. Baan J, vanderVelde ET, deBruin HG, et al. Continuous measurement of left ventricular volume in animals and humans by conductance catheter. Circulation 1984;70:812–823.

5. Chow LC, Dittrich HC, Shabetai R. Endomyocardial biopsy in patients with unexplained congestive heart failure. Ann Intern Med 1988;109:535–539.

6. Lie JT. Myocarditis and endomyocardial biopsy in unexplained heart failure: a diagnosis in search of a disease (letter). Ann Intern Med 1988;109:525–527.

7. O'Connell JB. The role of myocarditis in end-stage dilated cardiomyopathy. Tex Heart Inst J 1987;14:268–275.

8. Bowles NE, Richardson PJ, Olsen EGJ, Archard LC. Detection of coxsackie-virus-specific RNA sequences in myocardial biopsy samples from patients with myocarditis and dilated cardiomyopathy. Lancet 1986;1:1120–1122.

9. Bartle SH, Hermann HJ. Acute mitral regurgitation in man. Hemodynamic evidence and observations indicating an early role for the pericardium. Circulation 1967;36:839–851.

10. Maron BJ, Gottdiener JS, Arce J, Rosing DR, Wesley YE, Epstein SE. Dynamic subaortic obstruction in hypertrophic cardiomyopathy: analysis by pulsed Doppler echocardiography. J Am Coll Cardiol 1985;6:1–18.

11. Topol EJ, Traill TA, Fortuin NJ. Hypertensive hypertrophic cardiomyopathy of the elderly. N Engl J Med 1985;312:277–283.

12. Lorell BH, Paulus WJ, Grossman W, Wynne J, Cohn PF. Modification of abnormal left ventricular diastolic properties by nifedipine in patients with hypertrophic cardiomyopathy. Circulation 1982;65:499–507.

13. Siegel RJ, Criley JM. A comparison of ventricular emptying with and without a pressure gradient in hypertrophic cardiomyopathy. Br Heart J 1985;53:283–291.

14. Criley JM, Siegel RJ. Obstruction is unimportant in the pathophysiology of hypertrophic cardiomyopathy. Postgrad Med 1986;62:515–529.

15. Pollick C, Rakowski H, Wigle ED. Muscular subaortic stenosis: the quantitative relationship between systolic anterior motion and the pressure gradient. Circulation 1984;69:43–49.

16. Thompson R, Ahmed M, Pridie R, Yacoub M. Hypertrophic cardiomyopathy after aortic valve replacement. Am J Cardiol 1980;45:33–41.

17. Siegel RJ, O'Connor B, Mena I, Criley JM. Left ventricular function at rest and during Raynaud's phenomenon in patients with scleroderma. Am Heart J 1984;108:1469–1476.

18. Doherty NE, Feldman G, Maurer G, Siegel RJ. Echocardiographic findings in systemic lupus erythematosus. Am J Cardiol 1988;61:1144.

19. Siegel RJ, Shah PK, Fishbein MC. Idiopathic restrictive cardiomyopathy. Circulation 1984;70:165–169.
20. Yamaguchi H, Ishimura T, Nishiyama S, et al. Hypertrophic nonobstructive cardiomyopathy with giant negative T waves (apical hypertrophy). Ventriculographic and echocardiographic features in 30 patients. Am J Cardiol 1979;44:401–412.
21. French WJ, Siegel RJ, Cohen AH, Laks MM. Yield of endomyocardial biopsy in patients with biventricular failure. Chest 1986;90:181–184.
22. Schoenfeld MH, Supple EW, Dec WG, Fallon JT, Palacios IF. Restrictive cardiomyopathy versus constrictive pericarditis: role of endomyocardial biopsy in avoiding unnecessary thoracotomy. Circulation 1987;75:1012–1017.
23. Cherian KM, John TA, Abraham KA. Endomyocardial fibrosis: clinical profile and role of surgery in management. Am Heart J 1983;105:706–709.
24. Isner JM, Carter BL, Bankoff MS, Konstam MA, Salem DN. Computed tomography in the diagnosis of pericardial heart disease. Ann Intern Med 1982;97:473–479.
25. Gertz MA, Skinner M, Connors LH, Falk RH, Cohen AS, Kyle RA. Selective binding of nifedipine to amyloid fibrils. Am J Cardiol 1985;55:1646.
26. Gertz MA, Falk RH, Skinner M, Cohen AS, Kyle RA. Worsening of congestive heart failure in amyloid heart disease treated by calcium channel-blocking agents. Am J Cardiol 1985;55:1645.

32

The Patient with Known or Suspect Pericardial Disease

Stephen Keim, M.D.
C. Richard Conti, M.D.

INTRODUCTION

The patient with known or suspected pericardial disease offers a challenge for the clinician, who must be prepared to integrate both invasive and noninvasive data in order to obtain a secure diagnosis. The pericardium, by virtue of its extravascular location, is poorly visualized with standard angiographic techniques, and pericardial dysfunction must be surmised from the resulting hemodynamic effects. Sonography or more sophisticated technology (e.g., computed tomography (CT) scan, magnetic resonance imaging (MRI)) must be utilized in order to directly visualize the pericardial structures. These diagnostic procedures, however, only infer hemodynamic significance. Thus, neither approach is wholly sufficient to direct effective therapy, and both may need to be repeated during the course of treatment. Symptoms due to pericardial abnormalities in these patients are often masked by a more virulent extrapericardial disease process. Diagnosis requires the recognition that pericardial disease may be associated with a large number of primary disease entities. Physical examination and simple laboratory studies (e.g., chest x-ray and ECG) may be misleading, or nonspecific. The purpose of this chapter is to provide the reader with a multifaceted and integrated approach to pericardial disease that uses cardiac catheterization studies in addition to noninvasive studies.

PERICARDIUM: ANATOMY, EMBRYOLOGY, AND PHYSIOLOGY

To best use these laboratory studies a brief review of the anatomy and physiology of the pericardium is in order. The function of the pericardium is poorly understood, but it is present in various forms in all vertebrates (1, 2). The adult human pericardium is formed from the embryonic fusion of the mesodermal epimyocardial mantle and the pleuropericardial mantle (3). They join to form a thick fibrous sac that fuses with the adventitia of the great vessels and is firmly attached to the diaphragmatic aponeurosis (parietal layer). A more delicate, compliant visceral pericardial layer is directly attached to the epicardium. A potential space exists between these two layers that normally contains a small amount of fluid. The purpose and origin of the fluid is ill-defined, but it represents more than cardiac lymph fluid (2).

The pericardium has been ascribed several functions; however, it must be remembered that congenital or acquired absence of the pericardium usually is unnoticed, unless recognized on a chest x-ray done for other reasons. As a membrane, the pericardium behaves similarly to other serosal surfaces. As such, the composition, as well as production and disposition of the fluid, are under local cellular and hydrostatic forces. The supportive fibrous pericardium is a rigid constraint that prevents overdilation of the ventricles during acute stress and ensures an optimal relationship of filling pressures among all four chambers of the heart. Its thickness acts as a barrier against infection and tumor spread from contiguous structures. The pericardium does elicit systemic responses to pharmacologic and nerve stimulation (e.g., nicotine) (4).

The relatively poor understanding of the normal pericardial functions notwithstanding, the importance of the structure in pathological states has been appreciated for centuries (1, 2) (Table 32.1). Pericardial dysfunction can be divided into primary disease of the pericardium and secondary processes (e.g., tumor). Most important overall are the hemodynamic effects caused by the diseased structure.

PERICARDIAL EFFUSION

Accumulation of pericardial fluid need not necessarily imply pericardial disease, nor does the finding of fluid mean normal composition, as it may represent blood, chyle, or pus. When pericardial disease is present, chest pain may be the most prominent symptom and can be perceived in the middle thorax or in the shoulders (5). Usually, a simple effusion is clinically asymptomatic, and those symptoms that are present reflect the primary disease process.

Noninvasive Assessment

Commonly, cardiomegaly found on chest roentgenogram will be the first clue to the possible presence of chronic pericardial effusion. Electrocardiographic abnormalities consistent with pericarditis and pericardial effusion include P-R segment depression, ST segment elevation, and electrical alternans. Atrial arrhythmias, especially atrial flutter, are seen in patients with pericarditis, but sinus tachycardia is most frequently observed.

Echocardiography

As many as 5% of the general population have detectable pericardial effusion by sonography. M-mode echocardiography can detect small amounts (15 to 20 cc) of fluid (6), but two-dimensional echocardiography adds specificity, since pericardial fluid can be mistaken for fat or pleural fluid. This is especially true in

M-mode scanning, where a posterior clear space is visualized. The two-dimensional finding of echo-free space, anteriorly and posteriorly, in the parasternal short- and long-axis views (see Fig. 32.1) is more specific, but spatial resolution is still limited (7, 8). M-mode echocardiography combined with the two-dimensional technique, has made echocardiography the reference standard for assessment of pericardial fluid and pericardial thickening. Quantitative echocardiographic techniques allow for serial testing of fluid accumulation as a marker for effective therapy (6).

CT Scan and Magnetic Resonance Imaging

Both CT scanning with contrast and MRI are sensitive (7, 8) and specific methods for detecting thickened pericardium, but neither allows for real-time imaging (9, 10). With both techniques the pericardium appears as a thick line between the myocardium and pericardial fat. Improved spatial resolution allows the

Table 32.1.
Etiology of Pericardial Effusion

  I. Idiopathic
 II. Infectious
     A. Viral (Coxsackie B, Echo virus)
     B. Bacteria (tuberculosis, staphylococcal, gonoccocal)
     C. Fungal (histoplasmosis, *candida*)
III. Metabolic
     A. Uremia
     B. Myxedema
 IV. Drug induced
     A. Minoxidil
     B. Hydralazine
     C. Procainamide
  V. Autoimmune
     A. Systemic lupus erythematosus
     B. Scleroderma
     C. Rheumatoid arthritis
     D. Rheumatic pancarditis
     E. Postinfarction (Dressler's syndrome, thrombolysis)
 VI. Volume overload (chronic congestive heart failure)
VII. Trauma (penetrating injury, aortic dissection)
VIII. Neoplastic
     A. Pericardial metastasis (melanoma, breast carcinoma)
     B. Local invasion (lung cancer, lymphoma)

distinction to be made between pleural fluid and pericardial cysts from pericardial effusion (see Fig. 32.2). Better tissue characterization, especially with MRI, may provide unique insights into pathologic processes (10).

Invasive Assessment

Once pericardial effusion is detected, the consultant is frequently asked how to pursue further evaluation. This usually means directly obtaining pericardial fluid, tissue, or both. Pericardiocentesis and pericardial biopsy are not trivial procedures. The risk must be balanced with the benefit, especially in the asymptomatic patient. The techniques of pericardiocentesis and biopsy are discussed elsewhere (see Chapter 6). Pericardial fluid volume generally follows the course of the primary disease, and only if information derived from the fluid or pericardium would alter therapy, or when tamponade is present, should pericardiocentesis be performed. The approach to invasive assessment of pericardial effusion is determined by which procedure(s) is contemplated (e.g., fluid only, biopsy only, or both). There are no controlled data to conclusively support when acquisition of tissue is superior to fluid alone. An exception may be tuberculous pericarditis (11, 12). We are unaware of a comparison of cell block cytological analysis with direct tissue biopsy specimen to diagnose malignancy. If tissue is to be obtained, the subxyphoid pericardotomy approach is preferred.

For simple pericardiocentesis the catheterization laboratory serves well as a procedure room (see Chapter 6 for a discussion of techniques). Because of the availability and accuracy of noninvasive studies, neither catheterization nor blind pericardiocentesis should be done simply to determine if an effusion is present. If a cardiac catheterization is necessary to exclude cardiac tamponade or constrictive pericardial disease, assessment of the effusion and even pericardiocentesis can be performed at the same time. When effusion is present, the tip of a right atrial catheter, will generally lie some distance from the border of the cardiac silhouette during fluoroscopy. If angiography is done, the effusion will separate the edge of contrast from the radiolucency of the lung, and the contour of the right atrial border will change from convex to straight. In addition, techniques such as pericardioscopy can be performed that may be helpful for identifying tumor, foreign bodies, or loculated effusion (13, 14). Flexible fiberoptic pericardioscopy permits visualization from all pericardial surfaces and makes it

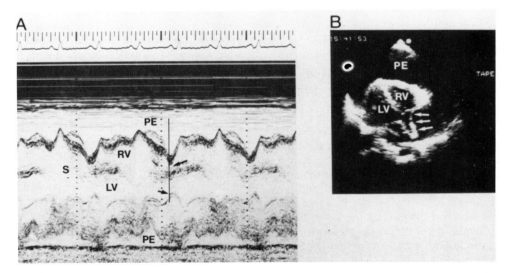

Figure 32.1. *A*, M-mode echocardiogram to show the interventricular septum(s), right ventricle (*RV*), left ventricle (*LV*), and the large anterior and posterior clear spaces that are pericardial effusion (*PE*). Note the diastolic posterior motion or collapse of the RV wall (*line*). *B*, a four-chamber view of a PE indicating collapse of the right atrial wall (*arrows*). *S*, septum. (From Quinones MA. Echocardiography in adult heart disease. Baylor College of Medicine Cardiology Series, 1985;7:4.)

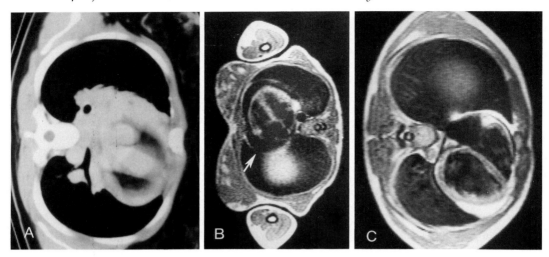

Figure 32.2. *A*, CT scan of patient with lymphomatous involvement of the pericardium that is noticeably thickened and not clearly separated from the myocardium. *B*, A MRI scan indicating a simple pericardial effusion. Note the thin parietal pericardium (*arrow*) and the normal sized cardiac chambers. *C*, A MRI scan of thickened parietal pericardium with associated fluid representing a patient with effusive constrictive pericarditis due to tuberculosis.

possible to biopsy selective sites (15). Corticosteroids can be injected into the pericardial space to treat uremic or idiopathic recurrent pericarditis (16, 17). Sclerosing agents (e.g., tetracycline) can also be infused via a small catheter to palliate recurrent malignant pericardial effusions (18, 19). A pigtail catheter may be introduced over a guidewire if chronic infusion or drainage is necessary.

CARDIAC TAMPONADE

Pericardial fluid may accumulate rapidly or to such an extent that cardiac function is impaired. The thick inelastic fibrous pericardium may expand or "creep" over a period of time, accommodating liters of slowly accumulating pericardial fluid. It follows that if noncompressible fluid fills a rigidly encased space shared by a vented, hollow structure, there will be an exponential rise in fluid pressure that will cause the pressure to rise in the hollow structure. When the hollow structure is the heart, the distending pressure rise is under physiologic limits, so eventually the hollow viscus will collapse. Many animal and human experiments have documented these findings of cardiac tamponade (1, 2, 20). Thus, the **essential hemodynamic abnormality of pericardial tamponade is a rise in intrapericardial pressure to equal the diastolic pres-**

sure in the heart so that diastolic filling is impaired. Thus, in tamponade ventricular transmural pressure is very low.

All pericardial effusions, as well as thoracic and pericardial masses, can alter cardiac filling. Clinically, these patients may be subdivided into two groups. First, there are those who develop pericardial effusions rapidly, resulting in **Beck's triad of decreasing arterial pressure, increasing jugular venous pressure, and a small quiet heart.** This catastrophic event usually occurs because of traumatic perforation of the heart, postinfarction myocardial rupture, or as a result of an ascending aortic dissection. These patients require diagnosis and therapy promptly and concomitantly. Second, others may develop effusions gradually. This condition usually allows time for definitive diagnosis and planned treatment. In a series of patients with gradually developing cardiac tamponade, 80% were tachypneic, 77% had tachycardia and 77% had a paradoxical pulse, 64% had a systolic blood pressure <100 mm Hg, and only 34% had diminished heart sounds (21). A recent study concluded that a paradoxical pulse >12 mm Hg and a drop >9% in systolic blood pressure during inspiration had an accuracy of 92% and 97%, respectively, in predicting moderate-to-severe tamponade. A paradoxical pulse >25 mm Hg was predictive of severe tamponade (22). Of note, neoplastic and uremic diseases accounted for nearly two-thirds of the cases. A paradoxical pulse may not develop if left ventricular diastolic pressures exceed the pericardial pressure, as in left ventricular failure. Orthopnea is common in tamponade and may reflect transmitted pericardial pressure to the left atrium and elevation of pulmonary venous pressure in the absence of left ventricular systolic dysfunction (2). Jugular venous pressure elevation, with a characteristically prominent x descent and absent y descent, correlates well with right atrial pressure tracings. On occasion, when there is hypovolemia, there may be a mismatch in the pericardial pressure and central venous pressure ("low pressure tamponade").

Noninvasive Assessment

Both chest roentgenograms and fluoroscopy lack sensitivity for assessing pericardial tamponade. Ungated CT scans and MRI correlate poorly with hemodynamic findings. Newer gated methods promise higher sensitivity since wall motion abnormalities caused by tamponade can be detected. Radionuclide studies have not successfully differentiated hemodynamically important effusions from those that do not impair hemodynamic function. MRI and cardiac ultrasound do help distinguish tamponade from right ventricular infarction and superior vena cava compression that may mimic tamponade. M-mode ultrasound shows exaggerated respiratory variations of ventricular filling and cardiac output (23). These signs include decreased left ventricular posterior wall excursion (24), decrease in E to F slope (25), and right ventricular end-diastolic expiratory collapse (26). Also identified is a marked displacement of the anterior right ventricular wall in late diastole (27). Several two-dimensional echocardiographic findings correlate well with hemodynamic findings. A cross-sectional picture of the right atrium, showing collapse lasting more than one-third of the cycle length, has a sensitivity of 94% and a specificity and predictive value of 100% (28). Right atrial collapse occurs at lower pericardial pressures than does right ventricular collapse, but both occur before a drop in systolic blood pressure, and both have predictive values of 100% (29).

Doppler waveform analysis can document the pulsus paradoxus and altered venous flow patterns, but adds little to the diagnosis of cardiac compression.

Invasive Assessment

Definitive assessment of the possible hemodynamic significance of some pericardial effusions requires cardiac catheterization and pericardiocentesis. Most patients with cardiac tamponade require drainage of the fluid. Although there is little information in the literature to support treatment of tamponade by volume infusion or inotropic agents, both may be helpful temporizing therapies until pericardiocentesis. The merits of performing **diagnostic pericardiocentesis** in the catheterization laboratory have been mentioned. Fluoroscopic documentation of catheter placement is often necessary because of altered pressure tracings. Right atrial catheterization with a stiff catheter can show a discrepancy between the atrial wall marked by the tip of the catheter and fluoroscopic border of the heart, confirming the existence of a large effusion. This simple procedure is often overlooked. Pressure tracings reveal the characteristic elevated right atrial pressure with preserved systolic atrial filling or x descent. The y descent is replaced by a gradually upsloping pressure wave, as diastolic filling is impeded by pericardial pressures. With inspiration the venous pressure usually falls slightly in tamponade but rises in constriction. In tamponade, as opposed to constrictive pericarditis (discussed below), the increased intrapericardial pressure is exerted upon the heart throughout the entire cardiac cycle with only momentary relief during ventricular ejection. In very severe acute tamponade, venous return may be completely impeded throughout diastole when cardiac volume and intrapericardial pressure are both maximal. Depending upon the severity of tamponade, right ventricular systolic pressure may rise slightly in mild-to-moderately severe cases. With severe compression it is proportional to the reduction in stroke volume. However, right ventricular diastolic pressure will be elevated and equal to the right atrial and pericardial pressures. Pulmonary artery diastolic pressure is also elevated to the same level as the right ventricular diastolic pressure with a diminished pulse pressure and it may be difficult to distinguish pulmonary artery from right ventricular pressure. At times, only the location of the catheter tip by fluoroscopy will allow identification of these pressures. Left ventricular systolic pressure is reduced proportional to the severity of compression, and diastolic pressure is elevated to equal the right ventricular diastolic pressure.

Right heart catheterization should be combined with catheterization of the pericardial sac. Pericardial pressure should be measured and is **always elevated** in tamponade and should be within 2 mm Hg of the right atrial and right ventricular diastolic pressures to confirm the diagnosis. Cardiac tamponade occurring in patients with severe left ventricular dysfunction may cause diagnostic problems, as tamponade will occur when intrapericardial pressures equal right atrial pressure. In these cases the right atrial pressure will remain somewhat elevated after pericardiocentesis.

Angiographic studies may show atrial collapse and small hyperactive ventricular chambers. This should reduce stroke volume through the Frank-Starling effect, but activation of the sympathetic nervous system and increased circulating catecholamines also stimulate contraction. Coronary angiography may demonstrate overt coronary compression in diastole (30).

Data Evaluation, Interpretation, and Decision-Making

If tamponade is present, pericardiocentesis can produce striking immediate hemodynamic changes (see Fig. 32.3) and may be lifesaving. Both the right atrial and pericardial pressures should fall after pericardiocentesis, and pericardial pressure should be clearly less than right atrial pressure and near or less than atmospheric pressure. The right atrial waveform returns towards normal with reappearance of a normal diastolic pressure fall or *y* descent. The early diastolic dip in ventricular pressures will return towards normal inasmuch as myocardial function permits it. Systolic aortic pressure increases, as do pulse pressure and cardiac output. Simultaneous echocardiography will demonstrate rapid normalization of chamber expansion.

The decision to leave the right heart and

pericardial catheters in place upon leaving the catheterization laboratory is dependent on findings in a given patient. It is imperative to repeat measurements when fluid has been removed to exclude concomitant constrictive physiology (see below). Right atrial pressure may be followed from a balloon flotation catheter to check for evidence that pericardial fluid may be rapidly reaccumulating. Serial echocardiograms are probably sufficient for the patient who is unlikely to reaccumulate quickly. In patients with effusions due to uremia or carcinomatous pericarditis, the pericardial catheter can be left in place, and therapeutic and sclerosing agents can be instilled. Patients who have recurrent effusions in the absence of uremia or cancer may be considered for pericardiectomy, although not all agree on this last recommendation (31, 32).

CHRONIC CONSTRICTIVE PERICARDITIS

In constrictive pericarditis, the pericardium restricts diastolic expansion. The causes of constrictive pericarditis may be similar to those of pericardial effusion with some exceptions (e.g., radiation) (Table 32.1). It is not understood why, with similar diseases, some patients will resolve their effusions and others will develop a chronic inflammatory process with pericardial thickening and cardiac compression. Pericardial constriction is commonly seen after tuberculous pericarditis (11, 33). Rheumatoid arthritis is the most commonly associated autoimmune disease (34), and constriction is rare with drug-induced pleuropericarditis of the lupus variety and in rheumatic heart disease (35). It has been described as a late sequela of Dressler's syndrome and hemopericardium of any cause (36, 37). As thrombolytic therapy comes into more widespread use, constrictive pericarditis may become an important late sequela. Idiopathic constrictive pericarditis is the most common type of pericarditis seen today. This is a slowly progressive disorder whose signs and symptoms may suggest volume overload.

Once constrictive pericardial disease is established, it does not disappear, even though the primary disease is cured. Since many manifestations are dependent on the blood volume status of the patient, symptoms

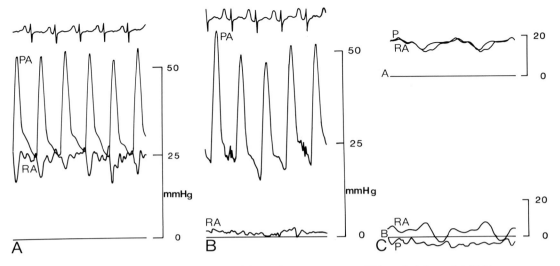

Figure 32.3. *A,* Simultaneous recordings of the pulmonary artery (*PA*) and right atrial (*RA*) pressures in a patient with scleroderma. Note the elevated PA and RA pressures. *B,* After pericardiocentesis there is a marked decrease in RA pressure. *C,* Simultaneous recording of pericardial (*P*) and RA pressures. Note the elevation and equalization of the pressures prior to pericardiocentesis (top) and lowering and separation of the pressures postpericardiocentesis (bottom).

may wax and wane. The usual clinical presentation to the consultant is refractory edema, often with ascites. The most striking single physical finding in these patients is jugular venous distention. A hypovolemic patient may have a paucity of physical findings, but jugular venous distention usually is persistent.

Noninvasive Studies

Chest roentgenogram may reveal slightly enlarged or normal heart size and clear lung fluids. Pericardial calcification suggests pericardial constriction but is not diagnostic. Electrocardiographic findings are nonspecific (1), but atrial fibrillation is often found. Careful blood pressure measurements may reveal pulsus paradoxus.

Cardiac ultrasound can characterize the hemodynamic effects of constriction and thickened pericardium. The M-mode echocardiogram may reveal middle and late diastolic flattening of the posterior left ventricular wall (38) and early diastolic notching of the intraventricular septum (39), reflecting the abnormal filling pattern of the left ventricle secondary to restricted free wall motion (40). These abnormalities correlate well with the hemodynamics of restricted cardiac motion. Premature opening of the pulmonic valve

reflects increased right ventricular diastolic pressures (41).

Two-dimensional echocardiography offers a better noninvasive assessment of restrictive physiology than M-mode. Strands of fibrin may be seen coursing from the visceral to the thickened parietal pericardium, which is suggestive of effusive-constrictive pericarditis. A dilated inferior vena cava without respiratory variation with normal-sized right atrium and ventricle is a reliable sign suggesting constriction. Doppler study of the aortic outflow can provide documentation of pulsus paradoxus (41). CT scan and MRI probably offer better diagnostic sensitivity and specificity for detecting a thickened pericardium. CT and MRI may add information about tissue characterization, as well as disclose other mediastinal pathology that may aid diagnosis (10).

A most difficult problem involves distinguishing restrictive cardiomyopathy from constrictive pericarditis (see Chapter 31). Invasive and noninvasive laboratory findings favoring either constriction or restriction are summarized in Table 32.2. In addition, patients with long-standing constrictive pericarditis may have myocardial dysfunction due to the same process that produced pericardial disease or due to myocardial atrophy. It has been suggested that the cross-sectional area

Table 32.2.
Laboratory Findings That May Help Differentiate Chronic Pericardial Constriction from Restrictive Cardiomyopathy

Test	Results Suggesting	
	Constriction	Restriction
Chest x-ray	Calcified pericardium	No calcium visible
Echocardiogram	Thickened pericardium Normal systolic wall motion Normal wall thickness	Normal pericardium Wall motion may be reduced Increased LV[a] wall thickening
CT scan	Thickened pericardium Calcified pericardium	Normal pericardium
MRI	Thickened pericardium	Normal pericardium with uniform signal intensity Wall may be thickened

Catheter laboratory
  Right and left heart
  Catheterization
	Equilibration of RV and LV diastolic pressures
	"Square root" sign
		LVEDP may be > RVEDP

Coronary angiography	Diastolic compression of coronary arteries Coronary artery "crinkling" Increased space between coronary arteries and cardiac silhouette	Normal coronary arteries and normal relationship to epicardial silhouette
Endomyocardial biopsy	Normal	Fibrosis, amyloid, etc.

[a] LV, left ventricular; RV, right ventricular; LVEDP, left ventricular end-diastolic pressure; RVEDP, right ventricular end-diastolic pressure.

change of the left ventricle during early diastole, measured by two-dimensional echocardiography, can help distinguish constrictive from restrictive disease (42), corroborating the earlier catheterization study of Tyberg et al. discussed below (43). This method makes no correction for heart rate and is labor intensive; therefore, it is not thought to be practical. Doppler analysis of mitral valve flow has also been suggested but as of yet has not proven useful. CT scanning has been useful in some cases (44), but endomyocardial biopsy should generally be performed.

Invasive Assessment

Catheterization, both left and right heart, is usually undertaken to evaluate the hemodynamics of constriction, to help differentiate it from myocardial disease, and to assess other problems (e.g., coronary artery disease (CAD)), should surgery be required. None of the hemodynamic findings are specific. Certain patients may require volume infusion to elicit so-called "occult" constriction. The characteristic hemodynamic feature of constriction is elevated right atrial pressure associated with a prominent y descent recorded on pressure tracings. This finding helps to differentiate constriction, where limitation to diastolic filling of the ventricle is not present in very early diastole (prominent y descent), from tamponade, where there is limitation to all phases of diastolic filling. There is also near equalization of right and left ventricular filling pressures that is usually recorded from the right atrial and pulmonary artery occlusive pressures. The characteristic diastolic filling pressure tracing that "dips and plateaus" ("square root sign") may be present (see Fig. 32.4). The dip is due to emptying of the right atrium across a normal tricuspid valve without impaired filling of the ventricle in early diastole. The plateau is due to rapid rise in filling pressure, as filling of the ventricle is

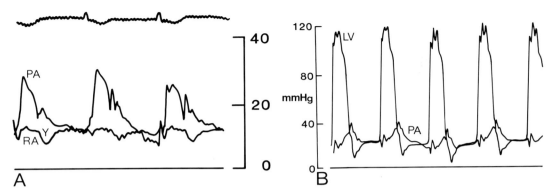

Figure 32.4. *A*, Note the normal pulmonary artery (*PA*) pressure with elevation of the right atrial (*RA*) pressure with a prominent *y* descent. *B*, Simultaneous, left ventricular (*LV*) and pulmonary arterial pressure tracings demonstrating the *square root sign* ventricular filling pattern.

restricted by the constricting pericardium. Right ventricular diastolic pressure is elevated, and the systolic pressure is normal to low. Pulmonary hypertension is said not to occur in pure constrictive pericarditis. Wise and Conti demonstrated that a pulmonary artery pressure to right atrial pressure ratio of <3.5 correctly differentiated their patients with constrictive pericarditis from those with cardiomyopathy (45).

Angiography is an important part of the catheterization procedure. The right atriogram may show straightening of the right atrial border, which is suggestive of constriction. Quantitative analysis of left ventricular angiograms shows that rapid ventricular filling occurs throughout the first half of diastole in patients with constriction (43). In contrast to restrictive cardiomyopathy ventricular filling occurs only very early in diastole and then slows. Digitized analysis of the left ventricular angiogram is now available in many clinical cardiac catheterization laboratories for this diagnostic test. Coronary angiography is probably warranted in all patients since the arteries can be compressed by the pericardium and unsuspected atherosclerotic disease may be present (46). There may be an increased distance between the coronary arteries and the cardiac silhouette, confirming the presence of a thick pericardium. A coronary artery segment may be compressed in diastole (47). Increased crinkling of the coronary arteries has also been described.

Sometimes, noninvasive testing, hemodynamic measurements, and angiography will all fail to distinguish convincingly that the process is either pericardial or myocardial. Use of right or left ventricle endomyocardial biopsy may be helpful. Nonspecific fibrosis is often found and is not helpful. However, specific stains may reveal abnormalities, such as amyloid, or entirely normal myocardium may be found. The distinction is important because constrictive pericarditis can be surgically corrected. Unfortunately, in some cases precise diagnosis may not be apparent with diagnostic procedures short of thoracotomy.

"Sero-effusive" constrictive pericarditis is a term sometimes applied to patients with hemodynamic abnormalities intermediate between constrictive pericarditis and cardiac tamponade. The problem arises when pericardial effusion causes increased intrapericardial pressure in patients with a thickened pericardium. Before removal of pericardial fluid, hemodynamic findings of tamponade predominate with pulsus paradoxus. After removal of fluid, however, the right atrial pressure remains abnormally elevated and shows absence of respiratory variation and prominent *y* descent, all findings of constriction.

Data Interpretation and Decision-Making

Certainly, the majority of causes of important constriction can be identified through multiple noninvasive studies confirmed by catheterization laboratory techniques. Surgery in patients who have occult constriction or who are relatively asymptomatic is usually delayed. Catheterization may also reveal patients with previously unsuspected myocardial dysfunction or combinations of both constriction and myocardial disease who would be less likely to respond well to surgery. If the pericardium is removed, it should be noted that the ventricular filling pressures frequently do not return to normal immediately. It may take weeks or months for them to trend downward. Thus, a postoperative patient may require diuretics and inotropic support. These observations support the suggestion that some residual myocardial dysfunction is present in many cases with pericardial constriction.

CONGENITAL OR ACQUIRED, COMPLETE OR PARTIAL ABSENCE OF THE PERICARDIUM

Congenital defects of the pericardium are not infrequent and usually are diagnosed at autopsy. Complete absence of the pericardium is responsible for a cardiac silhouette that is shifted leftward on chest x-ray and has a "Snoopy" dog appearance. It may be associated with a variety of other congenital anomalies, including patent ductus arteriosus (48), atrial septal defect (48), mitral stenosis (49), and tetralogy of Fallot (50).

Echocardiography can reveal abnormal septal motion, presumably due to the unrestrained heart (51, 52). CT scanning and MRI are the most sensitive in detecting the absence of the pericardium. At cardiac catheterization no resting hemodynamic abnormalities are usually found in cases with isolated pericardial absence. There are case reports of atrial entrapment or compression of coronary arteries, and sudden death has occurred in patients with **partial absence** due to strangulation of cardiac structure or compression of the coronary arteries (1, 2). Surgical removal of the pericardium is usually not associated with any residual problems. Certainly postthoracotomy tamponade and constriction are recognized complications. When the pericardium is removed completely to relieve symptoms of partial absence, the patient experiences little residual effect.

References

1. Fowler NO. The pericardium in health and disease. Mount Kisco, NY: Futura, 1985.
2. Shabetai R. The pericardium. New York: Grune & Stratton, 1981.
3. Sadler RW. Langman's medical embryology. 5th ed. Baltimore: Williams & Wilkins, 1985.
4. Holt JP. The normal pericardium. Am J Cardiol 1970;26:455-465.
5. Goss CM, ed. Gray's anatomy. 29th ed. Philadelphia: Lea & Febiger, 1973.
6. Horowitz MS, Schultz CS, Clifford S, Stinson EB, Harrison DC, Popp RL. Sensitivity and specificity of echocardiographic diagnosis of pericardial effusion. Circulation 1974;50:239-247.
7. Yousem D, Traill TT, Wheeler PS, Fishman EK. Illustrative cases in pericardial effusion misdetection: correlation of echocardiography on CT. Cardiovasc Interv Radiol. 1987; 10:162-167.
8. Ansari A, Rholl AO. Pseudopericardial effusions: echocardiographic and computed tomographic correlations. Clin Cardiol 1986;9:551-555.
9. Sechtem U, Tscholakoff D, Higgins CB. MRI of the normal pericardium. AJR 1986;147:239-244.
10. Sechtem U, Tscholakoff D, Higgins CB. MRI of the abnormal pericardium. AJR 1986;147:245-252.
11. Hageman JH, Esposo ND, Glenn WW. Tuberculosis of the pericardium, along ROM analysis of forty-four proved cases. N Engl J Med 1964;270:327-332.
12. Schepers GW. Tuberculis pericarditis. Am J Cardiol 1962;9:248-276.
13. Little AG, Ferguson MK. Pericardioscopy as an adjunct to pericardial window. Chest 1986;89:53-55.
14. Wong KKS. Use of a flexible choledochoscope for pericardioscopy and drainage of a loculated pericardial effusion. Thorax 1986;42:637-638.
15. Kondos GT, Rich S, Levitsky S. Flexible fiberoptic pericardioscopy for the diagnosis of pericardial disease. J Am Coll Cardiol 1986;7:432-434.
16. Fowler NO, Harbin AD. Recurrent acute pericarditis: follow-up study of 31 patients. J Am Coll Cardiol 1986;7:300-305.
17. Rutsky EA, Rostand SG. Treatment of uremic pericarditis and pericardial effusion. Am J Kidney Dis 1987;10:2-8.
18. Sheppard FA, Morgan C, Evans WK, Ginsberg J, Watt D, Murphy K. Medical management of malignant pericardial effusion by tetracycline sclerosis. Am J Cardiol 1987;60:1161-1166.
19. Patel AK, Kosolcharoen PD, Nallasivan M, Kronke G, Thomsen J. Catheter drainage of the pericardium. Chest 1987;92:1018-1021.
20. Metcalfe J, Woodbury JW, Richards V, Burwell S. Studies in experimental pericardial tamponade. Circulation 1952;5:518-523.
21. Guberman B, Fowler N, Engle P, Gueron M, Allen J. Cardiac tamponade in medical patients. Circulation 1981;64:633-640.
22. Curtiss EI, Sudhakar R, Uretsky B, Cecchetti A. Pulsus paradoxus: definition and relation to the severity of cardiac tamponade. Am Heart J 1988;115:391-398.
23. Wayne VS, Bishop RL, Spodick DL. Dynamic effects of pericardial effusion without tamponade. Br Heart J 1983;51:202-204.
24. Feigenbaum H, Zaky A, Waldhunsen JA. Use of ultrasound in the diagnosis of pericardial effusion. Ann Intern Med 1966;65:443-452.

25. Nanda NC, Gramick R, Gross CM. Echocardiography of cardiac valves in pericardial effusion. Circulation 1946;54:500-504.
26. Schiller NB, Botvinick E. Right ventricular compression as a sign of cardiac tamponade: an analysis of echocardiographic ventricular dimensions and their clinical implications. Circulation 1977;56:774–779.
27. Armstrong WF, Shilt BF, Helper D, Dillon JC, Feigenbaum H. Diastolic collapse of the right ventricle with tamponade: an echocardiographic study. Circulation 1982;65:1491–1496.
28. Gillan LD, Guyer D, Gibson TC, King ME, Marshall J, Weyman A. Hydrodynamic compression of the right atrium; a new echocardiographic sign of cardiac tamponade. Circulation 1983;68:292–301.
29. Kronzon I, Cohen ML, Winer HE. Diastolic atrial compression: a sensitive echocardiographic sign of cardiac tamponade. J Am Coll Cardiol 1983; 2:770–775.
30. O'Rourke RA, Fischer DP, Escobar EE, Bishop US, Rapaport E. Effect of acute pericardial tamponade on coronary blood flow. Am J Physiol 1967; 212:549–552.
31. Piehler JM, Pluth JR, Schaff HV, Danielson GK, Orszulak TA. Surgical management of effusive pericardial disease. J Thorac Cardiovasc Surg 1985;90:506–516.
32. Jansen EW, Vincent JG, Fost JA, Tavilla E. Treatment of pericardial fluid. J Thorac Cardiovasc Surg 1986;91:795–796.
33. Sagrista-Sauleda J, Permanyer-Miralda G, Soler-Soler J. Tuberculous pericarditis: ten year experience with a prospective protocol for diagnosis and treatment. J Am Coll Cardiol 1988;11:724–728.
34. Thadani U, Iveson J, Wright V. Cardiac tamponade, constrictive pericarditis and pericardial resection in rheumatoid arthritis. Medicine 1975;54:261–270.
35. Roberts W, Spray T. Pericardial heart disease: a study of its causes, consequences and morphologic features. In: Spodick DH, ed. Cardiovascular clinics. Philadelphia: FA Davis, 1976;7:11–65.
36. Kutcher MA, King SB, Alimuruna BN. Constrictive pericarditis as a complication of cardiac surgery: recognition of an entity. Am J Cardiol 1982;50:742–748.
37. Cohen MV, Greenberg MA. Constrictive pericarditis: early and late complication of cardiac surgery. Am J Cardiol 1979;43:657–661.
38. Pool PE, Seagren SC, Abassi AS, Charuzi Y, Kraus R. Echocardiographic manifestations of constrictive pericarditis: abnormal septal motion. Chest 1975;68:684–688.
39. Voelkel AG, Pietro DA, Holland ED, Fischer ML, Parisi AF. Echocardiographic features of constructive pericarditis. Circulation 1978;58:871–875.
40. Wann LS, Weyman AE, Dillon JC, Feigenbaum H. Premature pulmonary valve opening. Circulation 1977;55:128–133.
41. Lewis BS. Echocardiography in constrictive pericarditis — another test or diagnostic advance? J Int Cardiol 1983;2:532–536.
42. Pandian NG, Skorton D, Kieso RA, Kerber RE. Diagnosis of constrictive pericarditis by two-dimensional echocardiography: studies in a new experimental model and in patients. J Am Coll Cardiol 1984;4:1164–1173.
43. Tyberg TI, Goodyer AV, Hurst V, Alexander J, Langou R. Left ventricular filling in differentiating restrictive amyloid cardiomyopathy and constrictive pericarditis. Am J Cardiol 1981;47:791–796.
44. Isner J, Carter B, Baukoff M, et al. Differentiation of constrictive pericarditis from restrictive cardiomyopathy by computed tomographic imaging. Am Heart J 1983;105:1019–1025.
45. Wise DE, Conti CR. Constrictive pericarditis. In: Spodick DH, ed. Cardiovascular clinics: pericardial diseases. Philadelphia: FA Davis, 1976;7:197–210.
46. Miller JE, Mansour KA, Hitcher CR. Pericardectomy: current indications, concepts and results in a university center. Ann Thorac Surg 1982;34:40–45.
47. Goldberg E, Stein J, Berger M, Berdoff RL. Diastolic segmental coronary artery obliteration in constrictive pericarditis. Cathet Cardiovasc Diagn 1981; 7:197–202.
48. Broadbeat JD, Callahan JA, Kincaid OW. Congenital deficiency pericardium. Chest 1966;50:237-241.
49. Fischer JD, Ehrenhaft JL. Congenital pericardial defect. JAMA 1964;133:78–81.
50. Hippona FA, Coumary AB. Congenital pericardial defect associated with tetralogy of Fallot. Circulation 1964;29:132–135.
51. Payvandi MN, Kerber RE. Echocardiography in congenital and acquired absence of the pericardium. Circulation 1976;53:86–92.
52. Ruys F, Paulus W, Stevens C, Brutsaert D. Expansion of the left atrial appendage is a distinctive cross-sectional echocardiographic feature of congenital defect of the pericardium. Eur Heart J 1983;4:738–741.

33

The Patient with Known or Suspect Disease of the Aorta

Tomas D. Martin, M.D.
Carl J. Pepine, M.D.
James A. Hill, M.D.
Charles R. Lambert, M.D., Ph.D.

INTRODUCTION

Patients with known or suspect disease of the aorta in most cases require aortography and often cardiac catheterization studies for optimal management. In this chapter we will review the anatomic and pathophysiologic consequences of these diseases. We will integrate information obtained at the bedside with that obtained from the noninvasive laboratory so that data obtained at the time of catheterization may be more effectively used. A variety of invasive and noninvasive techniques have been used to facilitate the diagnosis of aortic disease. The standard by which all other diagnostic modalities have been measured is contrast aortography. Cardiac catheterization with contrast aortography provides clear multiplane visualization of the heart and aorta and all of its branches and allows assessment of the pathophysiologic consequences of aortic disease (see Chapter 14). At the present time, prior to surgical intervention, all patients with known or suspect disease of the aorta require catheter assessment with contrast aortography whenever possible. Newer noninvasive techniques, such as echocardiography, high-resolution computed tomography (CT), cine-CT, and more recently, magnetic resonance imaging (MRI), may provide important additional information helpful in clarifying a diagnosis. Each of these

diagnostic modalities has a place in the evaluation and treatment plan of patients with diseases of the aorta but none has replaced contrast aortography.

Diseases of the aorta may be either congenital or acquired. Each of these can be subdivided into several more specific groups. In the congenital category, the major abnormalities include: coarctation of the aorta, interrupted aortic arch, and supravalvular aortic stenosis. Acquired diseases of the aorta include four major types: traumatic, aneurysmal (degenerative, atherosclerotic, inflammatory, and mycotic), dissection, and occlusive. Occlusive disease of the aorta is primarily that of aortoiliac disease. This spectrum of aortic disease generally falls under the category of peripheral vascular disease and, therefore, will not be discussed in this chapter. Marfan's syndrome will be discussed separately, as it is a heritable disorder with extensive cardiac and aortic manifestations.

CONGENITAL ANOMALIES

Coarctation

Natural History and Pathophysiology

Coarctation of the aorta, defined as a localized narrowing of the aorta usually secondary to a localized thickening of the aortic wall, comprises 5 to 8% of all congenital cardiac anomalies (1, 2). Coarctation most commonly occurs in the preductal or postductal area (Fig. 33.1); however, it has been found in all areas of the aorta including the abdomen. Pathologically there is an abnormal ridge of posterior aortic media protruding into the lumen to cause an eccentric narrowing just distal to the origin of the left subclavian artery. Isolated coarctation, if left untreated, generally has a poor prognosis, often leading to death before the age of 40. Death is usually secondary to chronic hypertension and its complications (cardiac failure, stroke, etc.), bacterial endocarditis, or aortic rupture (precoarctation or postcoarctation). For these reasons the precise diagnosis must be pursued in patients with clinical findings suggesting coarctation. Bicuspid aortic valve, patent ductus arteriosus, ventricular septal defects, and mitral valve abnormalities are frequent, associated findings.

Clinical Findings

The clinical presentation varies. Approximately one-half of these patients present in infancy with signs and symptoms of cardiac failure often associated with other cardiac anomalies. In older patients, particularly adults, the coarctation is usually asymptomatic. It may be suspected when routine examination discloses upper extremity hypertension and decreased or absent femoral pulses and occasionally from a chest x-ray (3). Sometimes patients will complain of claudication. A thrill in the suprasternal notch and

systolic ejection murmur may be present. Chest x-rays may reveal cardiomegaly, increased vascular markings, rib notching, and/ or a hypoplastic aortic knob with a dilated poststenotic segment. The electrocardiogram may be normal or show left ventricular hypertrophy in older children. Echocardiography allows evaluation of the cardiac chambers and the septum along with the mitral and aortic valves. Pulsed Doppler echocardiography may localize the coarctation, and continuous wave Doppler can be used to estimate the pressure gradient across the coarctation. More recently, CT and MRI have been shown to accurately define the anatomy of coarctation (4) (Fig. 33.2).

Catheterization Findings

Catheter assessment with contrast aortography and cardiac catheterization remains the definitive diagnostic test in most centers. Aortography not only defines the coarctation accurately but also the anatomy of the arch and its branches and collaterals, as well as the aortic valve (Fig. 33.3). Catheter assessment should also provide information relative to the hemodynamic importance of the coarctation along with measurement of the gradient across the narrowing. Right and left heart catheterization also provide clear delineation of cardiac anatomy and any associated anomalies. In adults over 35 years of age, coronary angiography is also indicated. The information obtained by these studies is mandatory, as it dictates the therapeutic course, including the exact procedure to be performed for correction, timing of correction, and which, if any, associated anomalies are to be corrected or palliated simultaneously.

Data Integration, Decision-Making, and Catheter Intervention

Data from the noninvasive and invasive tests should provide enough information to make an accurate diagnosis and determine whether or not other cardiovascular anomalies exist. From these data a treatment plan can be devised. Correction is mandatory in all patients; however, the timing of the correction varies according to the patient's clinical condition. Patients with severe hypertension and/or congestive heart failure require correction as

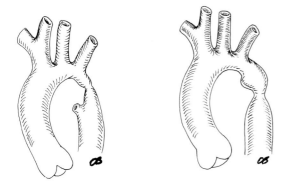

Figure 33.1. Preductal and postductal coarctation.

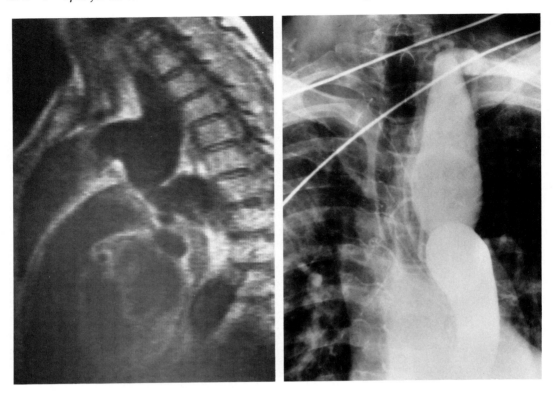

Figure 33.2. *Left,* MRI in the oblique plane demonstrating coarctation of the aorta with pre- and poststenotic dilatation and aneurysmal dilatation of the left subclavian artery. *Right,* Aortogram demonstrating identical findings. (From Akins EW, Carmichael MJ, Hill JA, Mancuso AA. Preoperative evaluation of the thoracic aorta using MRI and angiography. Ann Thorac Surg 1987;44:499-507.)

early as possible. Those with minimal symptoms can have correction delayed until they reach between 4 and 10 years. Most coarctations are repaired by one of a variety of surgical procedures, all of which have good results (5–8). **Percutaneous transluminal balloon angioplasty** is an option which has been reported to provide good early results. Balloon angioplasty has also been used for restenosis following surgical correction (9). Briefly, diameters of the coarctation and ascending and descending aorta are measured using the catheter diameter as a calibration reference. A 3-cm-long balloon angioplasty catheter is chosen so that the balloon outer diameter is approximately 2.5 times the coarctation segment diameter or the maximal ascending or descending aortic diameter, whichever is smallest. The balloon is advanced over a guidewire which is looped in the ascending aorta to help stabilize the balloon. The balloon position is localized using low pressure (about 2 atm) inflation so that the waist caused by the coarctation segment is at midballoon (Fig. 33.4). The balloon is inflated until the waist disappears (usually 5 to 6 atm). A repeat aortogram is recorded. The pressure gradient may not change or even increase for a short period of time after the procedure, but after several months it is generally reduced. The coarctation to ascending aortic diameter ratio increases significantly.

Aneurysms have been noted in a significant number of patients several months to years after dilation of native wedge-type coarctation (10, 11). In one report 43% of patients developed evidence of aneurysm formation at or immediately distal to the balloon dilation site, raising serious concerns about the long-term safety and efficacy of this procedure. The exact role, therefore, for catheter balloon dilation compared with operative correction remains unsettled (12).

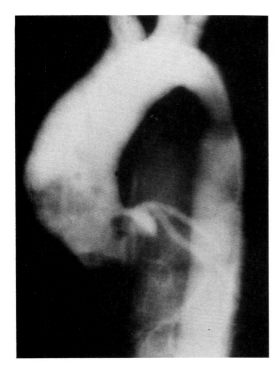

Figure 33.3. Aortogram revealing coarctation of the aorta, dilatation of the asecending aorta, domed bicuspid but competent aortic valve, and normal aortic arch.

Interrupted Aortic Arch

Natural History and Pathophysiology

Interrupted aortic arch is similar to coarctation of the aorta except it is a much more severe form with either total disconnection of the ascending and descending aorta or only a fibrous remnant connecting them. Three types have been described (Fig. 33.5): interruption distal to the left subclavian with all the branches of the arch arising from the ascending aorta; interruption between the left common carotid and the left subclavian, the left subclavian arising from the descending aorta; and interruption between the innominate artery and the left common carotid, the left common carotid and subclavian arising from the descending aorta. The first two types account for most instances. Ventricular septal defects and a patent ductus arteriosus are commonly associated, as are other more complex anomalies, such as truncus arteriosus or transposition of the great arteries.

In all of these circumstances, the pulmonary artery via a patent ductus arteriosus generally provides blood flow to the descending aorta and its branches. Because the right heart provides blood to the lower body and the left heart provides blood to the upper body, differential cyanosis may be observed. When a ventricular septal defect is present, left-to-right shunting may occur at the ventricular level and right-to-left shunting at the ductus level. How severe this is depends on the resistance in the descending aorta. Occasionally, a patent ductus arteriosus is absent. In this circumstance, blood flow to the lower extremities is dependent on the formation of collaterals via the intercostal and internal mammary arteries, as in severe coarctation.

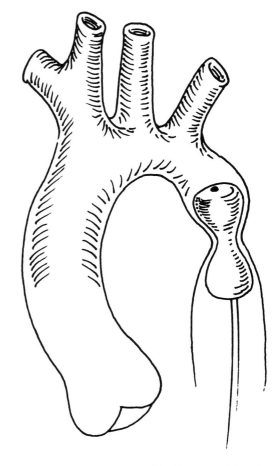

Figure 33.4. Diagram of balloon position for balloon angioplasty of coarctation.

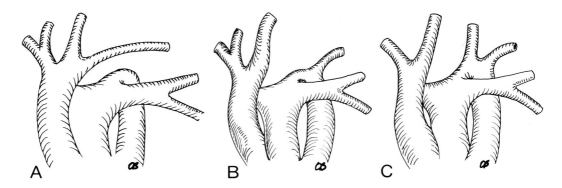

Figure 33.5. Types of interrupted aortic arch. *A,* Interruption distal to the left subclavian artery. *B,* Interruption between the left common carotid and left subclavian arteries. *C,* Interruption between the innominate and left common carotid arteries.

Clinical Findings

In the most common form, that of a patent ductus and ventricular septal defect in conjunction with an interrupted arch, congestive heart failure occurs early in life, and presentation is in the newborn period. Cyanosis may be observed, depending on the adequacy of mixing in the right ventricle and pulmonary artery, but is variable. Left untreated, survival is limited, with most infants dying within the first several months of life. When this condition is associated with other anatomic abnormalities, the course may be quite different. In the absence of shunting, cyanosis does not occur and survival may be prolonged well into adulthood.

The ECG generally exhibits right ventricular hypertrophy particularly in infants with varying degrees of left ventricular hypertrophy. The chest x-ray will differ depending on the presence or absence of intracardiac shunts. When intracardiac shunting exists and the ductus is patent, the cardiac silhouette will be enlarged and the lung fields variably congested depending on how much of the shunted blood preferentially flows into the patent ductus. When no shunts exist, the x-ray will resemble that of coarctation of the aorta. The echocardiogram is helpful to rule out other cardiac abnormalities and to differentiate this condition from aortic atresia. MRI, as in coarctation, provides good visualization of the aorta and may add significantly to the noninvasive findings; however, at present, there is not enough experience with MRI and this anomaly.

Catheterization Findings

As with any catheterization procedure in the patient with congenital heart disease, it is extremely important to completely assess the abnormalities present. The details of the techniques are discussed in Chapter 27. In the patient with interrupted aortic arch, the descending aorta can be entered either retrogradely through the femoral artery or via the left subclavian if the interruption is proximal to it or antegrade through a patent ductus if one is present. The ascending aorta can be entered either retrogradely through the right subclavian (axillary or brachial) artery or antegradely via the inferior vena cava, across the atrial septum, and out the aortic valve. Angiography should be performed in two planes in order to accurately assess the anatomy of the aortic arch. A steep left anterior oblique or lateral view will provide the most information to guide surgical correction.

Data Integration, Decision-Making, and Catheter Intervention

Once the appropriate diagnosis is made, the treatment is surgical correction if possible. A detailed discussion of surgical management of this congenital abnormality is beyond the scope of this chapter. At present there is no procedure for therapeutic catheter intervention.

Supravalvular Aortic Stenosis

Natural History and Pathophysiology

Supravalvular aortic stenosis is generally a congenital aortic defect that is one of three types. The hourglass configuration is most common and is associated with thickening of the media and intimal fibrous proliferation. A second type involves formation of a membrane just above the aortic valve with a central orifice and is associated with a normal size aorta. This is the least common type. The final type is tubular hypoplasia of the ascending aorta just above the sinuses of Valsalva. Associated with all of these types is dilation and tortuosity of the coronary arteries presumably because they are exposed to chronic high pressure from the systolic pressure generated in the left ventricle. The coronary arteries may also be obstructed, particularly in the ostial region secondary to aortic medial proliferation or adherence of the aortic cusp to the aortic wall near the site of supravalvular stenosis (Figs. 33.6 and 33.7). Premature coronary atherosclerosis is common. This abnormality may also coexist with other congenital abnormalities, commonly pulmonary branch stenosis. Prognosis, as in valvular aortic stenosis, is related to the degree of stenosis present (13).

Clinical Findings

This condition frequently has a familial predisposition and may be associated with mental retardation and characteristic facial features including a small chin, wide mouth, malocclusion, wide set eyes, and a broad forehead. Clinically, these patients generally present with the same manifestations as those with valvular aortic stenosis but earlier in life. Patients with the hypoplastic type are unlikely to reach adulthood because obstruction tends to be more severe. Physical findings are similar to valvular aortic stenosis except for the absence of an aortic ejection click and another often well-preserved right carotid pulse.

The ECG in this condition is similar to that in valvular aortic stenosis, with varying degrees of left ventricular hypertrophy. If significant pulmonary stenosis is present, right ventricular hypertrophy may also be present. The chest x-ray in supravalvular aortic stenosis differs from valvular aortic stenosis in that poststenotic dilation is not present. Doppler echocardiography will often demonstrate the anatomic abnormality, as well as functional assessment of the severity of the stenosis.

Catheterization Findings

Cardiac catheterization will demonstrate a pressure gradient across the obstruction. Angiography of the aorta or left ventricle will

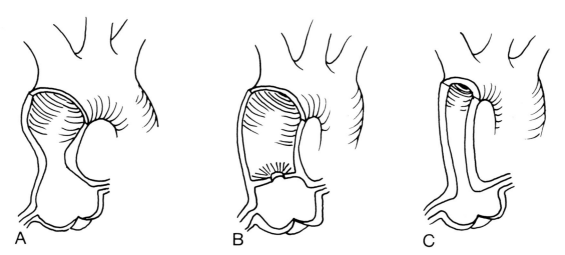

Figure 33.6. Types of supravalvular aortic stenosis. *A,* Hourglass type. *B,* Membranous type. *C,* Hypoplastic type.

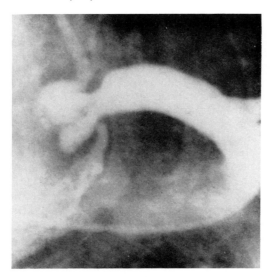

Figure 33.7. Cineangiographic frame of aortogram demonstrating hourglass type of supravalvular aortic stenosis and ostial stenosis of the left coronary artery.

localize the obstruction and guide surgical management (Fig. 33.7). This should be performed using standard views for evaluating the ascending aorta. Selective coronary angiography may be necessary if a suggestion

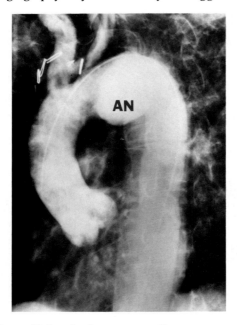

Figure 33.8. Aortogram revealing aneurysmal dilation (*AN*) in the proximal descending thoracic aorta secondary to a chronic transsection.

of myocardial ischemia or coronary obstruction is present and they can not be adequately visualized by aortography. It is also necessary to rule out significant pulmonary stenosis with subsequent abnormalities of right ventricular function.

Data Integration, Decision-Making, and Catheter Intervention

By integrating the results of both the noninvasive and invasive examinations a definitive diagnosis can be made and a therapeutic course chosen. Surgical correction with good results can be accomplished in most cases except when the ascending aorta is severely hypoplastic or atretic. In these cases the results from correction are poor. Catheter intervention is not recommended.

ACQUIRED DISEASE

Traumatic Aortic Disruption

Etiology, Natural History, and Pathophysiology

Trauma to the aorta may result from blunt or penetrating injury; however, this section will be devoted primarily to blunt aortic disruption. Acute transsection of the thoracic aorta most commonly occurs at the level of the ligamentum arteriosus or isthmus and is most commonly due to rapid deceleration. It is suspected that rapid deceleration results in a tearing of the relatively mobile arch and very proximal descending thoracic aorta away from the descending thoracic aorta, which is firmly attached to the paraspinous tissues. This injury causes rapid exsanguination into the free pleural space in most patients. Therefore, acute traumatic disruption of the thoracic aorta should be suspected in any patient who has sustained significant, blunt chest trauma, especially those who have undergone rapid deceleration. In one large autopsy series, 85% of patients with blunt aortic injury died before arriving at a hospital. In the small group of patients that survive, the injury is initially contained by periaortic tissues; however, rupture into the pleural space may occur at any time. It has been estimated that of those who reach a hospital alive, 10% die within 1 hr, 30% within 6 hr, and 40% within 24 hr (14). Those who survive the early posttraumatic period will usually develop aneurysmal dilation of the level of transsection (Fig. 33.8) and should be treated the same as any other aneurysm, as will be discussed later.

Clinical Findings

The posttraumatic clinical picture seen in patients with aortic tears is extremely variable, ranging from moribund and comatose to virtually asymptomatic. Clinical findings that are suggestive of a severe chest injury include bruises and/or abrasions to the chest wall, palpable rib and/or sternal fractures, chest wall crepitance, and decreased or absent breath sounds primarily on the left side, suggestive of a hemothorax. Patients will occasionally have decreased femoral pulses and blood pressure, but this is not usual.

The noninvasive evaluation should consist of an upright plain chest x-ray with a nasogastric tube in place and an ECG. The most common x-ray finding is a widened mediastinum (>8 cm at the level of the aortic knob), and the most sensitive is deviation of the esophagus (as seen by the nasogastric tube) to the right. Other findings on the plain chest x-ray are as follows:

1. Loss of the aortic knob;
2. Depression of the left mainstem bronchus >140°;
3. Left hemothorax or pneumothorax;
4. Rightward deviation of the trachea;
5. Left apical capping;
6. Anterior displacement of the trachea (lateral view);
7. Loss of the aortopulmonary window (lateral view);
8. Fractured first and/or second rib.

The ECG will probably be normal unless the patient has also sustained a cardiac contusion, in which case anterior ST segment and/or T wave changes may be present.

CT scanning with contrast has been recommended by some surgeons for use in patients suspected of having traumatic aortic disruption; however, this test is not 100% specific. Since the mortality from this injury in the early posttrauma period is so high, we feel there is no place for further noninvasive studies and that assessment with contrast aortography should be performed as soon as possible.

Catheterization Findings

The best approach is via the femoral artery. The right femoral artery is preferable, as some surgeons will utilize some type of bypass or shunt during the repair, and often times the left femoral vessels are used for retrograde perfusion. Passage of the catheter retrograde past the aortic injury is not associated with any increased morbidity. Angiography should be performed in at least two planes (i.e., anterior-posterior, lateral, and/or oblique). Injury to the aorta most commonly occurs at the isthmus; however, injury may occur in any portion. Since all patients with acute traumatic injuries of the aorta have suffered trauma of great force, the incidence of injury to other organs is very high. Of special concern are associated abdominal injuries, such as liver, spleen, and/or kidney, all of which may be easily delineated by abdominal aortography. Therefore, a total aortogram is necessary in all patients.

Data Integration, Decision-Making, and Catheter Intervention

Again, if the mechanism of injury and the immediate noninvasive studies are at all suggestive of an aortic injury, immediate angiography is mandatory. Aortography should give precise definition and localization of any aortic injury. Once the diagnosis is made, immediate surgical repair should be pursued. No therapeutic catheter intervention is available for this injury.

Aneurysmal Disease

Etiology, Natural History, and Pathophysiology

Aneurysmal disease of the aorta, especially of the abdominal aorta, is common and occurs in more than 6% of patients over the age of 65 (15). An aneurysm is any dilation of the aorta greater than two times the normal diameter. The etiology of aortic aneurysms in most cases is degeneration of the media of the vessel wall leading to weakening and subsequent dilation. Degenerative diseases of the aorta include cystic medial degeneration, myxomatous degeneration, and atherosclerotic degeneration. Atherosclerosis may produce aneurysmal dilation and/or occlusive disease.

Mycotic disease and the different types of inflammatory disease (Takayasu's arteritis, giant cell, granulomatous, and rheumatoid) also may produce aneurysms of the aorta due to degeneration of the aortic wall. Therefore, aneurysmal disease in general will be discussed in this section, as it is beyond the scope of this chapter to discuss each etiology in detail. Chronic aortic dissection may also become aneurysmal and will be discussed in the section devoted to dissection.

Aortic aneurysms may occur in isolated or multiple segments of the aorta (contiguous or separate) or encompass the entire aorta from the aortic valve to the iliac bifurcation (Fig. 33.9). Aneurysms of the ascending aorta and transverse aortic arch are usually secondary to cystic medial degeneration or myxomatous degeneration. Left untreated, ascending, transverse, and/or descending thoracic aortic aneurysms will progress, leading to aortic insufficiency (Fig. 33.10), compression of the airway, esophagus, pulmonary artery, and/or great veins. They may also rupture into the pericardium, pleura, or mediastinum. Progression with rupture leads to death in most cases. It was once thought that thoracic aortic aneurysms rarely ruptured. However, in several studies, the rupture rate of untreated thoracic aneurysms ranged from 46 to 74% with a median interval of only 2 years between detection and rupture (16-18).

Thoracoabdominal aneurysms are defined as aneurysms which involve segments of the descending thoracic aorta and abdominal aorta in continuity. These have been divided into four groups or types (19). Type I includes aneurysms that involve the entire descending thoracic aorta and upper abdominal aorta. Type II involves most of the descending aorta and most of the abdominal aorta. Type III involves the distal descending thoracic aorta and most or all of the abdominal aorta, and type IV is confined to the abdominal aorta and involves the segment associated with visceral vessels. These aneurysms are included with the thoracoabdominal aortic aneurysms, as the diagnosis, treatment, and associated complications are similar. The most common etiology of thoracoabdominal aneurysms is atherosclerotic degeneration, and these aneurysms are commonly associated with hypertension. The natural history of types I and II are similar to that previously discussed for

other thoracic aortic aneurysms. Types III and IV are similar to the abdominal aortic aneurysms, as will be discussed later.

Infrarenal abdominal aortic aneurysms are the most common aneurysms seen and treated (Fig. 33.11). As stated previously, as many as 6.5% of patients over age 65 will develop an abdominal aortic aneurysm and the frequency is increasing (15). This increased frequency is most likely secondary to increased awareness of the disease, improved diagnostic modalities, and the larger numbers of patients reaching older ages. Infrarenal abdominal aortic aneurysm repair accounts for 0.8% of general surgical operations and 10% of vascular operations (20). The etiology is variable; however, atherosclerotic degeneration is by far the most common. The natural history of all abdominal aneurysms is one of progression, with rupture reported to occur in 50% of patients within 1

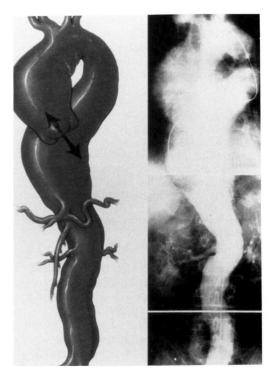

Figure 33.9. Diffuse aortic ectasia or megaaorta with aneurysmal dilation from the aortic root to the iliac artery origins along with aortic insufficiency. (From Crawford ES, Crawford JL. Diseases of the aorta. Baltimore: Williams & Wilkins, 1984:52.)

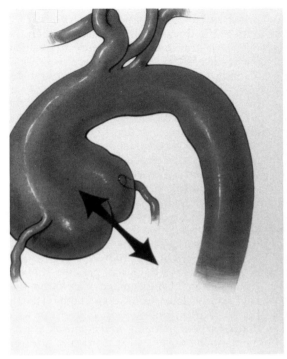
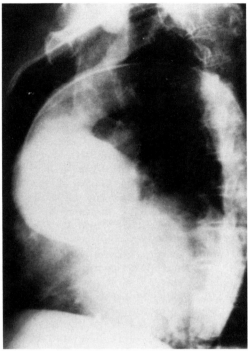

Figure 33.10. Aneurysmal dilation of the ascending aorta and sinuses of Valsalva resulting in massive aortic insufficiency. (From Crawford ES, Crawford JL. Diseases of the aorta. Baltimore: Williams & Wilkins, 1984:9.)

year of diagnosis and in over 90% within 5 years (21). The size of the aneurysm has been used as a predictor of rupture with an aneurysm >6 cm carrying a 43% incidence of rupture and an accompanying mortality of 90% (22). Smaller aneurysms, however, are not benign, as those <6 cm have been found to have an incidence of rupture of almost 20% with a 55% mortality. One autopsy series of patients dying from ruptured abdominal aortic aneurysms found that one-third had aneurysms ≤5 cm (23).

Clinical Findings

Clinical presentation of thoracic aortic aneurysms varies and is dependent on the site, size, and extent of the aneurysm. Most are asymptomatic until they reach sizable proportion, when symptoms, such as chest or back pain, stridor, dysphagia or hoarseness, occur. Signs or symptoms of aortic insufficiency may be present if the aneurysm involves the ascending aorta and aortic annulus. Often the first symptoms are those of rupture or

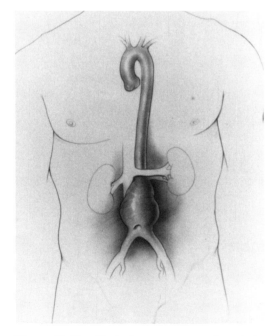

Figure 33.11. Typical appearance of an infrarenal abdominal aortic aneurysm.

impending rupture, and many patients die suddenly with no real symptoms.

Most patients with abdominal aortic aneurysms are asymptomatic at the time of presentation, with one recent series of 666 patients reporting 81% asymptomatic (20). The diagnosis in 70 to 75% of these patients is usually suspected when a pulsating mass in the abdomen is noted by the patient or physician or when calcification shadows are seen on abdominal roentgenograms. When symptoms are present, they usually consist of varying degrees of abdominal, flank, and/or back pain. The diagnosis is usually made on physical examination, with an abdominal ultrasound being an easy, reliable confirmatory test.

Thoracic aortic aneurysms are often initially suspected in the asymptomatic patient by enlargement of the mediastinal silhouette on plain roentgenograms (Fig. 33.12). When this occurs, noninvasive study of the aorta is indicated. Echocardiography is a good initial study to assess the heart and its function, the cardiac valves, and the root of the aorta. Echocardiography of the distal ascending, transverse arch and descending thoracic aorta, however, is of questionable value because of the technical limitations provided by the intrathoracic structures. CT scan of the thorax with contrast has been the definitive noninvasive procedure to evaluate aortic disease (Fig. 33.13); however, more recently, multiple reports have suggested that MRI is as good or better for delineation of aortic abnormalities (24-32). Included in the advantages of MRI are: (*a*) excellent soft issue contrast, (*b*) intravascular contrast occuring without need for contrast medium, (*c*) intrinsically three-dimensional, (*d*) gated images defining cardiac structure and function with excellent resolution, and (*e*) the ability to select tomographic planes in virtually any orientation (Fig. 33.14). At our institution, Akins et al., in a prospective preoperative evaluation of thoracic aortic aneurysms using MRI, found excellent correlation between MRI and angiography (24). In 25% of patients studied, clinically useful information was found that was not available from angiography. Limitations of MRI include the inability to provide definitive hemodynamic and anatomic assessment of the aortic valve, coronary arteries, and arch vessels. Also, severe vessel tortuosity may lead to misinterpretation of the extent of fusiform aneurysms.

Due to the ease and accuracy of abdominal ultrasound and the asymptomatic course, it is

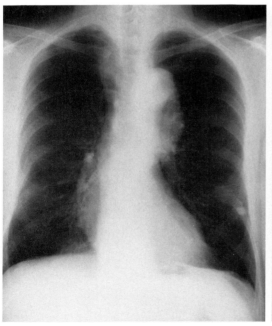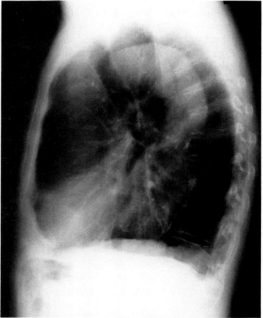

Figure 33.12. *A* and *B,* Chest x-ray showing widened mediastinal silhouette and enlarged descending thoracic aorta in a patient with a thoracoabdominal aortic aneurysm.

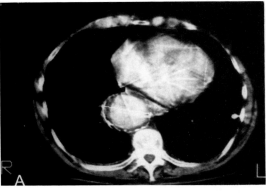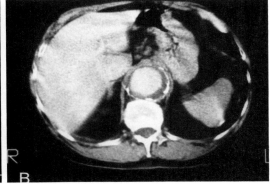

Figure 33.13. CT scan of the chest (*A*) of patient in Figure 33.12 revealing extension of the aneurysm into the abdomen (*B*). Note that both the location and the size of the aneurysm are delineated.

reasonable that patients in the susceptible age group (>50 years) have a yearly screening abdominal ultrasound. If there is a question of extent, either proximal or distal, CT and MRI have proven to be extremely useful.

Catheterization Findings

As we have stated previously, the best approach for aortography is usually via the femoral arteries. Due to the high incidence of associated aortic disease in patients with thoracic aortic aneurysms we recommend total aortography. Total aortography can be performed by using three separate injections of 50 cc each of contrast material. This will allow biplane chest and abdominal aortograms to be performed along with an oblique view of the thoracic aorta. These views should provide clear visualization of any aortic aneurysm.

Routine use of angiography in patients with abdominal aortic aneurysms confirmed by abdominal ultrasound, CT scan, or MRI and in those who have no history suggestive of either mesenteric and/or peripheral vascular occlusive disease is probably not indicated. If there is any question, however, regarding the aneurysm or the presence of occlusive disease, then angiography should be performed with biplane films of the abdominal aorta, mesenteric and renal vessels, iliacs, and femorals obtained.

Data Integration, Decision-Making, and Catheter Intervention

In patients with documented aneurysms of the thoracic aorta, there are several features

that must be delineated. First, and foremost, is the extent of the aneurysm. In a patient with an ascending aortic aneurysm, it must be determined if the aneurysm is isolated to the ascending aorta or if there is involvement of the aortic arch and/or coronary ostia and sinuses. If the aneurysm is isolated to the supracoronary aorta and does not involve the arch, the repair is relatively simple and involves replacement of that segment alone, utilizing routine cardiopulmonary bypass. If the aneurysm extends into the arch in part or in whole, then a more complicated surgical procedure is necessary. This includes profound hypothermia and circulatory arrest with reimplantation of the great vessels. This procedure is also necessary if the aneurysm is isolated to the aortic arch. If the aneurysm extends proximally to the coronary ostii and sinuses of Valsalva, again, a more complicated procedure is indicated. This requires reattachment of the coronary ostii to the graft or coronary artery bypass. The extent and severity of associated cardiac disease, primarily aortic valvular disease and/or coronary artery disease, along with myocardial function must also be determined. Cardiac catheterization is mandatory in all patients with ascending aortic aneurysms, as it provides not only visualization of the aneurysm but also assessment of the aortic valve. Aortic valvular insufficiency is frequently associated with these aneurysms. When significant aortic valvular disease is present, the valve must be replaced. This can be done separately or with a composite valve graft and reimplantation of the coronary ostia. Associated coronary artery disease requires that any coronary artery bypass grafts be implanted into the aortic graft.

For patients with aneurysms of the descending thoracic aorta, knowledge of the extent of involvement is also extremely important, as it again determines the operative approach. If the aneurysm extends into the distal arch, then cardiopulmonary bypass with profound hypothermia and circulatory arrest, as reported by Crawford et al. (33), may be necessary. If it extends distally into the very distal thorax or upper abdomen, then a thoracoabdominal approach is necessary (Fig. 33.15). Evaluation of the abdominal aorta is extremely important in patients with

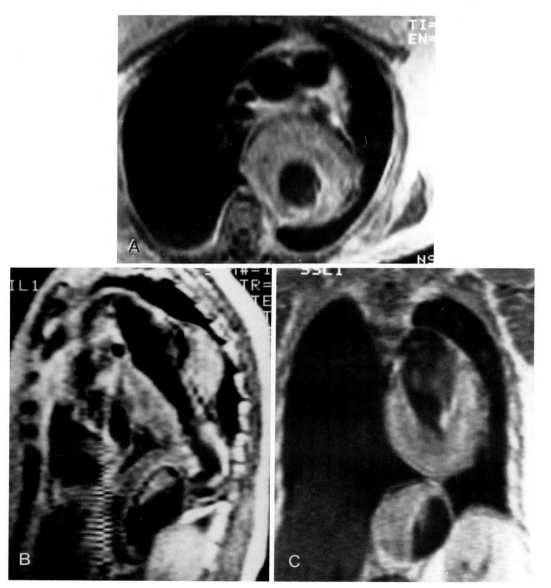

Figure 33.14. MRI in the axial (*A*), coronal (*B*), and sagittal (*C*) planes accurately defining the full extent and size of a large thoracoabdominal aneurysm. (From Akins EW, Carmichael MJ, Hill JA, Mancuso AA. Preoperative evaluation of the thoracic aorta using MRI and angiography. Ann Thorac Surg 1987;44:499-507.)

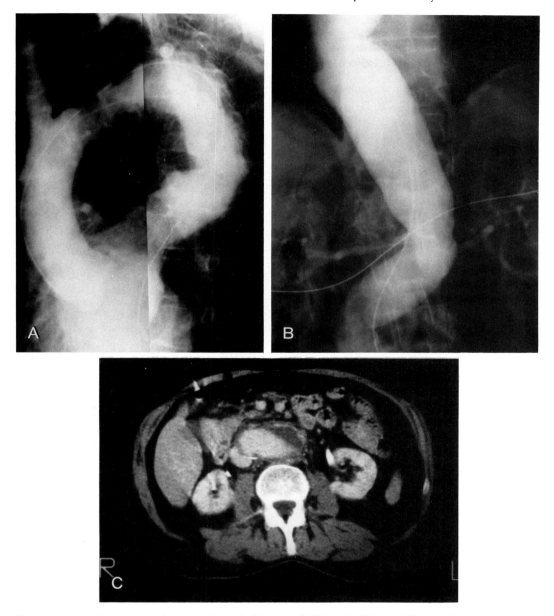

Figure 33.15. Aortogram (thoracic (*A*) and abdominal (*B*)) and CT scan (*C*) revealing extension of a known descending thoracic aortic aneurysm into the upper abdomen requiring a thoracoabdominal incision for correction.

aneurysms of the descending thoracic aorta, as 25% of these patients will have simultaneous abdominal aortic aneurysms (21). Again coronary artery anatomy must also be evaluated at catheterization, and if significant coronary artery disease is present, then aorta-to-coronary artery bypass must be considered. Left ventricular function is also assessed with cardiac catheterization. Patients with poor ventricular function have a significantly higher morbidity and mortality. Indeed, if ventricular function is extremely poor, they may be deemed inoperable, as they are not likely to tolerate cross-clamping of the aorta or other aspects of the repair.

Once the diagnosis of a thoracoabdominal aneurysm is suspected, optimal evaluation should include both invasive and noninvasive studies. Computed tomography and MRI provide the best information regarding size, extent, and differentiation between dissection and nondissection (24, 25, 28, 30, 31). However, most authorities still agree that catheter assessment with biplane aortography is mandatory, as 20% of these patients will have associated atherosclerotic occlusive disease of the visceral vessels, renal arteries, and/or the distal aorta and iliacs. Atherosclerotic occlusive disease of these vessels may necessitate correction at the time of aneurysm repair (21). In patients with severe mesenteric and/or renal occlusive disease, bypass or endarterectomy may be considered, and if severe peripheral vascular occlusive disease is present, then resection of the aneurysm should be coupled with an aorta biiliac or bifemoral bypass.

Of particular concern is the very high incidence of cardiac disease in these patients. Of the 666 patients reviewed by Johnston and Scobie (20), 45% had a history of myocardial infarction, angina, and congestive heart failure and/or electrocardiographic evidence of ischemia or old infarction, and 6.5% had previous coronary artery bypass. In those who had a myocardial infarction <6 months prior to surgery, congestive heart failure (recent or remote), class III or IV angina or unstable angina within the last 6 months, or significant valvular disease (aortic, mitral, or both), a mortality of 16% or greater was seen. Therefore, a very thorough preoperative cardiac evaluation, directed at assessing the coronary arteries and left ventricular function should be performed.

Aortic Dissection

Etiology, Natural History, and Pathophysiology

Aortic dissection is one of the most frequent and serious forms of aortic disease. Acute dissection results from a tear in the intima of the aorta that subsequently leads to destruction and separation of the media from the adventitia by an advancing column of blood under high pressure. The etiology of the initial intimal tear is variable and is usually associated with chronic hypertension and preexisting disease of the aortic wall such as arteriosclerosis, medial degeneration, aortitis, or trauma. Acute dissections begin in the ascending aorta in 55 to 65% of patients, in the descending aorta in 20 to 30%, in the transverse arch in 10 to 15%, and in the abdominal aorta in <2% (34-36).

Two classification systems have been proposed in the past 20 years (Fig. 33.16) (37-39). DeBakey and colleagues first classified aortic dissections into types I, II, and III (37, 38). Type I has the initial intimal tear in the ascending aorta with the dissection continuing through the arch and descending thoracic aorta and into the abdominal aorta (Fig. 33.17). Type II begins in the ascending aorta but ends at the left subclavian artery (Fig. 33.18), and type III begins in the very proximal descending thoracic aorta and continues distally. The Stanford classification groups DeBakey type I and II into category A and DeBakey type III into category B (39). This classification is based solely on whether the ascending aorta is involved (category A) or not involved (category B) and does not take into consideration the site of the initial intimal tear.

Dissection can progress proximally, distally or both; however, the distal dissection is

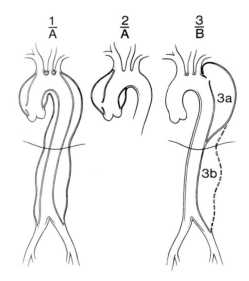

Figure 33.16. Classifications of aortic dissections, DeBakey types 1, 2 and 3 and Stanford types A and B. See text for discussion. (From Crawford ES, Crawford JL. Diseases of the aorta. Baltimore: Williams & Wilkins, 1984:174.)

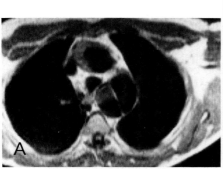

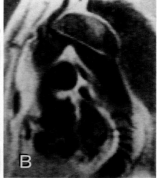

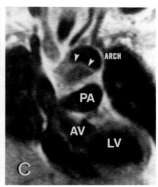

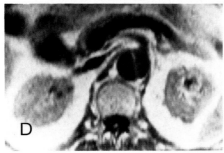

Figure 33.17. MRI revealing a DeBakey type I dissection with involvement of the ascending aorta (*A*), aortic arch (*B* and *C*) and extension of the dissection into the abdomen (*D*). *ARCH*, aortic arch; *AV*, aortic valve; *LV*, left ventricle; *PA*, pulmonary artery. (From Akins EW, Hill JA, Carmichael MJ. MR imaging of blood pool signal variation with cardiac phase in aortic dissection. J Comput Assist Tomogr 1987;11:543-545.)

usually much greater. Retrograde dissection rarely occurs when the tear is in the descending thoracic aorta and virtually never occurs when it begins in the abdominal aorta. Retrograde dissection commonly occurs when the dissection begins on the inner ascending aortic wall and involves 50% of the circumference. DeBakey type I and II (Stanford type A) dissections start in the ascending aorta and/or arch and usually course along the greater curve and upper descending thoracic aorta. Type III (Stanford type B) dissections usually start in the descending thoracic aorta and tear along the left posterior lateral surface. Ninety percent of these, along with the distal extent of DeBakey type I dissections, extend distally along the left posterior lateral surface of the aorta and into the left iliac. This is of particular importance to the angiographer; as the false lumen is commonly entered when catheterization via a left femoral approach is used.

Left untreated, the natural history of aortic dissections is ominous, with a 50 to 90% mortality in the acute phase (39). Patients who survive acute dissection are then at a significant risk of developing chronic fusiform aneurysms from dilation of the outer wall of the false lumen. Again, left untreated, 25% of chronic dissections will progress to rupture at the site of the intimal tear. Therefore, in DeBakey types I and II dissections, death is usually secondary to rupture into the pericardium with acute pericardial tamponade, and death from a ruptured type III is most often from exsanguination into the mediastinum or free left pleural space.

Clinical Findings

The classic symptom of an acute dissection is severe, unbearable retrosternal or left-sided chest pain that radiates straight to the back. It is often described as tearing or wrenching in nature and is often associated with diaphoresis, dizziness, and syncope. This pain is not relieved by nitroglycerin and is often refractory to intravenous narcotics. Acute dissections are often associated with sustained or intermittent hypertension or hypotension. Transient or persistent loss of blood pressure and/or pulses in any aortic branch may occur and is dependent on the extent and path of the dissection. Clinically, this may present in many forms including ischemia of one or more extremities (the left arm and/or left leg being the most common). Loss of cerebral blood flow will present as either a transient ischemic attack or a completed stroke, and loss of critical spinal cord blood will result in paraplegic or paraparesis. Mesenteric ischemia may also occur and present as abdominal pain with or without distention. This is an ominous sign, as the mortality is high if bowel infarction occurs. Again, any of these clinical findings may be transient or permanent and are totally dependent upon the course of the dissection.

Echocardiography is useful and accurate in evaluating the root of the aorta and the status of the aortic valve, along with providing cardiac function data. Over the last 5 years CT has been considered the most reliable noninvasive modality for assessing aortic dissections. However, there have been recent reports showing the efficacy of MRI (24, 25, 28, 30, 31). In one report, MRI supplemented the angiographic assessment of the type A aortic involvement when these abnormalities were missed by contrast angiography (24). The high contrast between the signal from the intimal flap and the low signal present in rapidly flowing blood facilitates detection of an aortic dissection. This allows demonstration of false lumen patency, which may be especially important in making the diagnosis.

Catheterization Findings

The extent of the disease is best determined by aortography in the anterior-posterior, lateral, and oblique projections with injections into both the true and false lumen. The true lumen is best entered from a right brachial artery approach and the false lumen from the left femoral artery. This is especially true in type I and III dissections, as the path of dissection is usually into the left iliac and femoral arteries. It is often very difficult to catheterize both the true and false lumen and often requires tremendous effort, persistence, and patience from the angiographer. It is likely that both lumens cannot be entered via a single approach, and one should not hesitate to try several catheterization sites. In patients with type I and II dissections, it is extremely important to visualize the coronary arteries and aortic valve and, if possible, to visualize the tear in the ascending aorta, as the surgical procedure performed is dependent on this information. An example of aortography performed from the right femoral artery with injection into the false lumen of a DeBakey type I aortic dissection is given in Figure 33.19.

Data Integration, Decision-Making, and Catheter Intervention

Early in the evaluation of many patients with aortic dissection, the exact diagnosis may

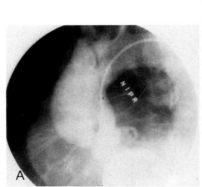
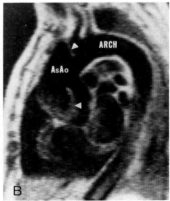

Figure 33.18. Aortogram (*A*) and MRI (*B*) sections in a patient with a DeBakey type II aortic dissection where the dissection is limited to the ascending aorta and proximal aortic arch. *AsAo,* ascending aorta; *ARCH,* aortic arch; *NIPR,* nitroprusside. (From Hill JA, Lambert CR, Akins EW, Carmichael MJ. Ascending aortic dissection: detection by MRI. Am Heart J 1985;110:894-896.)

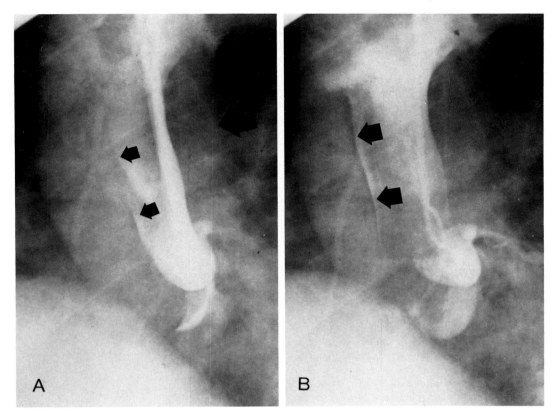

Figure 33.19. Systolic (*A*) and diastolic (*B*) frames during aortography (left anterior oblique) in patient with a DeBakey type I aortic dissection. The injection is into the false lumen and illustrates movement of the intimal flap (*small arrows, A* and *B*). The medial extent of the aorta is marked by the *large arrow* in the systolic frame (*A*). The diastolic frame is shown in *B*.

not be apparent. Acute myocardial infarction is frequently considered (40). This can be excluded in most patients with the initial electrocardiogram; however, as many as 23% will have electrocardiographic abnormalities consistent with myocardial ischemia or infarction. Therefore, in patients with suspected aortic dissection, further evaluation is warranted if their condition permits. If the patient is hemodynamically unstable, however, either from pericardial tamponade or continuing hemorrhage, immediate operative intervention is indicated. Patients who are stable should have pain controlled with intravenous narcotics, and have systolic pressure decreased to 120 mm Hg or less with intravenous nitroprusside and β-blockade. Once stabilized, contrast aortography should be performed, as it is considered the definitive diagnostic test.

Information that must be obtained from aortography and any noninvasive studies include (*a*) site of initial tear; (*b*) extent of the dissection; (*c*) status of all major aortic branches; and (*d*) status of the aortic valve and coronary arteries (primarily in type I and II dissections). With this information an adequate treatment plan can be developed. With type I and II dissections that do not involve the aortic valve or coronary arteries, treatment is supracoronary replacement of the ascending aorta and/or the aortic arch under profound hypothermia and circulatory arrest. If the aortic valve and coronary arteries are involved, then a composite valve graft must be utilized with either reimplantation of the coronary ostia to the graft or ligation of the coronary ostia followed by autogenous vein bypass.

The treatment of acute type III dissections is controversial with the operative mortality reported to be between 8 and 40%. Therefore, in the opinion of the authors, aggressive medical treatment should be instituted. If hypertension can be controlled and there are no signs of impending rupture, no surgical intervention may be necessary, as only 15 to 25% will progress to chronic aneurysms and/or rupture (35, 36, 39). These patients should all be followed closely with CT scan or MRI evaluation at least every 6 months, and subsequent aneurysms should be approached in the same manner as the nondissecting aneurysms.

OTHER

Marfan's Syndrome

Etiology, Natural History, and Pathophysiology

Marfan's syndrome is a heritable connective tissue disorder with well-known skeletal, ocular, and cardiovascular manifestations (41). Aortic aneurysms and dissections occur as a result of cystic medial necrosis, with these and other cardiovascular manifestations occurring in 98% of patients (42). The natural history of these manifestations is quite ominous. Ninety-five percent of these patients die of cardiovascular complications with 50% succumbing at an average age of 32 years (43).

Clinical Findings

Various skeletal manifestations are seen in virtually all patients with Marfan's syndrome and include long extremities, fingers and thumbs, extremely lax joints, sternal and spinal deformities, including pectus excavatum or caranatum and kyphosis or scoliosis, and very narrow highly arched palates (Fig. 33.20). Approximately 70% of these patients will have ocular problems including myopia and lens subluxation. The most common cardiovascular abnormality is fusiform aortic aneurysms, most frequently in the ascending aorta. Others include acute dissections, aortic aneurysms secondary to chronic dissections, cardiac valve abnormalities (most commonly "floppy" mitral valve), and occasionally peripheral arterial aneurysms. The clinical findings with each of these have been described previously.

All patients with known Marfan's syndrome should be followed clinically at frequent regular intervals. Annual chest x-ray should be performed, and if there is any question concerning the aorta, then either a CT scan or MRI should be performed to rule out aneurysm formation or dissection. Echocardiography is also an excellent test for following any known or suspected valvular disease as well as for following proximal aortic root size.

Catheterization Findings

The catheter findings will vary according to the pathologic manifestation of the disease and have been discussed previously. All patients with Marfan's syndrome, however, should undergo cardiac catheterization for evaluation of coronary anatomy and pathology as well as valvular disease if surgical correction is deemed appropriate by noninvasive

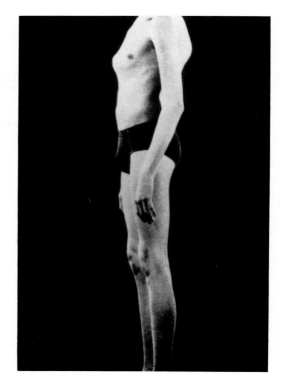

Figure 33.20. The classical physique of a patient with Marfan's syndrome: tall and thin, arm span greater than height, sternal and spine deformities typifying the skeletal manifestations. (From Crawford ES, Crawford JL. Diseases of the aorta. Baltimore: Williams & Wilkins, 1984:52:215.)

studies. Many operators prefer to utilize brachial cutdown allowing direct arterial repair in patients with Marfan's syndrome. An example of aortography in such a patient is given in Figure 33.21, illustrating annuloaortic ectasia commonly seen in Marfan's syndrome.

Data Interpretation, Decision-Making, and Catheter Intervention

In Marfan's syndrome any evidence of aortic or cardiac pathology necessitates careful evaluation and follow-up. This includes complete noninvasive evaluation and catheter assessment if indicated. Early correction of aortic and/or cardiac abnormalities is mandatory, as the mortality from these conditions is high. One surgical series reported that 63% of late deaths theoretically could have been prevented had more aggressive treatment been undertaken (42). Data integration, decision-making and catheter intervention techniques for each of the cardiovascular complications of

Marfan's syndrome have been discussed in the previous chapters. The only difference is to recognize that these patients have multiple systemic manifestations of their disease and that each area must be examined completely.

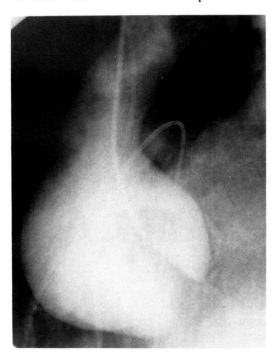

Figure 33.21. Cineframe from aortogram (left anterior oblique) from the right brachial artery in a patient with Marfan's syndrome illustrating annuloaortic ectasia.

References

1. Fyler DC, Buckley LP, Hellenbrand WE, Cohn HE. Report of the New England Regional Infarct Cardiac Program. Pediatrics 1980;65:375–461.
2. Keith JD. Coarctation of the aorta. In: Keith JD, Rower RD, Vlad P, eds. Heart disease in infancy and childhood. 3rd ed. New York: Macmillan, 1978:736–760.
3. Glancy DL, Morrow AG, Simon AL, Roberts WC. Juxtaductal aortic coarctation. Analysis of 84 patients studied hemodynamically, angiographically and morphologically after age 1 year. Am J Cardiol 1983;51:537–551.
4. Akins EW, Schuster JD, Victorica BE. Cardiovascular MRI in the pediatric patient (abstr). Southeastern Ped Cardiol Soc 1987;September 24–26.
5. Lababidi Z. Neonatal transluminal balloon coarctation angioplasty. Am Heart J 1983;106:752–753.
6. Singer MI, Rowen M, Dorsy TJ. Transluminal aortic balloon angioplasty for coarctation of the aorta in the newborn. Am Heart J 1982;103:131–132.
7. Lock JE, Bass JL, Amplatz K, Fuhrman BP, Castaneda-Ziniga W. Balloon dilatation angioplasty of aortic coarctations in infants and children. Circulation 1983;68:109–116.
8. Cooper RS, Ritter SB, Bolinko RJ. Balloon dilatation angioplasty: nonsurgical management of coarctation of the aorta. Circulation 1984;70:903–907.
9. Kan J, White RI, Mitchell Se, Farmlett EJ, Donahoo JS, Gardner TJ. Treatment of restenosis of coarctation by percutaneous transluminal angioplasty. Circulation 1983;68:87–94.
10. Marvin WJ, Mahoney LT, Rose EF. Pathologic sequence of balloon dilatation angioplasty for unoperated coarctation of the aorta in children (abstr). J Am Coll Cardiol 1986;7:117A.
11. Pellegrino A, Deverall PB, Anderson RH, et al. Aortic coarctation in the first three months of life: an anatomopathological study with respect to treatment. J Thorac Cardiovasc Surg 1985;89:121–127.
12. Cooper RS, Ritter SB, Rothe WB, Chen CK, Griepp R, Golinko RJ. Angioplasty for coarctation of the aorta: long-term results. Circulation 1987;75:600–604.
13. Martin MM, Lammer JH, Shaffer E, Dick M, Bove EL. Obstruction to left coronary artery blood flow secondary to obliteration of the coronary ostium in supravalvular aortic stenosis. Ann Thorac Surg 1988;45:16–20.
14. Parmley LF, Mattingly TW, Manion WC, Jahnke EJ. Nonpenetrating traumatic injury of the aorta. Circulation 1958;17:1086–1101.
15. Reigel MM, Hollier LH. Surgical repair of abdominal aortic aneurysms. In: Cardiac surgery: state of the art reviews. Sugery of the aorta. Philadelphia: Harley and Belfas, 1987;1:453.

16. Bickerstaff LK, Pairolero PC, Hollier LH, et al. Thoracic aortic aneurysms: a population based study. Surgery 1982;92:1103–1108.

17. Joyce J, Fairbairn J, Kincaid O, Juergens J. Aneurysms of the thoracic aorta: a clinical study with special reference to prognosis. Circulation 1964; 29:176–181.

18. Pressler V, McNamara JJ. Thoracic aortic aneurysm: natural history and treatment. J Thorac Cardiovasc Surg 1980;79:489–498.

19. Crawford ES, Crawford JL, Safi HJ, et al. Thoracoabdominal aortic aneurysms: preoperative and intraoperative factors determining immediate and long-term results of operation in 605 patients. J Vasc Surg 1986;3:389–404.

20. Johnston KW, Scobie TK. Multicenter prospective study of nonruptured abdominal aortic aneurysms. I. Population and operative management. J Vasc Surg 1988;7:69–81.

21. Crawford ES, Crawford JL. Aneurysms of degenerative origin. In: Diseases of the aorta. Baltimore: Williams & Wilkins, 1984:134–166.

22. Szilagyi DE, Smith RF, DeRusso FJ, et al. Contribution of abdominal aortic aneurysmectomy to prolongation of life. Ann Surg 1966;164:678–699.

23. Karmody AM, Leather RP, Goldman M, et al. The current position of nonresective treatment for abdominal aortic anerysm. Surgery 1983;94:591–597.

24. Akins EW, Carmichael MJ, Hill JA, Mancuso AA. Preoperative evaluation of the thoracic aorta using MRI and angiography. Ann Thorac Surg 1987;44:499–507.

25. Amparo EG, Higgins CB, Hricak H, Sollitto R. Aortic dissection: magnetic resonance imaging. Radiology 1985;155:399–406.

26. Amparo EG, Higgins CB, Shafton EP. Demonstration of coarctation of the aorta by magnetic resonance imaging. AJR 1984;143:1192–1194.

27. Glazer HS, Gutierrez FR, Levitt RG, Lee JK, Murphy WA. The thoracic aorta studied by MR imaging. Radiology 1985;157:149–155.

28. Geisinger MA, Risius B, O'Donnell JA, et al. Thoracic aortic dissections: magnetic resonance imaging. Radiology 1985;155:407–412.

29. Von Schulthess GK, Higashino SM, Higgins SS, Didier D, Fisher MR, Higgins CB. Coarctation of the aorta: MR imaging. Radiology 1986;158:469–474.

30. Goldman AP, Kotter MN, Scanlon MH, Ostrum B, Paramesivarau R, Perry WR. The complementary role of magnetic resonance imaging, Doppler echocardiography, and computed tomography in the diagnosis of dissecting thoracic aneurysms. Am Heart J 1986;111:970–981.

31. Hill JA, Lambert CR, Akins EW, Carmichael MJ. Ascending aortic dissection: detection by MRI. Am Heart J 1985;110:894–896.

32. Dinsmore RE, Liberthson RR, Wismer GL, et al. Magnetic resonance imaging of thoracic aortic aneurysms: comparison with other imaging methods. Am J Radiol 1986;146:309–314.

33. Crawford ES, Coseli JS, Safi HJ. Partial cardioplumonary bypass, hypothermic circulatory arrest, and posterolateral exposure for thoracic aor5tic aneurysm operation. J Thorac Cardiovasc Surg 1987;94:824–827.

34. Miller DC, Stinson EB, Oyer PE, et al. Operative treatment of aortic dissections: experience with 125 patients over a sixteen year period. J Thorac Cardiovasc Surg 1979;78:365–382.

35. Crawford ES, Crawford JL. Aortic dissection and dissecting aortic aneurysm. In: Diseases of the aorta. Baltimore: Williams & Wilkins, 1984:168–214.

36. Ergin MA, Lausman SL, Griepp RB. Acute dissections of the aorta. In: Cardiac surgery: state of the art reviews. Surgery of the aorta. Philadelphia: Harley and Belfas, 1987;1:377–392.

37. DeBakey ME, Henly WS, Cooley DA, et al. Surgical treatment of dissecting aneurysms of the aorta: analysis of seventy-two cases. Circulation 1961;24:290–303.

38. DeBakey ME, Hemly WS, Cooley DA, et al. Surgical management of dissecting aneurysms of the aorta. J Thorac Cardiovasc Surg 1965;49:130–149.

39. Daily PO, Trueblood HW, Stinson EB, et al. Management of acute aortic dissections. Ann Thorac Surg 1970;10:237–247.

40. Levinson DC, Edmeades DT, Griffith GC. Dissecting aneurysm of the aorta — its clinical, electrocardiographic, and laboratory features: report of 58 autopsied cases. Circulation 1950;1:360–387.

41. Marfan AB. Un cas de deformation congenitale des quartres membres, plus pronouncee aux extremities, caracterisee par l'allongement des os avec un certain degre d'amincussement. Bull Sox Chir Paris 1896;13:220–225.

42. Crawford ES, Crawford JL. Marfan's syndrome. In: Diseases of the aorta. Baltimore: Williams & Wilkins, 1984:215–248.

43. Murdock JL, Walker BA, Halperin BL, Kugma JW, McKusic VA. Life expectancy and causes of death in the Marfan's syndrome. N Engl J Med 1972; 286:804–808.

Index

Page numbers in *italics* denote figures; those followed by "t" denote tables.